MASSAGE FOR ORTHOPEDIC CONDITIONS

MASSAGE FOR ORTHOPEDIC CONDITIONS

Thomas Hendrickson, DC

Institute of Orthopedic Massage

Illustrations by Kim Battista

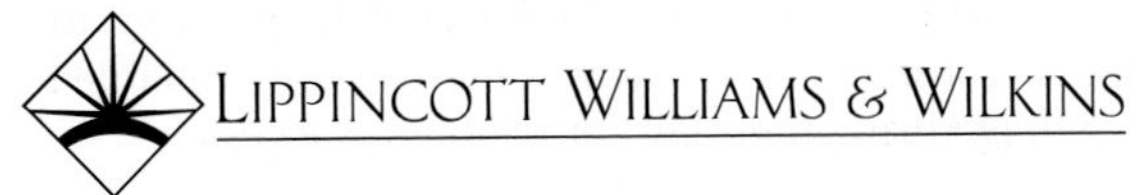

Editor: Peter Darcy
Managing Editor: Eric Branger
Marketing Manager: Christen DeMarco
Production Editor: Jennifer D. Weir
Cover Illustration: Terry Watkinson
Compositor: Graphic World
Printer: RR Donnelley

351 West Camden Street
Baltimore, Maryland 21201

530 Walnut Street
Philadelphia, Pennsylvania 19106

The publisher is not responsible (as a matter of product liability, negligence, or otherwise) for any injury resulting from any material contained herein. This publication contains information relating to general principles of medical care which should not be construed as specific instructions for individual patients. Manufacturers' product information and package inserts should be reviewed for current information, including contraindications, dosages and precautions.

Printed in China

Library of Congress Cataloging-in-Publication Data

Hendrickson, Thomas.
Massage for orthopedic conditions / Thomas Hendrickson.
p. ; cm.
Includes bibliographical references and index.
ISBN-13 978-0-7817-2287-2
ISBN-10 0-7817-2287-X
1. Massage. 2. Orthopedics. I. Title.
[DNLM: 1. Massage--methods. 2. Orthopedics. WB 537 H498m 2002]
RD732 H46 2002
616.7′0622--dc21

2001050742

The publishers have made every effort to trace the copyright holders for borrowed material. If they have inadvertently overlooked any, they will be pleased to make the necessary arrangements at the first opportunity.

To purchase additional copies of this book, call our customer service department at **(800) 638-3030** or fax orders to **(301) 824-7390.** For other book services, including chapter reprints and large quantity sales, ask for the Special Sales department.

For all other calls originating outside of the United States, please call **(301) 714-2324.**

Visit Lippincott Williams & Wilkins on the Internet: **http://www.lww.com.** Lippincott Williams & Wilkins customer service representatives are available from 8:30 am to 6:00 pm, EST, Monday through Friday, for telephone access.

07 08
5 6 7 8 9 10

DEDICATION

To Lauren Berry, RPT, for his generosity in selflessly passing on his wealth of knowledge, and to my parents, Bill and Jean Hendrickson, for their love and encouragement.

PREFACE

This book was written to fulfill the need for advanced training in massage therapy specializing in the management of musculoskeletal pain and dysfunction. It is intended as a textbook for massage therapists, as well as for chiropractors, physical therapists, osteopaths, physical therapy and orthopedic assistants, athletic trainers, and other health care providers.

The demand for safe and effective treatment of pain and disability is growing rapidly as the population seeks alternatives to drugs and surgery. In addition, an increasing number of people are experiencing musculoskeletal pain and dysfunction. Many factors can be cited for this, such as a more active elderly population, the popularity of recreational sports, the increased number of people using computers, and the growing numbers of people involved in car accidents.

The medical community has recognized that much of the pain and disability suffered by their patients involve soft tissue injury and dysfunction. Yet, at a 1987 symposium of the American Academy of Orthopedic Surgeons entitled "The Mechanisms of Injury and Repair of the Musculoskeletal Soft Tissue," experts addressed the limitations of orthopedic medicine in treating soft tissue injuries. They concluded that strains and sprains of the musculoskeletal soft tissue not only cause significant pain and impairment, but also are often poorly diagnosed and inadequately managed. Most massage schools have not provided adequate training in the assessment and management of soft tissue injuries, and chiropractors, osteopaths, and physical therapists often have had little or no training in advanced massage techniques for musculoskeletal pain and dysfunction in their degree programs.

Massage for Orthopedic Conditions provides a scientific basis for massage and manual resistive techniques and a rational, step-by-step guide to the assessment and management of the most common orthopedic conditions. The therapeutic protocol described in this text is called "Orthopedic Massage" (OM) and includes massage strokes, soft tissue and joint mobilization, and manual resistive techniques. As several other practitioners also use this term, "Orthopedic Massage" refers only to the method of treatment described in this text.

These techniques are based on 30 years of clinical experience and the latest scientific developments in the management of soft tissue injuries and dysfunction. This book began as a training manual for the 200-hour OM certification program at the Institute of Orthopedic Massage in Kensington, California. The techniques have been refined each year for the past 20 years of teaching and have been clinically tested with tens of thousands of patients.

The Therapeutic Contributions of Orthopedic Massage

The therapeutic protocols described in this text can provide reproducible results of functional improvement for most orthopedic conditions, including increased range of motion and decreased pain. In line with the modern goals of rehabilitation, OM helps normalize musculoskeletal function rather than merely provide symptomatic relief.

These techniques are designed to manage conditions related to orthopedics, for example, low back pain, neck stiffness and pain, rotator cuff and knee injuries, and many other conditions, such as arthritis, frozen shoulder, and tennis elbow. The techniques are applicable whether the pain or dysfunction is acute or chronic, or whether the condition arose from an injury, cumulative stress, or degenerative condition.

OM also enhances th [illegible] dancers and athletes, and assists an [illegible] chieve optimum health. In additio [illegible] benefits of traditional massage, su [illegible] d increased circulation, OM has sev [illegible] t goals. OM dissolves adhesions and [illegible] nective tissue. It helps normalize muscle function by reducing hypertonicity in the muscles and strengthening inhibited and weak muscles. It normalizes the position of the soft tissue and releases its torsion. It helps restore normal joint function by restoring natural lubrication, range of motion, and normal biomechanics. It releases entrapped peripheral nerves. And it facilitates normal neurological function through re-education of the nervous system through muscle energy technique (MET), a system of manual therapy that uses active participation of the client.

The Unique Aspects of Orthopedic Massage

This text introduces a new theoretical model of soft tissue alignment developed by my mentor, Lauren Berry, RPT. Berry was a mechanical engineer and physical therapist who theorized that muscles, tendons, ligaments, and all soft tissues have a normal position relative to the joint that they affect. He taught manipulations in very specific directions, transverse to the line of the fiber, to realign the soft tissue and help normalize the function of the soft tissue and its associated joint.

Massage for Orthopedic Conditions also introduces a new style of massage therapy that I developed called wave mobilization. This unique style of performing the massage strokes is based both on the science of ergonomics and the practice of Tai Chi, a Chinese internal martial art. In this book, I describe the ergonomics of giving a massage, including the functional position of the hand and the resting position of each joint, to teach the therapist how to use his or her body most efficiently. This text also describes the rational basis and provides step-by-step instructions for how to develop and use this internal energy or "chi" in your massage strokes instead of relying only on muscular effort.

OM is not only an efficient and remarkably effective technique for the management of the majority of orthopedic conditions, it is also deeply relaxing for both the client and therapist. OM allows the therapist to use minimal muscular effort and solves the problem of overuse injuries within the field of massage therapy. The Chinese call this use of minimal effort the "wu wei," the path of effortless effort. For the therapist, the effort of giving a massage is refreshing and energizing, akin to taking a walk. Tai Chi emphasizes internal strength, postulating that we can develop our inner life force, or chi, and learn to transmit it to others. It teaches that softness will dissolve hardness. After nearly 30 years of performing massage therapy, I am using dramatically less physical effort in my treatments and achieving more profound results.

This method of massage is also unique because the treatment can be given through clothing. This has allowed me to provide treatments to a diverse patient population, including Tibetan lamas and elderly patients in third-world countries where it would be inappropriate to have clothing removed for their therapy. Dramatic clinical results can be achieved even across ethnic, cultural, and language barriers.

In addition to describing a new method of massage, this book also describes the fundamentals of taking a history and performing an assessment. To gain their rightful place as a member of the health care team, massage therapists must know how to gather objective information, properly assess an injury or dysfunction, determine if massage is contraindicated, how to communicate that information to other health-care providers and insurance companies, and know when to refer.

The Development of Orthopedic Massage

The development of OM was influenced by many practitioners over a 30 year period. I began studying massage in 1972 as part of a teacher's training course in yoga and immediately began to appreciate the healing power of touch. In 1974 I completed a year-long training in Shiatsu massage with Riuho Yamada, a Zen priest and Shiatsu master. Master Yamada's treatments had tremendous power, which I believe resulted not only from his technical skill, but also from his life-long practice of meditation. I realized that his effectiveness was not related to how hard he worked, but to combining his internal energy with outward movements. This insight has been reinforced throughout my years of training and practice.

In 1976, I participated in an intensive, 4-month residential training program in Lomi work. Lomi work was developed by Robert Hall, MD, et al., and synthesizes the work of Ida Rolf (Rolfing), Fritz Perls (Gestalt therapy), and Randolph Stone (Polarity therapy). Life-long postural habits and emotional patterns are often dramatically changed. The deep tissue and Shiatsu approaches are limited, however, when treating soft tissue injuries.

The greatest influence in my career came in 1978 when I met Lauren Berry, RPT. By then, Lauren had been a healer for more than 50 years. He began his training with a Finnish doctor who taught him massage and manipulation. As a physical therapist and mechanical engineer, Lauren traveled all over the world studying healing. Lauren had a very pragmatic "nuts and bolts" approach. He used manipulation of the soft tissue and joints to correct mechanical dysfunctions in the body. People traveled from all over the country to be treated by this legendary healer. I trained with Lauren for 4 years. My last year was an apprenticeship, in which I assisted him in treating thousands of people. His work had not been previously documented, and I felt deeply honored when he permitted me to record his method of manipulating the joints. "The Berry Method, Volume I: The Joints," was published in 1981. Unfortunately, Lauren died shortly after completing the first volume, so the planned second volume on soft tissue was never realized.

Lauren's contributions to the treatment of soft tissue injuries were original and invaluable. He theorized that all of the soft tissues in the body have a specific position relative to the neighboring soft tissue and its associated joints, and that massage must be applied in specific directions to correct its positional dysfunction. Lauren observed predictable patterns of soft tissue malposition over the entire body, and developed a system of manipulation to correct those dysfunctional positions.

I began a 4-year chiropractic training program in 1982, concurrently training massage therapists in methods of advanced soft tissue therapy. Training massage therapists in Lauren's techniques presented me with two challenges. First, much of Lauren's method involved high-speed joint manipulation, which is not within the scope of practice for massage therapists. His techniques also involved quick manipulations of the soft tissue, which is incompatible with a relaxing massage. I realized that my work was to change the joint manipulations into gentle mobilizations, and transform his quick soft-tissue manipulations into massage strokes, while maintaining their therapeutic effectiveness.

The second challenge was to create a treatment that was as relaxing as it was therapeutic. Lauren's students debated about how hard one needed to work to be effective. Some students believed that a very deep, often painful touch was necessary to be effective, while others believed that a gentle touch was more effective. It was my personal goal to be as gentle as possible without sacrificing therapeutic results.

Over years of clinical practice and teaching I developed the concept of "interfascicular torsion" to describe the microscopic adhesions and abnormal twists I could feel with my hands. I observed that these torsional dysfunctions in the soft tissue were winding the body into abnormal spirals and developed techniques to unwind these segments.

As I developed my techniques for working on the spine, I placed my patients in a side-lying fetal position. This position was comfortable even for the patient with acute low back pain and it also allowed me to stand upright during the treatment, rather than lean over the table. As tai chi teaches that water will dissolve stone, I began experimenting with a rounded, wave-like stroke, transverse to the fiber. I also applied the principles of tai chi and moved my whole body into each stroke and practiced keeping my body relaxed and supple. Rocking my patients in rhythmic oscillations created a wave-like movement in my patient's entire body. These rocking movements had a quieting and calming affect on my patients. Also, I became more relaxed internally and began to notice an expansion of my own energy field. The therapy I was giving became an opportunity to develop my own internal energy.

My chiropractic education emphasized the role of the nervous system in both health and dysfunction or injury, and the vast reflex connections between the soft tissue, joints, and central nervous system. I also gained an appreciation of the profound neurophysiological effects of mobilization of the spine and joints of the extremities. As I began to incorporate joint mobilization techniques into my soft-tissue work, I achieved better results with less effort. These were not the high-speed, low-amplitude thrusting techniques associated with the chiropractic adjustment, but rather techniques involving gentle, rhythmic, oscillating movements of the joints.

Moving the joint while massaging the surrounding soft tissue has several effects: one, it helps reduce hypertonicity in the muscles; two, it helps normalize joint function by stimulating the normal lubrication of the synovial membrane, articular cartilage, and discs within the joint; three, it helps in pain management by stimulating the mechanoreceptors; and finally, it creates a profound relaxation response.

My work is also influenced by the insights of James Cyriax, MD, the modern developer of transverse friction massage. Cyriax's work has many parallels with Berry's, as both approaches work transverse to the line of the fiber. Cyriax theorized that brisk, transverse strokes at sites of injury restore the normal parallel alignment of the collagen fibers, which can become distorted after an injury. He focused his soft tissue therapy on critical junction sites, i.e., where a muscle interweaves with its tendon (myotendinous junction), where the tendon interweaves with the periosteum of the bone (tenoperiosteal junction), and at the attachment sites of ligaments, but did not address the function of the entire soft tissue complex. For example, transverse massage techniques on a lesion in the supraspinatus helps resolve that lesion, but does not address postural distortions, muscle weakness or hypertonicity, and positional dysfunctions in the neighboring soft tissue. OM incorporates some of the friction techniques of Cyriax, but in a unique style. OM mobilizes the associated joint with the friction strokes, which dramatically reduces the discomfort associated with transverse friction massage.

Another tremendous influence in the evolution of my work came from Vladimir Janda, MD, and Karel Lewit, MD, two physicians from the Czech Republic. These remarkable pioneers in manual therapy have made major contributions to the assessment and treatment of soft tissue injury and dysfunction. Janda discovered predictable patterns of muscle dysfunction, in which some muscles become weak and inhibited and others become short and tight in response to pain or joint dysfunction. Lewit and Janda also developed methods of treatment in the tradition of proprioceptive neuromuscular re-eduction (PNF), which requires the client's resistance to pressures applied by the therapist. Some texts, including this one, call these techniques muscle energy techniques (MET). OM incorporates the insights of Janda into each chapter and uses MET within the massage session to reduce muscle hypertonicity, facilitate or strengthen weak or inhibited muscles, re-educate muscles in their normal firing patterns, help normalize joint function, and help restore normal neurological function. MET can change chronic pain patterns and has proved extremely effective clinically.

Revelations have also come from my study of healing with Muriel Chapman, DO, and Rosalyn Bruyere. I learned from each that gentle touch itself is healing. I noticed in my clinical practice that with patients in severe pain effective clinical results could be achieved even if I used very light pressure. I have come to realize that one of the most important goals of the therapist in the clinical setting is to create an experience with touch in which the client feels completely safe, completely comfortable. This induces a state of relaxation and trust in the client that allows for the healing of not only the physical pain, but also provides an environment for the healing of the emotional and psychological components.

OM is intended to be a nurturing experience for both the therapist and client. One of the hallmarks of OM is that the client should be able to completely relax into the massage strokes. In the healthy individual, all of the massage strokes described in this text should feel comfortable to receive. If the massage stroke is painful, it indicates that the area is injured or dysfunctional, and requires that the therapist adjust the pressure of the massage strokes to ensure the client's comfort.

Each session is also an opportunity for the therapist to create an environment of kindness for the client. It is important to realize that anyone experiencing pain or dysfunction is emotionally vulnerable, perhaps worried, depressed, or anxious. Whether the client is out of shape, non-compliant or irritable, the therapist should aspire to be non-judgmental. The massage session gives us an opportunity to practice loving kindness. There is no greater calling.

Organization and Features

The book is divided into two sections. The first section should be read before performing the massage techniques described in the second section. The first section has two chapters. Chapter 1 describes the scientific and theoretical foundations for OM. It reviews the fundamentals of neuromusculoskeletal anatomy, describing the structure and function of all the soft tissues in the body, the mechanics of dysfunction and injury, the mechanical and neurological consequences of these dysfunctions and injuries, and, finally, how this information can guide the massage therapist in the most effective therapy.

Chapter 2 is divided into two parts. The first part provides an overview of clinical assessment, including taking a history and how to perform a fundamental orthopedic examination. The process of performing an objective examination is given in detail, including the assessment of active and passive range of motion, isometric testing, special tests, and palpation. This is followed by a summary of examination findings for the most common categories of orthopedic dysfunctions and injuries.

The second part of chapter 2 is an overview of the techniques used in this book. The essential stroke of OM, called wave mobilization, is described in detail, and exercises are provided to practice this stroke on a client or fellow student. A description of the second fundamental aspect of OM, MET, follows. The neurological basis of MET is described, as well as exercises to practice the six different styles of MET used in this text. A summary of the clinical effects of OM, mobilization, and MET are described. Finally, guidelines for the treatment of patients in acute or chronic pain are described in detail, as well as contraindications for massage therapy, and when to refer your client to another provider.

The second section of the book is divided into eight chapters and describes specific techniques for particular regions of the body. Each chapter provides an overview of the anatomy of the region, the structure and function of all the soft tissues, the most common orthopedic injuries and dysfunctions, and the protocol for the treatment of each of these conditions. Each chapter also describes a basic assessment of the region for the massage therapist and provides a step-by step guide for how to perform the MET and massage strokes for that area of the body. The strokes are divided into Level I and Level II. Level I strokes are massage strokes that can be performed on anyone, whether the client is symptomatic or not. These strokes bring the area to its highest level of functioning. Level II strokes are used as needed to supplement Level I strokes if pain or dysfunction is present in the region. They are typically deeper strokes and often work on sensitive attachment points, which is unnecessary for most clients.

Each technique chapter has a variety of features that were specifically designed to enhance the reader's learning experience:

- The easy-to-reference, bulleted format allows students to "keep their place" in the text and encourages students to practice the techniques with a partner as they read.
- Muscle anatomy and kinesiology are organized into tables for easy reference.
- Consistent organization reinforces basic concepts and fosters retention of fundamental information. For example, anatomy sections are divided into *structure, function, dysfunction and injury,* and *treatment implications* subsections. Similarly, muscle energy technique sections are divided in to *intention, position,* and *action* subsections.
- A "Caution" icon (⚠) highlights contraindications and precautions that the massage therapist should be aware of before performing a particular technique.
- The Study Guide section at the end of each chapter lists concepts and objectives that the reader should master for both the Level I and Level II techniques.
- References and Suggested Readings point the reader to articles and books that provide more information about anatomy, kinesiology, assessment, and the science of injury and repair.
- A case study describing the assessment and management of an orthopedic condition using an actual patient concludes each technique section.

How To Use This Book

It is essential that the student read chapters 1 and 2 first and practice the exercises described in chapter 2 before attempting the techniques described in chapters 3–10. At the training program at the Institute of Orthopedic Massage, the MET and Level I strokes are learned in the first semester and the assessment and Level II strokes are learned in the second semester. The MET is listed in the section before the massage strokes for convenience and easy reference, but in clinical practice the MET and massage strokes are interspersed throughout the massage session. The massage strokes are described very precisely and in a specific sequence. The student is encouraged to "follow the recipe" exactly as it is described. It is natural to feel insecure when you are learning something new. Be patient and kind with yourself. As you master the techniques over time, you will naturally create your own unique style of performing this method. It is akin to learning to play the guitar. First, learn the exact way to form the chords and the sequence of how the chords change in familiar songs. Then, use these skills to create your own music. Enjoy the rewards of learning something new, and have faith that with dedication and practice you will help relieve the suffering of all whom you touch.

Feedback and Further Information

Feedback from clinicians, students, or schools with constructive ideas of how to improve this text is appreciated. You may also contact the Institute of Orthopedic Massage for information about classes in the techniques described in this text.

Thomas Hendrickson, DC
Institute of Orthopedic Massage
406 Berkeley Park Boulevard
Kensington, CA 94706
Online at www:orthopedicmassage.com
E-mail: iom@dnai.com
Phone: (510) 524-3107
Fax: (510) 524-8242

ACKNOWLEDGMENTS

Although this is a single-authored text, I have had invaluable help from the teachers and teaching assistants at the Institute of Orthopedic Massage for nearly 20 years. They have carefully read the text year after year and made thoughtful suggestions both in how to best describe and teach these techniques, and in how to convey the scientific information most clearly. I would especially like to thank Tom Stinnett, Regina Callahan, Mila Gelman, Peter Rothe, Tiffany Turley, Leslie Peterson, and Elizabeth Roache. I would like to give a special appreciation to Jaymi Devans and Sarah Hammond. Jaymi carefully cross-referenced all the information and provided a selfless devotion to the editing of this book that helped me immeasurably. Sarah provided meticulous attention in proof-reading the manuscript. To the students at the Institute of Orthopedic Massage, who have continually challenged me with their questions and manifested great patience in studying from a work in progress. To Deborah Bates, for years of help in the design of the original training manual. To my office manager, Claudia Moore, whose grace and good humor make the running of the office and the Institute look easy.

I would also like to thank my editor Kathleen Scogna at Lippincott Williams & Wilkins and Kim Battista for her beautiful illustrations.

And finally, this book would never have been created if not for the inspiration and teaching of my mentor, Lauren Berry, RPT.

CONTENTS

SECTION I:

OVERVIEW OF THEORY AND TECHNIQUE

The Theoretical Foundations of Orthopedic Massage

Introduction to Orthopedic Massage

GENERAL OVERVIEW

The goal of orthopedic massage (OM) is to induce a change in the structure and function of the neuromusculoskeletal soft tissue to promote healing of the whole person. As most pain and disability in the body involves the soft tissues, it is important to understand their structure, function, dysfunction and injury, and the specific treatment goals for orthopedic conditions.

Body Composition: Mainly Fibers and Fluids

The soft tissue includes the skin; fascia; muscles; tendons; ligaments; cartilage; bursae; joint capsules; nerves; and the vascular, lymphatic, and synovial fluids. These tissues are mainly composed of fibers and fluids; even the bones are mineralized fibers. These fibers give the body its form and are akin to the framework of a house. They provide the tension to keep the body upright and transmit the forces that create movement. Most of the fibers run parallel to each other and are arranged in a spiral, at both the microscopic and macroscopic levels. The spiral orientation of the fibers has a specific direction for each joint.

The human body is approximately 70% water, which is contained in the fluids of the body. These fluids include the blood, lymph, synovial fluid, cerebrospinal fluid, and interstitial fluids (the fluids surrounding the cells). Like the Earth's oceans, the water within the body moves in waves. These waves are created by three pumps: the heart, the respiratory diaphragm, and the muscles.

Spirals, Waves, and the Human Body

We live in a spiral universe. Our local galaxy, the Milky Way, forms a spiral (Fig. 1-1). The spiral is a fundamental shape in the movement of air currents over the surface of the Earth (Fig. 1-2). Water, which covers 71% of the Earth's surface, moves in a spiral pattern, not only

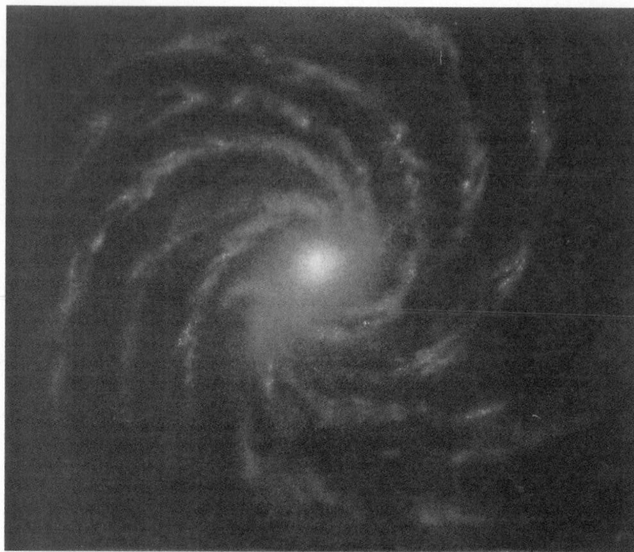

Figure 1-1. The galaxy we live in has a spiral shape. (Reprinted with permission from Kaufman W. Universe, 3rd Ed. New York: WH Freeman, 1991.)

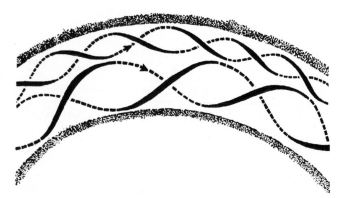

Figure 1-3. Spiraling movements within moving water. (Reprinted with permission from Schwenk T. Sensitive Chaos. New York: Schocken Books, 1976.)

as it snakes its way across the land, but also as it spirals internally in the form of secondary currents within the moving water (Fig. 1-3).

The spiral is also an essential pattern in the body and is present at many levels. Microscopically, tendons, ligaments, joint capsules, and the fascia of muscles are composed of parallel fibers of collagen. Each collagen molecule is a triple helix spiral (Fig. 1-4). Visually, the gross structure of a tendon is also a spiral (Fig. 1-5).

Muscles are composed of parallel fibers organized in spirals. The levator scapula, for example, forms a spiral from its attachments on the scapula to the cervical spine (Fig. 1-6). Actin and myosin are the two basic proteins that compose muscle fiber. Each actin filament is a double helix that is composed of two strands that spiral around each other, and myosin contains globular heads that are arranged in a spiral. Soft tissue is organized around the joint in a spiral. DNA, the code of instructions for cellular reproduction, is also a double helix spiral (Fig. 1-7).

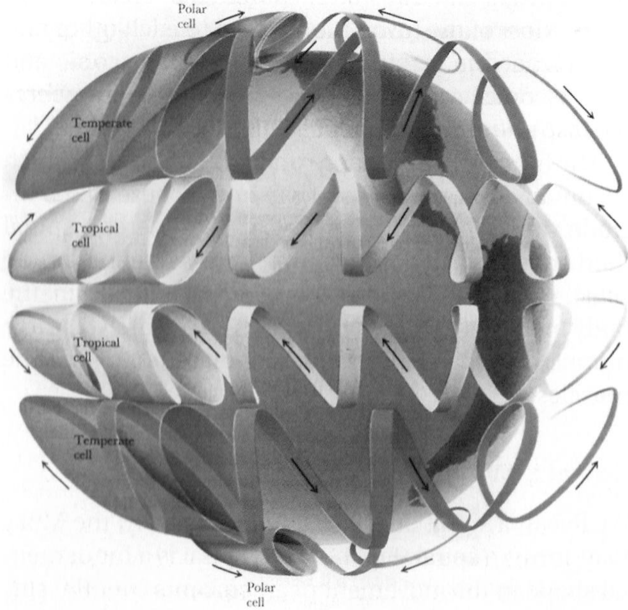

Figure 1-2. Spiraling circulation patterns of the air currents of the earth's atmosphere. (Reprinted with permission from Kaufman W. Universe, 3rd Ed. New York: WH Freeman, 1991.)

Soft-Tissue Alignment Theory

This book introduces a new theoretical model of massage therapy: *Muscles, tendons, and ligaments have a normal position relative to the neighboring soft tissue and to the joint that they affect.* Lauren Berry, RPT, a physical therapist and mechanical engineer, introduced this concept and also theorized that dysfunction and injury to a joint creates abnormal positions or misalignment in the soft tissue surrounding the joint. This misalignment occurs microscopically in the normal

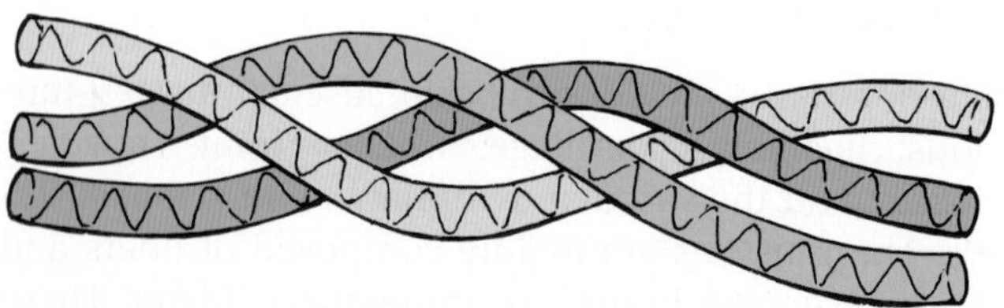

Figure 1-4. Triple helix spiral structure of collagen.

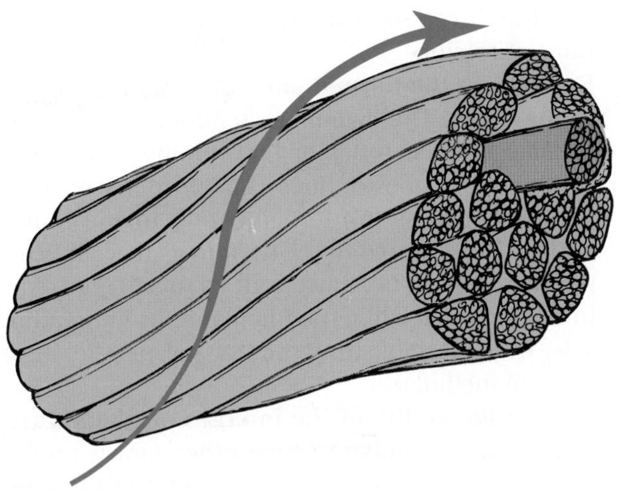

Figure 1-5. Arrangement of collagen fibers in a tendon shows its spiral orientation.

spiral alignment of collagen, and macroscopically in the gross position of a muscle, tendon, or ligament. For example, in a slumped posture the anterior deltoid rolls down and forward into an abnormal position. This abnormal alignment has mechanical and neurologic consequences.

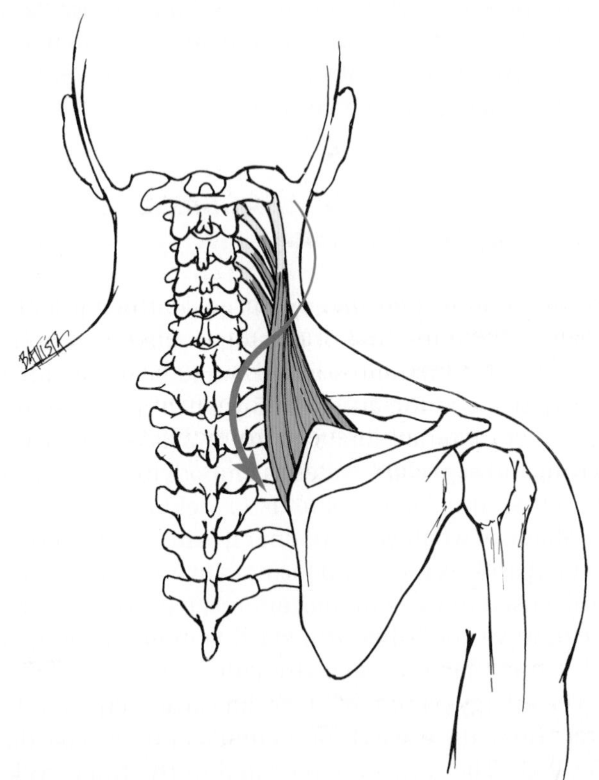

Figure 1-6. Levator scapula muscle shows the spiral orientation of the muscle from its origin to its insertion.

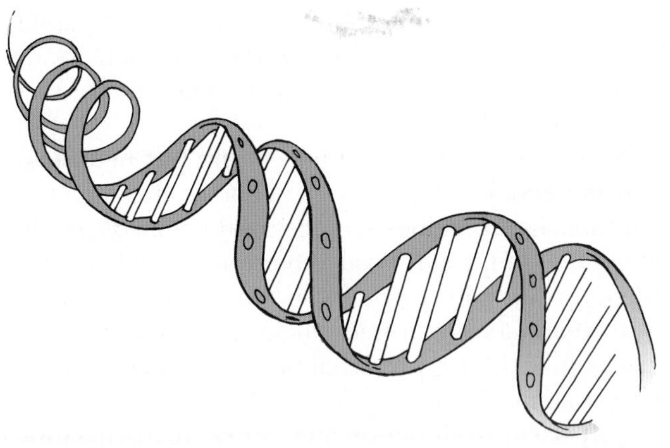

Figure 1-7. Spiral structure of DNA.

MECHANICAL AND NEUROLOGIC CONSEQUENCES OF SOFT-TISSUE DYSFUNCTION AND INJURY

Muscles, tendons, and ligaments can misalign. Soft-tissue injury and dysfunction changes the normal alignment of the soft tissue relative to the neighboring soft tissue and joint.

Muscles, tendons and ligaments can develop an abnormal torsion (twist). If the soft tissue develops an abnormal position owing to dysfunction or injury, it introduces an abnormal torsion or twist into the tissue. The abnormal twist decreases the water content of the tissue, leading to adhesions and abnormal function in the soft tissue and associated joint.

The fibers lose their normal parallel alignment. Mechanical injury of the soft tissue on the microscopic level represents a tearing apart of the collagen fibers. Because the fibers are repaired by new collagen deposited in a random orientation, they lose their normal parallel orientation, and the bundles of fibers or fascicles lose their ability to slide relative to each other. Therefore, the fascicles of collagen fibers in the tendons, ligaments, and joint capsules have a decreased ability to slide relative to each other, and adhesions are formed. These adhesions also prevent the normal broadening of the muscle fibers that occurs during muscle contraction.

Fluids stagnate, decreasing mobility of the cells. An initial outcome of dysfunction and injury to the body is a decrease in the normal flow of fluids, creating a loss of the primary circulatory rhythm. The rhythmic pumping of fluids in waves of movement is altered. The swelling after acute injury prevents normal fluid exchange. Sustained muscle contraction and adhesions in chronic dysfunction and injury also creates stagnation in the tissue. Stagnation reduces the tissue's ability to repair itself owing to decreased cellular activity, decreased nutrition, and the accumulation of waste products.

Soft-tissue dysfunction and injury has neurologic consequences. A vast network of nerves are embedded within collagen. Adhesions, loss of the normal parallel alignment of the soft-tissue fibers, abnormal position, torsion, and fluid stagnation not only cause pain, but also create abnormal neurologic reflexes in the muscles, joints, arteries, internal organs, and central nervous system (CNS).

Soft-tissue dysfunction and injury creates dysfunction in the joint. Abnormal position and torsion of the soft tissue also create abnormal forces moving through the joint, creating joint dysfunction and potential degeneration. Joint dysfunction and degeneration cause irritation to the sensory nerve receptors in the soft tissue surrounding the joint. This irritation can create neurologic reflexes that inhibit (weaken) or create hypertonicity in the surrounding muscles, leading to abnormalities of coordination and balance.

An example of the mechanisms of soft-tissue injury and dysfunction may be illustrated with an irritation or injury of the knee. An injury to the knee typically causes the joint to be held in a sustained flexion. This position pulls the soft tissue on the medial and lateral aspects of the knee into an abnormal posterior alignment. This misalignment creates an abnormal torsion in the muscles, tendons, and ligaments on the medial and lateral aspects of the knee, a shortening of the myofascia in the hamstrings in the back of the knee, and a weakening of the medial quadriceps. The increased torsion causes a decreased flow of cells and fluids in the area, leading to a decreased ability for repair.

ESSENTIAL TREATMENT GOALS OF ORTHOPEDIC MASSAGE

The treatment goals of OM are fully described in Chapter 2, Assessment and Technique. Some of the goals are similar to those of other forms of massage, but several specific treatment goals are unique to this method of massage:

- **Reposition the soft tissue.** One of our most fundamental intentions in OM is to reposition the soft tissue. We accomplish this by resetting the soft tissue in a specific direction for each joint.
- **Reintroduce the normal spiral orientation to the tissue.** The text describes the abnormal torsion patterns in the soft tissue surrounding each joint, and the direction of the strokes to unwind the abnormal torsion.
- **Reestablish the normal parallel alignment of soft-tissue fibers.** The ligaments, tendons, and muscles are like braided ropes or long phone cables, with tubes within tubes of fibers. Lauren Berry, RPT, applied techniques from engineering to the human body. He discovered that a twist in a steel cable or a phone cable can be "unwound" by rocking the structure back and forth perpendicular to its longitudinal axis, thus reestablishing the normal parallel alignment of the fibers.
- **Restore the ability of the bundles of fibers (fascicles) to slide relative to each other.** OM is applied perpendicular (transverse) to the line of the fibers almost exclusively. This dissolves abnormal adhesions, broadens the fibers, and increases lubrication.
- **Stimulate cellular activity and create electric currents to repair and regenerate the body.** Massage applied transverse to the fibers creates a mechanical tension or pulling force on the fibers that creates a piezoelectric effect, which means that mechanical energy is transformed into electrical energy. The piezoelectric effect increases cellular activity and repair of the tissue as well as proper alignment.
- **Restore the movement of the fluids.** OM strokes are applied in rhythmic cycles of compression and decompression, while rocking the body in oscillating waves. This technique not only restores the natural rhythmic movement of the body's fluids, but also creates a profound relaxation.

A NEW METHOD OF MASSAGE: WAVE MOBILIZATION

To accomplish these treatment goals, the author has created a new method of massage called wave mobilization. This method is based on 20 years of clinical experience and the author's 25 years of practice of tai chi. Tai chi was developed by the Taoists who observed nature and especially water as embodying the essence of their spiritual path. Water is so yielding that it takes the shape of whatever container it is in, yet so powerful that it dissolves rocks and forms canyons. The massage stroke used in wave mobilization is patterned after an ocean wave and is performed using internal energy, or chi, rather than muscular strength.

The energy pattern of an ocean wave is circular. The direction of the waves is perpendicular to the coastline (Fig. 1-8). The waves are repeated in rhythmic cycles, which cause the water to ebb and flow on the shore.

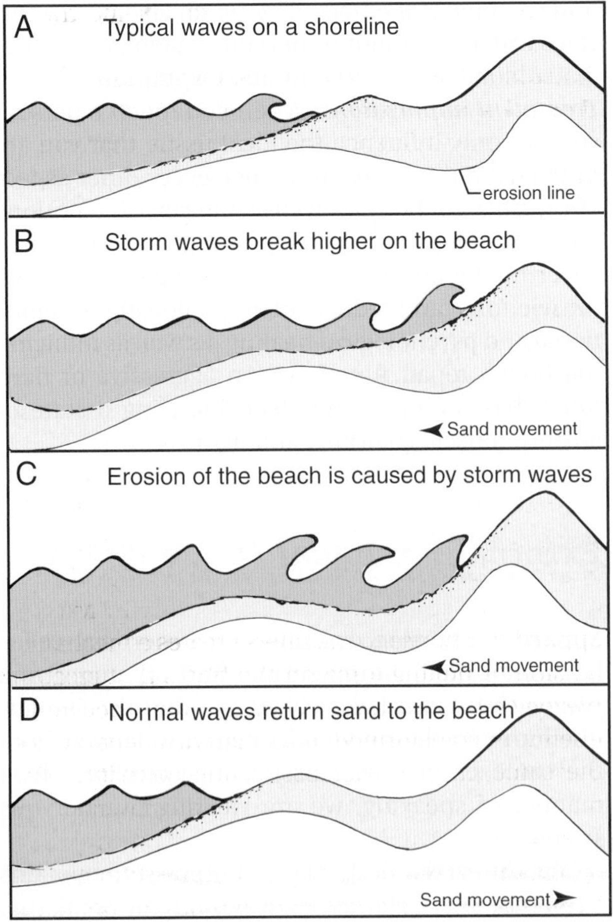
A Typical waves on a shoreline
erosion line
B Storm waves break higher on the beach
Sand movement
C Erosion of the beach is caused by storm waves
Sand movement
D Normal waves return sand to the beach
Sand movement

Figure 1-8. Wave mobilization stroke is modeled after the pattern of ocean waves. The ocean wave moves a molecule of water in a circular pattern. The waves move perpendicular to the shoreline, creating a digging motion.

Just as strong waves can dissolve a shoreline, massage applied in specific rhythmic cycles, perpendicular to the line of the fiber can dissolve adhesions and reintroduce normal motion in the tissue.

The massage strokes of OM are performed while mobilizing the body in rhythmic oscillations, like the ebb and flow of the ocean. The massage strokes are applied in a specific direction to reposition the soft tissue to its normal alignment and to remove the abnormal twist, or torsion, from the tissue. The strokes are applied perpendicular (transverse) to the line of the fiber to dissolve abnormal crosslinks and microscopic adhesions between the fibers and the fascicles. Dissolving these adhesions allows the fibers and fascicles to slide relative to each other, promotes the normal broadening of the muscle fibers, and helps realign the normal parallel orientation of the fibers. We perform the strokes in cycles of compression and decompression to restore the normal waves of movement of the fluids within the body.

MUSCLE ENERGY TECHNIQUE

OM also incorporates another treatment modality called muscle energy technique (MET). MET is a method of active resistance by the client against a force applied by the therapist. The author has developed a unique method of incorporating MET into the massage treatment. The clinical effects of MET are fully described in Chapter 2.

Because MET uses voluntary effort from the client to contract muscles, higher brain functions can be used to reprogram neurologic patterns of habitual muscle tension or muscle inhibition and weakness, helping to restore normal muscle function. MET dramatically transforms the role of the massage therapist from a practitioner who gives a treatment to someone to a practitioner who works with someone. The active participation of the client with the therapist can dramatically change chronic pain patterns.

MET also stimulates the synthesis of new cells to repair injured tissue, helps realign and strengthen connective tissue fibers, lengthens shortened tissue, increases the range of motion of the joints, and balances the strength of muscles crossing the joints to help evenly distribute the pressures moving through the joints.

Active contraction and relaxation of the muscles creates a spiral winding and unwinding of the soft tissue surrounding the joint. This tightening and relaxation of the soft tissue promotes the movement of the cells and fluids deep within the body to disperse stagnation, and promote the reoxygenation of the tissue, and the elimination of waste products.

ORTHOPEDIC MASSAGE PRINCIPLES

The development of OM was guided by three principles:

1. To translate the extraordinary clinical results of the soft-tissue manipulation techniques used by Lauren Berry, RPT, into massage strokes.
2. To create a massage style that is relaxing and nurturing, while maintaining superb clinical results.
3. To develop a massage technique that is also relaxing and energizing for the therapist. OM is performed by creating a wave of energy within the therapist by rocking his or her body from the back

foot to the front foot. This cyclical movement is coordinated with performing a massage stroke and then releasing the stroke in rhythmic cycles. Not only is this method profoundly relaxing and healing for the client, but it is also deeply relaxing and healing for the therapist.

BASIC ORGANIZATION OF THE BODY

The body's tissues are composed of three basic elements: cells, fibers and other intercellular substances, and body fluids.

Four Primary Types of Tissue

There are four primary types of tissue in adults:

- **Epithelium**—The epithelium consists of the skin, called the external epithelium, and the internal epithelium, which lines the internal organs and glands.
- **Connective tissue**—The connective tissue forms the structural framework of the body. It is the basic building block of soft tissue, including ligaments, tendons, joint capsules, and the fascia forming the structural framework of muscles. There are generalized types of connective tissue, including coverings of most organs and muscles and packing of most organs, and specialized types, including cartilage, bone, blood, and lymph.
- **Muscle**—The muscles are classified in three types: skeletal (also called voluntary muscle), smooth (intestinal tract and blood vessels), and cardiac (heart).
- **Nerve**—The nerves consist of long cells grouped in bundles. The nervous system includes the brain, spinal cord, peripheral nerves, and autonomic nervous system.

Body, Mind, and Emotions Form a Unified Whole

- It is important to realize that all of these tissues form an interrelated whole and that each tissue not only influences other tissues, but also affects a person's emotions and psychology. For example, when you massage a tight muscle, you are touching the skin, connective tissue, blood vessels, muscles, and nerve endings that communicate with every other part of the body. The touch stimulates sensory nerves that communicate to other muscles; to the neighboring joint; to the spinal cord; to the area of the highest centers of the brain that receives sensory information; and to the limbic area of the brain, which is the emotional center of the body. The touch also communicates with the autonomic nervous system, which regulates blood flow, heart rate, and respiration.
- ***Treatment implications:*** When you touch a person, you not only influence the local tissue that you are touching, but you also influence every other aspect of the physical body, as well as the client's emotions and psychology. A nurturing and gentle touch can lower the blood pressure, slow the heart rate, relax muscle tone, and reduce anxiety, allowing for emotional and psychological healing, as well as inducing the body's repair functions. An aggressive or hard touch has the opposite effect, inducing a state of anxiety, muscle guarding, and distress.

External Epithelial Tissue (Skin)

- ***Structure:*** The skin consists of a superficial cellular layer called the epidermis and an underlying connective tissue layer called the dermis. The epithelium and the nervous system are derived from the same embryologic tissue, the ectoderm. In a manner of speaking, we are wearing our nervous system.
  - The skin is the body's largest organ and contains blood vessels, glands, muscles, connective tissue, and nerve endings.
  - The skin contains four types of sensory nerve receptors called mechanoreceptors, which communicate with every other part of the body. The mechanoreceptors are sensitive to touch, pressure, movement, superficial proprioception (positional changes), pain, and temperature.
- ***Function:*** The skin provides sensation and protection, helps regulate water balance, and regulates temperature. The sense of touch is the first of the senses to become functional in embryonic life, followed by proprioception.
  - Sensory information from the skin communicates to the spinal cord where reflex (automatic, unconscious) connections are made to muscles, internal organs, and blood vessels. Skin pain can cause a contraction in the skeletal muscles or internal organs. A calming touch applied to the skin can reflexively relax muscles and internal organs.[1]
- ***Dysfunction and injury:*** Adhesions in the skin can develop after a blunt injury, cut, or surgery. As the superficial fascia in the dermis is connected to the underlying deep fascia covering the muscles, these adhesions decrease the ability of the tissue to stretch and thus limit joint function. Adhesions in the su-

perficial fascia can also entrap the cutaneous nerves, leading to pain, numbing, and tingling.

- *Treatment implications:* A nurturing touch is critical to promote healing. One hallmark of OM is that the massage strokes are applied with a gentle, nurturing touch. For much of the session the client is put in a fetal position and rocked in rhythmic oscillations that mimic the intrauterine heartbeat we all felt as developing embryos in the womb. This form of mobilization is profoundly relaxing.

Connective Tissue

As the name implies, connective tissue connects all the parts of the body. It consists of hard and soft tissues. Bone is mineralized connective tissue. It forms the structural walls for organs and blood vessels and binds joints together through ligaments and joint capsules. It gives shape to the body through broad sheets of fascia and the compartments, called septa, which contain the muscles. It transmits the pull of the muscles through the connective tissue surrounding the muscles and the tendons. As we will see, it is the connective tissue that is injured in the strains and sprains of muscles, tendons, and ligaments. Therefore, it is one of the primary tissues to be addressed in OM.

CONNECTIVE TISSUE COMPONENTS

Cells

- There are six different types of cells in ordinary connective tissue, but only the fibroblast is important for our consideration. Important cells of specialized connective tissue are the chondrocyte or cartilage cell and the osteocyte or bone cell.
  - **Fibroblasts**—Fibroblasts produce all of the components of connective tissue, including fibers and ground substance, and are active in inflammation and repair. These cells are found in ligaments, tendons, joint capsules, and fascia.
  - **Chondrocytes**—Chondrocytes or cartilage cells are found in the collagen matrix of cartilage. Chondrocytes synthesize new cartilage in the normal turnover of cells and in the repair of damaged cartilage.
  - **Osteocytes**—Osteocytes or the bone cells transport materials to maintain the structure of the bones and are active in the repair of bone.
- *Function:* The normal function of the cells and the creation of new cells (synthesis) are stimulated by movement. Cellular activity is also increased by the inflammatory process after an injury.
- *Dysfunction and injury:* Decreased movement or immobilization causes cells to break down tissue (lysis) and creates atrophy in the muscles, tendons, and ligaments, and osteoporosis in the bones.
- *Treatment implication:* Cellular activity is increased by mechanical stimulation, which includes massage, mobilization, and active muscle contraction called MET.

Fibers

The three types of connective tissue fibers are: reticulin, elastin, and collagen.

Reticulin is a meshlike network for support of organs and glands. Elastin is more elastic and is found in ligaments and the linings of arteries. Collagen is one of the main tissues that a massage therapist works with, and is described below.

- *Structure:* Collagen forms the gross structure of tendons, ligaments, joint capsules, fascia of muscles, cartilage, and bone. It gives tissues their shape and can be likened to the wood framing of a house. The collagen fibers are long, soft, white, tough fibers synthesized from fibroblasts, which make tropocollagen, a triple helical (spiral) structure (Fig.1-9).
  - Tropocollagen molecules line up side by side, overlapping, and are chemically bound together in a parallel arrangement by intermolecular crosslinks to form fibrils. These crosslinks give collagen great strength and stability.
  - The fibrils pack together to form a fiber, and the fibers are generally collected into bundles called fascicles.
  - The collagen fibers and fascicles are normally aligned in a parallel and longitudinal orientation. The greatest strength is found when the fibers and fascicles are oriented in this parallel and longitudinal alignment along the lines of mechanical stress.
  - Mature collagen resembles the structure of a rope, with small strands forming larger strands, all wound together in a spiral.
  - The individual fibers and the fascicle bundles normally can slide freely past one another.[2] The normal gliding of the collagen fibers is maintained by movement and the lubrication from the ground substance.
- *Function:* Collagen forms approximately 80% of tendons, ligaments, and joint capsules, and a large percentage of cartilage and bone. It forms the structural

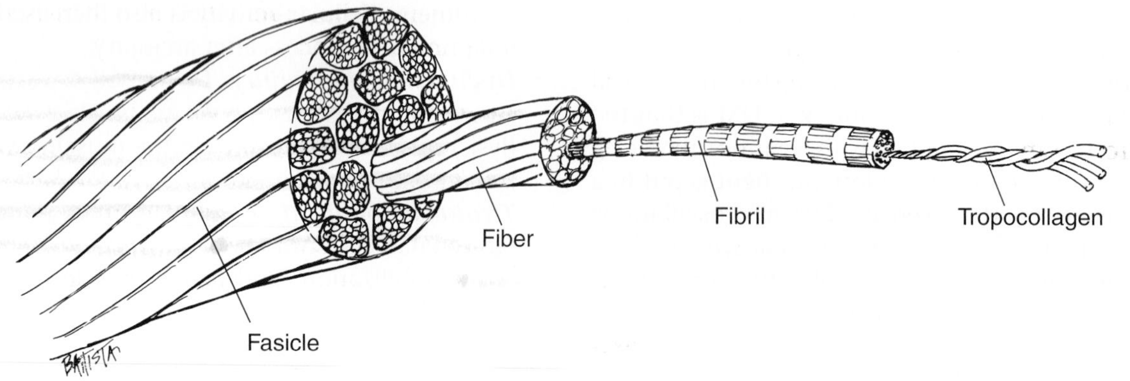

Figure 1-9. Collagen structure. Collagen fibers are organized in bundles called fascicles, which are designed to slide relative to each other in the healthy state.

support for the muscles; blood vessels; and nerve fibers, including those of the brain, the skin, and the internal organs.

- Collagen stabilizes the joints through the ligaments, the joint capsules, and the periosteum by resisting the tension or pulling force transmitted through the joints by movement or gravity.
- Collagen transmits the pulling force of muscle contraction through the fascia within the muscle and through the tendon.
- **Wolff's law** states that bone is laid down along lines of stress. This same law applies to soft tissue. Normal stresses, in the form of exercise, and the activities of daily living increase collagen synthesis and strengthens connective tissue.

■ ***Dysfunction and injury:*** Dysfunction to collagen is defined as either excessive mechanical stress or a lack of adequate stress to the tissue.

- *Excessive mechanical stress* is also called cumulative or repetitive stress. It creates excessive deposits of collagen, causing abnormal crosslinks and adhesions. The fibers pack closer together, and the lubrication is decreased, which decreases the ability of the fibers and fascicles to slide relative to each other. Cumulative stress is caused by three main factors.
  - **Posture:** Abnormal stresses, such as a forward-head posture (FHP) creates an excessive tension or pulling force on the soft tissues around the cervicothoracic junction, and this area feels thick owing to the excessive deposits of collagen.
  - **Dynamic activity:** The stress of repetitive gripping of a tennis racquet and the reactive force of hitting the ball causes a thickening of the collagen within the muscles of the elbow, wrist, and hand and at their attachment sites.
  - **Misalignment:** An example of misalignment is patellar-tracking dysfunction. The kneecap or patella is pulled laterally and rubs against the femur; this irritation creates excessive deposits of collagen.
- *Immobilization* or lack of use decreases collagen production, leading to atrophy in the connective tissue and to osteoporosis in the bone. Without movement the collagen is laid down in a random orientation, packing the fibers close together, forming adhesions. This atrophy and random orientation of the fibers creates weakness in the tissue and instability of the associated joint.
- *Injury:* An injury to collagen is a tearing apart of the collagen fibers microscopically or a complete disruption of the structure (see "Mechanics of Soft Tissue Injury", p. 34) Most soft-tissue injuries are injuries to collagen.
  - An injury creates an inflammatory response. During the repair phase of the inflammatory cycle, the fibrils and fibers are laid down in a random orientation, instead of in the normal parallel and longitudinal arrangement. This random weave decreases their strength. The fibers pack closer together, forming abnormal crosslinks and adhesions, thus preventing the normal gliding characteristics of the collagen.[2]
  - Adhesions are abnormal deposits of connective tissue between gliding surfaces. These adhesions can occur at every level of the soft tissue, from the ligament or tendon adhering to the bone, to adhesions between the fascicles, or the fibers themselves.
  - Adhesions decrease tissue extensibility. The tissue becomes less elastic, thicker, and shorter. The client will often feel stiff in the area of adhesions.

- ***Treatment implications:***
  - The goals of treatment of collagen are:
    - Stimulate the fibroblasts to repair the injured collagen.
    - Provide mechanical stimulation to realign the collagen fibers to their normal parallel alignment.
    - Lengthen shortened tissue.
    - Stimulate the fluids to increase the lubrication between the fibers and the fascicles and thus promote normal gliding.
    - Stimulate the fluids to promote nutrition, reoxygenation, and elimination of waste products.
  - It is essential to maintain motion for the collagen to align itself properly. Movement also promotes the normal sliding of the fascicles and helps maintain the normal interfiber distance. If the movements of daily life are inadequate to restore function, then the abnormal crosslinks in the collagen can be reduced through OM and MET.
  - *Orthopedic Massage:* OM involves performing massage strokes transverse to the collagen fibers. This dissolves abnormal crosslinks and adhesions; helps realign the fibers to their normal parallel array; and increases the lubrication between the fibers and the fascicles, promoting the normal gliding characteristics of the tissue. Stroking transverse to the fibers provides a mechanical tension or pulling force to the tissue, which stimulates cellular activity and promotes repair. It also creates an electrical current in the tissue caused by the piezoelectric effect (see below). Massage also creates heat in the tissue. As the collagen fibers are stretched with transverse massage strokes, energy is stored. After the massage stroke, the fibers are released, and the stored energy from stretching the tissue is released as heat. Heat is also produced by compression of the tissue, by the heat of the therapist's hands, by the friction of crossing the fibers back and forth, and by the mobilization of the body. This heat stimulates cellular activity and improves the lubrication of the fibers by making the ground substance more fluid (see "Ground Substance").
  - *Muscle Energy Technique:* MET involves the active contraction of the client's muscles against the resistance provided by the therapist. This contraction creates a tensile (pulling) force that increases collagen synthesis, helps realign the collagen fibers in their normal parallel array, dissolves abnormal crosslinks and adhesions, and lengthens shortened tissue. The work energy of active muscle contraction is also released as heat after the contraction is released and the muscle relaxes.

CAUTION: **The treatment of injuries requires special precautions: In the early stages after an injury, great care must be exercised by the therapist to use only gentle massage so as not to disturb the newly forming crosslinks. These normal crosslinks are essential to maintaining the strength of the tissue. Gentle isometric MET is used to help realign the developing fibrils, but excessive force of stretching is contraindicated in the first 2 weeks after an injury (see Chapter 2).**

Ground Substance

- ***Definition:*** Ground substance is a transparent, viscous fluid—much like raw egg whites in appearance and consistency—that surrounds all the cells in the body. Viscosity is the resistance to flow.
- ***Structure:*** The primary components of ground substance are glycoaminoglycans (GAGs) and water. GAGs act to draw water into the tissue and bind it. Water makes up approximately 70% of ground substance.
- ***Function:*** Ground substance acts as a source of nutrition and a medium to disperse waste products. It also acts as a lubricant and spacer between the collagen fibers, preventing the fibers from adhering to each other.[3] Ground substance has a thixotropic quality. **Thixotropy** is the quality of a substance to become more fluid when stirred and more solid when it remains undisturbed.[1] Massage therapy can change the viscosity of the ground substance from a gel to a fluid.
- ***Dysfunction and injury:*** Injury causes a decrease of the GAGs that bind water, which, in turn, decreases the lubrication and spacing provided by the ground substance. The fibrils and fibers pack closer together, leading to abnormal crosslinks and adhesions. This decreases the normal gliding of the fibers, fascicles, whole tendons, ligaments, joint capsules, and muscles relative to the neighboring soft tissues and bone. With disuse and immobilization, tissue fluids stagnate and nutrition is decreased, which inhibits repair. The tissues tend to cool, and the ground substance becomes thicker, more gellike, leading to greater stiffness,

decreased circulation and nutrition, and decreased lubrication.

- *Treatment implication:* Massage, mobilization, and MET can reintroduce motion into the tissue. Movement stimulates the synthesis of ground substance and GAGs, and promotes the circulation of blood, lymph, and ground substance, which contains a high percentage of water. This water can then bind to the GAGs, creating greater lubrication to the tissue. Movement also transports nutrients and promotes the exchange of waste products. As mentioned above, heat creates a change in the ground substance from being sluggish and thick to a more fluid state. MET creates heat through muscle contraction and the pulling and release of the fascial components. MET also promotes circulation deep within the body by means of the pumping action of muscle contraction, which affects the lymph and blood flow.

PROPERTIES OF CONNECTIVE TISSUE

Viscoelasticity

Viscoelasticity describes the mechanical behavior of soft tissue, which contains both elastic fibers and a fluid gel (ground substance).

- **Elasticity** is the ability of a tissue to be stretched and to return to its previous length. This is like a spring. Collagen has a wavelike crimp in it that lengthens when it is stretched a small amount and that springs back to its original length.
- **Viscosity** is the resistance of fluids to movement. The ground substance of soft tissue has the viscosity of egg whites. The degree of viscosity of a fluid depends on how quickly or how slowly it is moved. For example, if you move your hand slowly through water, little resistance is encountered. If you move your hand rapidly greater "fluid friction" is encountered.
- *Treatment implications:* If the ground substance of the soft tissue is thick, the massage strokes need to be slowed down. It is helpful to perform MET to thick tissue, which increases the heat in the tissue and helps make the ground substance less viscous (more liquid), which, in turn, decreases the friction of your strokes. If soft tissue is stretched slowly, then it will lengthen more easily. When a more rapid force is applied, soft tissues become stiff and more easily injured. This helps explain why rapid acceleration in a car accident is damaging to the soft tissue.

Piezoelectricity

- *Definition:* Piezoelectricity is the ability of a tissue to generate electrical potentials in response to mechanical deformation. Piezoelectricity is a property of most, if not all, living tissues.
- *Dysfunction and injury:* Adhesions create a resistance to normal electrical flow.[4] This decrease in electrical currents conducted in the connective tissues interferes with the normal repair and rejuvenation process.
- *Treatment implications:* Massage strokes mechanically deform the collagen fibers by compressing and crossing the fibers. This creates electric potentials, which help realign the collagen fibers in their normal parallel array. It also increases the negative charge in the soft tissue, which has a strong proliferative effect, stimulating the creation of new cells to repair the injured site.[5] MET provides mechanical stimulus that also generates piezoelectric currents.

THREE GENERALIZED TYPES OF CONNECTIVE TISSUE

Loose Irregular (Areolar)

- *Structure:* Loose, irregular connective tissue consists of a meshwork, like a spiderweb, of collagen and elastin fibers interlacing in all directions, and of an abundance of ground substance and cells.
- *Function:* Loose, irregular connective tissue suspends and binds structures together. Muscles, arteries, veins, nerves, and organs are all suspended from this type of tissue.
- *Dysfunction and injury:* Injury or cumulative stress can irritate or inflame a muscle or peripheral nerve, creating adhesions in the loose, irregular connective tissue. This inhibits the ability of these structures to slide freely within their connective tissue spaces.
- *Treatment implication:* Perform OM perpendicular to the line of the muscle or nerve. These scooping strokes dissolve these adhesions with the heat caused by tissue compression and friction, and by the mechanical pressure of stretching the tissue perpendicular to the line of the fiber. By taking the tissue into tension and then releasing it with the OM stroke, the abnormal crosslinks are reduced, and the soft tissues increase their extensibility and allow greater range of motion to the structure being suspended.

Dense Irregular

- *Structure:* Dense, irregular connective tissue forms thick bundles of collagen interweaving in three dimensions. There are few cells and little ground substance. It is found in the outer connective tissue sheaths of muscles and nerves, and in the dermis of the skin.
- *Function:* Because of the three-dimensional interweaving of the collagen, this tissue has considerable strength and can withstand forces from various angles.

Dense Regular

- *Structure:* Dense, regular connective tissue consists of parallel bundles of collagen fibers that form either thick bundles such as tendons and ligaments; broad, flattened tendons called aponeuroses; or flattened ligaments such as the outer layer of the synovial joint capsule. (For a discussion of the joint capsule, see "Joint Structure and Function").

TYPES OF CONNECTIVE TISSUE STRUCTURES

Tendons

- *Structure:* Tendons are a continuation of the connective tissue (fascia) within the muscle. This fascia is called a tendon after the muscle fibers end. The muscle and tendon are therefore best described as a unit, the **musculotendinous** unit, the **myotendon,** or the **myofascia.** The junction where the muscle fibers end and the connective tissue forming the tendon continues is called the **myotendinous junction.** The tendon attaches to the bone by interweaving to the connective tissue covering of the bone called the periosteum, and this attachment is called the **tenoperiosteal junction.**
  - Tendons are composed of long spiraling bundles of parallel collagen fibers, oriented in a longitudinal pattern along the line of stress, and embedded in a matrix of ground substance and a small number of fibroblasts.
  - Collagen molecules combine to form ordered units of microfibrils, fibrils, and fibers (Fig. 1-10). These fibers run parallel to each other and are contained in a bundle called a fascicle. Each fascicle is normally capable of sliding past the other fascicles in the healthy state.[6] A group of fascicles together forms the gross tendon.
  - Tendons and ligaments have a microscopic "crimp" or wavelike structure that acts like a spring and can withstand large internal forces.
  - Tendons may be a cordlike structure like the Achilles tendon; a flattened band of tissue like the rotator cuff; or a broad sheet of tissue called an aponeurosis, such as the origin of the latissimus dorsi.
  - Tendons are surrounded by a loose connective tissue sheath called a paratenon. In areas of high pressure or friction, such as where tendons rub over the bones of the wrist and ankle, the tendon sheath is lined with a synovial layer to facilitate gliding of the tendon (Fig1-11).
- *Function:* Tendons attach muscle to bone and transmit the force of muscle contraction to the bone, thereby producing motion of the joint. They also

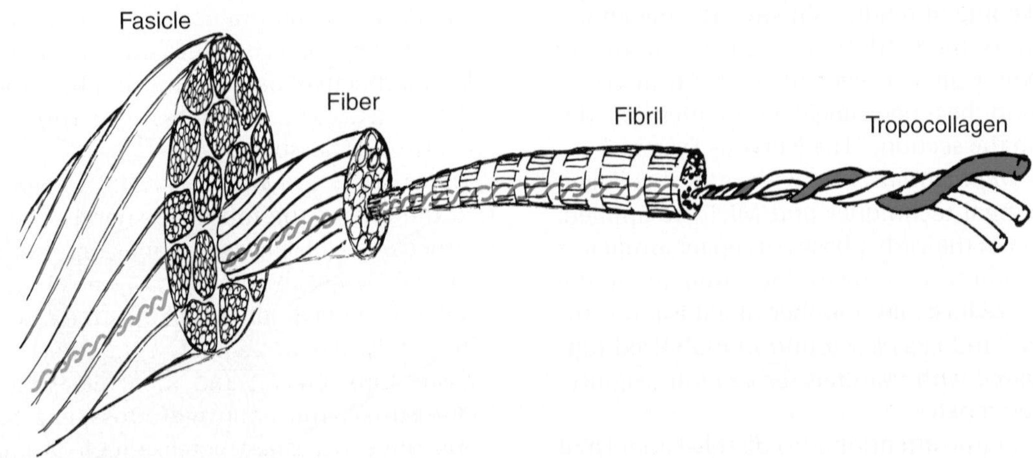

Figure 1-10. Longitudinal and parallel alignment of the collagen fibers and the crimp or wave within the fibers of a tendon and ligament.

help stabilize the joint and act as a sensory receptor through Golgi tendon organs (GTOs). (See "The Nervous System" section for more information on GTOs.) The crimp in the tendon imparts an elastic quality to the structure.

- *Dysfunction and injury:* An injury to the tendon is called a **strain** and typically represents a tearing of the collagen fibers at the musculotendinous junction, at the tenoperiosteal junction, or within the body of the tendon. The term **tendinitis** is used to describe injuries to the tendon portion of the muscle-tendon unit. Tendons are susceptible to fatigue and degeneration, leading to chronic inflammation, which is called **tendinosis.** Loss of normal motion in a tendon through injury or immobilization creates loss of collagen fibers (atrophy) and adhesions between the tendon and the surrounding structures, including the tendon sheath. This decreases the strength of the tendon.
  - Reid[7] has categorized tendinitis into five functional grades, depending on the symptoms reported by the patient.[7]
    - Grade I: Pain only after activity.
    - Grade II: Minimal pain with activity.
    - Grade III: Pain interferes with activity, but disappears with rest.
    - Grade IV: Pain does not disappear with rest; significant pain and swelling.
    - Grade V: Pain interferes with activities of daily living; chronic and recurrent pain; significant pain and swelling, signs of soft-tissue changes, and altered muscle function.
  - These injuries and dysfunctions are also categorized on the basis of the structures affected. **Tenosynovitis** is a roughening of the gliding surfaces within the tendon sheath, and **tenovaginitis** is a thickening of tendon sheath, creating an enlargement of the tendon that jams in the sheath (commonly called "trigger finger"). An injury to the tendon has neurologic consequences, described in the section, "The Nervous System."
- *Treatment implications:* As with other collagen injuries, manual techniques and MET are applied. Mobilization in the early phases of repair stimulates collagen synthesis, improves the strength of the tendon, and reduces the number of adhesions.[2] Increased DNA and cells are found in mobilized tendons compared with immobilized tendons, signifying increased repair.[8]
  - The therapeutic intention is to dissolve abnormal crosslinks and adhesions, increase the lubrication and nutrition by creating a thixotropic effect on the ground substance, help realign the developing collagen fiber in the early stages of repair, lengthen the tissue in the chronic phase if indicated, and restore neurologic function with MET. As with other collagen structures, great care must be taken in the early stages after an injury, as the collagen is fragile, and too much pressure may disturb the newly forming tissue. If the tendon has weakened through injury, immobilization, or disuse, exercise is necessary to strengthen the tissue.

Ligaments

- *Structure:* Ligaments are composed of dense, white, short bands of nearly parallel bundles of collagen fibers embedded in a matrix of ground substance and a small number of fibroblasts. The fibers are bound together in a fascicle (see Fig.1-10). They are both microscopically and grossly similar to tendons, except that they contain some elastic fibers, giving them greater elasticity. Ligaments are pliable and flexible.
  - There is a normal parallel sliding of fibers, and the fascicles are free to slide relative to each other in the healthy state.[2] They have a "crimp" or wavelike structure that acts like a spring, withstanding large internal forces (see Fig. 1-11).
  - All ligaments surrounding the joints contain specialized nerve endings, including proprioceptors and mechanoreceptors, which give information about posture and movement, and play an important role in joint function. The ligaments also have pain fibers.
- *Function:* Ligaments attach one bone to another, help stabilize the joint, help guide joint motion, pre-

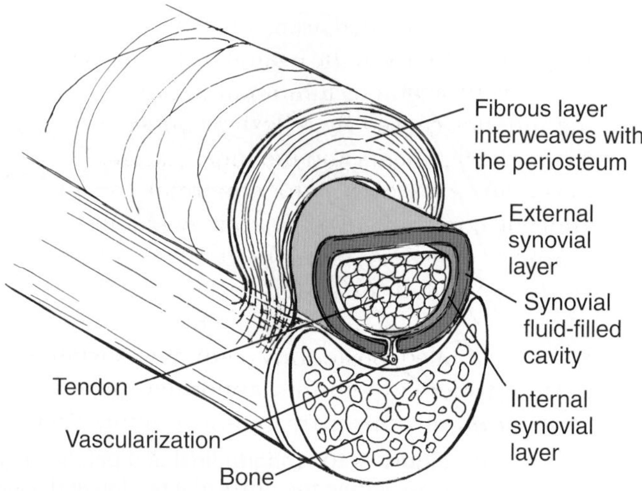

Figure 1-11. Tendon sheath structure.

vent excessive motion, and act as sensory receptors. Extrinsic ligaments are located over the joint capsule, whereas intrinsic ligaments are thickened portions of the capsule.

- Ligaments and tendons exhibit viscoelastic behavior. With normal motion, the ligament is stretched, and the crimp in the tissue straightens out. When the mild stretch is released, the ligament or tendon returns to its normal length. This describes the elastic nature of the tissue. If a stretch or force is slowly applied to a ligament over time, the tissue retains some of its new length, which describes its viscous behavior.
- A reflex connection exists between the ligaments of a joint and the surrounding muscles, which has instantaneous effects on muscle tone.[9]

- ***Dysfunction and injury:*** Ligament injuries are called **sprains,** and are a tearing of the collagen fibers.
  - Sprains are categorized into three grades, depending on the extent of the injury.
    - Grade I: Microscopic tearing of a few fibers. There is some pain, but no loss of stability.
    - Grade II: Gross tears, and some loss of structural integrity.
    - Grade III: Complete tearing through the body of the ligament or at its attachment. Frequently requires surgery.
  - Because of their functions to help stabilize the joint and as potent neurosensory structures, injuries to the ligaments can create profound disturbances to joint function.
  - Similar to the joint capsule, the ligaments might respond to an injury by becoming excessively stretched, creating joint instability, or they may become shortened, contributing to joint stiffness and loss of normal range of motion in the joint. Immobilization causes ligaments to atrophy and weaken owing to decreased collagen content.
  - Irritation or injury of the ligaments can cause a reflexive contraction or inhibition in the surrounding muscles caused by reflexive connections between the ligaments and the musculature.[10]
  - Ligaments can twist into abnormal torsion, a concept contributed by Lauren Berry, RPT. For example, after a knee injury, the knee often assumes a position of sustained flexion. The ligaments on the medial and lateral sides of the knee are pulled posteriorly with this sustained flexion, winding them into abnormal torsion.
- ***Treatment implications:*** Treatment of injured ligaments requires thorough assessment to differentiate whether the ligament is thick and fibrous owing to increased collagen, abnormal crosslinks, and adhesions, or if the ligament is too lax, owing to injury, immobilization, or disuse.
  - For ligaments that have developed adhesions, perform gentle scooping strokes transverse to the line of the fiber. If you palpate thickened, fibrous tissue in the chronic state, transverse friction massage (TFM), as described by Cyriax,[11] is effective in dissolving these adhesions and rehydrating the tissue.[11] The author has contributed a new method of applying TFM that dramatically reduces the pain associated with TFM.
  - If ligaments are too lax, exercise rehabilitation can stimulate the production of new collagen and help restore normal integrity to the ligament.
  - Abnormal torsion in the ligaments is corrected with OM strokes applied in a specific direction.
  - To help restore the neurologic function of the ligament, MET is used. As the muscle is connected to the ligaments with a neurologic reflex, isometric contractions to the muscles surrounding the ligaments can help restore neurologic communication.

Periosteum

- ***Structure:*** Periosteum is a dense, fibrous connective tissue sheath covering the bones. The outer layer consists of collagen fibers parallel to the bone and contains arteries, veins, lymphatics, and a rich supply of sensory nerves. The inner layer, called the osteogenic layer, contains osteoblasts—cells responsible for new bone formation.
- ***Function:*** The periosteum functions as follows:
  - The bone cells in the periosteum generate new bone during growth and repair when the periosteum is stimulated.
  - The periosteum interweaves with the joint capsule and ligaments, and stretching of the periosteum gives mechanoreceptor information regarding movement, position, and irritation of the joint.
  - The periosteum blends with the tendons, forming the tenoperiosteal junction, which provides the site where the muscle pulls on the bone for joint movement.
  - The sensory nerves in periosteum include pain fibers and nerves that are extremely sensitive to tension (i.e., a pulling force).[12]
- ***Dysfunction and injury:***
  - As the myofascia interweaves with the periosteum, repetitive stress can excessively stimulate the osteogenic layer to create bone spurs, a common problem with runners who develop heel spurs caused by the excessive or repetitive stress

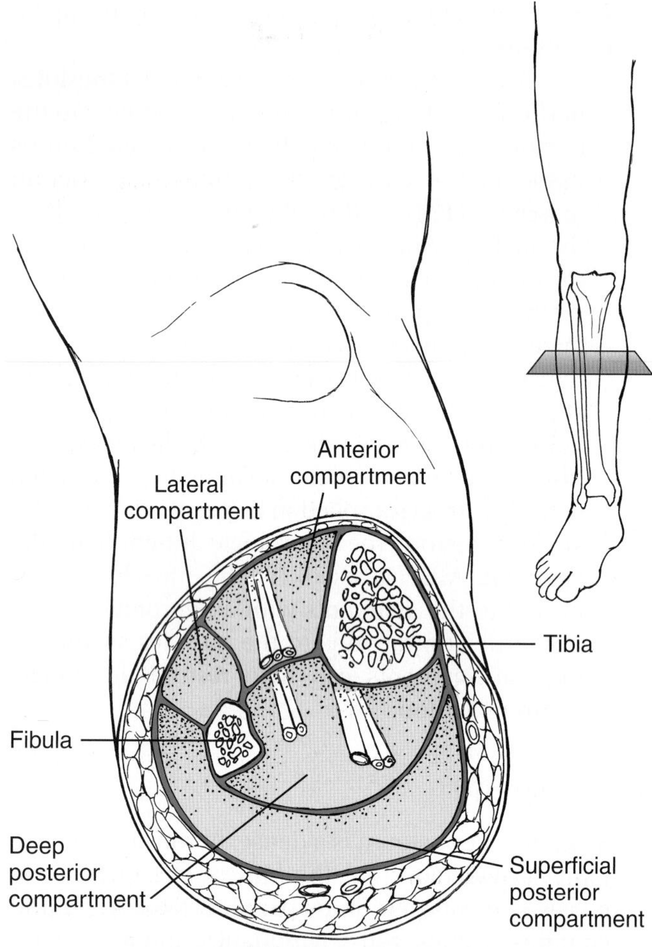

Figure 1-12. Deep connective tissue forms compartments in the body to organize muscle groups. This upward view is of the compartments of the right leg.

to the plantar fascia that interweaves with the periosteum of the heel.

- Excessive tension on the periosteum caused by an abnormal position of the joint increases collagen deposition, creating abnormal crosslinks and adhesions. Increased collagen deposition leads to stiffness and loss of normal motion in the joint and diminished function of the mechanoreceptors, potentially causing problems with balance and coordination.
- A common site of soft-tissue injury is at the tenoperiosteal junction. An acute tear or cumulative microtearing of the periosteum can cause the orientation of the collagen in the area to become random, leading to the development of the abnormal crosslinks and adhesions described above. Discomfort or pain can result when the muscle contracts and pulls on the adhesions in the periosteum.

- *Treatment implications:* The periosteum should feel smooth and glistening to the touch. If adhesions are palpated, first perform MET to the muscles that attach to the involved site. This increases the extensibility of the periosteum and the tenoperiosteal attachment. Adhesions are treated manually with back-and-forth OM strokes or brisk transverse friction strokes for chronic conditions. Although the primary direction of the strokes is perpendicular to the shaft of the bone and therefore perpendicular to the periosteum, strokes are performed in all directions because the interweaving tendons and ligaments form oblique angles to the bone.

Fascia

- *Structure:* Fascia is a fibrous connective tissue arranged as sheets or tubes; some are thick and dense; others are thin, filmy membranes. All fascia are connected in the body.
  - Superficial fascia lies under the dermis of the skin and is composed of loose, fatty connective tissue.
  - Deep fascia is a dense connective tissue that surrounds muscles and forms fascial compartments called **septa,** which contain muscles with similar functions (Fig.1-12). These compartments are well lubricated in the healthy state, allowing the muscles inside to move freely between each other, and relative to the fascial envelope.

PAIN AND SOFT TISSUE

Soft-Tissue Innervation

- *Structure:* Soft tissue has four basic categories of sensory (afferent) nerves: mechanoreceptors, chemoreceptors, nociceptors, and proprioceptors. These nerves provide connective tissue with an important neurosensory role. The terms mechanoreceptors and proprioceptors are sometimes used interchangably by some authors, although the proprioceptor is a subclass of a mechanoreceptor. These receptors are stimulated by some action, such as rotation of a joint, tension caused by muscle contraction, compression, or swelling. They are described more fully below in the section "Joint Structure and Function."
- *Function:*
  - Mechanoreceptors—sensitive to touch, pressure, and movement.
  - Proprioceptors—transmit changes in position and movement.

- Chemoreceptors—sensitive to the acid/base balance(pH), oxygen, etc.
- Nociceptors—transmit irritation or pain.

- ***Dysfunction and injury:*** Compression, irritation, or injury cause dysfunction in these sensory nerves. This topic is explored in the section, "The Nervous System."

Soft Tissue Is Pain Sensitive

A common source of musculoskeletal pain is from the deep somatic tissues. These include the periosteum, joint capsule, ligaments, tendons, muscles, and fascia. The most pain-sensitive tissue is the periosteum and the joint capsule. Tendons and ligaments are moderately sensitive, and muscle is less sensitive.[13]

Causes of Soft-Tissue Pain

Pain is caused by the stimulation of the nociceptor or pain receptor. These receptors are usually stimulated by chemicals such as bradykinin, serotonin, and histamine, which excite the nerve endings. Pain can be elicited by three different classes of stimuli: mechanical, chemical, and thermal. Basically, the soft tissue pain is caused by the chemicals released from an injury; from mechanical irritation caused by cumulative stress, which causes tissue damage and a microinflammatory environment; or from emotional or psychological stress, which causes hypertonic muscles, creating low oxygen and increased acids (Fig. 1-13). These basic categories can be expanded into the following six fundamental causes[14]:

- **Mechanical irritation** of the periosteum, joint capsules, bone, tissue around the blood vessels (perivascular tissue), ligaments, muscle and its fascia, and other soft tissues around the joint. Mechanical irritation develops from abnormal tension, compression, or torsion (twisting) of the soft tissue. Abnormal alignment of the joint creates mechanical irritation of the soft tissue surrounding the joint.
- **Injury** that creates inflammation and ischemia (low oxygen). This generates a chemical irritation of the pain fibers in the periosteum, joint capsules, bone, perivascular tissue, ligaments, synovial tissue, muscle and its fascia, and other soft tissues around the joint.
- **Neurogenic pain** caused by the irritation of sensory nerves, which then release chemicals (neuropeptides) from the nerve endings. These chemicals irritate the pain fibers in the periosteum, joint capsules, bone, perivascular tissue, ligaments, synovial tissue, muscle and its fascia, and other soft tissues around the joint (see "The Nervous System").
- **Reflex hypertonicity** of muscle, induced and maintained by proprioceptive and nociceptive sensory nerves. This creates stagnation in the tissue and decreased oxygen (ischemia), which causes pain.
- **Nerve entrapment** caused by soft-tissue swelling, adhesions in the connective tissue, or sustained muscle contraction. Entrapment of the nerve creates congestion and fluid stagnation. This reduces the flow of the axoplasm within the nerve, leading to altered sensation (paresthesia). Entrapment also reduces oxygen to the nerve because of stasis of the blood flow and leads to pain.
- **Psychological or emotional exaggeration** (enhancement) of pain and muscular hypertonicity. Pain is also an emotional and psychological experience and can be exaggerated by many factors, such as history of pain and social conditioning.

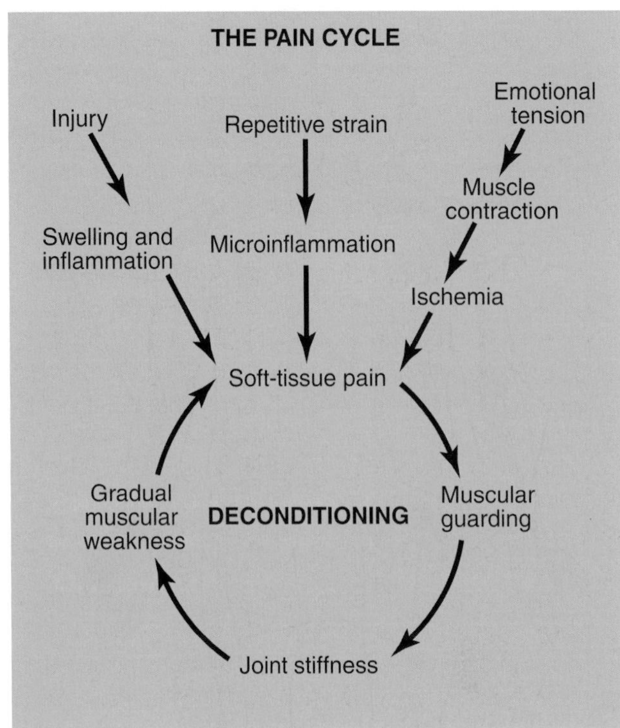

Figure 1-13. Soft-tissue pain cycle. Chronic pain leads to gradual weakness and deconditioning.

Referred Pain

- Pain that originates in deep somatic tissue is usually referred into specific patterns called **sclerotomes** (Fig.1-14). Sclerotomes are "those deep somatic tis-

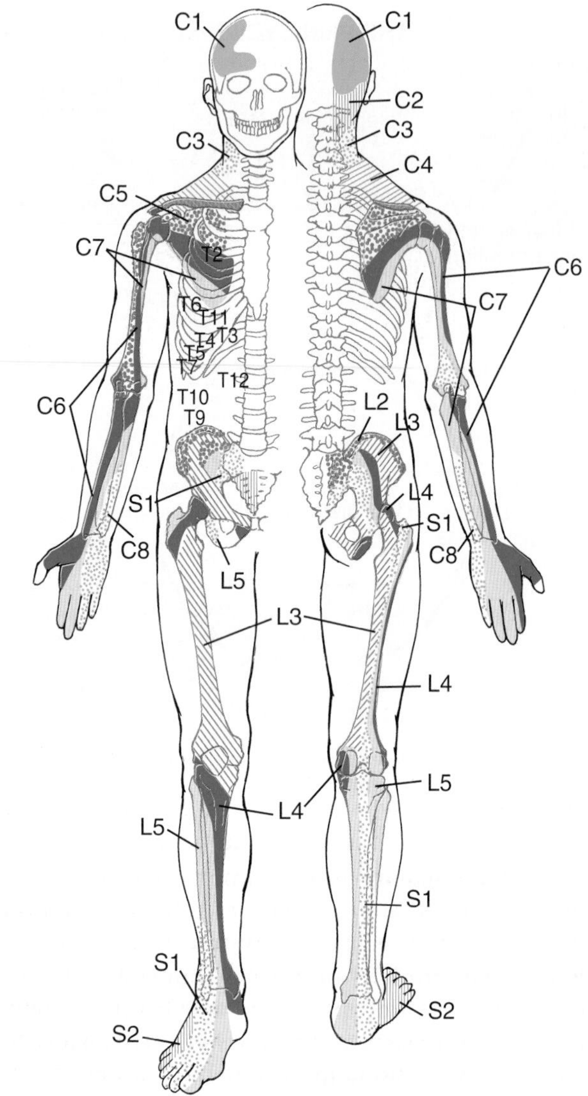

Figure 1-14. Irritation or injury of fascia, ligaments, tendons, joint capsules, or other connective tissues refers pain into regions innervated by the same spinal nerve. The pathways are called sclerotomes.

sues (fascia, ligaments, capsules, and connective tissue) that are innervated by the same spinal nerve."[13] The extent of the radiation depends on the intensity of the irritation to the tissue.

- When a tissue of a particular sclerotome is irritated, the pain may be perceived as originating from any and all of the tissue innervated by the same nerve.

Quality of Pain from Deep Somatic Tissues

- Deep somatic tissue pain is called **sclerotomal pain,** or deep somatic pain, and is described as deep, aching, and diffuse, as opposed to sharp, well-localized pain that comes from the skin or from irritation of a nerve root.
- A nerve root irritation can manifest as both **dermatomal pain** (i.e., sharp and well localized on the skin, as paresthesia [altered sensation, numbing, and tingling]) and as deep, aching sclerotomic pain.[13] For further discussion of dermatomes, see Chapter 3, "Lumbosacral Spine," and Chapter 5, "Cervical Spine."
- Sclerotomal pain is often associated with autonomic disturbances, such as sweating, pallor, and feelings of nausea and being faint.
- Pain of sclerotomal origin and from the viscera send impulses to the limbic and hypothalamus areas of the brain (the emotional centers) and may be responsible for emotional reactions of anxiety, fear, anger, and depression.

Pain-Gate Theory of Melzak and Wall and Its Relation to Massage

- The pain-gate theory proposes that there are two main factors that determine how pain is perceived:
  - First, it depends on the balance between mechanoreceptor information and pain fiber information. Touch, vibration, and joint and muscle movement stimulate mechanoreceptors, causing a decrease in the pain information received by the brain.
  - Second, the brain inhibits or enhances a reaction to pain. Athletes in intense competition can ignore an injury, and fear and anxiety can exaggerate pain.
- ***Treatment implication:*** Orthopedic massage moves the entire region of the body being worked on, as well as the local tissue, to stimulate a large number of mechanoreceptors, rather than pressing only at the site of the injury or dysfunction and keeping the rest of the body passive. This dramatically reduces the discomfort of working on these deep somatic tissues.

Muscle Structure and Function

GENERAL OVERVIEW

Muscle Structure

- There are approximately 250 skeletal muscles, and they are responsible for all of the body movements (Fig.1-15).

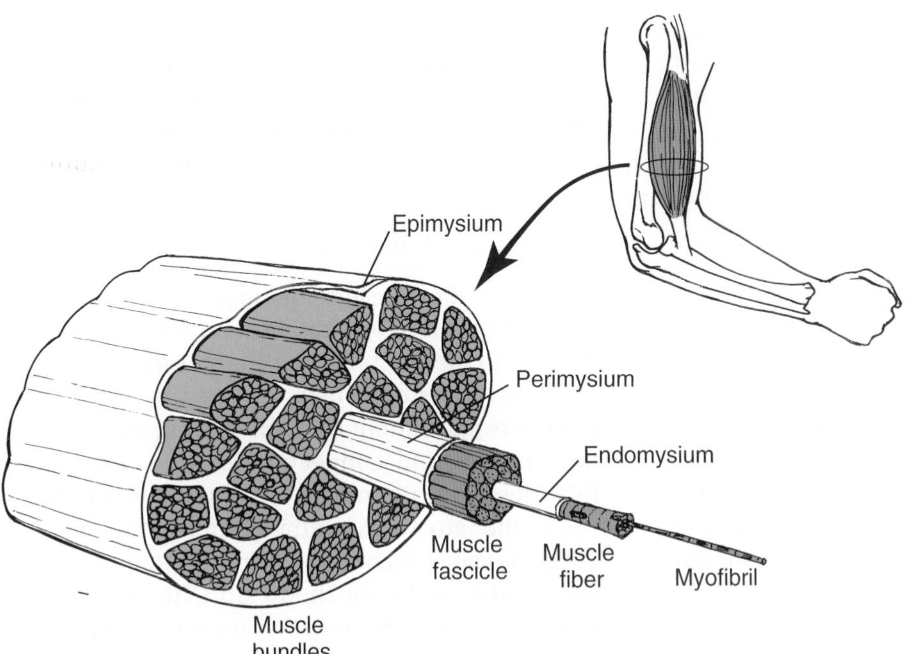

Figure 1-15. Anatomy of a muscle showing the layers of the connective tissue.

- ***Structure:*** The structural unit of skeletal muscle is the muscle fiber, which is a long, thin, threadlike cell.
  - The fibers are arranged in parallel, like collagen, and are collected in bundles called **fascicles.**
  - Each fiber is composed of many myofibrils.
  - The myofibril is composed of thousands of strands of proteins, also arranged in parallel, called myofilaments that are further divided into two kinds, actin and myosin, the basic proteins of contraction. Microscopically, the actin is arranged in a spiral.
  - There are two types of skeletal muscle fibers:
    - One is called the **extrafusal fiber,** and is under voluntary control. This is the typical muscle fiber.
    - The second is called an **intrafusal fiber** or **muscle spindle,** and lies embedded within the other fibers. This fiber functions as a sensory nerve receptor, and operates without conscious control.
  - In addition to the muscle fiber, every muscle contains satellite cells, which help regenerate muscle fibers in the event of injury to the muscle fiber.

Muscle Function

- **Movement**—Muscles are responsible for all the movements of the body.
- **Proprioception**—There are four types of nerve receptors in muscles (see below), that give the CNS information about the length, tension, pressure, movement, and sense of joint and body position in space.
- **Protection**—Muscles are connected to the nerves in the skin, and the nerves in the neighboring joint's capsule and ligaments through neurologic reflexes; therefore, if the skin or joint is irritated or injured, the muscle may go into a reflexive spasm (called "splinting"), or into inhibition (weakness).
- **Pump**—The muscles are called a musculovenous pump because the contracting skeletal muscle compresses the veins and moves blood toward the heart.[12] This contraction and relaxation of the muscles is essential to normal health in that it is used to eliminate the body's waste products and to bring in nutrition, including oxygen.
- **Pain receptors**—Muscles have pain receptors (nociceptors) that fire with chemical or mechanical irritation.
- **Posture and Stability**—Muscles are called dynamic stabilizers of the joints because they actively hold the joints in a stable position for posture and movement.

Muscle Connective Tissue

- ***Structure:*** The muscle fibers are so interwoven with connective tissue that a more accurate term for the muscle is **myofascia.** Three layers of connective tissue surround and support a muscle (see Fig. 1-15):
  - Epimysium, a fascia of fibrous connective tissue that surrounds the entire muscle.

    - Perimysium, a dense CT that surrounds each fascicle.
    - Endomysium, a loose CT that surrounds each individual fiber.
- *Function:*
    - The connective tissue of muscle transmits the pull of the contracting muscle cells and gives the muscle fibers organization and support.
    - The collagen fibers of these three layers of CT form the tendon, which attaches the muscle to the bone. The tendon fibers interweave with the CT of the periosteum, joint capsule, and ligaments.
    - All of these connective tissue layers are lubricated in the healthy state. Muscles as a whole are designed to slide relative to each other, and each fascicle within the muscle is also capable of sliding relative to the other fascicles in the healthy state.
- *Dysfunction and injury:* An injured muscle is called a pull or **strain.** A mild strain typically involves an injury to the connective tissue, i.e., the collagen, and not to the muscle fiber[15] (See "Dysfunction and Injury", above).
- *Treatment implication:* OM dissolves abnormal crosslinks and adhesions in the connective tissue that prevent the normal gliding of muscle fascicles. MET stimulates cellular activity for regeneration in the tissue and helps realign the connective tissue to its normal parallel alignment. Contract-relax (CR) MET can stretch the myotendon and postisometric relaxation (PIR). MET will lengthen the fascia within the muscle (see "Muscle Energy Technique" in Chapter 2).

Viscoelastic Property of a Muscle and Its Fascia

- Tension in a muscle and its fascia is created by active and passive elements. The passive elements include the collagen fibers and ground substance, and the active components include the contractile proteins, actin and myosin, and the nerves.
- The connective tissue fibers of the muscle compose the **elastic** component. As described previously, the collagen fibers of the fascia of the muscle become the tendon. This fascia has a crimp or wavelike structure, similar to a spring. The tissue can be stretched within its normal limit and return to its resting length, much like a spring can be pulled and released. When you stretch the fascia or pull on the fascia when you contract a muscle, energy is being stored, like pulling a spring. The energy is released as heat when the stretch or muscle contraction is released.
- Since muscle contains ground substance, it demonstrates **viscous** behavior. It becomes thicker and stiff when it is stretched quickly, is cold, or is immobilized. It becomes more fluidlike if the myofascia is stretched slowly or when it is warmed-up.

The Body as a Tensegrity Structure

- Muscle is the tension member of the body that transmits the force of muscle contraction to the connective tissue to move the body and dynamically stabilize its posture. The bones are the compression members and cannot keep the body upright without the muscles and connective tissue. Lauren Berry, RPT, describes the muscles and the connective tissue as the "guy wires" of the body. In other words, it is the tension members of the structure, not the bones, that hold the body upright. Buckminster Fuller[15a] coined the word "tensegrity" to describe this type of structure. The strength and stability of a tensegrity structure, like the human body, depends on the soft tissues, including the muscles, and all the connective tissues, including the tendons, ligaments, and joint capsules.
- One of the fundamental contributions of Lauren Berry is that he theorized that these soft tissue guy wires can become misaligned. These distortions decrease the stability in a joint and create imbalances in the forces moving through the joint, leading to accelerated degeneration. This concept is explored later in the chapter.

Role of Muscle in Movement and Stability

- **Agonist**—The muscle(s) that contracts to perform a certain movement are called the agonist(s). This muscle is also called the prime mover. For example, the biceps is an agonist for elbow flexion. All movements in the body are accomplished by more than one muscle.
- **Antagonist**—The muscle(s) that performs the opposite movement of the agonist are called the antagonist(s). The triceps is the antagonist for the biceps, because the triceps extends the elbow.
- **Co-contraction**—When the agonist and antagonist are working simultaneously, they are co-contracting. For example, when you make a fist, the flexors and extensors of the wrist are co-contracting to keep the wrist in a position that ensures the greatest strength of the fingers. Typically, however, when the agonist is working, the antagonist is relaxing.
    - **Sherrington's law of reciprocal inhibition** states that there is a neurologic inhibition of the antago-

nist when the agonist is working. When we contract the biceps to flex the elbow, the triceps is being neurologically inhibited (relaxed), which allows it to lengthen during elbow flexion. Co-contraction is an exception to this rule.

- **Synergist**—The muscle(s) that works with another muscle to accomplish a certain motion. The term "synergist" includes stabilizers (i.e., muscles that support a joint to allow the prime mover to work more efficiently) and neutralizers (i.e., muscles that prevent a certain motion as the agonist is working).

Tonic and Phasic Muscles

- ***Structure:*** The muscles of the body may also be divided on the basis of which muscles have primarily a stabilizing role, and which muscles have primarily a role in movement. These categories are controversial because most muscles can function in both roles. However, it has been proved clinically useful because muscles react to pain in predictable ways, discussed below in the section, "Dysfunction Due to Impaired Muscle Function".
  - **Tonic (postural)**—Muscles that play a primary role in maintenance of posture, and, therefore, function essentially as stabilizers are called tonic or postural muscles.
  - **Phasic**—Muscles whose primary roles are quick movement are phasic muscles.
- ***Dysfunction and injury:*** It has been found that tonic (postural) muscles react to stress by becoming short and tight, and that phasic muscles react to stress by becoming inhibited and weak.[16] Janda[17] has discovered that there are predictable patterns in which muscles tend to become tight and which muscles tend to become weak. His insights are incorporated throughout this text.
- ***Treatment implications:*** See the treatment implications discussed in the section, "Muscle Dysfunction."

Innervation

- Two types of motor (efferent) nerves supply each muscle:
  - **Alpha nerves**—The alpha nerves fire when we voluntarily contract a muscle.
  - **Gamma nerves**—The gamma nerves have voluntary and involuntary functions. They unconsciously help to set the tone of the muscle, in addition to its resting length, and function during voluntary activities for fine muscular control.
- Five types of sensory (afferent) nerve receptors supply each muscle. The sensory nerves are sensitive to pain, chemical stimuli, temperature, deep pressure, and mechanoreceptor information. Two specialized receptors, the muscle spindle and the GTO, detect muscle length and changes in length and muscle tension and changes in muscle tension (see the section, "The Nervous System" and Figure 1-22 for further discussion).
  - **Muscle spindle**—Muscle spindles detect the **length** of the muscle.
  - **Golgi tendon organ**—GTOs detect the **tension** in the muscle.

Three Types of Voluntary Muscle Contraction

- **Isometric**—In an isometric contraction, the muscle contracts, but its constant length is maintained. If, while sitting, you place your hand under your thigh and attempt to lift your leg off the chair, your biceps isometrically contracts, but there is no movement.
- **Concentric**—Concentric contraction is when a muscle shortens while it contracts (i.e., the origin and insertion move toward each other). As you bring a glass of water to your mouth, your biceps is shortening while it contracts.
- **Eccentric**—Eccentric contraction is when the origin and insertion move apart while a muscle contracts. As you lower the glass back to the table, your biceps is lengthening while it maintains some contraction.

Relation Between Muscle Length and Tension

A muscle develops its maximum strength or tension at its resting length or just short of its resting length because the actin and myosin filaments have the maximum contact (crossbridges). When a muscle is excessively shortened or lengthened it loses its ability to perform a strong contraction. A muscle can develop only moderate tension in the lengthened position and minimum tension in the shortened position. For example, if the wrist is maximally flexed, the ability to make a fist is diminished because the finger flexors are in a shortened position.

Involuntary Muscle Contraction By Voluntary Muscles

- Withdrawal reflexes, such as pulling away from a hot stove, involve instantaneous muscle contraction.
- Righting reflexes from the ligaments and joint capsule communicate to the muscle and stimulate in-

stantaneous muscle contraction for protection of the joint and associated soft tissue.

- Arthrokinetic reflexes describe unconscious muscle contraction of muscles surrounding a joint caused by irritation in the joint (see the section, "Function of the Joint Receptors.")
- Splinting or involuntary muscle contraction can be caused by a muscle injury.
- Emotional or psychological stress creates excessive and sustained muscle tension.
- The maintenance of posture involves unconscious muscle contraction.

MUSCLE INJURY

- A muscle injury is called a **strain,** or pulled muscle, and is usually a tear of the collagen in the connective tissue layers surrounding and imbedded within the muscle. Because of the development of abnormal crosslinks in the collagen and adhesions within the muscle's fascia, a muscle typically shortens and loses some of its extensibility after an injury.
- Muscle strains are classified in three grades, although it is difficult to assess the severity.[7]
  - Grade I: Mild injury, with minimal structural damage.
  - Grade II: Moderate injury, with a partial tear; significant functional loss occurs.
  - Grade III: Severe injury, a complete tear; complete loss of function occurs; may require surgery.
- *Areas of injury:* Usually occurs at the junction where the muscle and tendon meet, called the **myotendinous junction,** or where the tendon attaches to the periosteum of the bone, called the **tenoperiosteal junction.**
  - The myotendinous junction is stiffer than other areas of the muscle, making it the weakest link. For all muscles, failure consistently occurs near the myotendinous junction.[2]
  - Junction sites of ligament, tendon, and joint capsules are relatively avascular and have an increased stiffness. These junctions, therefore, are more prone to injury.[2]
- *Repair of Muscle Injury:* After a tear of the CT of the muscle, fibroblasts lay down collagen. If the tear is significant, adhesions form in the CT layers. After a tear of the muscle fiber, satellite cells help myoblasts develop into muscle fibers. The regeneration is usually complete in 3 weeks. Immobilization causes decreased cellular activity, decreased collagen in the fascia, and loss of muscle fibers (atrophy).
- *Treatment implications:* As discussed above, OM and MET minimizes adhesion formation, promotes the circulation, increases the lubrication, and promotes the proper alignment of the collagen fibers. Movement also stimulates the regeneration of new connective tissue and muscle fibers. MET promotes muscle regeneration that is stimulated by the longitudinal pulling force.[8] MET also promotes the normal parallel alignment of the connective tissue and muscle fibers. PIR and contract-relax-agonist-contract (CRAC) MET are used to lengthen the fascia within the muscle (See Chapter 2, Assessment and Technique).

MUSCLE DYSFUNCTION

Muscle Dysfunction: A New Concept in Orthopedics

- *Definition:* Muscle dysfunction is defined as sustained hypertonicity, sustained inhibition (weakness), abnormal position, or abnormal torsion in the soft tissue.

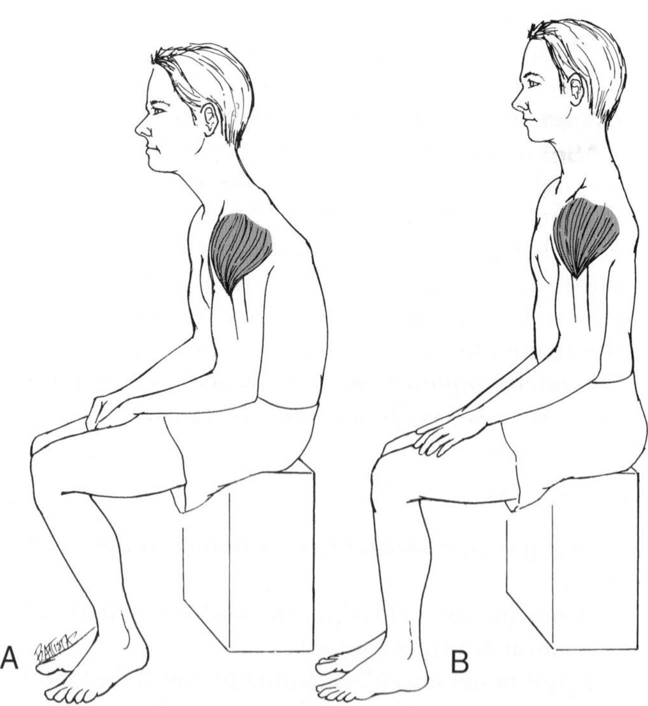

Figure 1-16. A. In a slumped, rounded-shoulder posture the fascicles of the anterior deltoid roll into an abnormal position and abnormal torsion. The muscle twists into an internally rotated position. **B.** In the normal upright posture, the fascicles of the deltoid are aligned in a superior direction.

Causes of Muscle Dysfunction

- Poor posture—Sitting or standing in poor posture creates cumulative stress.
- Static stress—Sitting or standing for long periods is fatiguing.
- Muscle injury—A muscle may become hypertonic owing to injury (strain), or it may become weak owing to injury or from posttraumatic atrophy.
- Joint dysfunction or injury—Injury or dysfunction may lead to a reflexive spasm or weakness in specific muscles around the joint (called the arthrokinetic reflex by Wyke.[18])
- Emotional or psychological stress—Anxiety and anger can create sustained muscle contraction, and depression can cause sustained weakness in the muscles.
- Chronic overuse—A muscle fails to relax after intense use, leading to ischemia and tension myositis (pain in the muscle caused by sustained contraction).
- Disuse—Deconditioned syndrome is a phenomenon in which a muscle is weakened owing to lack of use. This phenomenon precedes muscle atrophy.
- Viscerosomatic reflexes—An irritation or inflammation in a visceral organ can cause a muscle spasm. For example, a kidney infection can cause a spasm of the lumbar muscles.

Two Types of Muscle Dysfunction

Dysfunction Caused by Abnormal Position and Abnormal Torsion

- Lauren Berry, RPT, contributed a revolutionary concept in manual therapy. He theorized that all soft tissue has a specific position relative to the neighboring soft tissues, and that muscles, tendons, ligaments, bursae, and nerves can become malpositioned. This text describes the patterns of the abnormal position in the soft tissue, and the treatment to correct positional dysfunction.
  - Abnormal position in the anterior deltoid provides an example of positional dysfunction. In the rounded-shoulders posture, the anterior deltoid rolls or winds into a more anterior–inferior position relative to the shoulder joint (the glenohumeral joint). This abnormal position decreases the function of the muscle, and contributes to the dysfunction of the shoulder (Fig. 1-16).
- The author has developed this concept further, and theorizes that this malposition creates an abnormal torsion or twist in the muscle and fascia, including the fascicles and fibers, down to the microscopic level.
  - The normal alignment of a muscle to the joint is rarely along the central axis of the joint. Therefore, any sustained contraction of the muscle creates a torsion or twist to the ligaments and joint capsule surrounding the joint to which the muscle is attached.
  - This abnormal torsion is akin to taking a wet washcloth, holding both ends, and putting a twist in it. The twist causes the washcloth to lose its water content. Similarly, the abnormal torsion decreases the water content in the tissue. This decreases the interfiber distance and creates abnormal crosslinks and adhesions between the muscles, fascicles, and fibers, leading to stiffness and decreased function.
- ***Treatment implications:*** The muscle and fascia need to be stroked in a specific direction. In the case of the anterior deltoid, it needs to be stroked superiorly and posteriorly to restore its normal position and function and to release the torsion within the fascicles. This text describes each muscle's positional dysfunction, and the direction of the massage strokes necessary to correct it.

Dysfunction Caused by Impaired Muscle Function

- Janda[17] and Lewit[19] use the expression "functional pathology of the motor system" to describe unconscious reflexes from the central or the peripheral nervous system (PNS) that cause sustained hypertonicity or sustained weakness (inhibition) in the muscles. Pain always creates impaired function, but impaired function can take years to develop into pain.
- The most important signs of impaired muscle function according to Janda[20] are:
  - **Increased muscle tone (muscle hypertonicity)**—Muscles that are held in a sustained contraction are an important factor in the genesis of pain. Hypertonicity has many causes (see the section, "Patterns of Inhibition [Weakness] and Hypertonicity).
  - **Muscle inhibition (weakness)**—A muscle may be functionally weak, which creates joint instability and causes other muscles to become hypertonic in compensation.
  - **Muscle imbalance**—Muscle imbalance is a change in function in the muscles crossing a joint, in which certain muscles react to stress by getting short and tight and others become weak. This is an important factor in chronic pain syndromes because this imbalance alters the movement pattern of the joint.

- **Joint dysfunction**—Muscle dysfunction creates an uneven distribution of forces on the weight-bearing surfaces of the joint, predisposing it to degeneration and dysfunction of the proprioceptive nerves that provide critical information about the position and movement characteristics of the joint.
- **Abnormal muscle firing pattern**—Muscle dysfunction is often expressed by improper contraction. For example, hip abduction should be typically performed by the gluteus medius, but the tensor fascia lata often substitutes for this action because of a weak gluteus medius.

- ***Treatment implications:*** Impaired muscle function is best treated with MET. Having the client actively contract muscles in a precise and controlled way engages the higher brain centers, the sensory-motor cortex, to override unconscious patterns in the lower brain, and reeducates the reflexes between the muscle, joint, and spinal cord. Refer to "The Nervous System" section and to Chapter 2 for further discussion.

Patterns of Inhibition (Weakness) and Hypertonicity

- Janda[17] discovered clinically that muscles react to pain or excessive stress in two opposite ways in predictable patterns. He found that certain muscles tend to become overactive, short, and tight and described these muscles as having a postural or stabilizing function, similar to tonic muscles. He found that other muscles tend to become inhibited and weak. He noticed that most of these muscles were concerned with movement rather than stability; therefore, he grouped inhibited and weak muscles as phasic muscles. An example of muscle imbalance is what Janda[17] calls the **upper crossed syndrome** (Fig. 1-17). The terms postural and phasic have led to some confusion among clinicians and researchers, and more accurate terms have been suggested for these two groups: **tightness-prone** and **inhibition (weakness)-prone** muscles.[21]

In addition to the causes of muscle dysfunction listed previously, muscle injury, chronic pain, and inflammation create disturbances in normal muscle function and may stimulate a neurologic-based tightness or weakness in a muscle.

An important difference between the two muscle groups is that a small reduction of strength in an inhibition-prone muscle initiates a disproportionately larger contraction of the antagonist tightness-prone muscle.[19] Janda[17] notes that much of our work and recreational activities favor tightness-prone muscles getting stronger, tighter, and shorter as the inhibition-prone muscles become weaker and more inhibited. It is important, however, to realize that some muscles, such as the quadratus lumborum and the scalenes, can react with either tightness or weakness.

- **Muscles that tend to be tightness-prone** and react to pain or excessive stress with hypertonicity and eventual shortening are as follows:
  - Sternocleidomastoid, pectoralis major (clavicular and sternal parts), and minor, upper trapezius, levator scapulae, the flexor groups of the upper extremity, erector spinae, iliopsoas, tensor fascia lata, rectus femoris, piriformis, pectineus, adductors, hamstrings, gastrocnemius, soleus, and tibialis posterior.
- **Muscles that tend to be weakness-prone (inhibited)** and to react to pain by becoming neurologically inhibited and, therefore, weakening are as follows:
  - Deep cervical flexors, extensor group of the upper extremity, pectoralis major (abdominal part),

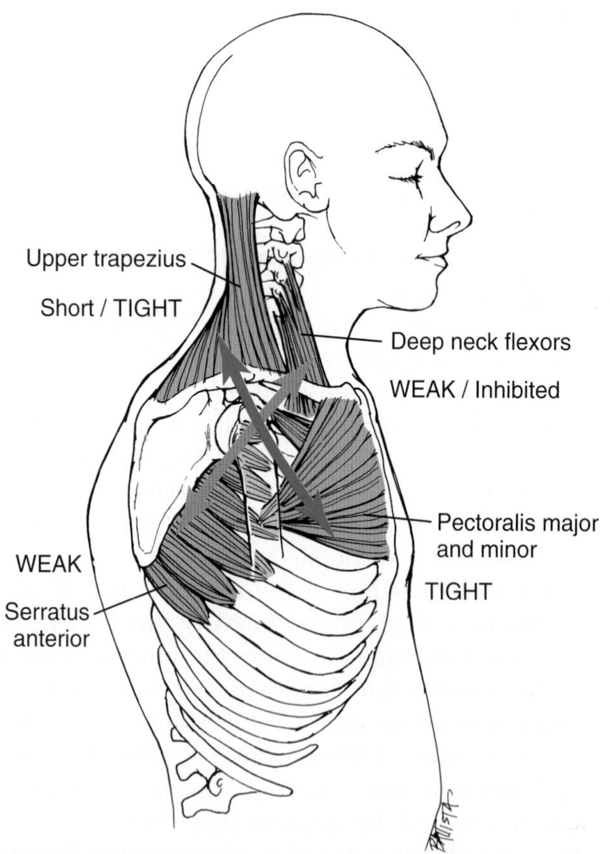

Figure 1-17. Upper crossed syndrome, a typical pattern of muscle imbalance. The upper trapezius and pectoralis major and minor are usually short and tight, and the deep neck flexors and serratus anterior and lower trapezius are typically weak and inhibited.

middle and lower trapezius, rhomboids, serratus anterior, rectus abdominus, internal and external obliques, gluteal muscles, vasti muscles (medialis, lateralis, and intermedius), tibialis anterior, and the peroneal muscles.

Consequences of a Hypertonic Muscle

- ***Definition:*** A muscle that is held in a sustained contraction is also called a hypertonic muscle. This means that the muscle is constantly working. This constant contraction has several effects.
  - The muscle consumes more oxygen and energy than a muscle at rest, and therefore contains more lactic-acid waste products, which irritate the nerves.
  - Circulation is decreased because the muscle is not performing its normal function as a pump. This leads to ischemia and decreased oxygen, again causing the pain receptors to fire.
  - The sustained tension in the muscle pulls on its attachments to the periosteum, joint capsule, and ligaments, creating increased pressure in the joint, loading the cartilage unevenly, and creating excessive wear in the joint and accelerated degeneration.
  - Hypertonic muscles can compress the nerves that travel between the muscles or, in some cases, through the muscle. This leads to decreased nerve function and to paresthesias or altered sensations, typically, a pins and needles feeling. A common example is the compression of the sciatic nerve by a hypertonic piriformis muscle.

Consequences of an Inhibited (Weak) Muscle

- A healthy muscle functions to dynamically stabilize the joint. A weak muscle creates instability. This leads to imbalanced forces moving through the joint and accelerates degeneration.
- Weakness contributes to poor posture, which creates areas of excessive tension and compression.
- Inhibition leads to loss of adequate motor control and to abnormal firing patterns in the muscle, leading to substitution of other muscles and abnormal joint movements.
- An inhibited muscle does not have adequate cycles of contraction, and therefore, the pumping of the vascular system and lymphatics is diminished.

Joint Structure and Function

JOINT TYPES

- ***Definition:*** A joint is the connection (articulation) between two bones or cartilage elements.
- Joints are classified by the type of tissue that unites the two bones.
  - Fibrous joint (synarthrodial)—A fibrous joint is united by fibrous tissue (e.g., sutures of the skull) that have little movement.
  - Cartilaginous joint (amphiarthrosis)—A cartilaginous joint is united by fibrocartilage (e.g., symphysis pubis) and the intervertebral discs of the spine and have slight movement.
  - Synovial joint (diarthrosis)—The most common joint in the body is the synovial joint. The bones are not united. The joint has a joint cavity filled with synovial fluid, and the two bones are surrounded by a joint capsule and characterized by having free mobility.

SYNOVIAL JOINT COMPONENTS

Joint Capsule

- ***Structure:*** The joint capsule is composed of two layers (Fig. 1-18A)(Fig. 1-18B). The outer layer is fibrous connective tissue and the inner layer is synovial tissue. The outer layer is reinforced with intrinsic and extrinsic ligaments. Intrinsic ligaments are thickenings within the body of the capsule, whereas extrinsic ligaments lie superficial to the capsule. Many of the tendinous insertions of muscles interweave with the joint capsule. For example, the multifidus, rectus femoris (reflected head), vastus medialis and lateralis, pectoralis major, teres major, biceps, triceps, and most of the forearm flexors all interweave directly with the capsule.
- ***Function:***
  - The outer layer helps to stabilize the joint, helps guide joint motion, and prevents excessive motion. It is innervated with a rich supply of nerves, including mechanoreceptors and pain fibers. The mechanoreceptors sense the rate and speed of motion, the position or proprioception, and have reflex connections to the muscles. Irritation or injury to the capsule can create muscle contractions, designed to protect the joint.

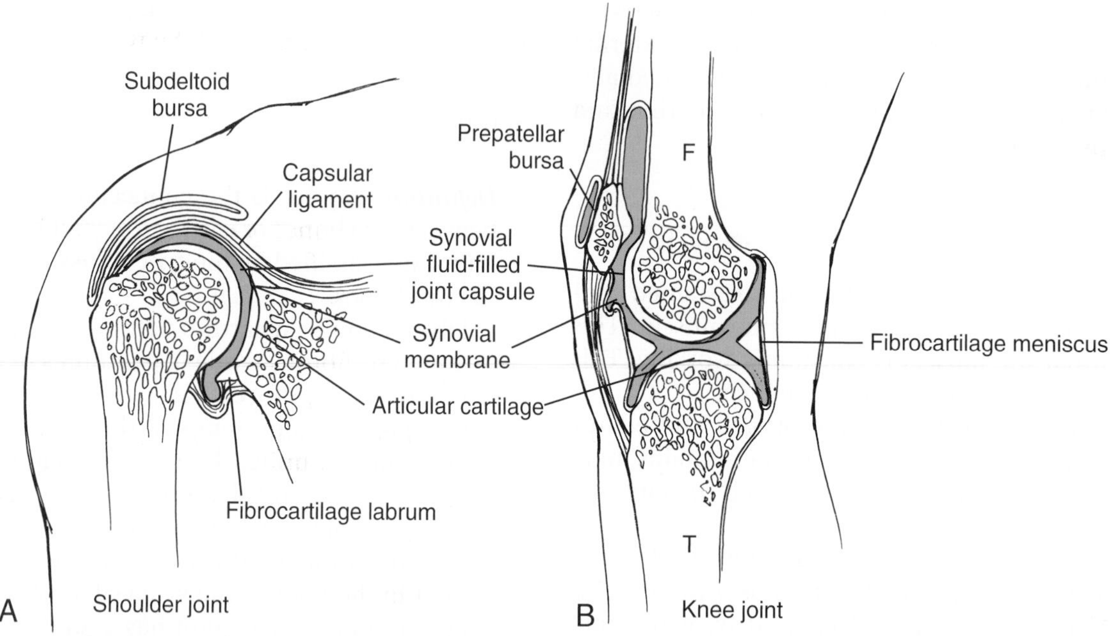

Figure 1-18. **A.** Typical synovial joint. **B.** Knee joint showing the fibrocartilage meniscus and bursae, which are additional features of a synovial joint.

- The inner layer of the joint capsule is a synovial membrane that secretes synovial fluid when it is stimulated by joint motion. Synovial fluid is a thick, clear, viscous fluid, much like egg white, that provides lubrication and nutrition. Maintaining joint motion is critical, as the joint dries out and degenerates if it is not moved.

- ***Dysfunction and injury:***
  - *Outer fibrous layer:* Fibrosis or thickening of the joint capsule is caused by an increased production of collagen and by a decrease in the ground substance. It occurs in three conditions: one, acute inflammation; two, chronic irritation or inflammation caused by imbalanced stresses moving through the joint; and three, immobilization.[13] A tight, fibrotic joint capsule results in abnormal movement between the joint surfaces, leading to excessive compression in certain areas of the cartilage and to accelerated degeneration of the joint.

The capsule and supporting ligaments may also be excessively stretched because of injury. If there is a loss of adequate motion owing to immobilization, the fibrous layer of the joint capsule atrophies because of a loss of collagen. This creates joint instability.

  - *The inner synovial layer:* The synovial membrane can become injured or dysfunctional because of acute trauma to the joint, cumulative stresses from chronic irritation caused by imbalanced forces moving through the joint, or immobilization. Joint swelling occurs during inflammation. The swelling typically causes abnormal muscle function controlling the joint. Immobilization, on the other hand, thickens the synovial fluid with disuse, and causes an eventual decrease in the amount of synovial fluid. This leads to adhesions between the capsule and the articular cartilage, tendon sheaths, and bursae, contributing to stiffness and consequent degeneration in the joint.

- ***Treatment implications:***
  - *For a fibrotic joint capsule:* MET is performed to the muscles of the associated joint. As the muscle's fascia interweaves with the joint capsule at the tenoperiosteal junction, isometric muscle contractions pull on the capsule and increase its extensibility. Mobilization is used to reduce intra-articular adhesions. The fibrotic capsule is treated with manual pressures on the capsule itself. The massage strokes are directed in all directions owing to the irregular alignment of the collagen. This stroke process is analogous to removing the tuck out of a sheet; you spread it in all directions to smooth it out.

To help restore length in the shortened capsule, PIR MET is performed. Because there are neurologic connections between the muscles and the capsule, a lengthening response can be induced with muscle contractions of the muscles of the associated joint. This has proved clinically effective, although the explanation is hypothetical.

- *For an atrophied or excessively stretched capsule:* A capsule that is too loose needs exercise rehabilitation, to help lay down new collagen fibers, restoring its normal length, and coordination and proprioception exercises to help restore neurological function.
- *For an acute, swollen joint capsule:* A swollen capsule is treated with isometric MET to use the muscle contractions to help pump the excess fluid out of the capsule. Pain-free, passive range of motion (ROM) is also used in the flexion/extension plane to act as a mechanical pump. If there is too little fluid in the joint, the MET and passive mobilizations of the joint help stimulate the synovial membrane, increasing synovial fluid, and therefore the lubrication and nutrition in the joint.

Ligaments

- Some extrinsic ligaments lie over the joint capsule and attach from one bone to the other, and some intrinsic ligaments are thickenings of the joint capsule. The ligaments are fully described in the section "Connective Tissue," above.

Cartilage

- ***Definition:*** Cartilage is a dense, fibrous connective tissue composed of collagen, ground substance, and chondrocytes or cartilage cells.
- ***Structure:*** Synovial joints have two types of cartilage: articular or hyaline cartilage and fibrocartilage.

Types of Cartilage:

- **Articular cartilage (hyaline cartilage):** Hyaline or articular cartilage covers the ends of bones and provides a smooth gliding surface for opposing joint surfaces. Articular cartilage is mostly water. It is elastic and porous, and functions like a sponge, in that it has the capacity to absorb and bind synovial fluid. Intermittent compression and decompression creates a pumping action, which causes the movement of synovial fluid in and out of the cartilage. Cartilage is self-lubricating as long as it moves. Articular cartilage creates new cells with use and deteriorates with disuse. It has no nerve or blood supply.

There are three normal ways that the synovial joint goes through cycles of compression and decompression: locomotion (walking, running), intermittent contraction of the muscles, and the twisting and untwisting of the joint capsule.[13]

- **Fibrocartilage:** Consists of dense, white fibrous connective tissue arranged in dense bundles or layered sheets. The fibrocartilage has great tensile strength combined with considerable elasticity. Fibrocartilage functions to deepen a joint space, such as the cartilage labrum or lip of the hip and shoulder; allows two bones to fit together better, such as the menisci of the knee; acts as a shock absorber, such as the intervertebral discs of the spine; and lines body grooves for tendons, such as in the bicipital groove for the long head of biceps.

- ***Dysfunction and injury:*** Damage to articular cartilage may be caused by an acute trauma or cumulative stresses. These stresses are often the result of imbalances in the muscles surrounding the joint, a tight joint capsule, or both. A tight capsule creates a high-contact area in the cartilage and decreased lubrication. Imbalanced muscles create altered weight distribution through the joint, causing excessive pressures on the cartilage and creating fatigue in the cartilage. The cartilage degenerates, beginning with fracturing of the collagen fibers (fibrillation) and depletion of the ground substance. An arthritic joint is a joint with degeneration of the cartilage.
- ***Treatment implications:*** It has been assumed that cartilage cannot repair itself, but as Kessler and Hertling[25] point out, recent studies show that cartilage cells (chondrocytes) can stay active and lay down new cartilage and that arthritis is "somewhat reversible if managed correctly." The joint must be moved to stimulate the synthesis of chondrocytes and the secretion of the synovial fluid. Mobilization in flexion and extension pumps synovial fluid into and out of the joint. Rhythmic oscillations and MET wind and unwind the joint capsule to pump the fluid into and out of the cartilage, rehydrating the cartilage. In the manual techniques, we wind and unwind the joint capsule and compress and decompress the area we are working on to promote fluid exchange.

Bursa

- ***Structure:*** Bursae are synovial-filled sacs lined with a synovial membrane that are found in areas of increased friction, such as the subdeltoid bursa between the deltoid muscle and the acromion process.
- ***Function:*** The function of a bursa is to secrete synovial fluid to neighboring structures, which decreases friction.

- *Dysfunction and injury:* A bursa is susceptible to acute and chronic conditions. Bursitis typically is caused by excessive friction of the muscles and connective tissue, tendons, and fascia that overlie the bursa. As there are pressure receptors in the bursa, a swollen bursa can be extremely painful. A chronic bursa can remain swollen or dry out, creating adhesions within the sac.
- *Treatment implications:* Lauren Berry, RPT, contributed an effective treatment for bursitis. The method involves a gentle, slow, continuous stroke over the bursa to help massage the excess fluid out. If a bursa has dried-out, the same strokes are applied more deeply to help stimulate the synovial membrane to secrete fluid.

Innervation

- Joints receive nerves from two sources: the articular nerves, which are branches of the peripheral nerve, and the branches of the nerves that supply the muscles controlling the joint.
- Many sensory receptors surround the joint. Although some of them are described as Ruffini endings and Pacinian corpuscles, these nerves can be categorized into four types.[18] These four types of joint receptors are located in the joint capsule, ligaments, periosteum, and articular fat pads (see the section, "The Nervous System").
  - **Type I**—A type I receptor is a mechanoreceptor that provides information concerning the static and dynamic position of the joint. Type I receptors are located in the superficial layers of the superficial joint capsule.
  - **Type II**—A type II receptor is a dynamic mechanoreceptor that provides information on acceleration and deceleration of movement. Type II receptors are found in the deep layers of the fibrous joint capsule.
  - **Type III**—A type III receptor is a dynamic mechanoreceptor that monitors the direction of movement, and has a reflex effect on muscle tone to provide a "breaking effect." Type III receptors are found in the intrinsic and extrinsic joint ligaments.
  - **Type IV**—A type IV receptor is a pain receptor (nociceptor). It is inactive under normal conditions. Type IV receptors are found in capsules, ligaments, and periosteum.

Function of the Joint Receptors

- Conveys information automatically to the CNS on the functional status of the joint and its surrounding soft tissue. This reflex control of the muscles surrounding the joint is called the arthrokinetic reflex.[17] The CNS creates contraction or relaxation of the muscles to protect the joint. The arthrokinetic reflex coordinates agonists, antagonists, and synergists around the joint for gross movements and fine muscular control.
- Controls posture, coordination, and balance.
- Controls the direction and speed of movement.
- Gives information about the position of the joint and body image.
- Reports pain in the joint when the joint is irritated or inflamed.

Joint Receptor Dysfunction and Injury (Irritation)

- Mechanical or chemical irritation (inflammation) of the joint receptors causes some muscles to become weak (inhibited) and some muscles to become short and tight (facilitated). As mentioned previously, Janda[17] has described the patterns of these muscle dysfunctions (see "Muscle Dysfunction").
- Irritation of the pain receptors and mechanoreceptors typically cause the flexors of the joint to become facilitated or hypertonic, and the extensors of the joint to become inhibited or weak.[22]
- Irritation of the joint receptors can also lead to profound abnormalities in posture; muscle coordination; and control of movement, balance, and awareness of body position.

SYNOVIAL JOINT FUNCTION, DYSFUNCTION, AND TREATMENT

Joint Stability

- For a joint to perform a full and painless range of motion, it must be stable. Otherwise, abnormal forces move through the joint, leading to excessive wear and tear on the articular surfaces. This stability is determined by several factors:
  - The **shape of the bones** that make up the joint. The hip joint sits deeply within the socket (acetabulum) of the pelvis; therefore, it is much more stable than the glenohumeral joint of the shoulder, because the fossa of the glenoid cavity is shallow.
  - **Passive stability** is provided by the ligaments and joint capsule. Because the ligaments and joint capsule do not have contractile fibers, their role is called passive.
  - **Dynamic stability** is provided by the muscles. As mentioned, it is important for the muscles that

cross a joint to be balanced, or the forces that move through the joint will create uneven stresses, leading to dysfunction and eventual degeneration of the cartilage.

Normal Joint Movements

- Normal joint movements open and close the joint surfaces, leading to compression and decompression of the cartilage. These movements also wind and unwind the joint capsule and ligaments, stimulating the lubrication and nutrition into the joint.
  - When a joint is in the **close-packed position,** the joint surfaces are most compressed, and the joint capsule and ligaments are tightest.
  - When a joint is in the **loose-packed position,** the joint is most open, and the joint capsule and ligaments are somewhat lax. Generally, extension closes the joint, and flexion opens the joint surfaces.
- John Mennell, MD,[23] has introduced the concept of **"joint play,"** which describes movements in a joint that can be produced passively (i.e., by the therapist) but not voluntarily. In most joint positions, a joint has some "play" in it that is essential for normal joint function.

Joint Dysfunction

- Mennell[23] also introduced the concept of **joint dysfunction** as a cause of pain and disability. He defines joint dysfunction as "a loss of joint play movements." This definition is the same as the chiropractic concept of **joint fixation.**

Joint dysfunction has many causes, including a meniscoidal entrapment in the facet joints of the spine, roughened surfaces of the joint cartilage, and degenerative joint disease, but there are two causes that massage therapy can effectively treat:

- Adhesions or shortening of the joint capsule or ligaments.
- Sustained contraction of the muscles surrounding the joint, muscle imbalances across a joint, and abnormal firing patterns of the muscles moving the joint. Korr[24] hypothesized that sustained muscle contraction may be the major factor in decreased mobility of the dysfunctioning joint.
- ***Treatment implications:*** Short and tight muscles must be lengthened and relaxed, and muscles that are weak and inhibited need to be reeducated to regain their normal firing pattern and strength. Muscles cannot be restored to normal if the joints they move are restricted, and the joints will not regain their normal movement characteristics if the muscles that move the joint are not relaxed and strong, and if the ligaments and joint capsule are not normalized. It is important to realize that a joint can have too much play owing to a loss of stability in the ligaments or muscles. These conditions are treated with exercise rehabilitation to strengthen and stabilize the area.

Joint Degeneration

- Most conditions called arthritis are in fact noninflammatory, and should be referred to as arthrosis, meaning joint degeneration. Osteoarthritis (OA) and degenerative joint disease (DJD) are typically used interchangeably to describe a chronic degeneration of a joint, although OA may be used to describe an inflammatory condition.

One common cause of joint degeneration is a loss of normal function of the joint. This altered function can occur as a result of a prior trauma or cumulative stress on the joint. The massage therapist can effectively address two main causes of altered function:

- Imbalanced muscles that move the joint, which leads to a loss of dynamic stability to the joint, creating uneven forces moving through the joint.
- Tight, fibrotic joint capsules and ligaments.

Joint Mobilization

- ***Definition:*** Joint mobilization is any active or passive attempt to increase movement at a joint.[25] Passive mobilization techniques are graded from one to four, and are usually performed as rhythmic oscillations. These movements are within the scope of practice for the massage therapist. Grade five is a high-velocity, low-amplitude thrust, and is not within the scope of the massage therapist.

  The goals of joint mobilization are to:
  - Restore the normal joint play that allows for normal joint motion.
  - Promote the exchange of cells and fluids in and out of the joint to promote joint repair and regeneration.
  - Stimulate normal lubrication in the joint by stimulating the synovial membrane and promoting rehydration of the articular cartilage.
  - Normalize neurological function by firing type III joint receptors and GTOs, resulting in a relaxation of the muscles surrounding the joint[26] (see the section, "The Nervous System").

- Decrease swelling, which can cause pain, decreased motion, and tissue stagnation.
- Reduce pain. As mentioned above, the pain-gate theory of Melzak and Wall states that mechanoreceptor stimulation overrides pain information in the brain, and suggests that joint mobilization in pain-free ranges can have an analgesic effect.[9]

The Nervous System

GENERAL OVERVIEW

The nervous system is anatomically and functionally connected throughout the entire body, but it may be structurally divided into the CNS and the PNS and functionally divided into the somatic or motor nervous system and the autonomic nervous system.[12] Although massage affects every part of the nervous system, massage for orthopedic conditions is focused on the somatic nervous system. (Fig. 1-19).

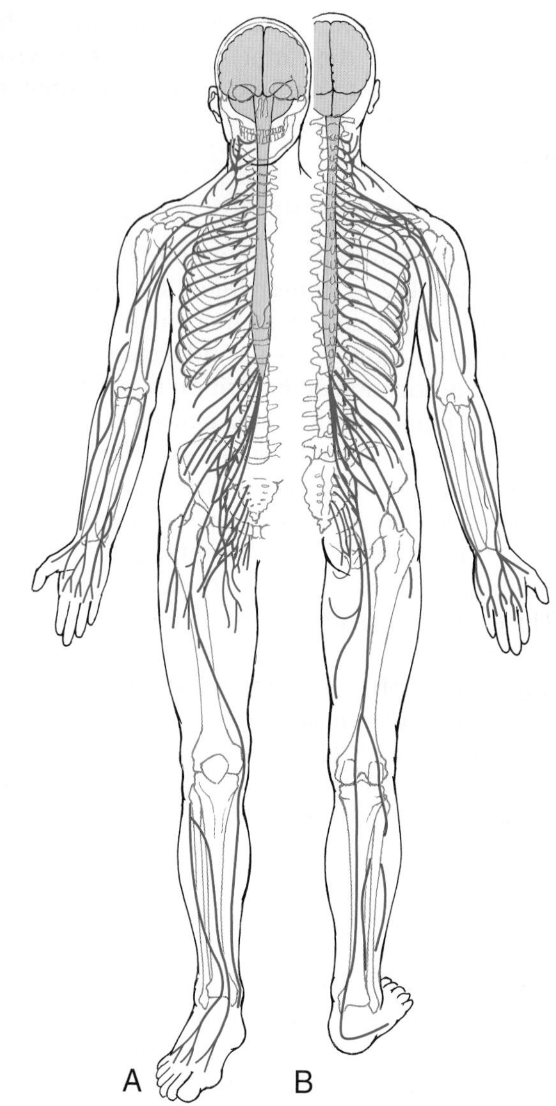

Figure 1-19. Overview of the somatic or motor nervous system, which includes the CNS and the PNS. The CNS includes the brain and spinal cord, and the PNS includes the cranial nerves (not shown) and the 31 pairs of spinal nerves that extend into the arms and legs. **A.** Anterior view. **B.** Posterior view.

Central Nervous System

The CNS consists of the brain and spinal cord.

The Brain

- ***Structure and Function:*** The brain is divided into three sections, the cerebrum, brainstem, and cerebellum. The cerebrum is the largest portion and the most recently developed part of the brain and is responsible for higher mental functions and personality. The frontal-lobe area of the cerebrum also contains the **motor cortex,** which controls voluntary movements.
  - Another area of the cerebrum is called the parietal lobe and contains the **sensory cortex,** which receives information about touch and proprioception. Some proprioceptive signals, however, go only to the spinal cord.
  - The limbic system and hypothalamus integrate emotional states, visceral responses, and the muscular system.[8] Emotions can alter muscular tone. States of anxiety create sustained increased tone (hypertonicity) and depression creates loss of muscle tone (hypotonicity).
  - The brainstem is the center for the automatic control of respiration and heart rate.
  - The cerebellum functions to control muscle coordination, muscle tone, and posture.

The Spinal Cord

- ***Structure and Function:*** The spinal cord is a continuation of the medulla portion of the brain and travels within the vertebral canal from the opening in the skull called the foramen magnum to the lumbar spine. After the cord ends at approximately the second lumbar vertebra it continues as a collection of nerve roots called the cauda equina.
  - The spinal cord is divided into gray matter, which contains the neuron cell bodies, and the white matter, which contains the nerve fibers. One portion of the cord receives information from the sensory receptors, and another portion transmits

motor information from the muscles. An interneuron communicates and amplifies information between the sensory and the motor portion of the cord.

- A reflex arc is the simplest communication between the sensory and the motor nerves. The classic example is the deep tendon reflex that occurs when you tap the quadriceps tendon. By tapping the tendon, the quadriceps automatically contracts. However, information from all four classes of sensory receptors—the mechanoreceptors, proprioceptors, chemoreceptors, and nociceptors—unconsciously send information to the cord, which stimulates countless automatic (reflexive) adjustments in the muscular system. Irritation of the sensory receptors can cause reflexive hypertonicity or reflexive inhibition (weakness) in the muscles (Fig. 1-20).
- The spinal cord becomes individual spinal nerves as they exit the vertebral column through openings between the sides of the vertebra called the intervertebral foramen. (See Chapters 3 to 5 for more information on the spinal nerves.)

- ***Dysfunction and injury:*** In addition to the voluntary control of movement, the CNS sends unconscious signals to the muscular system that cause sustained muscular contraction of which the person is unaware. It is a common clinical experience that a client has habitually contracted muscles, without any awareness that those muscles are tight. This condition is commonly experienced in the upper trapezius. For example, when the therapist touches this muscle, the client is often surprised that it is tight and tender. That the client is unconscious that the muscle is hypertonic represents a loss of sensory awareness.
    - Another common clinical experience is to find that the client has lost the ability to voluntarily contract a muscle that is held in an involuntary contraction. The therapist asks the client to contract a muscle against resistance and the client is unaware of how to engage that muscle. These conditions describe what Thomas Hanna[27] calls "sensory motor amnesia."
    - The muscles may be held in sustained tension due to overuse, poor posture, psychological or emotional stress. States of anxiety and anger, for example, can create sustained muscular hypertonicity. Emotional stress, such as depression, can also create a decrease in muscular tone and a loss of sensory motor communication.
- ***Treatment implications:*** MET is used to bring sensory awareness to the muscles, guiding the client to feel the muscles working. MET also educates the client to bring conscious awareness to the muscles as the client voluntarily contracts them. Using the higher brain through MET by having the client actively participate in muscle movement can alter unconscious habits of muscle tension and help normalize muscle function. To facilitate sensory-motor integration helps correct sensory-motor amnesia.

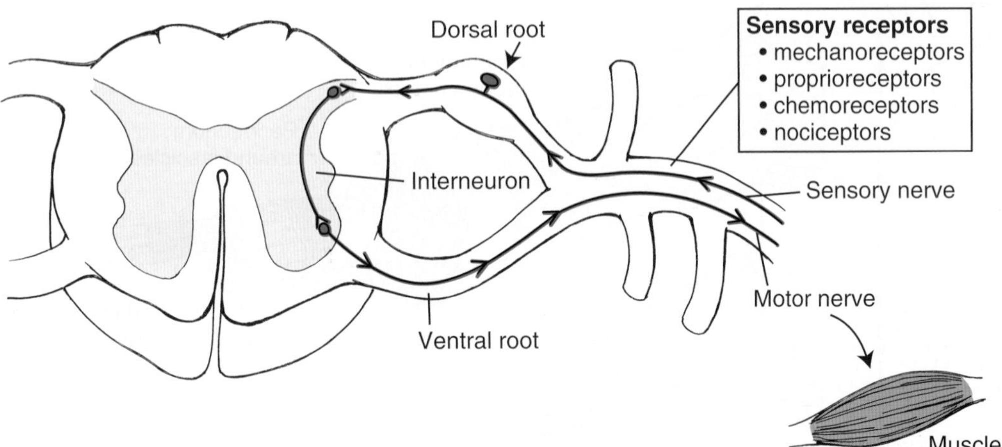

Figure 1-20. Reflex arc. The afferent or sensory nerves receive information from four broad classes of receptors: mechanoreceptors, proprioceptors, chemoreceptors, and nociceptors (pain receptors). The information is sent to the spinal cord and stimulates an interneuron and then the efferent or motor nerves. One motor nerve, the alpha nerve, innervates the extrafusal muscle fiber. Sustained sensory stimulation from mechanical irritation (muscle or joint dysfunction), injury, or emotional tension can create increased alpha stimulation and reflex muscle hypertonicity, or inhibit the alpha nerve activity and cause muscle inhibition and weakness.

As Lederman[8] points out, studies show that stroking an animal's back stimulates the limbic system, and leads to muscular relaxation. Massage can calm anxiety, and MET can engage the muscles to increase their tone in depressed clients.

Because the brain can alter muscle function, it is important that the therapist give the client an image of healing. You might say "I think you will feel a lot better" after your massage to create a positive image of healing, if this is a reasonable possibility.

Peripheral Nervous System

The PNS consists of 12 pairs of cranial nerves and 31 pairs of spinal nerves.

- *Stucture:* The structure of a peripheral nerve is similar to tendons and muscles and consists of long parallel fibers, arranged in bundles called fascicles (Fig. 1-21). The nerves are fluid-filled cells with three connective tissue coverings, the epineurium, perineurium, and endoneurium. Unlike tough electrical wires, they are soft structures that can be injured by compression and mechanical irritation.
  - The nerves are lubricated, and the fibers, fascicles, and gross nerves are designed to slide within the connective tissue spaces. When a muscle contracts and a joint moves, the nerve slides in the healthy state.
  - The spinal nerves begin from expansions of the spinal cord that form two nerve roots—the motor (anterior) root and the sensory (posterior) root.
- *Function:* The spinal nerves of the PNS have four main functional divisions.
  - **Somatic sensory nerves (afferent)**—The somatic sensory nerves relay information to the CNS concerning pain, temperature, touch, and pressure from the skin. It also conveys pain and proprioceptive information about position and mechanoreceptor information about movement from the muscles, tendons, ligaments, joint capsules, and periosteum.
  - **Somatic motor nerves (efferent)**—The somatic motor nerves relay information from the brain, through the spinal cord, and then to skeletal muscles.
  - **Visceral sensory**—These nerves are part of the autonomic nervous system (ANS) and send pain and pressure information from the internal organs to the CNS (see the section, "Autonomic Nervous System").
  - **Visceral motor**—The visceral motor nerves transmit impulses from the ANS to the involuntary

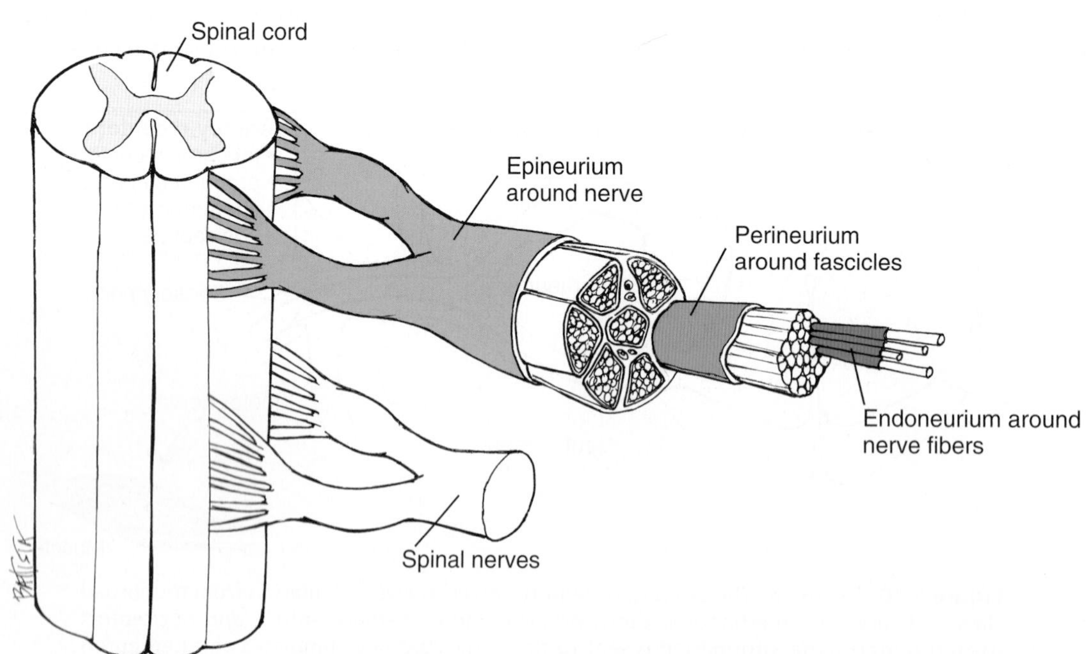

Figure 1-21. Peripheral nerve anatomy. The peripheral nerves begin as 31 pairs of spinal nerves, which then travel throughout the body. They are structured similarly to tendons, ligaments, and muscles, with long parallel fibers contained in bundles surrounded by connective tissue.

muscles, such as those found in internal organs, and glandular tissue.

- *Dysfunction and injury:* The peripheral nerves are susceptible to irritation because of compression or tethering (pulling) at the nerve roots in the area of the intervertebral foramen (IVF). They are also susceptible to compression and irritation in the extremities:
  - Nerves can become restricted or entrapped by adhesions in the connective tissue spaces through which the nerves travel. This restriction prevents the normal gliding of the nerve.
  - Nerves can become restricted or entrapped in the connective tissue spaces of hypertonic muscles.
  - Nerves can become compressed in fibro-osseous tunnels such as the carpal tunnel.
  - Nerves can become compressed, restricted, or irritated because of compression from the swelling or inflammation caused by overuse or injury.
- *Treatment implication:* Peripheral nerves are strong and resilient,[12] and they can be gently massaged without damage. Lauren Berry, RPT, insisted that all massage strokes on the peripheral nerves should be transverse (perpendicular) to the line of the nerve. This releases the adhesions in the connective tissue of the nerve itself and also releases the adhesions in the loose connective tissue that suspends the nerve. This method has proved a safe and comfortable treatment with excellent clinical results. The treatment to decompress the area of the nerve roots of the spine is addressed in each of the Chapters 3 to 5, and the manual release of peripheral entrapment of the nerves in the extremities is addressed in the subsequent chapters.

Autonomic Nervous System

- *Structure:* The ANS is the part of the nervous system that innervates the heart, blood vessels, diaphragm, internal organs, and the glands, and that influences every other part of the body, including the muscular system. There are two main divisions, the sympathetic and the parasympathetic.

Sympathetic Nervous System

- *Structure:* The cell bodies form a cord called the sympathetic trunk, which borders the vertebral column on both sides, and extends from the base of the skull to the coccyx.
- *Function and Dysfunction:* The sympathetic nervous system is responsible for the "fight or flight" response, and is active when a person is under stress. It releases adrenaline into the blood, causes constriction of the peripheral blood vessels, increases the heart rate, and inhibits the normal movement of the intestines (peristalsis) so that blood is available to the skeletal muscles.[12] When a person is under stress, there is an increased tension in the muscles because of the effects of the sympathetic nervous system.

Parasympathetic

- *Structure:* The cell bodies are located in the cranial and sacral regions.
- *Function and Dysfunction:* The parasympathetic nervous system is responsible for energy building, feeding, and assimilation. It is active when the body is at rest and recuperation. It causes a decrease in the heart rate, stimulates the normal movement of the intestines and promotes the secretion of all digestive juices. A person can be in parasympathetic override, which would contribute to lethargy and loss of normal drives. Most people in western cultures have an underactive parasympathetic nervous system, and an overactive sympathic nervous system.
- *Treatment implications:* One of the primary benefits of massage given in a relaxing manner is the stimulation of the parasympathetic nervous system. This induces a state of relaxation and promotes the healing and rejuvenation functions of the parasympathetic nervous system. To induce a relaxing, parasympathetic treatment, the therapist needs to have a gentle touch and a calming voice. The therapist's emotions and attitudes can be calming, by conveying acceptance and support to the client.

Somatic Nervous System

The somatic or motor nervous system includes the CNS and the PNS. Somatic sensory (afferent) nerves are the key components of this system.

- *Structure:* Somatic sensory nerves are specialized receptors that bring information from the periphery to the CNS about four specific categories of information.
  - **Touch and pressure from the skin**—Sensory nerve endings located in the superficial and the deep layers of the skin communicate light touch, deep pressure, temperature, and pain. These nerve endings provide only external information from the environment.
  - **Position (proprioceptors) and movement (mechanoreceptors)**—Proprioceptors and mechanore-

ceptors are located in muscles, tendons, and joints and communicate information about body position and movement (see below for more information, and refer to the section, "Joint Structure and Function").
  - **Oxygen and acid-base balance (chemoreceptors)**—Chemoreceptors are irritated when the body is inflamed and when a muscle is in a sustained contraction, which decreases the amount of oxygen in the tissue ("ischemia").
  - **Pain and irritation (nociceptors)**—Many irritants cause stimulation of the pain fibers, but pain is essentially caused by either mechanical irritation or the release of chemicals from injury to the tissue.
- ***Dysfunction and injury:*** All connective tissues and muscles have a supply of sensory nerve fibers that secrete neuropeptides such as Substance P when they are irritated. These neuropeptides interact with fibroblasts, mast cells, and other cells to create a neurogenic inflammatory response, called **neurogenic pain.**
- ***Treatment implications:*** The somatic sensory nerves are the principal means by which the massage therapist communicates with the client. Each touch and movement sends a message to the spinal cord and brain, which, in turn, communicates with every other part of the body, including the centers of the person's emotions and psychology. Working within the client's comfort is critical because this helps heal the whole person.

Sensory Receptors in Muscle

- As mentioned, five types of sensory (afferent) nerve receptors supply each muscle (Fig. 1-22). The sensory nerves are sensitive to pain, chemical stimuli, temperature, deep pressure, muscle length and the rate of muscle length changes, and muscle tension and the rate of change in tension.
  - Type Ia is a primary muscle spindle.
  - Type Ib is a GTO.
  - Type II is a secondary muscle spindle and includes paciniform and pacinian corpuscles, which are sensitive to deep pressure.
  - Type III are free nerve endings, sensitive to pain, chemicals, and temperature.
  - Type IV are nociceptors (pain receptors).
- Muscles also function as sensory organs through these sensory nerve endings, and information from the receptors has a profound influence on muscle activity. The two classes of sensory receptors that have a particular significance for the massage therapist are the muscle spindles and GTOs. They detect the length and tension in the muscle and tendon, set the resting tone of the muscle, adjust the tension in a muscle for coordination and fine muscular control, and protect the muscle and joint through reflexes that contract or inhibit the muscle automatically.

Muscle Spindles

- ***Structure:*** Muscle spindles are specialized muscle fibers called intrafusal fibers, located in a fluid-filled capsule embedded within each muscle. There are two types of muscle spindles: primary endings (Type Ia) and secondary endings (Type II). Primary endings respond to slow and rapid changes of muscle length, and secondary endings respond to slow changes in muscle length and are sensitive to deep pressure.
- ***Function:*** Muscle spindles detect changes in muscle *length*, so stretching a muscle will increase rate of discharge. The spindles also play a role in joint position, muscle coordination and fine muscular control, and proprioception.[28] Muscle spindles also help set the tone of a muscle. The more refined the function, the greater the concentration of muscle spindles. The greatest concentration of spindles is found in the lumbrical muscles of the hand[29] and then in the suboccipital muscles and in the muscles that move the eyes.
- ***Dysfunction and injury:*** States of anxiety or emotional or psychological tension can cause an increase in the firing rate of the spindle cells. This increase causes the muscle tone to be "set" to high, creating hypertonicity and stiffness.
- ***Treatment implications:*** If the spindle cells are set too high, then there are two ways to decrease the firing rate of a spindle cell and, therefore, cause the muscle to relax.
  1. Decrease the muscle length by bringing the origin and insertion toward each other. This method is emphasized in strain–counterstrain and positional-release techniques and is used in OM.
  2. Contract a muscle isometrically. This method causes the spindle activity to stop temporarily, allowing the muscle to be set to a new, more relaxed length.[30]

Golgi Tendon Organs

- ***Structure:*** GTOs are sensory receptors in the form of a slender capsule located along the muscle fiber at the musculotendinous junction.
- ***Function:*** GTOs are sensitive to changes in muscle *tension*. Originally, they were thought to have only a protective function to prevent damage to a muscle

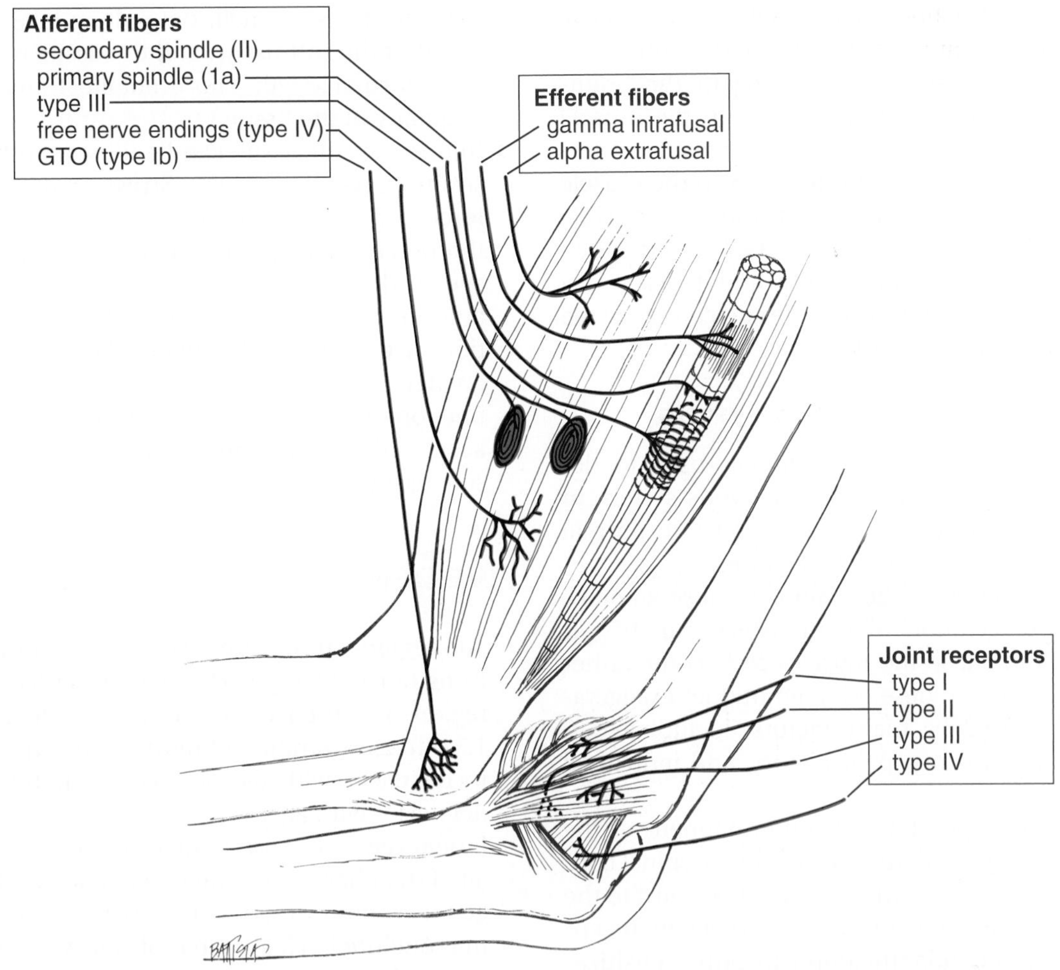

Figure 1-22. Muscle and joint receptors. The extrafusal fibers are innervated by alpha motor neurons, and the intrafusal fibers (muscle spindles) are innervated by gamma motor neurons. There are five classes of sensory nerves in a muscle, including the muscle spindle; GTO; free nerve endings (nociceptors or pain fibers); and receptors sensitive to deep pressure, temperature, and chemical stimuli. Muscle spindles are sensitive to muscle length and changes in length, and the GTOs are sensitive to muscle tension. Spindle cells and GTOs also give proprioceptive information regarding position of the body.

being forcefully contracted. Current research, however, suggests that the GTOs fire during minute changes in muscle tension.[31] This discharge of the GTO stimulates nerves at the spinal cord, called inhibitory interneurons, causing the muscle to relax.[31] Inhibitory interneurons communicate through the spinal cord to the brainstem and, therefore, do not reach conscious awareness.

As with spindle cells, GTOs are used for fine muscular control; they equalize the contractile forces of separate muscle fibers. Through practice these receptors help adjust muscular tension to the appropriate amount in the countless activities of daily living.[1]

- ***Dysfunction:*** Abnormal firing of the GTOs can set the resting tone of the muscle too high, creating hypertonicity.
- ***Treatment implication:*** MET is performed to reset the muscle to its resting length and tone. When a muscle voluntarily contracts isometrically, the GTOs increase their discharge, which has an inhibiting effect on the muscle, causing it to relax.

Motor Nerves in Muscles

- **Alpha motoneurons**—Originating in the motor cortex of the brain, alpha motoneurons innervate the contractile muscle fibers (extrafusal fibers). They are responsible for voluntary muscle contraction.

- **Gamma motoneurons**—Originating in the brainstem, gamma motoneurons innervate the muscle spindle (intrafusal fibers). These nerves carry unconscious information from the CNS to the muscle that sets the tone of muscle, and are responsible through voluntary muscle contraction for fine muscular control. States of anxiety and tension can cause increased spindle discharge and can cause the muscles to be stiff and hypertonic.[24]

Sensitization of the Nervous System

- ***Definition:*** The term *sensitization* is used to describe the phenomenon in the nervous system in which there is an exaggerated response to normal stimuli. There are two principal causes.
  - The limbic areas of the brain can cause an emotional exaggeration of pain, which can trigger the CNS to cause the muscles to become either too tight or too loose. This emotional exaggeration is caused by many factors, including culture, family history, pain history, and individual psychology.
  - The other cause of sensitization happens at the level of the spinal cord. The area in the spinal cord that receives information about pain is next to the receptive field for movement (mechanoreceptors). Chronic inflammation can cause sensitization of the mechanoreceptors such that normal mechanical stimuli (e.g., movement of a joint within a normal range) causes the mechanoreceptor to be a pain producer.[32]

Mechanics of Soft-Tissue Injury

ROLE OF COLLAGEN IN SOFT-TISSUE INJURY

- Soft tissues experience mechanical trauma by pulling (tension), compression, and shearing. As mentioned, connective tissue has unique deformation characteristics, referred to as its viscoelastic nature.
  - If the connective tissue is held in a sustained stretch for enough time, it retains some length after the force is removed. This gradual lengthening is called **creep** and describes its viscous quality.
  - If the stress is small, the pulling takes the crimp out of the soft tissue, and the tissue will return to its normal length. This event illustrates the elastic quality of the tissue.
- Injuries to soft tissue can be illustrated by a stress-strain curve (Fig. 1-23). **Stress** is defined as the force per area applied to the tissue, and **strain,** as the percent change in length. The degree of damage to the soft tissues is affected not only by the amount of stress, but also by the rate or acceleration of the stress. The higher the acceleration, the greater the damage. This explains the whiplash phenomenon, in which low speed (7 mph) but high acceleration (300 milliseconds) can damage the soft tissues.

FIVE DEGREES OF SOFT-TISSUE FAILURE

- **Toe region**—If the stress is small, the tissue returns to its normal length. This is represented by the toe region of the curve. Tissue may be loaded with a 1.5% to 2.5% strain and return to normal. This ability decreases with age, because the amount of crimp decreases with age.
- **Linear region**—If the strain is between 2.5% and 4%, all of the fibers have straightened out, and the collagen tears at its outermost fibers first, which is called microfailure.[33] This degree of injury is represented by the linear area of the curve. The tearing of collagen is like a rope that frays from its outer fibers to the center. The client complains of stiffness with this amount of tear.[13] Microfailure can occur within the normal physiologic range if there is repetitive stress on an already damaged structure.[34]
- **Progressive failure region**—A strain between 4% and 6% is called the yield point, at which point major tearing occurs.
- **Major failure region**—A strain of more than 6% involves many points of rupture.
- **Complete rupture**—An 8% strain causes the collagen fibers to tear completely apart.
- Even with microfailure, the cells, fibers, and ground-substance matrix are now damaged, and an inflammatory response is initiated. The injury also affects the sensory nerves in the connective tissue, which causes the profound neurological disturbances described above.
- Following the tear of the collagen fibers, repair and regeneration of the tissue is carried out through the process of inflammation and repair.

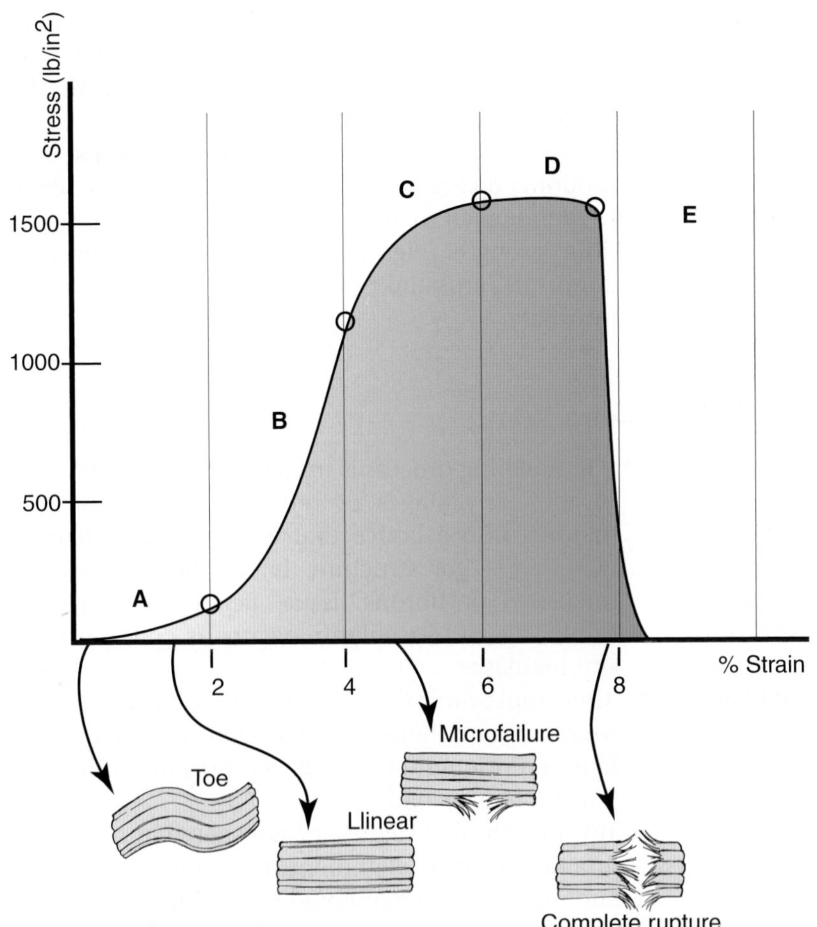

Figure 1-23. Stress–strain curve for a ruptured Achilles tendon. The five distinct regions are **(A)** toe region, **(B)** linear region, **(C)** progressive failure region, **(D)** major failure region, and **(E)** complete rupture.

Stages of Inflammation and Repair

FOUR CARDINAL SIGNS OF INFLAMMATION

- **Redness**
- **Heat**
- **Swelling**
- **Pain**

INFLAMMATION—THE BODY'S RESPONSE TO TWO TYPES OF IRRITANTS, LIVING AND NONLIVING

- **Living irritants**—Microorganisms, such as bacteria, are an example of a living irritant.
- **Nonliving irritants**—Trauma is the primary cause of inflammation. Joint dysfunction can irritate the cartilage and periarticular soft tissues, creating a microinflammatory environment, with the same cellular responses described in this chapter.

FUNCTIONS OF INFLAMMATION

- Protects the body from infection.
- Repairs damaged tissue by stimulating new cell growth, which then synthesizes new fibers for repair.

Two Types of Trauma

- **Direct**—blunt trauma from contact sports, car accidents, etc.
- **Indirect**
  - Acute—occurs with sudden overloading.

- Chronic or overuse—occurs as a result of repeated overload, frictional resistance, or both.
- Acute on chronic—occurs as a result of a sudden tear of a persistent lesion.

PHASES OF INFLAMMATION AND REPAIR

Vascular (Acute)

This type of inflammation typically lasts 24 to 48 hours. In some cases, however, it may last from 4 to 6 days.

- Dilation of the arteries, veins, and capillaries, causing redness and heat.
- Escape of blood plasma, causing edema (swelling).
- Increase in number of fibroblasts and macrophages. The fibroblasts increase in size and synthesize ground substance and collagen. This process begins within 4 hours of injury, and can last 4 to 6 days. Collagen initially forms a weak, random mesh of fibers.
- Pain is produced by the pressure from the swelling and by the chemical irritation that stimulates the pain receptors (nociceptors).

Regeneration and Repair

The process of regeneration and repair takes 2 to 6 days and lasts approximately 3 weeks.

- Scar tissue is highly cellular, and new capillaries are formed. The capillaries are laid down in a random orientation unless the area is mobilized.
- Fibroblastic activity and collagen formation increases.
- Immature connective tissue is less dense and therefore more easily injured. Pain does not indicate the level of repair, so care must be taken with the amount of pressure applied in a massage.
- In these early stages, collagen is laid down in a random, disorganized pattern, usually in a plane perpendicular to the long axis, and therefore has little strength (Fig. 1-24).[6] The collagen develops abnormal crosslinks leaving the tissue with less flexibility.

Remodeling

The remodeling process is from day 21 to day 60.

- In the early stages of remodeling, the collagen matures into a lattice that is completely disorganized in a gel structure. It can be palpated as thickened or fibrous tissue. Relative decrease in cellularity and vascularity occurs as collagen density increases.
- After approximately 2 months, fibroblastic activity decreases and there is less collagen synthesis.
- Random orientation of collagen provides little support for tensile loads.
- Two months to 2 years later, collagen may develop a functional linear alignment in response to stimuli and may become reoriented to the line of stress.
- Immobilization leads to significant adhesion formations; osteoporosis or loss of bone density; and to the atrophy of muscles, capsules, and ligaments.
- Chronic inflammation can result from repeated episodes of microtrauma, or chronic irritation to the tissue.

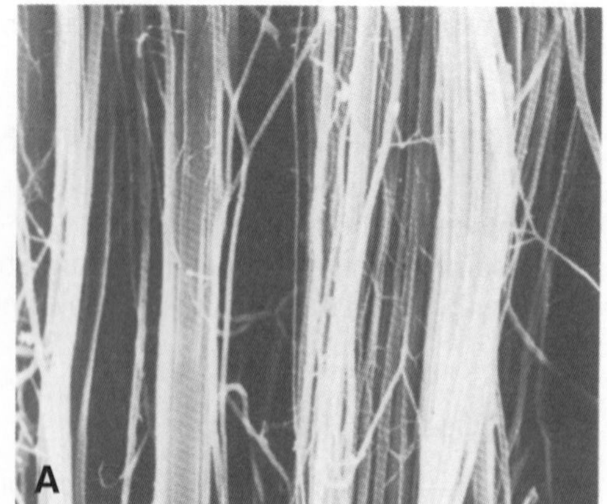

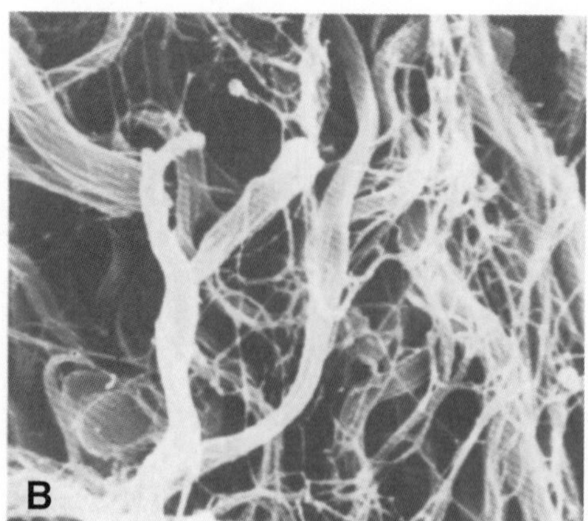

Figure 1-24. **A.** The normal longitudinal arrangement of a ligament. **B.** The random crossweave of the collagen fibers in the early stages of repair after an injury to the ligament. (Reprinted with permission from Woo S, Buckwalter J. Injury and Repair of the Musculoskeletal Soft Tissues. Park Ridge, IL: American Academy of Orthopedic Surgeons, 1988.)

Review of Neuromuscular Consequences of Inflammation

- Inflammation leads to stimulation of pain receptors that cause compensatory adaptations that either facilitate muscles, causing hypertonicity, or inhibit muscles, causing weakness.[35]
- Typically, with joint inflammation, the flexors of the joint become hypertonic, and the extensors become inhibited.[22]
- Chronic inflammation can cause sensitization of the mechanoreceptors, such that normal mechanical stimuli (e.g., movement of a joint within a normal range) cause the mechanoreceptor to be a pain producer.[32]

STUDY GUIDE

Level I

1. List the three basic elements and four primary types of tissue.
2. List the three connective tissue cell types discussed in the chapter and describe their function.
3. Describe the arrangement of collagen fibers and how collagen is affected in injury. Describe the treatment implications of this collagen change.
4. Describe the function and dysfunction of ground substance and define thixotropy and its relevance to massage therapy.
5. Describe why movement in the early stages of repair is indicated.
6. List the three connective tissue layers of a muscle, and list the most common sites of injury in the myofascia.
7. List the causes of pain from soft-tissue injury and dysfunction.
8. Describe a sclerotome and the quality of pain from those tissues.
9. Describe Janda's concept of soft-tissue dysfunction and its relevance to massage therapy.
10. Describe Lauren Berry's concept of soft-tissue dysfunction and its relevance to massage therapy.

Level II

1. Describe the pain-gate theory of Melzak and Wall and its relevance to massage therapy.
2. Describe six functions of a muscle.
3. Define a tensegrity structure and how this structure maintains stability.
4. Describe the functions of the following structures: muscle spindle, GTO, and alpha and gamma nerves.
5. List the eight causes of muscle dysfunction.
6. Describe how cartilage maintains its circulation and health.
7. Define the arthrokinetic reflex.
8. Describe two causes of joint dysfunction that OM can effectively treat.
9. Describe the differences between the sympathetic and the parasympathetic nervous systems and the implication for massage therapy.
10. Describe two types of sensitization in the nervous system.

REFERENCES

1. Juhan D. Job's Body. Barrytown, New York: Station Hill Press, 1987.
2. Woo S, An K-N. Anatomy, biology, and biomechanics of tendon, ligament, and meniscus. In: Simon S, ed. Orthopedic Basic Science. Park Ridge, IL: American Academy of Orthopedic Surgeons, 1994:45–88.
3. Engles M. Tissue response. In: Donatelli R, Wooden M, eds. Orthopedic Physical Therapy. New York: Churchill Livingstone, 1989:1–31.
4. Becker R. The Body Electric. New York: William Morrow, 1985.
5. Turchaninov R. Research and massage therapy: part 2. Massage and Bodywork 2001;Dec/Jan:48–56.
6. Woo S, Buckwalter J. Injury and Repair of the Musculoskeletal Soft Tissues. Park Ridge, IL: American Academy of Orthopedic Surgeons, 1988.
7. Reid DC. Sports Injury and Assessment. New York: Churchill Livingstone, 1992.
8. Lederman E. Fundamentals of Manual Therapy. New York: Churchill Livingstone, 1997.
9. Wyke BD. Articular neurology and manipulative therapy. Aspects of Manipulative Therapy. Edinburgh: Churchill Livingstone, 1985:72–80.
10. Freeman MAR, Wyke B. Articular reflexes at the ankle joint: an electromyographic study of normal and abnormal influences of ankle-joint mechanoreceptors upon reflex activity in the leg muscles. Br J Surg 1967;54: 990–1001.
11. Cyriax J. Textbook of Orthopedic Medicine: Diagnosis of Soft Tissue Lesions, vol 1, 8th Ed. London: Bailliere Tindall, 1982.
12. Moore K, Dalley A. Clinically Oriented Anatomy, 4th Ed. Baltimore: Lippincott Williams & Wilkins, 1999.
13. Lynch M, Kessler R, Hertling D. Pain. In: Management of Common Musculoskeletal Disorders, 3rd Ed. Baltimore: Lippincott, 1996:50–68.
14. Zimmerman M. Pain mechanisms and mediators in osteoarthritis. Semin Arthritis Rheum 1989;18:22–29.
15. Medoff R. Soft tissue healing. Ann Sports Med 1987; 3:67–70.

15a. Buckminster Fuller R. Synergetics. Collier Books, Macmillan, 1975.

16. Norkin C, Levangie P. Joint Structure and Function, 2nd Ed. Philadelphia: FA Davis, 1992.
17. Janda V. Evaluation of muscular imbalance. In: Liebenson C, ed. Rehabilitation of the Spine. Baltimore: Williams & Wilkins, 1996: 97–112.
18. Wyke B. Articular neurology—a review. Physiotherapy 1972;58: 94–99.
19. Lewit K. Manipulative Therapy in Rehabilitation on the Locomotor System, 3rd Ed. Oxford: Butterworth Heinemann, 1999.
20. Janda V. Function of muscles in musculoskeletal pain syndromes. Seminar notes. Seattle, April 18–19, 1999.
21. Bullock-Saxton J, Murphy D, Norris C, Richardson C, Tunnell P. The muscle designation debate: the experts respond. J Bodywork Movement Therapies 2000;4:225–241.
22. Young A. Effects of joint pathology on muscle. Clin Orthop 1987;219: 21–27.
23. Mennell J. Joint Pain. Boston: Little, Brown and Company, 1964.
24. Korr I. Proprioceptors and somatic dysfunction. J Am Osteopath Assoc 1975;74:638–650
25. Kessler R, Hertling D. Arthrology. In: Management of Common Musculoskeletal Disorders, 3rd Ed. Philadelphia: Lippincott, 1996:22–49.
26. Wooden M. Mobilization of the upper extremity. In: Donatelli R, Wooden M, eds. Orthopedic Physical Therapy. New York: Churchill Livingstone, 1994: 297–332.
27. Hanna T. Somatics. Menlo Park, CA: Addison-Wesley, 1988.
28. Lewis MM. Muscle spindles and their functions: a review. Aspects of Manipulative Therapy. Edinburgh: Churchill Livingstone, 1985: 55–58.
29. Wadsworth C. The wrist and hand. In: Malone T, McPoil T, Nitz A, eds. Orthopedic and Sports Physical Therapy, 3rd Ed. St. Louis: Mosby, 1997:327–378.
30. Pearson K, Gordon J. Spinal reflexes. In: Kandal E, Schwartz J, Jessell T, eds. Principles of Neural Science. New York: McGraw-Hill, 2000:713–736.
31. Guyton A, Hall J. Textbook of Medical Physiology, 10th Ed. Philadelphia: WB Saunders, 2000.
32. Mense S. Nociception from skeletal muscle in relation to clinical muscle pain. Pain 1993;54:241–289.
33. Kellett J. Acute soft tissue injuries—a review of the literature. Med Sci Sports Exerc 1986;18:489–500.
34. Carlstedt C, Nordin M. Biomechanics of tendons and ligaments. In: Nordin M, Frankel V, eds. Basic Biomechanics of the Musculoskeletal System. Philadelphia: Lea & Febiger, 1989:59–74.
35. Janda V. Pain in the locomotor system—a broad approach. Aspects of Manipulative Therapy. Edinburgh: Churchill Livingstone, 1985:148–151.

SUGGESTED READINGS

Corrigan B, Maitland GD. Practical Orthopaedic Medicine. London: Butterworths, 1983.

Greenman PE. Principles of Manual Medicine, 2nd Ed. Baltimore: Williams & Wilkins, 1996.

Janda V. Evaluation of muscular imbalance. In: Liebenson C, ed. Rehabilitation of the Spine. Baltimore: Williams & Wilkins, 1996:97–112.

Kessler R, Hertling D. Arthrology. In: Management of Common Musculoskeletal Disorders, 3rd Ed. Philadelphia: Lippincott, 1996: 22–49.

Lederman E. Fundamentals of Manual Therapy. New York: Churchill Livingstone, 1997.

Lewit K. Manipulative Therapy in Rehabilitation on the Locomotor System, 3rd Ed. Oxford: Butterworth Heinemann, 1999.

Lippert L. Clinical Kinesiology for Physical Therapy Assistants, 3rd Ed. Philadelphia: FA Davis, 2000.

Lynch M, Kessler R, Hertling D. Pain. Management of Common Musculoskeletal Disorders. Baltimore: Williams & Wilkins, 1996: 50–68.

Magee D. Orthopedic Physical Assessment, 3rd Ed. Philadelphia: WB Saunders, 1997.

Norkin C, Levangie P. Joint Structure and Function, 2nd Ed. Philadelphia: FA Davis, 1992.

Reid DC. Sports Injury and Assessment. New York: Churchill Livingstone, 1992.

Assessment & Technique

Assessment

GENERAL OVERVIEW OF ASSESSMENT

The clinical massage therapist has an expanded role compared with the therapist working in a spa environment. When working with a client who has pain, dysfunction, or disability, the therapist needs to take time at the beginning of the session to gather information from the client about any pain or decreased function. This process is called taking a history. It is also necessary to perform a brief examination. The history and examination form the two elements of the assessment.

The assessment helps identify what structures need to be worked on, creates a clear intention about your treatment goals, provides a baseline of objective information to measure the effectiveness of your treatment, helps prevent treating conditions that are contraindicated, and indicates to the massage therapist when to refer to a doctor or other health-care provider. The assessment is within the scope of a massage therapist and does not constitute making a diagnosis. A diagnosis determines the cause of a client's pain, dysfunction, or disability and is not within the scope of practice of massage therapists.

Two Parts of an Assessment

Subjective Examination
The subjective part of the examination is that information which the client reports to you. It requires asking the client about his or her chief complaint (i.e., the pain, dysfunction, or disability that led the client to seek treatment). This process is called taking the history of the chief complaint and is detailed below.

Objective Examination
The objective part of the examination includes the information that the therapist can observe or feel. It includes two aspects:

- Observation
- Examination

Recording Information

Providing massage therapy to clients who have pain, dysfunction, or disability requires that the therapist keep good records. Good record keeping provides the therapist with the information necessary to communicate with other health-care providers and forms an accurate record about what you were treating, the styles of treatment you used, and the effectiveness of your treatment.

This text describes the essentials of performing an assessment for the massage therapist. How extensive your assessment is depends on whether you are working under the direction of a doctor or another health-care provider or are working independently. In the former situation, it is the responsibility of the primary provider to take a thorough history, perform a complete examination, and inform the massage therapist regarding the client's condition. If you are working independently, it is your responsibility to take a history and perform an examination.

Subjective, Objective, Action (Assessment), and Plan (SOAP) Notes

The health-care community has developed a standard format to record information in the client's chart. These notes form a medical and legal record. If you are working independently, create a chart for each patient. If you are working under the direction of another provider, you will still need to take notes about your session. Some clinics want you to write your notes in the client's chart, whereas other clinics want you to verbally communicate to the primary therapist or to write your notes in a separate file that you keep with you.

There are four different categories of information that you want to record in your notes. These categories are remembered with the acronym "SOAP," which stands for subjective, objective, action (assessment), and plan.

- **Subjective**—The subjective information is the client's present complaint, that is, his symptoms. If the client does not have any symptoms, write down, "wellness treatment." To find out the details of the symptoms, use the format described below called "history of the chief complaint." Abbreviate "subjective" with the letter "s," with a circle around it.
- **Objective**—This information is a summary of the examination findings. These findings are called **signs,** that is, what the therapist can objectively observe. Abbreviate "objective" with the letter "o," with a circle around it.
- **Action** (Assessment)—In the realm of manual therapy, the letter "a" stands for the action taken, that is, what treatment was given. In the medical community, "a" stands for assessment. As a massage therapist, briefly describe what techniques you performed and on what major areas you worked. Often, a client says, "Whatever you did last time worked like a miracle," and unless the treatment approach was written down, the therapist may not remember what created such a positive response. Abbreviate "action" with the letter "a," with a circle around it.
- **Plan**—The plan is an outline of your treatment goals. How many treatments do you recommend? How often? What structures do you want to work on next session, and what tests do you want to perform? If you are working under the direction of a primary provider, you will not be making the decision about how many treatments, or how often, but recommendations from the massage therapist are important in the decision. Abbreviate "plan" with the letter "p," with a circle around it.

Progress Notes

- The notes in the client's chart are called progress notes. The first visit requires taking a history of the chief complaint, unless a primary provider has performed the examination. If you are working independently, keep a chart on the client to record the notes about your examination findings and the treatments performed. You only need to record the significant examination findings. If the only positive examination finding is a loss of approximately 50% of right cervical rotation in active range of motion (ROM) and that motion elicited a pain in the right scapular region, it is only necessary to write that finding.
- The first visit in which an established client presents with a new problem requires taking a history, however brief. Do not make the mistake of assuming that a client's chronic low back pain is the same as always, unless you specifically ask if there have been any new incidents, injuries, or symptoms. Since last seen, your client may have had an acute, low-back strain, and unless asked, may not tell you about it.
- The following four to six visits typically only require a brief notation regarding present symptoms, positive objective findings, the treatment you performed, and the plan for what you want to work on next time. If you are treating someone in acute distress, reassess the positive objective findings in each follow-up visit.

- The primary provider typically performs a reevaluation approximately every six treatments. If you are practicing independently, you will need to perform this examination yourself. This allows you to measure the effectiveness of your treatment by determining if there are gains in the functional status. Do not rely solely on a change in symptoms to measure progress. Improvement of function is the measure of effective treatment.
- This information will form your progress notes. That is, you should note if the condition is getting better, worse, or staying the same.

SUBJECTIVE EXAMINATION: TAKING A HISTORY

When you ask clients about the condition for which they seek treatment, this is called "taking a history." With experience, this part of your session becomes the foundation for the rest of your treatment. Gathering accurate information from the client on the nature of his or her complaint helps you determine the severity of the condition, if the condition is acute or chronic, if your treatment needs to be extremely gentle or if more vigorous work is indicated, if massage is contraindicated, and if a referral to another provider is indicated. The history becomes a critical aspect to your session. What follows are the essential points to cover in your questions. We will assume that the client is seeking treatment for pain, but the condition may be loss of motion, loss of strength, numbing or tingling, or various other symptoms.

Location

Ask the client to point to the area of complaint. A shoulder pain does not indicate where the pain is. Shoulder pain may mean the upper trapezius, the lateral humerus, or many other areas.

Onset

Did the condition (pain, loss of motion, etc.) arise suddenly or gradually? Was there an incident of injury? A gradual onset suggests an overuse syndrome, postural stresses, or somatic manifestations of emotional or psychological stresses. When you ask about the onset, you are gathering information about the recent episode of pain or dysfunction. A separate question addresses when the client first noticed this condition (see History of Area of Chief Complaint) and thus helps to determine any previous incident or injury prior to the current episode that involved this same region.

Frequency

How often does it hurt, or how often does the client notice the dysfunction or disability? Is it once a day, once a week, ten times a day, constant? The simplest types of sprains and strains to the muscles, tendons, and ligaments hurt when they are being used, and are relieved with rest. Constant pain is a "red flag"; that is, a symptom that is usually associated with a severe injury or pathology. Severe inflammation may hurt constantly, but so too, do tumors and fractures. A client with constant pain needs a referral to a doctor. Many people use the phrase "it hurts all the time" to mean that it hurts frequently, rather than that it hurts at every moment.

Duration

How long does it last when it hurts? The more serious the condition, the longer it will last.

Quality

Typical words used to describe the chief complaint:

- **Stiff, achy, tight**—These words are associated with muscles, tendons, ligaments, and joint capsules and their associated connective tissue and usually describe a simple tension or a mild overuse of the soft tissue. If an ache is more than mild, is frequent, and lasts a long time, it is more serious and represents inflammation. A thorough examination is required to rule out a more serious condition.
- **Sharp**—This describes a more severe injury to the musculoskeletal system or a nerve root condition. A muscle or ligament tear can be sharp when the muscle or ligament is used, but it is usually relieved at rest. A nerve-root inflammation can elicit a sharp pain, but the pain is often independent of movement. The protocols of how to distinguish these two conditions are described in the section, "Objective Examination."
- **Burning**—Burning pain is associated with nerve inflammation. It is safe to perform massage on a client with this type of pain, but the client typically needs a referral to a chiropractor or osteopath to assess the need for spinal manipulation.
- **Tingling, numbing**—These words describe a nerve compression, either near the spine or in the extremities.

- **Throbbing**—This is associated with acute inflammation and swelling, such as an acute bursitis. Gentle massage is indicated with mild, throbbing pain to help resolve the inflammation. Severe throbbing is a contraindication to massage.
- **Gripping**—This word is typically used to describe a serious condition, often a nerve root injury (see Chapter 3, "Lumbosacral Spine," and Chapter 5, "Cervical Spine."). If the client describes a mild gripping pain, gentle massage may be performed. Severe gripping pain is a contraindication to massage and requires a referral to a doctor.

Radiation

Is there pain, numbing, or tingling in the arms or legs? As mentioned in Chapter 1, "The Theoretical Foundations of Orthopedic Massage," there are two basic types of referred pain: sclerotomal, and dermatomal. Irritation or injury to the soft tissue can refer into the extremities, giving sclerotomal pain. However, when these conditions refer, the pain is diffuse and achy, rather than sharp and well localized. Sharp, well-localized pain in the extremities that hurts even at rest typically indicates a nerve root problem, and needs a referral to a chiropractor or osteopath.

Severity

Ask your clients to rate their pain on a 0 to 10 scale, with 10 being the worst pain ever experienced and 0 being no pain. The number 10 should be used for incapacitating pain (i.e., the client cannot work or perform household duties with pain that severe). Moderate pain, 5 to 9, interferes with a person's ability to perform work or household duties. That is, because of the pain, the client cannot do certain activities. Mild pain, 1 to 4, does not interfere with a person's activities of daily living (ADL).

Aggravating Factors

What activities make the condition worse? Moving, sitting, standing, walking, or resting? The most simple strains and sprains of the musculoskeletal system are irritated with too much movement and relieved by rest. When a condition hurts more with rest, it indicates either an inflammation or a pathology.

Relieving Factors

What activities make the condition better? Resting, moving, or applying ice or heat? As the soft tissue heals, it feels good to move the injured area. Stretching tight muscles, shortened ligaments, and joint capsules feels good, despite some mild discomfort. Acute injuries involving the soft tissue are painful with large movements and are relieved with rest.

Night Pain

Inflammation and tumors are worse at night. Constant, gripping pain that is worse at night is a red flag and needs a referral to a doctor. An area that hurts at night but is relieved with movement indicates inflammation.

Prior Treatments and Their Effects

Are you the first therapist to treat this condition? If so, you need to perform a careful history and examination to determine if massage is contraindicated and when to refer. It is also important to know if the client has had massage therapy before and whether it was helpful.

Progress

Is the client getting better, worse, or staying the same? If a client is getting worse, then use extra care in your history and examination to determine if a referral is indicated.

History of Area of Chief Complaint

Have there been any accidents, injuries, or surgeries to the area of complaint in the client's past? The longer the history, the more challenging the condition.

Medications

If a person has taken pain medication within 4 hours of your assessment and treatment, you need to be cautious, as the pain medication may be giving the client a false sense of comfort with the examination and depth of the therapist's work.

Diagnostic Studies Performed

Have there been x-rays, magnetic resonance imaging (MRI), etc., performed? Get a copy of the report for your file. Does the report indicate a severe condition?

OBJECTIVE EXAMINATION

Accurate examination requires that the therapist follow a specific sequence of procedures and apply those steps to the area of the body under examination. This ensures that all the relevant information is being gathered. Each chapter in this book describes the specific examination procedures for a particular region of the body. However, it is important to first understand the basic principles of the examination and why each aspect of the examination is performed.

Observation

- Posture—Notice the posture of the client in both standing and seated positions, and the posture or position of the area of complaint. For example, notice if the shoulder is held in an elevated or forward posture on one side.
- Redness, swelling—This indicates inflammation, and massage is contraindicated for red, hot, swollen tissue. The therapist needs to be extremely gentle in the area surrounding the redness and swelling. Perform reciprocal inhibition (RI) or contract-relax (CR) muscle energy technique (MET).
- Scars—Scars indicate either prior surgery or prior injury and reveal that the area is compromised. Ask the client to describe how he or she received the scar.
- Atrophy—An area of atrophy has either been deconditioned owing to lack of use, or indicates neurologic involvement. Simple atrophy can be a result of immobilization caused by prior fracture or lack of use due to pain. Complex atrophy is a long-standing condition that involves the damage or dysfunction of the nerve innervating the afflicted muscles. Do not work vigorously on an atrophied muscle. The area needs MET to reestablish the neurologic communication and exercise.

Motion Assessment

The next part of the examination is divided into two sections. In **active motion assessment,** the therapist asks the client to perform movements in specific directions. In **passive motion assessment** the therapist moves the client. Injuries and dysfunctions of the musculoskeletal system hurt when the injured area is moved, and more complex conditions, such as inflammation of the nervous system; systemic conditions, like heart disease; or pathologies, such as tumors, are not significantly affected by movement. If an area does not hurt at rest, but it does with movement, then the simplest of conditions—the sprains and strains of soft tissue—is indicated.

Active Movements

The following categories are noted by the therapist:

- ROM—Is the motion normal, decreased, increased? Determining normal ROM is more complex than it might seem. You need to consider the client's age and sex. There is less ROM as we age, and women typically have greater ROM than men. If the complaint is in the extremities, then begin with the noninvolved side, and always compare both sides.
    - **Decreased ROM** is caused by either pain or changes in the joint or soft tissue. If the loss of motion is not a result of pain, then the therapist needs to gather more information to determine whether the lack of motion is caused by adhesions in the joint capsule, spastic muscles, degeneration in the joints, or other causes.
    - **Increased ROM** that is significantly different from the other side indicates a moderate to severe injury to the ligaments, joint capsule, or both. Increased ROM on both sides compared with normal ROM suggests a generalized hypermobility syndrome and potential instability in the joints.
- **Pain**—If movement is painful, ask the client to describe its location, quality, and severity. The three stages of healing elicit pain at different ranges of the movement are as follows:
    - **Acute** conditions yield pain before the normal ROM.
    - **Subacute** conditions give pain at the end of that normal range.
    - **Chronic** conditions may elicit pain with overpressure at the end of active or passive motion.

Passive Movements

Passive motion is typically tested only if the client cannot perform full and pain-free active motion. James Cyriax, MD, has developed a system of soft tissue assessment called "selective tension" testing.[1] He made the simple but profound observation that muscles and tendons and their associated connective tissues can be accurately examined by means of isometric testing, since muscles are contractile tissues; and that noncontractile soft tissues, such as the joint capsule, ligaments, fascia, bursae, dura mater, and dural sheath are best tested with passive testing. This principle helps differentiate muscle strains from ligamentous sprains and therefore helps determine where and how to apply the treatment. These principles are developed further throughout this text. When performing passive motion on the client, note the following three categories:

- **ROM**—Passive ROM is typically greater than active ROM.

- **Pain**—Note the location, quality, and severity. Pain with passive motion at different ranges of the movement indicates a stage of healing that is the same as active motion.
  - **Acute** conditions yield pain before the normal ROM.
  - **Subacute co**nditions give pain at the end of the normal range.
  - **Chronic** conditions may elicit pain with overpressure at the end range.
- **End feel:** This term was developed by James Cyriax and is defined as the feeling transmitted to the therapist's hands as a slight overpressure is applied at the end of the joint's ROM.[1] The end-feel gives important information about the type of injury or dysfunction and the severity. For example, elbow flexion normally has a muscular end-feel as the biceps and other soft tissues are being compressed. A bony end-feel in elbow flexion would be abnormal, and would indicate a possible arthritis. Seven categories of end-feel are differentiated:
  - **Soft-tissue approximation**—A soft end-feel, as felt in flexing the elbow, as the biceps and forearm muscles are pressed together.
  - **Muscular**—A more rubbery feeling than a soft-tissue approximation, as felt in stretching the hamstrings.
  - **Bony**—An abrupt, hard end-feel, as felt in extending the elbow.
  - **Capsular**—A thick, tight feeling, similar to that of stretching leather, as felt in external rotation of the shoulder.
  - **Muscle spasm**—A tight, bound feeling, ending before the normal ROM, as felt in a muscle spasm. Palpation confirms the assessment.
  - **Springy block**—A feeling of the joint rebounding or springing, associated with a decreased ROM. A classic finding with a torn meniscus of the knee as the joint is brought to passive extension.
  - **Empty**—A pain that causes the client to stop further passive motion even though the therapist cannot detect any tissue tension or other resistance to the motion. Typical with a pathology, acute bursitis, or emotional guarding.

Isometric Testing

Isometric contraction is an assessment of the contractile structures (e.g., muscles, tendons, and their associated connective tissues) and the nervous system. These tests are performed as part of CR-MET (see "Muscle Energy Technique" p. 57). During the contraction the therapist notes two things, the **strength** of the resistance and whether the client experiences **pain.** Isometric testing yields three possible findings:

- **Strong and painless** contraction indicates a normal structure.
- **Painful** contraction indicates an injury or dysfunction in the tested muscle-tendon-periosteal unit.
- **Weak and painless** contraction may indicate one of nine possibilities:
  - The muscle is inhibited due to hypertonic antagonist.
  - The muscle is inhibited due to dysfunction or injury in a local joint that the muscle crosses.
  - Fixation or subluxation of a vertebra of the spine, causing irritation to the motor nerve and weakness in the muscles innervated by that nerve.
  - Nerve injury (e.g., rupture of a disc), which can create pressure on the nerve root, causing the muscle that the root innervates to weaken.
  - The muscle is deconditioned from lack of use.
  - An atrophied muscle from previous injury or disease.
  - Reflexive weakness caused by visceral imbalance, which is called the viscerosomatic reflex, and may be assessed by means of applied kinesiology (AK).
  - Stretch weakness describes a condition in which a muscle is kept in a habitually stretched position that causes it to weaken.
  - Tightness weakness, a condition in which a muscle is habitually short and tests weak, even if tested at its resting length.[2]

Palpation

This text assumes that the therapist has been trained in the fundamentals of palpation. See Hoppenfeld[3] and Chaitow[4] for textbooks on palpation.

As mentioned in Chapter 1, to touch another human being is an act of giving and receiving information. It conveys not only our skill, but also our sensitivity and compassion. Our touch is also a powerful assessment tool. Our hands receive information about the condition of the tissue under our fingers, as well as the client's general health, and emotional and psychological state.

A hallmark of orthopedic massage (OM) is that during palpation and performance of the massage strokes, the touch of the therapist is gentle, even though the pressure may be deep. The therapist wants to convey with touch that the client is completely safe physically and emotionally. The client should be able to relax completely under the therapist's touch.

Three Characteristics of Soft Tissue the Therapist Can Palpate

Three qualities of soft tissue that can be palpated inform the therapist about the state of health of the tissue.

- **Water content**—Healthy tissue is well hydrated without feeling boggy or swollen.
- **Fiber content**—Healthy soft tissue feels resilient and springy, in part owing to the fiber. Too little fiber and the tissue is atrophied; too much fiber indicates adhesion or scarring.
- **Temperature**—Heat is an indication of inflammation.

Four Categories of Feeling in Soft Tissue Based on Palpation

Based on the three characteristics of tissue, four categories may be used to differentiate between acute and chronic conditions. These categories therefore help guide the therapist in performing the massage:

- **Normal**—The soft tissue feels resilient, homogeneous, relaxed, and fluid without being watery.
- **Chronic**—The soft tissue feels fibrous, gristly, dry (decreased water), thickened, stiff, and tight.
- **Acute**—The soft tissue feels watery (edema), warm, or hot.
- **Atrophy**—The soft tissue feels mushy and flaccid owing to a loss of tone (i.e., decreased fiber content).

Assessment of Severity of Injury by Palpation

Pressing into tissue and taking out all the slack puts the tissue in tension. Normally, there is no pain with pressing into the soft tissue, only a sense of pressure.

- **Acute**—The client feels pain before tissue is in tension.
- **Subacute**—The client feels pain at tissue tension.
- **Chronic**—The client may feel pain with overpressure (i.e., pressing further into the tissue after the tissue is in tension).

PATTERNS OF SOFT-TISSUE AND JOINT DYSFUNCTION, INJURY, AND DEGENERATION

After performing the history and objective examination, gather all the pieces of information to form a picture of the client's condition. Patterns will emerge within the countless types of injuries and dysfunctions in the body. Knowing these patterns helps guide you in determining the type of injury or dysfunction and, therefore, helps create an appropriate treatment. It can be frustrating for the client and the therapist to assume that the client merely has tight muscles, when examination findings suggest a degeneration in the joint (arthritis). These categories overlap, and most clients present with several categories at the same time. Understanding what is being treated dramatically increases the effectiveness of the treatment.

We apply each of these patterns to each region of the body in the following chapters of this book. Remember that gathering objective information is part of an assessment and within the scope of practice for a massage therapist. To determine the cause of a client's pain is to make a diagnosis and not within the scope of practice for a massage therapist.

Arthritis or Osteoarthritis

The word *arthritis* means inflammation of a joint. In common language the word arthritis or **osteoarthritis (OA)** usually refers to chronic pain or stiffness in a joint. The more accurate term for chronic degeneration of the joint is arthrosis or **degenerative joint disease (DJD).** Following common usage, this text uses OA and DJD interchangeably and implies a chronic condition, unless specified otherwise. Joint degeneration refers to degeneration of the cartilage.

- Active and passive ROMs are decreased. If the joint is inflamed , then movements are painful, especially at the end of the normal range. Chronic degeneration often has crepitation (grinding sounds) with active and passive movement.
- Resisted (isometric) movements are usually painless.
- Passive motion elicits a bony end-feel in chronic conditions.

Capsulitis

Capsulitis is an inflammation of the joint capsule. As with arthritis, the term is often used for chronic conditions, as in adhesive capsulitis of the shoulder. Technically, chronic adhesions in the capsule are a **capsulosis.**

- Active and passive ROMs are decreased and painful, especially at the end of normal range.
- Resisted (isometric) contraction is usually painless.
- Passive motion reveals an empty end-feel if there is inflammation, and a thickened, leathery (capsular) end-feel if the condition is chronic.

Tendinitis

Tendinitis is a tear to the collagen fibers of a tendon, caused by an acute injury or cumulative overuse syndrome. This leads to inflammation of the tendon.

- Active motion may be limited and may be painful, depending on the extent of the injury.
- Passive stretching may be painful when the tendon is fully stretched.
- Isometric testing is typically strong but elicits pain at the site of the injury.

Muscle Strain

A **muscle strain** is a tear to the muscle and its associated connective tissue as a result of an acute episode or a cumulative overuse syndrome.

- Active motion may be painful and limited, depending on the extent of the injury.
- Passive movement is usually not painful except by fully stretching a muscle and putting overpressure at the end of normal range.
- Isometric testing is typically strong but elicits pain at the site of injury. Mild strains are not painful to isometric testing, unless the muscle is challenged repeatedly to a state of fatigue.

Ligament Sprain

A **ligament sprain** is a tear to the ligament and its associated connective tissue due to an acute episode or a cumulative overuse syndrome.

- Active ROM is decreased and painful.
- Passive motion elicits pain at the site of the injury.
- Isometric testing is not painful.
- Moderate to severe ligament sprains create hypermobility in the associated joint.

Bursitis

A **bursitis** is an inflammation of the fluid-filled bursal sac, typically a result of repetitive overuse of the muscle that overlies the bursa. This friction irritates the bursa, stimulating excessive fluid buildup and pain caused by the pressure within the bursa.

- Active ROM is decreased and painful.
- Passive motion that compresses the bursa elicits pain and is limited.
- Isometric contraction of the muscle overlying the bursa may be painful, depending on how acute the bursitis is. In an acute bursitis, isometric contraction of the muscle is painful.

Disc Lesion (Herniation, Bulge, Protrusion)

A disc injury is a tear of the fibrocartilage between the vertebrae of the spine. The tear may be contained, called an **internal derangement,** or there may be a displacement of the nucleus, causing the outer rim of the disc to bulge or protrude, called a **herniation.** This bulge often presses against the nerve roots, leading to pain, numbing, or tingling in the extremities.

- Observation often shows an antalgic posture (i.e., sustained lateral flexion), caused by the pain, in either the trunk or the cervical spine.
- Active and passive ROM is limited and painful, especially in extension.
- With cervical discs, isometric testing may reveal weakness in the muscles of the arm, hand, or both; with lumbar discs, a weakness in the muscles of the leg and foot may result.

Muscle Dysfunction

As mentioned in Chapter 1 in the section "Muscle Dysfunction" muscles may malfunction for various reasons. These dysfunctions are not tears of the tissue, but rather sustained tension, or sustained weakness in the muscle. Muscle imbalances cause uneven distribution of forces through the joint, and though typically painless, they lead to vulnerability in the tissue from fatigue and degeneration in the associated joint. Muscles may be weak (inhibited), or hypertonic (facilitated) because of reflex activity from joint dysfunction or injury, muscle injury, poor posture, and emotional stress.

- Active and passive ROM of the associated joint is often normal.
- Isometric testing is the best way to identify muscle weakness. Sustained muscle contraction is best identified by palpation.

Soft-Tissue Positional Dysfunction

Lauren Berry, RPT, contributed the concept of positional dysfunction of the soft tissue. The fascicles or bundles of fibers of the muscles, tendons, ligaments, and nerves can roll out of their normal position relative to the other fascicles. As a result, the entire muscle, tendon, ligament, and nerve can become displaced relative to the joint and neighboring soft tissues. The author has theorized that this displacement creates an abnormal torsion or twist in the tissue and decreased function. Positional dysfunction is caused by poor posture, joint injury or dysfunction, and emotional or psychological stress.

- Active and passive ROM of the associated joint is typically not painful.
- Isometric testing does not reveal positional dysfunction, although positional dysfunction of the muscle can create muscle weakness.
- Palpation reveals an increased tension in the soft tissue, chronic positional dysfunction leads to adhesions, and the tissue will feel thick and fibrous.

Joint Dysfunction (Joint Fixation or Subluxation)

Joint dysfunction is the loss of passive glide (joint play) of the joint surfaces. It is often asymptomatic. If the joint is painful, the pain is usually of sudden onset and is often sharp and well localized. If massage does not reduce muscle tension, then the underlying cause may be reflex activity from the joint dysfunction.

- Active and passive movements in one direction are decreased.
- Passive mobilization of the joint identifies loss of normal play in the joint.
- Isometric testing typically is not used to detect joint fixation, but muscles that are innervated with the nerves that emerge from the level of spinal fixation are often weak.

Nerve Entrapment or Compression Syndromes

Nerves are susceptible to compression within the spinal canal due to stenosis (narrowing); as they exit the spine through the intervertebral foramen, from protrusions of the intervertebral disc or bony spurs; and as they travel through muscles (e.g., through the scalenes) and fibro-osseous tunnels, such as the carpal tunnel. Typical symptoms include numbing and tingling (paresthesias), unless the nerve root is affected, in which case pain is the predominant symptom. Compression of the motor nerve root causes muscle weakness in the associated myotome.

- Increased compression of an already compressed nerve elicits or increases the symptoms. For example, Phalen's test compresses the median nerve and increases the symptoms of carpal tunnel syndrome. (See Chapter 10, "The Elbow, Forearm, Wrist, and Hand".)
- Stretching an entrapped or compressed nerve increases the symptoms. For example, the straight–leg-raising test (SLR) increases pain, numbing, or tingling in the leg if the lumbosacral nerve roots are irritated. (See Chapter 3.)
- Manually stroking across an entrapped nerve temporarily increases a numbing and tingling sensation.

General Overview of Orthopedic Massage and Muscle Energy Technique

This chapter introduces the fundamental principles of the techniques described in this book. Two different treatment modalities are used in this method of massage. The first is OM, a new style of massage therapy developed by the author, and the second is MET. Each of the subsequent chapters describes how to apply these two modalities to each region of the body.

OM was developed on the basis of three principles: (1) to translate the extraordinary clinical results of the quick, soft-tissue manipulation techniques used by the author's mentor, Lauren Berry, RPT, into massage strokes; (2) to create a massage style that is relaxing and nurturing, while maintaining superb clinical results; and (3) to develop a massage technique that is also relaxing and energizing for the therapist. These goals were realized with the development of a new massage stroke called **wave mobilization.**

The wave mobilization stroke was developed during the course of 20 years of clinical practice and the author's 25-year practice of Tai Chi. Although most of this style is new, OM also incorporates two other approaches in massage therapy, the longitudinal and spreading strokes of connective tissue massage and the transverse friction massage concepts of James Cyriax, MD.

In addition to this new style of massage therapy, the treatment approach described in this book includes MET, which has been successfully used by osteopaths, chiropractors, and physical therapists for decades. This method of therapy can dramatically change the role of the massage therapist from a practitioner who gives a treatment *to* someone, to a practitioner who works *with* someone. The active participation of the client with the therapist can change neurologic patterns that relate to the soft tissue and joint function, and dramatically change chronic pain patterns.

Orthopedic Massage

GENERAL OVERVIEW

A key to maintaining a healthy career as a massage therapist is to pay attention not only to *what* you are doing, but also to *how* you are doing it. It requires a balance in the therapist's attention between what is felt *in the client's body,* and what the therapist feels *in his or her body.* What is required is a continuous focus on relaxation for the client and the therapist. The relaxation response of the client creates the neurologic and emotional environment for healing, and to be relaxed as the therapist creates an internal environment of healing. In other words, giving a massage can promote healing in both the client and the therapist.

First Goal for the Therapist: Effortless Work

Massage is work. Effortless work is akin to taking a walk; it is relaxing and energizing. As in walking, learn to use the legs to perform most of the work in the massage. Balance the work required from the legs with the effortless quality of moving from the center of your body. Performing effortless work is based on two principles:

- **Proper ergonomics.**
- **Using chi (internal energy) in massage.**

Ergonomics for the Massage Therapist

Rule No. 1: Keep Your Joints in the Open (Resting) Position

The resting position of a joint is the position in its ROM at which the joint is under the least amount of stress.[5] As mentioned in Chapter 1, the human body is a tensegrity structure; that is, the muscles, tendons, and connective tissue (the myofascial system) are the tension members of the body. These tension members keep the body upright and provide the force that moves the bones. Bones and joints, however, are the compression members.

- The myofascial system is designed to perform the work of giving a massage, not the bones and joints.
- Giving a massage with the myofascial system providing the work requires the joints to be in the resting position and not in the closed-packed (tight) position.
- In the closed-packed position the fingers, wrist, elbow, and knee are all extended. In this position, the forces are applied to the joint, the joints are under maximum compression, and the ligaments and joint capsule are maximally tight. The repetitive stresses giving a massage load the cartilage of the joint and accelerate the degeneration of the joint.
- To achieve the open-packed (loose) position of the joints, the following posture is assumed (Fig. 2-1):
    - **Spine**—The spine is upright, midway between flexion and extension. Avoid excessive lordosis (swayback) by tucking your pelvis, keeping a slight curve in the lumbar spine.
    - **Temporomandibular joint (TMJ)**—The teeth are slightly apart. The top of the tongue is lightly touching the upper palate.
    - **Elbow**—The elbow is in approximately 70° of flexion. Always keep some flexion in the elbows, as this allows the muscles to absorb the pressure of pushing into the client.
    - **Wrist**—The wrist is in neutral position, midway between flexion and extension, or extended as much as 20°.
    - **Metacarpophalangeal (MCP) joints** (the knuckles)—The open position is slight flexion.
    - **Interphalangeal (IP)**—The open position is slight flexion.
    - **Knee**—The knees are in slight flexion.

Rule No. 2: Keep Your Wrist and Hand in the "Position of Function" as Much as Possible

In the position of function of the wrist and hand, the intrinsic and the extrinsic musculature are in balance and under equal tension. It is the position in which finger and thumb flexion can occur with the least effort.[2]

- Wrist— In a neutral position, midway between flexion and extension, or extended as much as 20°, with slight ulnar flexion.
- Fingers—The knuckle joints (MCP joints), and the joints of the fingers are all in slight flexion.

An easy way to determine the position of function of the hands is to stand in a relaxed posture, with the arms hanging at the sides. The wrist and hands automatically assume the resting position (Fig. 2-2A). If the elbows are flexed approximately 70°, they are now re-

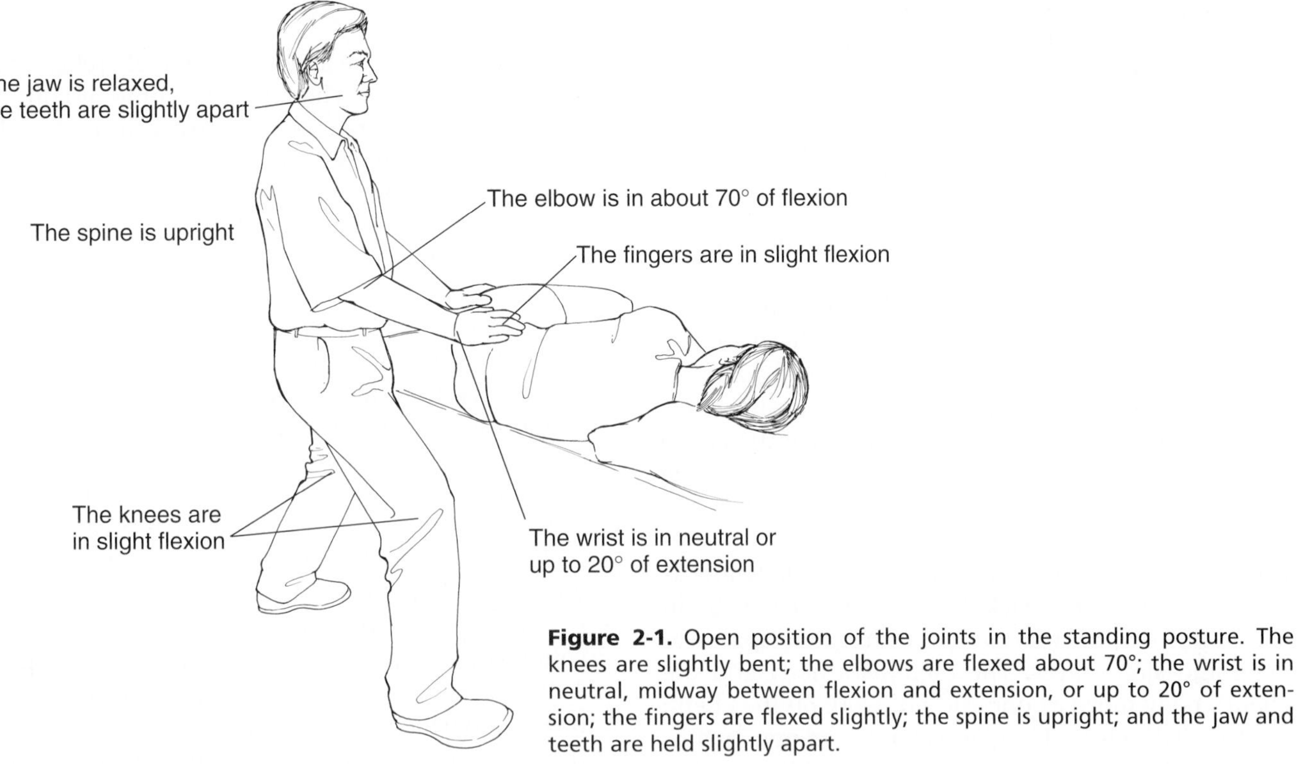
The jaw is relaxed,
the teeth are slightly apart
The spine is upright
The elbow is in about 70° of flexion
The fingers are in slight flexion
The knees are
in slight flexion
The wrist is in neutral or
up to 20° of extension

Figure 2-1. Open position of the joints in the standing posture. The knees are slightly bent; the elbows are flexed about 70°; the wrist is in neutral, midway between flexion and extension, or up to 20° of extension; the fingers are flexed slightly; the spine is upright; and the jaw and teeth are held slightly apart.

laxed and open, the best position for performing the massage (Fig. 2-2**B**).

Use of Chi (Internal Energy) in Your Massage

Chi is a Chinese word that means life force (literally, breath). It is a fundamental concept of Taoism, a religion that was founded in China by Lao Tzu, who is said to have been born in 604 B.C. Literally, Tao means "the way," and it means the way things are, the way to live one's life, and the essence or source of the universe.

The Taoists observed nature and especially water as embodying the essence of the Tao. Water is so yielding that it takes the shape of whatever container you put it in, yet it is so powerful it dissolves rocks and forms canyons.

Taoists believe that you can actually draw chi from the universe, and they developed exercises such as t'ai chi ch'uan, and chi gung to build a person's chi. The expression of this energy in daily life was to practice the path of "wu wei," which can be translated as "effortless effort." The goal is to combine two seemingly incompatible conditions, activity and relaxation. This effortless effort is supple, never forced or strained.

From tai chi we learn that "the motion should be rooted in the feet, released through the legs, controlled

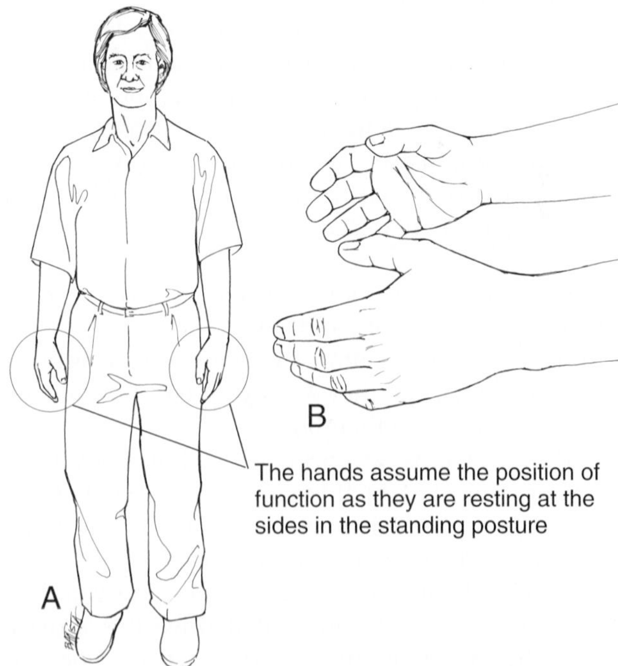
B
The hands assume the position of
function as they are resting at the
sides in the standing posture
A

Figure 2-2. A. An easy way to determine the position of function of the hands is to stand in a relaxed posture, with the hands hanging at the sides. **B.** The hands automatically assume a resting position, also called the position of function. If the hands are kept in this position and the elbows are flexed, the hands remain in the best position for performing a massage, open and relaxed. Try to keep your hands and wrists in this position as much as possible while performing the massage.

by the waist, and manifested through the fingers."[6] The therapist bends the knees and imagines the legs extending into the earth as roots, drawing water up through the center of the foot. It rises up the legs, into the belly and the heart, and then moves out from the heart, into the arms and hands as waves of healing energy (chi).

All parts of the body should move together, so that there is not only an economy of motion, but also a concentration of power and increased effectiveness. First move the body weight backward onto the back leg, gathering chi, like water ebbs back to the ocean. Release the chi by moving the whole body forward, similar to an ocean-wave flowing forward. Use the entire mass of the body to rock the client and perform the stroke. Rock the client forward as you perform the massage stroke, and let the client rock back as you release the stroke, or gently pull the client back slightly as you move your body back. Perform this rocking in an oscillating rhythm that varies from quick ripples to deep and slow waves. The therapist's body and the client's body move as one. Do not work *on* the client; work *with* the client. Imagine a cloud of energy streaming through your hands and through your client, rather than pressing on the client.

The therapist's muscles should remain relaxed, and the joints should remain open (i.e., in some flexion), as this allows the energy to flow. Tightening your muscles constricts your chi. Remain supple and relaxed, maintaining a slow and even breath from the belly.

To summarize, keep the following points in mind when using chi in massage:

- Relax your entire body—the hands, wrists, arms, shoulders, back, belly, and jaw.
- Minimize muscular effort. Effort is often felt as invasive by clients, and they resist your effort by tensing somewhere else in their body.
- Move your hands by moving your whole body. Even if your stroke is 1-inch long, rock your whole body into that stroke. This moves the mass of your body into the area where you are working.
- The pelvis should face the area you are working. The legs are the "engines" that drive the strokes, and the pelvis is the steering wheel. Point it straight into the strokes.
- Breathe from your belly. Make sure that your breathing is relaxed, and that the sensations in your body are comfortable.
- Keep your hands soft and relaxed. Imagine a stream of energy moving through your hands.

Therapist–Client Relationship

- The client should be able to completely relax when receiving this work. There may be some discomfort when tight or injured areas are worked on, but the massage should not be painful.
  - To achieve client relaxation, especially in the case of a first-time client, it is helpful to make statements such as, "I may touch some sore or painful areas as I work. If you cannot completely relax into my massage, please tell me and I will lighten up the pressure. I have found that the greatest therapeutic results come when you are comfortable and completely relaxed."
- Clients need to allow their body to rock when stroked. Instruct them to avoid bracing or tensing their body in any way or holding their breath.
- If clients tense, pull away, or hold their breath, then you are working too hard.
- If an area is tender, then lighten your pressure, soften your hands, and slow down.
- This work should relax the whole person, not just the muscle on which you are working.
- If an area still remains too painful for manual work, use reciprocal inhibition or CR-MET (see section "Muscle Energy Technique") to reduce the hypertonicity, or work in another area.
- To increase the effectiveness of the therapy, ask clients to participate in the session with their conscious attention. During manual techniques, ask the client to place their attention on the muscle you are trying to relax. Guide them mentally by saying, "feel this muscle relaxing." During MET, ask the client to become consciously aware of when a muscle is contracting and when it is relaxing. Bringing conscious attention to the therapy engages the client's higher brain functions and dramatically increases the effectiveness of the therapy because of changes effected in the central nervous system (CNS).
- Create a mental image of healing for the client. It can be dramatically helpful to say, "I think that you are going to feel a lot better" if you believe that it is a reasonable possibility. It is important not to create false hope, but it is equally important to help create a mental image of healing.

Client Position

- To minimize your reach, bring the client as close to the edge of the table as comfortable. In the side-

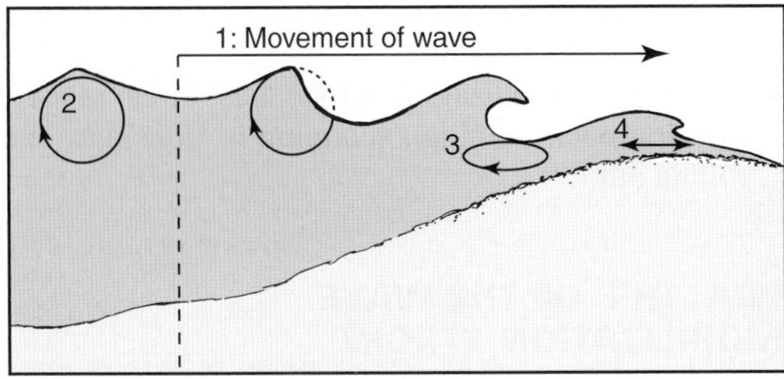

Figure 2-3. Ocean wave characteristics. ***1.*** The waves move perpendicular to the shoreline and perpendicular to the ground. ***2.*** A water molecule moves in a circular pattern by the passage of a wave. ***3.*** As the water becomes more shallow, the waves become flatter and more elliptical. ***4.*** Just above the sea floor the wave does not move in a circular pattern, but forward and backward.

lying position, the legs are tucked into a fetal position, and the arms are flexed in a similar "prayer position."

- It is essential that the client remain in a neutral position in the side-lying position. That is, the client's shoulder and hips should be aligned vertically over each other and not rotated forward or backwards. If the client is not in the neutral position, then he cannot be rocked easily.

Therapist Positions

- Four basic positions are described in this text. The four positions refer to the direction of the therapist's pelvic region. They are described relative to the massage table. The head of the massage table is where the client's head is positioned. The three standing positions are given for teaching purposes, as it is assumed that the therapist is facing his or her work, whatever the exact angle.
  - 45° headward.
  - 45° footward.
  - 90° to the table. In this position the therapist is facing the table.
  - Sitting.

Table Height

As OM is performed by keeping the knees slightly bent, the table height is lower than usual. The proper table height is determined by first having the therapist stand with her side next to the table. With the arms in a relaxed position hanging at the sides and the fingers hanging down, the top of the table should be at the tip of the fingers.

WAVE MOBILIZATION STROKE

The author has developed a new type of massage stroke called wave mobilization. The stroke was developed using the insights of the Taoists on the nature of water.

Nature of Water

- Water is so supple it will take the shape of whatever container it occupies.
- It is so powerful that it will dissolve rocks to form canyons.

Ocean Waves: Wave Mobilization Stroke Model

- Ocean waves move perpendicular to the shoreline (Fig. 2-3).
- The energy that moves through the ocean moves the water in a circular motion.
- As the ocean wave approaches more shallow water, the interaction with the bottom slows the wave making it more elliptical and flatter.[7]
- Waves just above the sea floor move back and forth instead of in a circular motion.
- Ocean waves ebb and flow in rhythmic cycles.
- Strong waves, such as storm waves, create a rounded digging motion that erodes the beach (Fig. 2-4).

Wave Mobilization Stroke Qualities

- The wave mobilization stroke has two aspects: (1) mobilization or rocking the client's body in an oscillating rhythm and (2) applying a massage stroke into the client's body as the body is being mobilized.

First Intention: Mobilize (Rock) the Body

- The strokes are applied in an oscillating rhythm like the ebb and flow of the ocean. The frequency varies from brisk back-and-forth strokes applied to thick and fibrous tissue to slow and gentle strokes applied to an acute injury. The typical frequency is between 50 and 70 cycles per minute. This frequency has been found to be the most relaxing. Studies have found that babies are rocked to sleep most effectively when this frequency of rocking is used.[8]

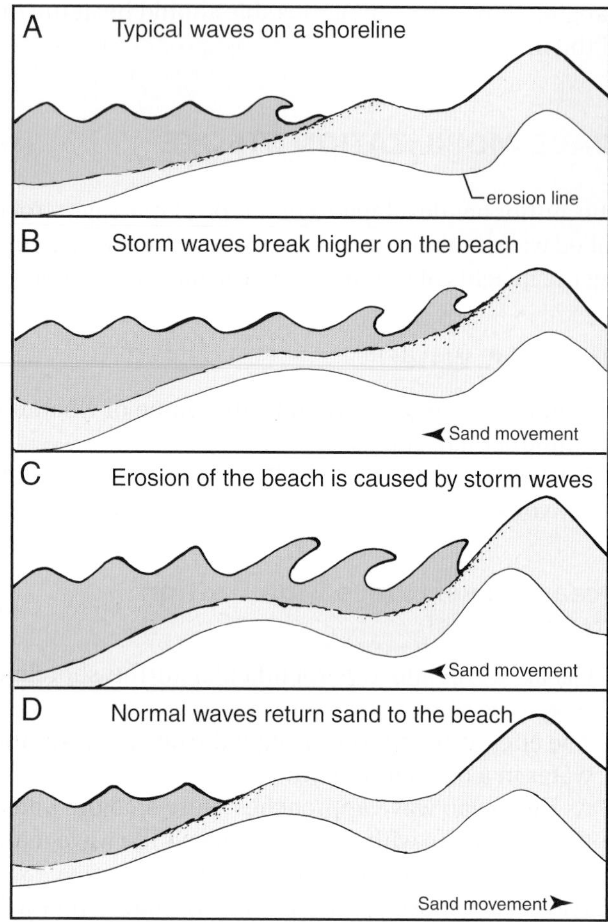
A Typical waves on a shoreline
erosion line
B Storm waves break higher on the beach
Sand movement
C Erosion of the beach is caused by storm waves
Sand movement
D Normal waves return sand to the beach
Sand movement

Figure 2-4. Strong waves, such as storm waves, create a digging motion that erodes the beach.

- Mobilize the whole segment where you are working. Rock the client's body with each stroke, rather than focusing only on what your fingers or thumbs are touching.

Second Intention: Apply a Wavelike Stroke into the Soft Tissue

- The stroke is transverse (perpendicular) to the line of the fiber of the soft tissue.
- Just as water molecules are displaced in a circular pattern by the ocean wave, we want to displace the tissue in a circular pattern. The stroke is a circular scooping motion, applying one half of a circular motion as you scoop down into the soft tissue.
- The stroke becomes flatter, more elliptical, if you encounter greater resistance in the tissue, or if the tissue is near the bone.
- For tissue that is next to the bone we apply back and forth flatter strokes or transverse friction strokes. This is akin to the back and forth movement of water against the sea floor.
- The wave mobilization stroke has three phases: drawing back (ebbing), scooping in (flowing), and rolling out.

PRACTICE OF THE WAVE MOBILIZATION STROKE

The following description takes the therapist step-by-step through the wave mobilization stroke. The description is followed by an exercise in working with a fellow therapist to practice the stroke.

Beginning Posture to Perform the Wave Mobilization Stroke

- Take a "bow stance" by placing your heels together, with the feet 45° from the midline (Fig. 2-5A).
- Bend your knees slightly. Place all of your weight on your right foot and move your left foot shoulder

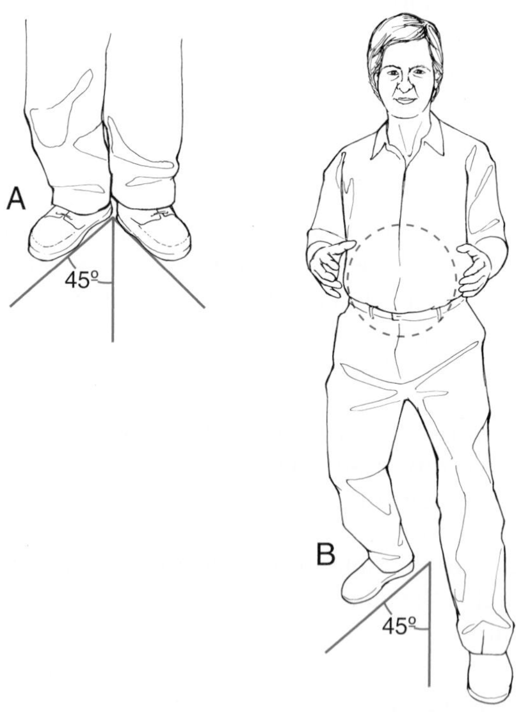
A
45º
B
45º

Figure 2-5. A. Basic standing posture to perform the wave mobilization stroke involves being in a "bow" stance. To begin, place the heels together with the feet spread apart 45° from the midline. **B.** The bow stance, with the hands holding a golden sphere of energy. The back leg continues to face 45° from the midline. The front foot faces in the same direction as the pelvis. The knees are over the toes.

width apart and then approximately 12 inches in front of you. Turn the left foot to face the same direction as your pelvis, and not 45° from the midline as is the right foot (Fig. 2-5**B**).

- Your hips continue to face forward. Move your weight forward, with about 70% of it on the left foot. Your left knee should be over the left toes.
- Hold a "golden sphere of energy" in front of your belly. The hands are relaxed, approximately 1 foot apart. The wrists are straight; the elbows flexed approximately 70°. The fingers and thumb are in slight flexion, the position of function.
- Your whole body—hands, arms, shoulders, back, belly, jaw, face—is relaxed, but not limp. Rather, you are alert and awake. Tuck your chin slightly to lengthen the neck and to keep your head upright.

First Movement: Drawing Back or Gathering Chi

- Inhale and move 70% of your weight onto your back leg, gathering your chi (Fig. 2-6). Keep your trunk on one level as you move back. Your trunk does not rise up nor sink down, and it does not tip from side to side. The only exception to this is if you are working on a large client or a client whose muscles are particularly thick. Let your body sink down approximately 1 inch by bending the knees a little more as you move your weight onto your back leg.
- As you move your weight back, your hands rise up slightly in a rounded motion, as if you are moving over a ball.

Second Movement: Move Forward or Scoop in or Sinking Chi

- As you begin to exhale, begin to move your whole body forward and allow the hands to sink in another rounded motion (Fig. 2-7). The hands remain in the position of function.
- As your body moves forward, imagine your hands sinking into the tissue, as a wave of energy moves through water.

Third Movement: Roll Through or Dispersing Chi

- During the finishing portion of the stroke lighten the pressure, allowing your hands to rise up. Imagine rolling your hands through the tissue, as if your thumbs are rolling over the lip of a bowl (Fig. 2-8). This movement is akin to the curling action of the ocean wave as it breaks.
- At the end of the stroke, your left knee should be over your left toe. The end of the body movement should be coordinated with the end of the stroke. Therapists commonly make the mistake of stopping their body movement while continuing the stroke

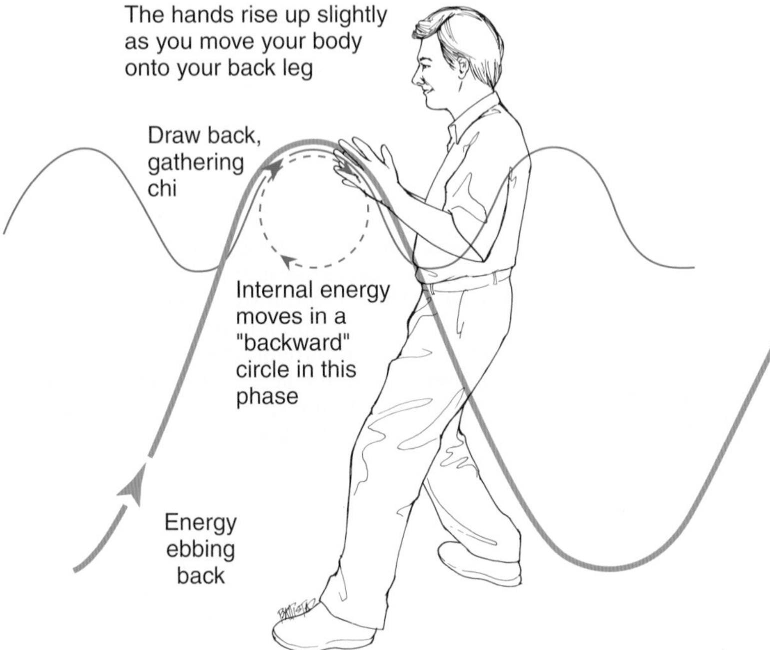
The hands rise up slightly as you move your body onto your back leg
Draw back, gathering chi
Internal energy moves in a "backward" circle in this phase
Energy ebbing back

Figure 2-6. The first movement of the wave mobilization stroke is called "drawing back, gathering chi." The first part of all the massage strokes performed in the standing posture is to move approximately 70% of the body weight onto the back leg. This movement is essential because it allows the therapist to move the whole body into the massage stroke. If you are working on a particularly tense client or on a large body, allow the body to sink down approximately 1 inch by bending the knees a little more as you move your weight onto your back leg.

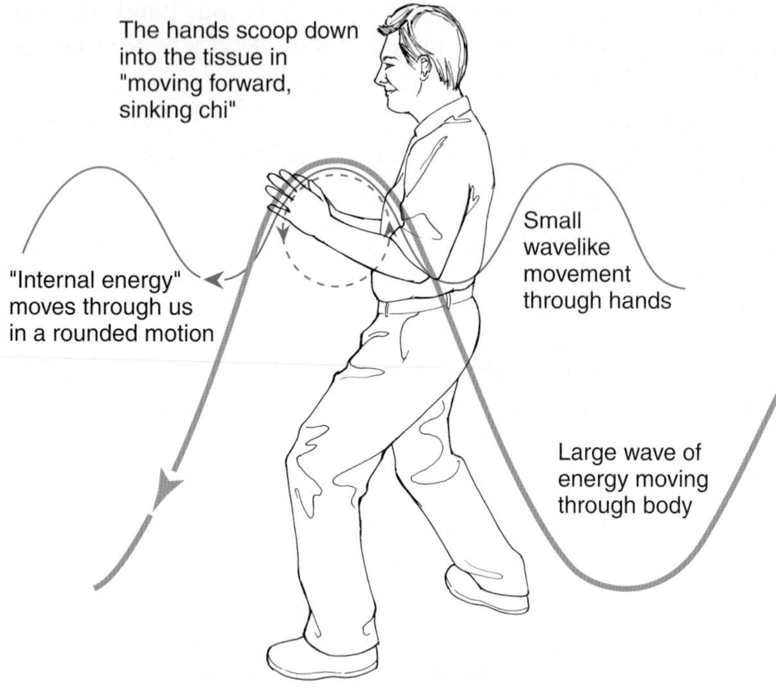
The hands scoop down into the tissue in "moving forward, sinking chi"
"Internal energy" moves through us in a rounded motion
Small wavelike movement through hands
Large wave of energy moving through body

Figure 2-7. The second movement, which is called "moving forward, sinking chi." The whole body moves as one piece. The legs, pelvis, and arms all move together. The hands remain in a position of function. As the body moves forward, the hands press into the tissue. The greater the resistance in the tissue, the more elliptical (flatter) the stroke. As mentioned in Figure 2-6, when working on tight areas, you have allowed your body to sink down approximately 1 inch in the first movement. If you are in this lower position, the second movement involves elevating the body approximately 1 inch as you move forward. When working on most clients, the therapist's body remains on a level plane as it moves forward and backward.

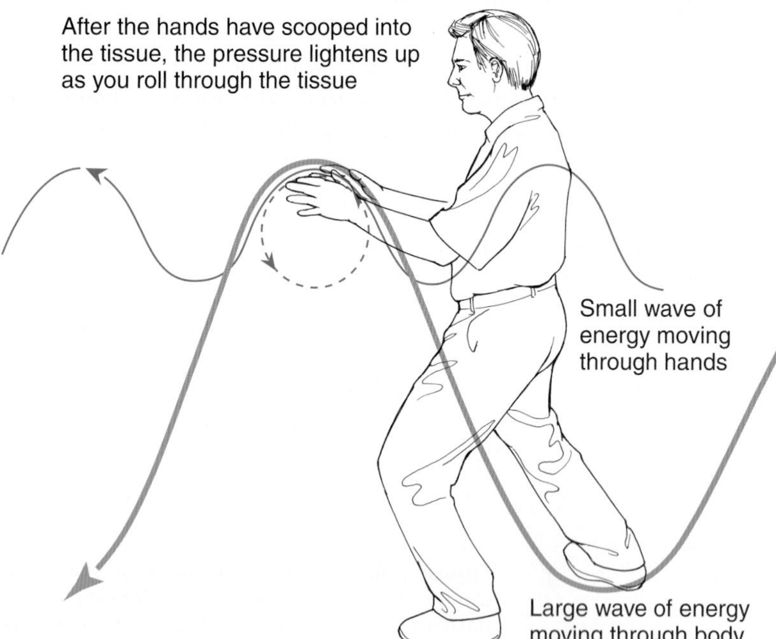
After the hands have scooped into the tissue, the pressure lightens up as you roll through the tissue
Small wave of energy moving through hands
Large wave of energy moving through body

Figure 2-8. The third movement, which is called "roll through, dispersing chi." After the hands have pressed into the tissue during the second movement, the finishing portion of the stroke involves rolling through the tissue. The pressure lightens, and you feather out the tissue, as if you are rolling over the lip of a bowl. This is akin to the breaking of the wave.

with their hands. This, however, creates excessive work for the muscles of the hands and arms.

PRACTICING WITH A FELLOW THERAPIST

- *Intention*: The following description of how to perform the basic wave mobilization stroke can be applied to any area of the body. For demonstration purposes, this practice stroke is applied to the muscles of the thenar pad at the base of the thumb. It is described in the context of a classroom situation with a fellow therapist, who will assume the role of the client for practice purposes.
- *Client Position*: The client sits on the massage table with a pillow on the lap and the right hand resting on the pillow with the palm up. The therapist assumes the bow stance (see "Beginning Posture to Perform the Wave Mobilization Stroke") with the pelvis facing perpendicular to the thenar pad. The therapist then places both thumbs on the thenar pad and holds the dorsal surface of the shaft of the thumb.

First Movement: Drawing Back or Gathering Chi

- Inhale and move 70% of your weight onto your back leg, gathering your chi (Fig.2-9A). Keep your trunk on one level as you move back.

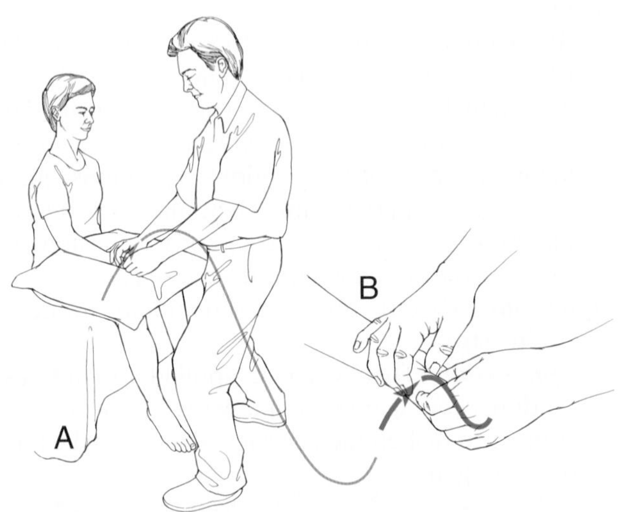

Figure 2-9. A. Standing position to practice the wave mobilization stroke on the thenar eminence. During the first movement, move your weight back onto your back leg. **B.** During the first movement, draw the skin back and rotate the shaft of the thumb slightly toward the palm.

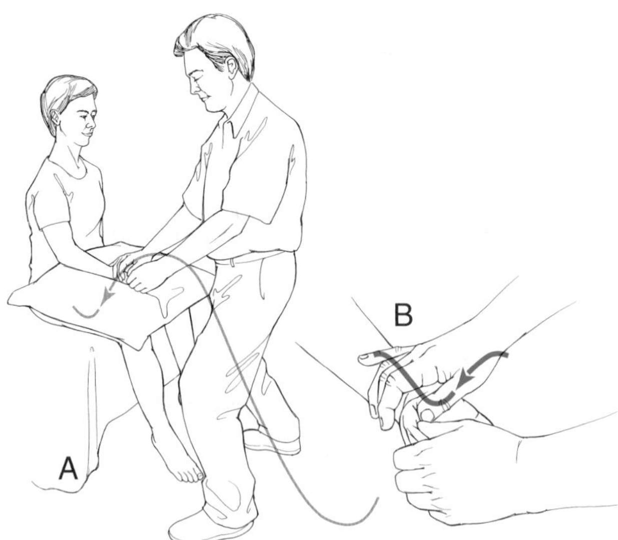

Figure 2-10. A. During the second movement, the whole body moves forward. As the body moves forward, the mass of the body moves the therapist's thumbs into the soft tissue of the client's thenar pad. The pelvis faces the direction of your stroke. Keep the entire body relaxed. **B.** Both thumbs sink into the soft tissue of the thenar eminence, in a rounded scooping motion, perpendicular to the shaft of the thumb. Work only within the client's comfortable limit. The fingers stabilize the shaft of the client's thumb in the sinking portion of the stroke, rather than mobilize it.

- As you move your weight back, draw the skin back approximately 1 inch and rotate the shaft of the thumb slightly toward you (Fig. 2-9B).

Second Movement: Move Forward or Scoop in or Sinking Chi

- As you begin to exhale, begin to move your whole body forward (Fig. 2-10A). Let the body movement move the thumbs into the muscles of the thenar pad in a rounded scooping motion (Fig.2-10B). Gently squeeze your fingers to stabilize the back of the client's thumb, which allows the therapist's thumbs to sink into the muscles.

Third Movement: Roll Through or Dispersing Chi

- The finishing portion of the stroke involves moving the body, thumbs, wrists, and arms together. As the body continues to move forward, the thumbs perform a rounded scooping motion approximately 1 inch long, rolling a wave of pressure through the tissue as if rolling over the lip of a bowl (Fig. 2-11A). The stroke does not slide over the skin. At the same

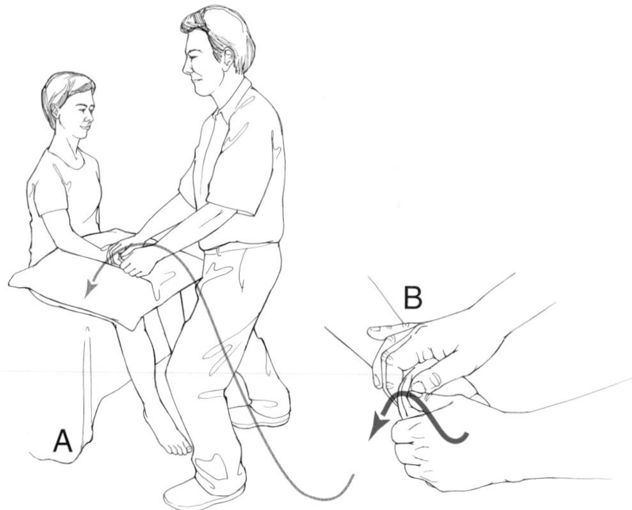

Figure 2-11. A. During the finishing portion of the stroke, the therapist's body continues to move forward. If the body stops moving, the hands should stop also. **B.** The finishing portion of the stroke involves decreasing the pressure of the stroke and feathering out the client's soft tissue, as if rolling over the lip of a bowl. You may feel the soft-tissue fibers rolling under your thumbs.

time you are performing the stroke, gently mobilize the client's thumb by rotating it away from the palm (laterally) (Fig. 2-11B). The body continues to move forward until the stroke is finished.

- Release the pressure on the skin, place your thumbs on a slightly different spot, and move the body as you pull the skin back approximately 1 inch to perform the stroke again. Practice for several minutes, and then perform the same strokes on the other hand.

Perform the Strokes in an Oscillating Rhythm

- An essential feature of the wave mobilization strokes is the rhythm. Just as the continuous rhythm of the ocean waves is soothing, these strokes are profoundly relaxing if they are performed rhythmically. Although the treatment of a chronic ligament condition requires rapid strokes compared with the slow strokes of an acute muscle condition, try to make the transition from brisk strokes to slower strokes as smooth as possible. As mentioned, the most relaxing treatment is achieved if the strokes are performed at a frequency of approximately 50 to 70 strokes per minute. See the section "First Intention: Mobilize (Rock) the Body."

MASSAGE STROKES OVERVIEW

Four Types of Transverse Strokes

Nearly all the strokes in OM are applied transverse to the line of the fiber. Some exceptions are described below in the section "Two Basic Longitudinal Strokes."

- *Type one*: The fundamental wave mobilization stroke is a short, rounded, scooping stroke, approximately 1 inch in length. As mentioned, the stroke becomes flatter and more elliptical as resistance is encountered in the tissue (see "Ocean Waves: Wave Mobilization Stroke Model"). This stroke does not slide over the surface of the skin, but moves through the skin.
  - *Application*: This stroke is typically applied to the muscle bellies and the associated fascia throughout the entire body. It may be applied to all the soft tissue, including the tendons, ligaments, and nerves.
- *Type two*: Short, back-and-forth strokes. These strokes may be applied slowly or with medium speed. They are slower than a type three stroke.
  - *Application*: These strokes are applied to myotendinous junctions, tenoperiosteal junctions, areas of thickening within the muscle belly, tendons and tendon sheaths, and ligaments. It is a deeper stroke than a type one stroke but not as deep as the type three stroke.
- *Type three*: Short, brisk, transverse friction strokes. These strokes are flat and not rounded or elliptical. The speed of the stroke is also an essential feature.
  - *Application*: Type three strokes are popularly known as transverse friction massage (TFM), pioneered by James Cyriax, MD. They are designed to dissolve fibrosis and are typically applied to attachment sites of the tendons, ligaments, joint capsule, and periosteum. They may also be applied more superficially to dissolve adhesions in the skin, dermis, and superficial fascia.
- *Type four*: A short, brisk, unidirectional, rounded scooping stroke.
  - *Application:* This stroke is applied to muscles, tendons, and ligaments to unwind abnormal torsion, or to realign the fascicles in the muscle, tendon, or ligament.

Two Basic Longitudinal Strokes

These strokes are classic, connective tissue strokes in the tradition of Ida Rolf. They are designed to lengthen fascia that has shortened and thickened. Although postisometric relaxation technique (PIR) (see "Muscle Energy Technique," below) is effective in lengthening the muscle and its deep fascia, it often is necessary to apply longitudinal strokes to stretch the fascia that forms the superficial sleeve around a structure or that forms the deep fascial compartments. For example, the crural fascia of the anterior compartment of the leg is a thick structure and often requires deep longitudinal strokes to lengthen the fascia. These strokes are applied only as needed, as they can be uncomfortable.

- A long, continuous, stroke that slides over the skin.
  - ***Application***: These strokes are applied at various depths. Superficially, they are designed to lengthen the superficial fascia and to dissolve adhesions between the fascia and the surrounding structures. These strokes may be applied to the deep fascia to lengthen the coverings of the muscles (epimysium), separate muscles that have adhered to each other, or dissolve adhesions between the muscle and the muscle's fascial compartment.
- A slow, deep stroke that does not slide over the skin.
  - ***Application***: These strokes are applied to localized adhesions ("knots") within the muscle that do not respond to either the transverse strokes or the MET. As these strokes are typically uncomfortable, they are applied only after the other techniques have been tried.

Stroke Direction

- The direction of the strokes is described in two ways: (1) in one specific direction, for example, from medial to lateral and (2) back and forth in a particular plane.
  - For clarification, when the instructions are given to perform types two and three transverse strokes that move back and forth in a specific plane of the body, it is easier to describe the stroke direction in common terms, such as the medial to lateral plane, rather than to use the exact anatomic plane or axis. The correspondence of the common terms to the anatomic terms are as follows:
  - Transverse strokes in the anterior to posterior plane are also referred to anatomically as the horizontal or transverse plane. Strokes back and forth in the medial to lateral plane are anatomically referred to as the coronal plane, and back and forth strokes in the superior to inferior plane, are anatomically referred to as the sagittal plane.

Guidelines for Stroke Application

- The client must be able to relax completely into the strokes to have the greatest clinical benefit. The intention is to engage the parasympathetic nervous system, which regulates healing and regeneration within the body. To engage this part of the nervous system, the client needs to be able to relax completely.
- The strokes are performed rhythmically, without sudden changes in speed.
- The more acute the condition, the lighter the strokes and the more gentle the rocking. In chronic conditions, deeper strokes and greater rocking may be applied.
- The more watery the tissue, the lighter the stroke. The more fibrous the tissue, the deeper the stroke.
- The closer we are to the attachment point, the shorter the stroke. The more the stroke is in the muscle belly, the larger the amplitude and the broader the stroke.
- Mobilize the entire segment where you are working, not just the tissue under your hands. If you are working on the biceps, mobilize the arm with each stroke in a rhythmic, rocking motion (oscillation). This stimulates the mechanoreceptors and makes the strokes much more comfortable.
- Oscillate the body back and forth rhythmically. This mimics the interuterine rhythm of the mother's heartbeat we felt as babies in the womb. It is profoundly relaxing. In the extremities this oscillation also winds and unwinds the joint capsule, compressing and decompressing the joints and stimulating the secretion of synovial fluid, which is the joint's normal lubricant. If the joint is swollen, this oscillation pumps out the excess fluid.
- Keep your hands as relaxed as possible, even though you may be working deeply.
- Perform gentle, passive mobilization to the joints to hydrate the joints, induce normal realignment of healing fibers, and heal mechanoreceptor function.

Muscle Energy Technique

- ***Definition***: MET is a procedure that involves a voluntary contraction of a patient's muscle in a precisely controlled direction, at varying levels of intensity, against a distinctly executed counterforce applied by the therapist.[9]
- ***History***: The origins of MET began during the 1940s by Kabat,[9a] who developed techniques of active patient participation to strengthen muscles that were neurologically impaired. He called these types of

muscular reeducation techniques proprioceptive neuromuscular facilitation (PNF). During the 1950s, Fred Mitchell, Sr, DO, and other osteopaths applied these techniques to mobilize joints and called it "muscle energy technique." MET has been refined by many practitioners, including Philip Greenman,[9] Karel Lewit,[10] Vladimir Janda,[11] and Leon Chaitow.[12] It is important to realize that although MET has been used by osteopaths to move a vertebra through a specific restriction barrier,[13] these techniques can be also applied to the soft tissue.

- ***Application for massage therapists***: It is not the goal of the massage therapist to move a vertebra in a specific direction. For the massage therapist, MET is used to treat the soft tissue and nervous system. Because MET uses voluntary effort, we are using the highest part of the CNS to reprogram involuntary patterns in the muscles. A secondary effect is that active muscle contraction helps mobilize the joints. MET has many clinical uses, which are described below.

CLINICAL USES

- To decrease sustained contraction in hypertonic muscles and to lengthen shortened fascia within the muscles.
- To increase the extensibility and to reduce the sensitivity of the periarticular tissue (the soft tissue surrounding the joint).[14] As the ligaments, joint capsule, and periosteum interweave with the fascial expansion of the muscles at the tenoperiosteal attachments, muscle contraction places a stretch on the connective tissues around the joint.
- To strengthen a weakened muscle or group of muscles. Isometric contraction provides increased tonus and performance due to increased muscle fiber participation.
- To reestablish normal movement patterns. If a muscle is weak, then other muscles substitute for its action. MET can reeducate the muscle to perform its normal action.
- To reduce localized edema as the muscles are the pumps of the lymphatic and venous systems.
- To mobilize restricted joints and increase their ROM. These techniques are helpful prior to chiropractic or osteopathic adjustments.
- To provide pain management through reciprocal inhibition and mechanoreceptor stimulation.
- To facilitate sensory-motor integration, which brings the client's awareness to areas of habitual contraction and corrects what Thomas Hanna[14a] calls "sensory motor amnesia."
- To reduce trigger points in a fast and painless way.[11,14,15]
- One form of MET, CR, involves isometric contraction. Voluntary isometric contraction is used not only to reduce muscle hypertonicity but for assessment purposes.[18] We note whether the muscle is weak, painful, or strong and painless (see "Isometric Testing").

USING MUSCLE ENERGY TECHNIQUE (MET) TO INDUCE NEUROLOGIC AND MECHANICAL RELAXATION IN A MUSCLE

Neurologic Basis of MET

Although the practice of MET has a large following among osteopaths, chiropractors, and physical therapists, there is still debate in the literature about how MET works. Some authors focus on the Golgi tendon organs (GTOs),[12] whereas others focus on the muscle spindle.[13] The essential neurologic role of muscle spindles can be summarized as follows:

- MET employs the conscious, voluntary contraction of isolated muscles. Isolated voluntary contraction of a muscle is different from the muscle contraction used in most daily activities. Because higher brain centers are used to isolate muscle contraction, unique neurologic effects are achieved compared with those accomplished in functional activities.
- Remember that there are two types of muscle fibers, extrafusal and intrafusal. The extrafusal fibers provide the force of muscle contraction and are innervated by alpha motor nerves. The intrafusal fibers, also called muscle spindles, are innervated by gamma nerves, and act as sensory receptors to help regulate the length and tone of a muscle.
- During sustained muscle contraction in which muscles are unconsciously or involuntarily tightened, gamma motor neuron activity is thought to be abnormally set to a higher gain or firing rate. This keeps the muscle's tone too high (hypertonic) and its resting length abnormally short.
- Voluntary isometric contraction shortens the muscle belly, slackening the intrafusal fibers and unloading the muscle spindle, turning it off temporarily (Fig. 2-12).[16] As isolated voluntary isometric contraction requires only alpha motor nerve

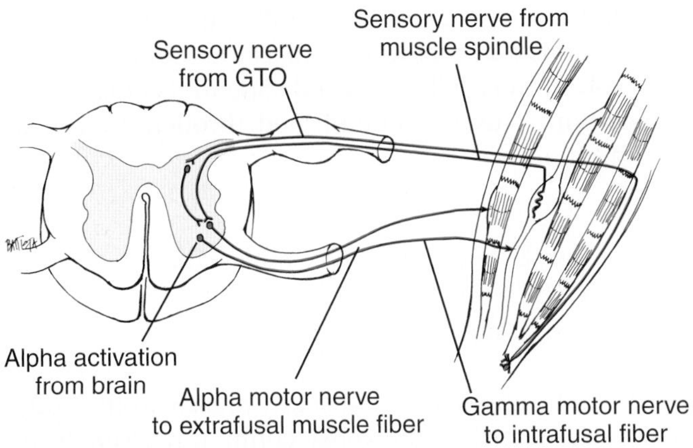

Figure 2-12. Voluntary isometric contraction stimulates the alpha motor neurons, causing contraction of the extrafusal muscle fibers. This causes a relaxation of the intrafusal fibers, temporarily silencing the muscle spindles. This pause in spindle activity causes a relaxation of muscle tone.

activity, the gamma motor nerve is not firing to the muscle spindle.

- As the muscle relaxes after voluntary isometric contraction, the alpha motor nerve turns off and the muscle belly lengthens. During this relaxation phase, the gamma motor nerves begin to fire to reset the muscle's resting tone. Theoretically, because the gamma motor nerves have just been turned off, the new rate at which they are firing has been reduced, decreasing the resting tone of the muscle.
- Sherrington's law of reciprocal inhibition states that when a muscle (agonist) contracts, it has an inhibiting effect on the opposing muscle, the antagonist.

Mechanical Basis of Muscle Relaxation Using MET

- Muscles that are in an adaptive, shortened position or held in a sustained contraction have an increased stiffness. Relaxation after isometric contraction increases muscle temperature and reduces this stiffness because of the thixotropic property of muscle.[17]

USING MUSCLE ENERGY TECHNIQUE TO LENGTHEN MUSCLES AND REDUCE TRIGGER POINTS

- Muscle contraction increases muscle temperature because the stored energy from the contraction is released as heat as the muscle relaxes. The increase in temperature increases the elasticity and extensibility of the connective tissue (fascia of the muscle-tendon unit) and decreases the viscosity of the ground substance.
- When a muscle contracts isometrically, the muscle fibers shorten, and the connective tissue lengthens to keep the muscle at the same length. This lengthening dissolves abnormal crosslinks in the collagen, allowing more normal gliding of the fibers and permitting the muscle to be stretched to a new length.
- The muscle spindles are allowed to be set to a new length–tension relation after an isometric contraction, as described above.
- The pain and dysfunction associated with trigger points is relieved when the muscle is restored to its full length.[14]

THERAPEUTIC PRINCIPLES OF MUSCLE ENERGY TECHNIQUE

There are many styles of MET. The style listed below has proved most effective clinically.

- The most important principle is that MET should never be painful. If it is even mildly painful, stop. The therapist should then attempt to use less pressure until a resistance that is comfortable to the client is found.
  - If it is still painful, use RI (see "Reciprocal Inhibition"). If a contraction still elicits pain, work with any muscle related to the associated joint that is not painful. For example, if resisted internal and external rotation of the shoulder are painful, try resisted adduction, flexion, or extension.
- Perform MET on the hypertonic or shortened muscles first, as those tissues inhibit their antagonists. After you have released the hypertonic muscles, use MET to strengthen the weakened muscles.
- The muscle is typically positioned in its mid-range position, halfway between its fully stretched and its fully relaxed position. This position is the most accurate measure of its strength and is usually the most comfortable position. If a muscle cannot be placed at its mid-range position, it is placed at its pain or resistance barrier.
- The therapist instructs the client to resist the pressure that the therapist exerts. This is important, as the therapist wants to be in complete control of the effort that the client is exerting. Otherwise, some clients believe that their strongest effort is what is required, and they may strain or overwhelm the therapist. The therapist might say, "I am going to try to move you in a certain direction.

Your job is to resist me and not let me move you. Tell me if there is anything more than a slight discomfort. It should not be painful." Then the therapist applies pressure gradually.

- The therapist typically applies only modest pressure that requires only 10 to 20% of the client's strength to resist the therapist's force. In acute conditions, only a few grams of pressure is required to make a neurologic change. In chronic conditions, as much as 50% effort may be applied to create more heat and a greater stretch on the connective tissues.
- The client resists the therapist's effort for 5 to 10 seconds in acute conditions, and the therapist may have them hold longer for chronic conditions. Gently tap on the muscle that is being contracted to bring sensory awareness to an area of unconscious hypertonicity. The therapist might say, "Feel this muscle working," as it contracts, and then "Feel this muscle relaxing" as it relaxes.
- This contract (resist)-relaxation cycle typically is repeated 3 to 5 times, but it may be repeated as many as 20 times in chronic conditions.
- It is often helpful to add a contraction to the opposite muscle (antagonist) after the contraction of the agonist. This is especially helpful after PIR, as it not only adds a deeper level of relaxation, but "sets" the involved muscle in a relaxed state in its lengthened position. This is accomplished through reciprocal inhibition.

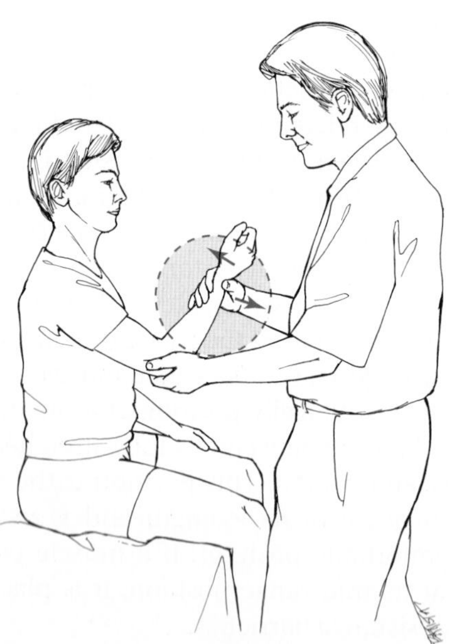

Figure 2-13. CR- and RI-MET can be demonstrated with the biceps and triceps muscles. During CR-MET, the therapist holds the distal forearm and instructs the client to "not let me move you" as the therapist attempts to pull the forearm slowly and gently toward him (extend the elbow). To perform RI-MET on the biceps, the therapist instructs the client to "not let me move you" as the therapist attempts to push the forearm away from him (flexing the elbow). In resisting, the client contracts the triceps, the antagonist of the biceps.

MUSCLE ENERGY PROCEDURES: USING BICEPS HYPERTONICITY AS AN EXAMPLE

MET can be applied to almost any muscle in the body. This text describes the most commonly used techniques in each region of the body. MET is specific, and the direction of the resistance must be precise to be effective.

Contract Relax (CR)

- *Intention*—The purpose in applying CR is to achieve relaxation in hypertonic muscles, to bring sensory awareness to a muscle, and to assess weakness or pain in the muscles.
- *Position*—The therapist places the client's elbow into a resting position, halfway between full flexion and full extension, or until a resistance barrier is felt (Fig. 2-13).
- *Action*—The therapist holds the forearm and stabilizes the elbow and gives the client the following instructions: "Don't let me move you" while attempting to pull the elbow into extension. Once the therapist has educated the client, he or she may simply say "resist" or "hold," but in the beginning it is often confusing for the client if the therapist only says "hold." If the therapist says "Don't let me move you" the client does not have to think about the exact direction or what muscle is working.
- Client resists the therapist's pressure for 5 to 10 seconds. Make sure the client is not holding his/her breath.
- Tell the client "Relax." Wait a few seconds until he or she is completely relaxed.
- Repeat the CR cycle 3 to 5 times or until you feel the muscle relax.

Reciprocal Inhibition (RI)

- *Intention*—RI is used in acute conditions. If contraction of a muscle is painful even with minimal effort from the client, RI on the muscle that has the opposite action, that is, the antagonist of the painful muscle, sends a neurologic message to the agonist to inhibit its contraction. RI is also useful to alternate with the CR-MET or at the end of a series of PIR procedures. This reinforces the relaxation after the CR and sends a message to the agonist to relax in its more lengthened state after a PIR technique. In the following example, we assume that the biceps is hypertonic and painful with any isometric contraction.

- *Position*—The therapist extends the client's elbow until the resistance barrier or just before pain is felt (see Fig. 2-13).
- *Action*—The therapist says to the client, "Don't let me move you" and then presses on the distal forearm and attempts to flex the elbow. This contracts the triceps, reciprocally inhibiting the biceps.
- The therapist instructs the client to relax, waits a few seconds, and then repeats the cycle 3 to 5 times.

Postisometric Relaxation (PIR)

- *Intention*—The purpose in applying PIR is to lengthen shortened muscles and the associated fascia and to relieve trigger points. The finger flexors are used as an example, as they are typically short and tight.
- *Position*—Client is supine with the elbow extended; the forearm supinated, with the wrist over the edge of the table. The therapist places his or her fingers on the palmar surface of the client's fingers and the stabilizing hand on the client's distal forearm.
- *Action*—The therapist slowly and gently presses the client's fingers into extension until just before the stretch elicits pain or until the therapist feels a resistance to stretch in the muscle and fascia (Fig. 2-14A). The therapist then instructs the client, "Don't let me move you," and has the client resist as he or she slowly presses on the fingers for approximately 5 to 10 seconds, attempting to press the fingers toward greater extension (Fig. 2-14**B**).
- The therapist tells the client, "Relax," and waits a few seconds until the client is completely relaxed.

- After the client relaxes, the therapist slowly and gently presses the fingers until just before the stretch elicits pain or until a resistance to stretch is felt in the muscle and fascia.
  - Starting from this new barrier, the therapist repeats the contract (resist), relax, lengthen, contract cycle 3 to 5 times.
  - If the therapist cannot increase the stretch, the client should be told to resist for 20 to 30 seconds at the comfortable resistance barrier for several cycles, and then the stretch should be attempted again. Sometimes an increase in the ROM can be achieved only one degree at a time.

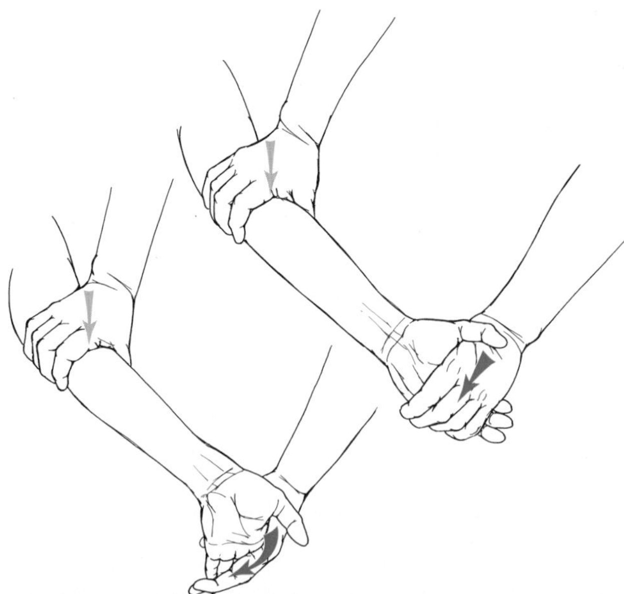

Figure 2-14. PIR-MET is easily demonstrated with the finger flexors. The client is supine with the elbow extended. The therapist places one hand on the fingers and slowly presses the fingers into their comfortable limit of extension. Next, the therapist instructs the client to "not let me move you" while slowly and gently pressing on the fingers. After approximately 5 seconds, the therapist relaxes for a few seconds, and then presses the fingers into further extension to their comfortable limit. This contract, relax, lengthen cycle is repeated several times.

Contract-Relax-Antagonist Contract

- *Intention*—The intent in using contract-relax-antagonist-contract (CRAC) cycle is to stretch adhesions, lengthen the connective tissue, and reduce hypertonicity in muscles. The CRAC technique adds an RI to the PIR technique by having the client actively contract the antagonist. This contraction has an inhibitory effect on the stretched muscle, and it is effective for stretching chronically shortened muscles. This technique is for chronic conditions only. The gastrocnemius serves as an example.
- *Position*—The client is supine. The therapist places one hand on the client's knee. The other hand holds the heel, and the forearm rests on the ball of the foot (Fig. 2-15).
- *Action*—The client actively pulls the foot into dorsiflexion, and the therapist keeps contact with the

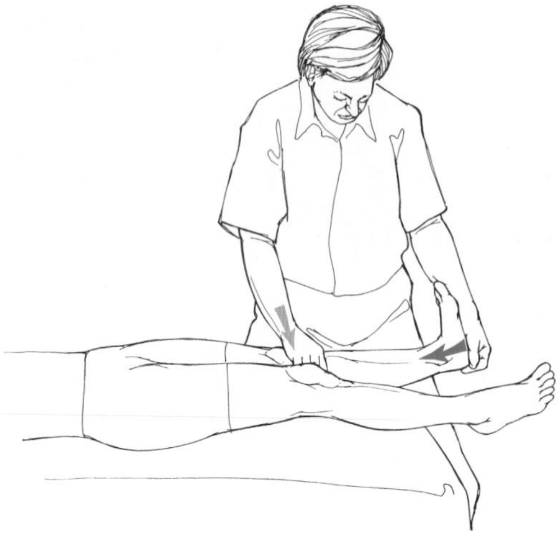

Figure 2-15. CRAC-MET can be demonstrated with the gastrocnemius muscle. The client is supine with the knee extended. The therapist places one hand on the heel and rests the forearm on the ball of the client's foot. Next, the therapist instructs the client "Do not let me move you" while slowly and gently pressing his or her forearm into the ball of the client's foot for approximately 5 seconds. The therapist relaxes for a few seconds, and then instructs the client to actively pull the foot toward the head, dorsiflexing the ankle and lengthening the gastrocnemius. The CRAC cycle is repeated several times.

forearm against the ball of the foot. The therapist instructs the client to relax in this position. The therapist then instructs the client, "Don't let me move you," and has the client resist as the therapist slowly leans his or her body weight toward the head of the table, pressing the forearm against the ball of the client's foot, attempting to pull the foot further into dorsiflexion. The therapist holds for 5 seconds, and instructs the client to relax. Next, the therapist tells the client to actively pull the foot into dorsiflexion (headward) until a new resistance barrier is encountered.

- The therapist repeats the CRAC sequence 3 to 5 times per session or as needed. The sequence is then repeated on the client's other side.

Eccentric Contraction

- *Intention*—The intent in using eccentric contraction (EC) is to dissolve adhesions and lengthen the connective tissue. This procedure must be done with care, as excessive force may irritate the soft tissue. It is contraindicated on deconditioned or frail clients or on clients who have had joint replacements. This technique is for chronic conditions only. The biceps is used as an example.
- *Position*—The therapist extends the elbow until just before the stretch elicits pain or until a resistance to the stretch in the muscle and fascia is felt (see Fig. 2-13).
- *Action*—The therapist says to the client, "Don't let me move you," while he or she attempts to pull the elbow into extension. The therapist may use a moderate force, having the client resist with approximately 50% of his or her maximum effort for 5 to 10 seconds. Next, instruct the client to "Keep resisting, but now let me move you very slowly." The therapist overcomes the client's resistance by pulling the elbow into further extension, while the client is attempting to pull the elbow into flexion.
- The therapist instructs the client to relax and repeats the procedure 3 to 5 times, beginning at the new resistance barrier, and moving the elbow to its greatest extension in the pain-free range.
- Eccentric MET should be incorporated into practice with only light resistance at first.

Concentric Muscle Energy Technique

- *Intention*—If muscles are weak, concentric muscle energy technique (C-MET), can help restore proper neurologic firing patterns and increase muscle tone. This technique must be done as a precise and controlled movement, with emphasis on isolating the muscle contraction to a precise

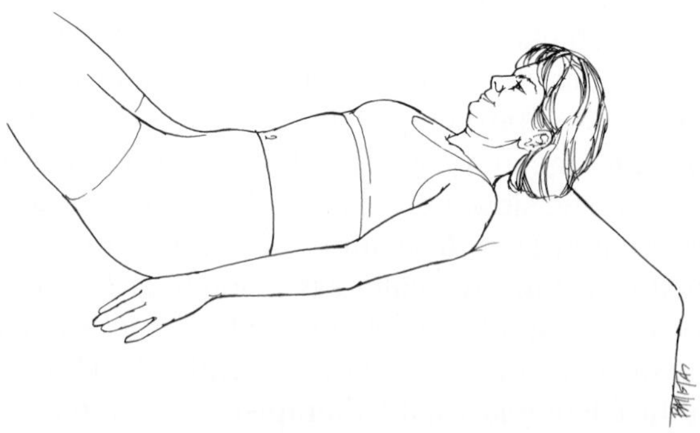

Figure 2-16. A demonstration of concentric MET may be performed on the deep cervical flexors and hyoid muscles. These muscles are often weak, and substitution for their action is performed by the sternocleidomastoid (SCM) and scalenes. With the client laying on her back on the table, with knees bent and feet on the table, instruct the client to lift his or her head slowly off the table a few inches by tucking his or her chin and rotating it toward his or her throat.

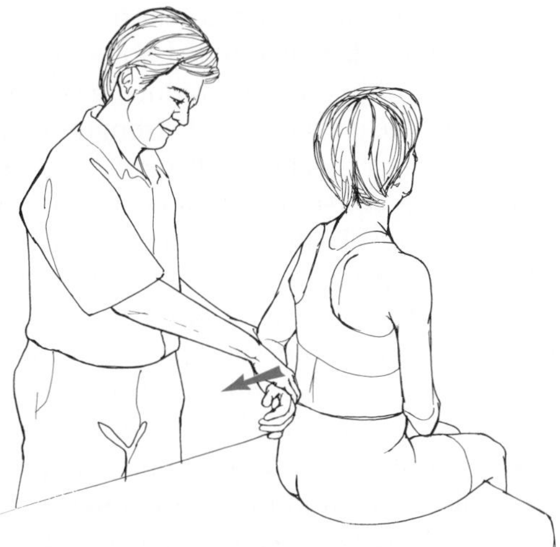

Figure 2-17. To increase the range of internal rotation of the shoulder joint, have the client sit on the table and place the back of one hand on his or her back. The therapist places his hand between the client's hand and the back. The therapist instructs the client to "not let me move you" while slowly and gently attempting to pull the arm away from the back for approximately 5 seconds. The therapist relaxes for a few seconds, and slowly and gently pulls the hand further away from the back until it is uncomfortable or a resistance barrier is felt. Again, the therapist instructs the client to "not let me move you" while slowly and gently attempting to pull the arm further away from the back, increasing the internal rotation of the glenohumeral joint.

action rather than on strength. We will assume that the deep neck flexors and hyoid muscles are weak but not painful. This technique should not be performed if the client is experiencing acute neck pain.

- *Position*—The client is supine. The client bends her knees and brings her feet flat on the table (Fig. 2-16).
- *Action*—The client is asked to slowly raise her head off the table a few inches to look towards his or her feet by first tucking her chin. The therapist watches to see whether the head is extending on the neck (i.e., if the chin is jutting away from the throat) or the head is being flexed with the neck and the chin moves closer to the throat. If the deep neck flexors are of normal strength, then the chin moves toward the throat and not up to the ceiling. If the deep cervical flexors are weak, the sternocleidomastoid (SCM) and scalenes substitute for the deep cervical flexors, extending the head and jutting the chin toward the ceiling.
- This action is repeated several more times. The client should perform this movement as an exercise until the muscles are strong and the client is using the muscles in a precise and controlled way.

Muscle Energy Technique to Increase the ROM in Joints

- *Intention*—The intent in using MET is to increase the ROM of a joint. As the ligaments, joint capsule, and periosteum interweave with the fascial expansion of the muscles at the tenoperiosteal attachments, muscle contraction places a stretch on the connective tissues around the joint. Isometric contraction can increase the extensibility of the soft tissue surrounding the joint.[14] Neurologically, it is not well understood why voluntary muscle contraction affects the joint capsule, but Freeman and Wyke[19] and others have documented that reflexes exist between muscles and ligaments. All of the styles described above may be used to increase the ROM of a joint, rather than to focus on affecting the muscle and its associated fascia. It can be confusing, however, for the therapist to attempt to determine which muscles are involved if there is a decrease in the ROM of a joint. Therefore, do not think of muscles; simply determine the direction of decreased motion, and have the client resist your attempts to move the joint into the restricted direction. This approach has proved valuable for capsular adhesions. Decreased internal rotation of the shoulder is used as an example.
- *Position*—Client is sitting and places one hand on the lower back (Fig. 2-17). If this is difficult, the hand is placed on the sacroiliac joint (SIJ) or greater trochanter area. The therapist holds one hand on the elbow and the other hand on the distal forearm.
- *Action*—The therapist says to the client, "Don't let me move you," as he or she attempts to pull the client's hand away from the lower back, that is, attempts to move the shoulder into greater medial rotation. Hold for 5 seconds. The client then relaxes for a few seconds during which the therapist pulls the client's hand slowly away from the lower back until just before the stretch elicits pain or until a resistance to stretch is felt in the fascia. This is usually only approximately 1 inch. If the stretch is painful, the therapist releases the pull until it is comfortable again. This action is repeated 3 to 5 times.

- Remember that when working with joints, even a slight change in the ROM can translate into a significant change of function.

SUMMARY OF THE CLINICAL EFFECTS OF ORTHOPEDIC MASSAGE AND MUSCLE ENERGY TECHNIQUE

- Increases the synthesis of new cells to promote repair and healing of injured or compromised tissue.
  - Crossing transverse to the fiber in the soft tissue creates a tensile (stretching) force on the collagen, which increases the activity of the fibroblasts and leads to the synthesis of collagen and ground substance.
  - All cells in the body are stimulated to increase their activity with mechanical stimulation. The longitudinal pulling force of active muscle contraction of MET increases muscle regeneration through synthesis of satellite cells.
  - The normal functioning of the cells depends on movement.
- Promotes fluid exchange of blood, lymph, synovial fluid, and interstitial fluids (ground substance) to increase the nutritional exchange and oxygenation of the tissue, as well as the elimination of waste products.
  - Healthy repair depends on the free movement of the fluids of the body, which carry the cells, fibers, and nutrition for repair. Stagnation in the tissue leads to poor repair and the accumulation of waste products.
  - Massage and mobilization facilitate circulation, which decreases swelling and tissue congestion.
  - Massage and mobilization help normalize the articular synovial fluid by one of two effects: stimulation of the synovial membrane through joint mobilization or stimulation of excess fluid release by mobilization of the joint in a flexion and extension pumping action.
  - Winding and unwinding of the joint capsule and joint mobilization rehydrate the articular cartilage.
  - Rhythmic oscillations (rocking movements) promote circulation and decrease joint swelling.
  - Compression and decompression of the OM strokes act like a pump to increase and decrease the pressure within the tissue, promoting the exchange of fluids.
  - Compression from the massage strokes creates heat, which creates a thixotropic effect on the ground substance, increasing its water uptake.
  - MET through muscle contraction can stimulate the circulation deep within the body (down to the bone) and within the joint, reducing swelling.
- OM and MET help realign and strengthen connective tissue fibers, especially collagen.
  - Crossing transverse to the fiber imparts tension (stretch) to the elastic component (collagen), like pulling on a spring or crossing the string of a musical instrument. When the stretch is released, the energy imparted into the stretched fiber is released as heat. Heat promotes lubrication and nutritional exchange at the microscopic level.
  - Crossing transverse to the fibers spreads the fibers, dissolving abnormal crosslinks and adhesions, resulting in a greater ability of the tissue to lengthen and an increase in the ROM of the joints.
  - CR-MET creates tensile forces (pulling or stretching) that increase collagen synthesis, resulting in greater tissue strength. It also provides a pulling force through muscle contraction that elongates the connective tissue and helps realign the collagen fibers into their normal parallel alignment.
  - PIR or CRAC-MET provides stretching to the connective tissue that dissolves abnormal crosslinks in the fascia within the muscle, allowing for greater length and elasticity in the tissue.
- Normalize the function of the muscles.
  - OM and MET reduce muscle hypertonicity.
  - MET increases the length of the fascia within the muscle and the myotendon.
  - Isotonic and CR-MET strengthens a weakened muscle or group of muscles.
  - PIR-MET can reduce or eliminate trigger points.
- Normalize positional dysfunction.
  - OM and MET realign tissue that has developed an abnormal torsion or twist.
  - OM and MET corrects interfascicular torsion by unwinding the abnormal torsion.
  - OM and MET help realign the collagen fibers into their normal parallel alignment.
- Establishes normal neurologic function in the soft tissue through manual techniques and MET.
  - OM and MET decrease adhesions that entrap nerve fibers and decrease neurologic flow.
  - MET helps normalize the arthrokinetic reflex, reducing reflex facilitation or inhibition.
- Facilitates sensory-motor integration by bringing the client's conscious awareness to areas of habitual contraction or weakness, correcting what Thomas Hanna calls "sensory motor amnesia."
- Mobilizes restricted joints and helps promote healthy cartilage.

- Mobilization and OM promote the exchange of synovial fluid into and out of the joint by winding and unwinding the joint capsule.
- Mechanical stimulation through massage, mobilization, and muscle contraction (MET) stimulates the synthesis of chondrocytes and cartilage repair.
- Massage, mobilization, and MET decrease adhesions, allowing for increased ROM in the joints.

- Provides pain management.
  - Mobilization increases mechanoreceptor stimulation, which reduces pain sensations because of the pain-gate and reoxygenation of the tissue.
  - Massage, mobilization, and MET decreases swelling in the tissues and joints by promoting fluid exchange.
  - Massage, mobilization, and MET increase circulation which increases the oxygenation in the tissues and the elimination of lactic acid and other waste products, which are pain producers.
- Creates a piezoelectric effect.
  - Stretching the fibers by longitudinal or transverse strokes creates a piezoelectric current that increases synthesis of new cells and the creation of electrical potentials that realign the fibers.
- Massage, mobilization and MET creates an electromagnetic field effect.[20]
  - The cells, fibers, and fluids in the body are a "liquid crystal" that emits a biomagnetic field. Collagen is a semiconductor that, when stimulated (piezoelectric effect) through movement, massage, or manipulation, generates an electric field. Electric currents emit a magnetic field.
  - Living systems respond to external energy fields, and biomagnetic fields are emitted from the hands of the therapist.
  - Energetic pulses precede action, so healing intention from the therapist is critical.

Treatment Considerations for Soft-Tissue Injuries

ACUTE PHASE (0–4 DAYS)

Treatment Considerations: Movement, Ice, Compression, and Elevation

Remember movement, ice, compression, and elevation or "MICE." Traditionally, the acronym for treatment of acute injuries has been "RICE," the letter "r" indicating "rest" as the first recommendation. Lederman[8] suggests that the acronym should be changed to MICE.

- Movement—Pain-free movement is now recommended for most soft-tissue injuries in the early stages of rehabilitation. Severe injuries require rest, but immobilization leads to adhesions, weakening of the connective tissues, osteoporosis, decreased nutrition in the area, and sluggish lymphatics. Pain-free movement of the injured area supplies healthy stimulation to the tissue to stimulate the synthesis of new cells needed for healing. Even micromovements (i.e., millimeters of movement) promote nutritional exchange and cellular regeneration, and help realign the healing fibers.
- Ice—Apply ice for 20 minutes, every 2 waking hours, until the heat and swelling decrease. A simple rule for when to use ice or heat is: if the area is painful even at rest, use ice. If it does not hurt at rest, use heat to promote circulation.
- Compression—There are many styles of compression, from ace bandages to air casts.
- Elevation—Elevating an area promotes venous return.

Treatment Considerations: Orthopedic Massage and Muscle Energy Technique

- The first *goals in treating an injury in the acute phase* are as follows: to reduce the swelling; to promote nutritional and cellular exchange; to induce a relaxation response; to reduce hypertonicity; and to increase pain-free motion. Treatment is designed to encourage the body to form a strong but mobile repair at the site of injury and to ensure painless restoration of normal function.
- Palpate the area to determine the amount of heat and swelling. A hot area indicates acute inflammation, and massage is contraindicated, as pressure may disturb the healing fibers. Massage may be performed on an area that is warm, as the inflammation is resolving. The more watery the tissue, the lighter your strokes.
- Keep your hands relaxed, your touch gentle, and your pace slow when working with an acute injury. There are two kinds of discomfort that a client can feel while being worked on. The first is a discomfort that "hurts good" because something is being touched that is uncomfortable but feels good to be touched. The client can completely relax into this kind of "good hurt." The second is a discomfort that does not feel good. The client pulls away, tenses, tightens, or holds his or her breath. This is nontherapeutic touch.

- When working with acute injuries, the rocking portion of the wave mobilization stroke needs to be slow and of small amplitude. It is akin to a small, gentle wave in a protected bay on a calm day.
- Passive movements (mobilization) in the pain-free range should begin as early as tolerated, to prevent adhesions.[21] Studies indicate that limited, immediate mobilization improves repair.[22] Any movement is beneficial that does not cause symptoms.
- Gentle massage transverse to the healing fibers keeps the developing scar mobile. Transverse massage to muscle fibers imitates the normal broadening that occurs during muscle contraction and restores mobility by dissolving microscopic adhesions. Gentle massage transverse to the line of the fiber on tendons, ligaments, capsules, and other soft tissues dissolves the adhesions in the connective tissues.[1]
- CR and RI-MET performed with light resistance help restore proper neurologic function, promote nutritional exchange by use of the muscular pump, and promote the normal parallel alignment of the healing fibers. PIR, CRAC, and eccentric MET are contraindicated, as stretching disturbs the newly formed tissue.
- As the body is more than 70% water, even slight pressure (e.g., grams) sends waves of movement through the body. Field effects from the electromagnetic radiation from the therapist's hands have healing properties.

SUBACUTE PHASE (REPAIR PHASE) (4 TO 21 DAYS)

Treatment Considerations: Advice for the Client

- As new tissue is fragile, clients must use caution when beginning an exercise program to avoid re-injury. Movements are expanded within pain-free range to prevent adhesions from developing and to help realign the healing fibers.
- Exercise programs should begin with active ROM, muscle strengthening exercises within tolerance, and submaximal isometric exercises.[23]

Treatment Considerations: Orthopedic Massage and Muscle Energy Technique

- The *goals in treating an injury in the subacute phase* are as follows: to help promote the repair and regeneration process; to help realign the developing fibrils; to release the torsion within the tissue; to reposition the soft tissue along normal lines of stress; to dissolve abnormal crosslinks and adhesions; to improve flexibility and strength; and to help restore normal neurologic function.
- The remodeling of the healing tissue is easier to effect in the early stages of repair. However, the collagen fibers that are repairing the injured area are fragile. It is important that the massage strokes should remain fairly light, otherwise you run the risk of breaking down these immature collagen fibers. The depth of the massage may be increased slightly during the subacute phase, but always within the client's comfort level.
- MET, including CR and RI, is performed to help restore proper neurologic function, promote nutritional exchange by using the muscular pump, and promote alignment of the healing fibers.

REMODELING PHASE (DAYS 21 TO 60)

There are *two possible outcomes* after soft tissue has been injured or has been chronically dysfunctioning. They require different treatments.

- ***One***: The area is *unstable* from soft-tissue damage, weak muscles and ligaments, inhibitory reflexes from the involved joint or the spine, deconditioning, or atrophy.
- ***Two***: The area is *stiff and contracted* from soft-tissue adhesions, joint damage, hypertonic muscles, shortened ligaments, or facilitatory reflexes from the involved joint or the spine that cause the muscles to be hypertonic.

Treatment Goals for an Unstable Area: Orthopedic Massage and Muscle Energy Technique

- As a massage therapist, you have *two treatment goals:* (1) to identify any areas that remain hypertonic, as hypertonic muscles have an inhibiting effect on their antagonists, due to the law of RI and (2) to perform CR and C-MET on weak muscles to help strengthen them and promote lymphatic circulation and nutritional exchange.
- The therapist's *goal in providing treatment* is to strengthen the supporting muscles and the related soft tissues. The client is encouraged to perform resistive isotonic exercises. Most of the treatment is accomplished by the client's own efforts, and they need to take an active role in their rehabilitation to restore normal function. Unless you are fluent in exercise therapy, refer these clients to a physical therapist, personal trainer, or chiropractor who special-

izes in rehabilitation to guide them in strengthening and stabilization exercises.

Treatment Goals for an Area That Is Stiff and Contracted: Orthopedic Massage and Muscle Energy Technique

- The therapist's *goals in providing treatment* are to dissolve the adhesions, lengthen the scar tissue, realign the soft tissue, rehydrate the joints, and restore normal neurologic function.
- As the soft tissue feels thick and fibrous, OM may be performed at an increased depth to release the tissue down to its attachments to the bone. PIR, CRAC, and eccentric MET may be used to lengthen the connective tissue, dissolve adhesions, increase the ROM in the joint, and help restore normal neurologic function. Joint mobilization is performed to rehydrate the joint, promote the exchange of fluids to increase the nutrition to the area, and promote the exchange of waste products.
- For help in maintaining benefits of the massage therapy, a daily exercise program is encouraged. This exercise program should include exercises to stretch tight areas and to strengthen weak areas, as well as exercises of balance and coordination to help restore neurologic function.

CHRONIC PAIN OR DYSFUNCTION REQUIRES A COMPREHENSIVE PROGRAM OF REHABILITATION

- It is important to remember that continuing problems to the nervous system from soft-tissue injury can manifest as problems in coordination, balance, movement, posture, weakness, hypertonicity, and stiffness. Your recommendations for treatment should include balance and coordination exercises, as well as posture training and strength and flexibility training.

CONTRAINDICATIONS TO MASSAGE THERAPY: RED FLAGS

Red flags consist of signs and symptoms that are rarely encountered in benign (nonpathologic) forms of pain. Your goal is to quickly identify those clients who might have a pathologic condition in which massage therapy might be contraindicated and to distinguish them from the vast majority of clients who would benefit from massage therapy.

History Questions for the Client to Rule Out Serious Pathology

- Do you have constant pain that is worse at night and not relieved by any position? (Tumors and infections, as well as significant inflammation, are often worse at night.)
- Do you have constant writhing or cramping pain? (Rule out tumor and infection)
- Do you have intense local pain that developed after a recent, significant trauma? (Rule out fracture)
- Do you have any fevers? (Rule out infection)
- Do you have a history of cancer or other serious medical problems?
- Do you have any unintended weight loss? (Often associated with cancer)
- Do you have bowel or bladder control problems? (May indicate pressure on spinal cord)
- Do you have significant, unexplained lower limb weakness? (May indicate pressure on spinal cord or significant nerve-root compression)

If a client answers yes to any of the above questions, it is important that a doctor evaluate him. If your client has severe pain, has a red flag, and has not been seen by a doctor prior to his office visit to you, refer that client out for evaluation prior to your session.

If the client is in moderate pain, that is, the pain is interfering with work or ADLs and has red flags, you may treat the client if he can comfortably lie on your table in the fetal position without pain.

If the client is in pain in the fetal position, refer him to a doctor before you provide treatment. If the client can lie on your table in the fetal position comfortably, use the MET and the massage strokes slowly and gently. Only work within pain-free limits. At the end of the session, inform the client that you recommend that a doctor evaluates him. You could say, "I need to have more information to treat you effectively." Or you might say, "There are many causes of pain, and I recommend that you see a doctor to make sure you don't have a more serious injury." If your client has mild pain and a red flag, you can safely provide treatment, but he or she needs to be referred to a doctor also.

Conditions in Which Deep Pressure Is Contraindicated

OM uses a wide range of pressures that the therapist may apply to the client and includes the practice of the "laying of hands" that uses the electromagnetic field from the therapist's hands as the therapeutic modality.

With this in mind, there are no contraindications to the laying of hands. It takes years of practice in the art of massage to know the proper amount of pressure to apply to a particular condition. However, deep pressure is contraindicated in certain conditions:

- Osteoporosis
- Disc herniation
- Pregnancy
- Inflammation

GUIDELINES FOR REFERRING CLIENTS

In addition to knowing the red flags that indicate when massage is contraindicated, it is important to know that certain conditions are best treated in conjunction with other practitioners. A good clinician knows when to refer to other health-care providers for further evaluation or treatment. Throughout this text, it is indicated when a referral is recommended. The three providers most often referred to include

- A medical doctor (MD) to diagnose a client who has a red flag and to rule out a pathologic condition.
- A doctor of chiropractic (DC) or doctor of osteopathy (DO) to evaluate and provide adjustment, or manipulation for the spine and the extremities.
- A registered physical therapist (RPT) or specialist in exercise rehabilitation (e.g., personal trainer, Pilates trainer, yoga instructor).

Listed below are symptoms that typically indicate the need for a referral. As the vast majority of pain and dysfunction in the body is a problem of function and not pathology, most of the referrals are to specialists in problems of functional disturbance (chiropractors and osteopaths), and not to specialists in disease and pathology (medical doctors).

- Clients with radiating pain and/or numbing or tingling in the arms or legs.
- Any chronic pain (not soreness) should be evaluated.
- Sharp localized pain, as distinguished from an ache, that does not improve in 3 days should be assessed.

OVERVIEW OF TREATMENT

General Treatment Guidelines

- OM sessions typically last 1 hour, although the length of the session can vary greatly. Chiropractic doctors have effectively used these techniques in 15-minute sessions prior to the adjustment. Massage therapists can be effective in 30-minute sessions.
- Treatments are typically given weekly for 4 to 6 weeks to treat most conditions. A client in acute distress may be treated more frequently. Clients in chronic pain may have weekly treatments for several months, and then graduate to two times per month for several months, then once a month, and so forth until the point of maximum medical improvement (MMI) has been reached. This is the point at which there are no further gains in the subjective or objective findings. Treatment frequency is then determined by how well the client can maintain his or her functional gains. In chronic conditions, OM and MET can help support functional gains.
- The client should be evaluated approximately every six treatments to determine the need for continuation of care. The goal in reevaluating is to identify subjective and objective improvement, gather objective examination findings for future treatments, and assess the need for a referral if there is little or no improvement.
- OM is also designed for health enhancement (wellness care), and improvement in sports, dance, and recreation. Many clients elect to be treated on an ongoing basis.

Treatment Protocol for the Acute Client

- It is important to determine the severity of your client's condition to determine your treatment protocol. Once you have ruled out red flags through your history questions and determined that your client is a candidate for massage therapy, perform the assessment.
- Begin your work on the noninvolved side in injuries or dysfunctions of the spine, as it is not only easier for the client, but a relaxation response is transferred from one side of the body to the other.
- As mentioned, tell your client that she or he should be able to completely relax into the massage and MET.
- In work on the spine, begin the session with gentle rocking movements of the whole body, as described in the first series of strokes in Chapter 3. This helps you make contact with your client in a noninvasive way and determine the level of guarding. If the client's body is resistant to the rocking, slow down, until you feel a relaxation response. You might say in a gentle voice, "Allow me to move your body. This rocking is like putting a baby to sleep. Just relax."

- Once the client is more relaxed, you may elect to perform CR- or RI-MET if the muscles are extremely tender and hypertonic. Typically, spend only a few minutes at a time with MET, and then perform more strokes. Alternate the MET with the strokes throughout the session.
- The greater the client's distress, the lighter the strokes. Rock the client slowly, and with a small amplitude. Small, gentle movements can be soothing and help disperse swelling. Large, brisk movements can be irritating.
- Remember that the relief of pain does not mean the restoration of normal function. Once the pain is resolved, assess the area again to ensure that the ROM is normal and that the length and strength of the muscles in the region are balanced.

Treatment Protocol for the Chronic Pain Client

- A general treatment for most chronic pain clients typically involves a "spinal session," that is, performing Level I strokes on the lumbosacral, thoracic, and cervical areas of the spine. Then focused work is performed on the specific area of complaint.
- The strokes are usually applied more deeply, as it is necessary to dissolve adhesions in the soft tissue. We often perform manual work in areas that are uncomfortable and need to remind the client that he or she should be able to completely relax into the massage strokes, even if they are uncomfortable. Otherwise, ask the client to always let you know if he or she cannot relax into what you are doing.
- Perform MET throughout the session, interspersing it with the strokes.
- Mobilize the client with bigger movements in areas of fibrosis and perform only small amplitude mobilizations in areas of instability.
- Instruct your client in correct posture. The cumulative stresses from poor posture can create chronic tension patterns that can be the source of a client's pain.
- It is essential that chronic pain clients have proper exercise instruction that includes strength and stabilization training, in addition to instruction in coordination and balance.
- Rehabilitation has two categories: passive care and active care. **Passive care** is care that is done to the client, including massage therapy. **Active care** is that care that the client does on his or her own. It is now well recognized that activity decreases the disability associated with chronic pain.[24]

Clients That Are Reactive to Treatment: Side-Effects

- If a client develops **side-effects** of increased pain after your session, assume that you worked too hard for too long in an area. Massage therapists are often enthusiastic, which can lead to working too hard, especially when learning a new technique. If your client is mildly sore for a day or two, as if she or he went to a new exercise class, that is considered normal. This soreness is often associated with the first sessions. Moderate to severe discomfort after a session or the next day may mean that your treatment was much too vigorous.
  - All interventions have potential side-effects. This is well known and easily accepted in allopathic medicine when a patient develops side effects to a drug. It is not as easily accepted when a client has side-effects to massage or physical therapy, or to chiropractic or any other manual intervention. The goal of the therapist is to minimize side-effects, as it is unreasonable to assume that your treatments will never have side-effects. The more experienced the practitioner, the fewer the side-effects.
- You may be missing an underlying joint problem. For example, if the joint is inflamed and you work too hard, your client may have increased pain the day after the treatment.
- You may be missing underlying emotional distress. Massage can change habits of muscle function and posture, and even a positive change can be unconsciously sensed as a distress to that person's homeostasis. Inquire if your client is experiencing a period of high stress.
- You may be missing an underlying pathology. Even if your client's symptoms do not fall into the category of the red flags, there may be a subclinical pathology.

Clients That Are Unresponsive to Therapy

If your client does not show some improvement to your treatments after a trial of four sessions, there are several possible causes:

- Your client may be deconditioned or atrophied and lack enough muscle tone to hold the changes that you introduce. He or she may lack proper exercise habits to support the changes you make in these sessions.
- Poor posture places stress on the system that can undermine your therapy. You can perform brilliant work to help reestablish normal function in the neck

and shoulders that is undone between your sessions as the client sits in front of the computer all week with poor posture.

- You may not have enough experience and may need to refer your client to a more advanced practitioner.
- An underlying joint problem, pathology, or emotional problem may exist.
- The personality match between the client and the therapist may be poor. If the client is not improving under your care and you do not suspect the need for further assessment, refer your client to another practitioner.
- The client needs a different kind of treatment. Although OM is extremely effective for most neuromusculoskeletal conditions, your client may need another style of massage therapy, such as trigger point therapy, myofascial release, Active Release Technique, Feldenkrais, or Rolfing, to name a few.

STUDY GUIDE

Assessment and Technique: Level I

1. Describe the three characteristics of the tissue to palpation.
2. Describe the four categories of tissue palpation that help us differentiate an acute from a chronic problem.
3. Describe the stages of inflammation and repair and the treatment considerations for each stage.
4. Describe the open position of the joints and its implication for a massage therapist.
5. Describe the position of function of the wrist and hand, and why it is important for the massage therapist.
6. List four principles of using chi in your massage.
7. Name three qualities of ocean waves that are similar to the wave mobilization stroke of OM.
8. Describe why pain-free movement is typically recommended in the early stages of rehabilitaion.
9. List six clinical uses of MET.
10. Define RI, CRAC, and PIR-MET, and describe how to increase the ROM of a joint with MET.

Assessment and Technique: Level II

1. Describe the parts of an assessment.
2. Define the acronym "SOAP."
3. List four questions that will help determine if massage is contraindicated (the "red flags").
4. List six categories of information that you want to gather in taking a history.
5. Describe the two most important categories of information from an active motion assessment.
6. List five different reasons a muscle tests weak to isometric challenge.
7. Describe the clinical effects of OM.
8. Describe the hypothesis how muscle energy technique relaxes a hypertonic muscle.
9. Define the acronym "MICE."

REFERENCES

1. Cyriax J. Textbook of Orthopedic Medicine: Diagnosis of Soft Tissue Lesions, vol 1, 8th Ed. London: Bailliere Tindall, 1982.
2. Norkin C, Levangie P. Joint Structure and Function. 2nd Ed. Philadelphia: FA Davis, 1992.
3. Hoppenfeld S. Physical Examination of the Spine and Extremities. New York: Appleton-Century-Crofts, 1976.
4. Chaitow L. Palpation Skills. New York: Churchill Livingstone, 1998.
5. Magee D. Orthopedic Physical Assessment. 3rd Ed. Philadelphia: WB Saunders, 1997.
6. Lo B, Inn M, Amaker R, Foe S. The Essence of T'ai Chi Ch'uan. Berkeley, CA: North Atlantic Books, 1985.
7. Garrison T. Oceanography. 3rd Ed. Pacific Grove, CA: Brooks/Cole/Wadsworth, 1999.
8. Lederman E. Fundamentals of Manual Therapy. New York: Churchill Livingstone, 1997.
9. Greenman PE. Principles of Manual Medicine. 2nd Ed. Baltimore: Williams & Wilkins, 1996.

9a. Voss D, Ionta M, Myers B. Proprioceptive Neuromuscular Facilitaion, 3rd ed. Philadelphia: Harper and Row, 1985.

10. Lewit K. Manipulative Therapy in Rehabilitation on the Locomotor System. 3rd Ed. Oxford: Butterworth Heinemann, 1999.
11. Janda V. Evaluation of muscular imbalance. In: Liebenson C, ed. Rehabilitation of the Spine. Baltimore: Williams & Wilkins, 1996:97–112.
12. Chaitow L. Muscle Energy Techniques. New York: Churchill Livingstone, 1996.
13. Mitchell F. Elements of Muscle Energy Technique. In: Basmajian J, Nyberg R, eds. Rational Manual Therapies. Baltimore: Williams & Wilkins, 1993.
14. Lewit K, Simons D. Myofascial pain: relief by postisometric relaxation. Arch Phys Med Rehabil 1984; 65:452–456.

14a. Hanna T. Somatics. Reading, MA: Addison-Wesley Publishing, 1988.

15. Liebenson C. Manual resistance techniques and selfstretches for improving flexibility/mobility. In: Liebenson C, ed. Rehabilitation of the Spine. Baltimore: Williams & Wilkins, 1996.
16. Kandel E, Schwartz J, Jessell T. Principles of Neural Science. 4th Ed. New York: McGraw-Hill, 2000.
17. Pitman M, Peterson L. Biomechanics of skeletal muscle. In: Nordin M, Frankel V, eds. Basic Biomechanics of the Musculoskeletal System. Philadelphia: Lea & Febiger, 1989:89–111.

18. Kendall F, McCreary E, Provance P. Muscles: Testing and Function. 4th Ed. Baltimore: Williams & Wilkins, 1993.
19. Freeman MAR, Wyke B. Articular reflexes at the ankle joint: an electromyographic study of normal and abnormal influences of ankle-joint mechanoreceptors upon reflex activity in the leg muscles. Br J Surg 1967; 54:990–1001.
20. Oschman JL. What is healing energy? Part 6: Conclusions: is energy medicine the medicine of the future. Journal of Movement and Bodywork Therapies 1998;2:46–60.
21. Kellett J. Acute soft tissue injuries—a review of the literature. Med Sci Sports Exerc 1986;18:489–500.
22. Woo S, Buckwalter J. Injury and Repair of the Musculoskeletal Soft Tissues. Park Ridge, IL: American Academy of Orthopedic Surgeons, 1988.
23. Kisner C, Colby LA. Therapeutic Exercise. 3rd Ed. Philadelphia: F.A. Davis Company, 1996.
24. Liebenson C. Rehabilitation of the Spine. Baltimore: Williams & Wilkins, 1996.

SUGGESTED READINGS

Basmajian J, Nyberg R, eds. Rational Manual Therapies. Baltimore: Williams & Wilkins, 1993.

Chaitow L. Palpation Skills. New York: Churchill Livingstone, 1998.

Greenman PE. Principles of Manual Medicine. 2nd Ed. Baltimore: Williams & Wilkins, 1996.

Hoppenfeld S. Physical Examination of the Spine and Extremities. New York: Appleton-Century-Crofts, 1976.

Kendall F, McCreary E, Provance P. Muscles: Testing and Function. 4th Ed. Baltimore: Williams & Wilkins, 1993

Lederman E. Fundamentals of Manual Therapy. New York: Churchill Livingstone, 1997.

Liebenson C. Rehabilitation of the Spine. Baltimore: Williams & Wilkins, 1996.

Magee D. Orthopedic Physical Assessment. 3rd Ed. Philadelphia: WB Saunders, 1997.7

SECTION II:

CLINICAL APPLICATION

Lumbosacral Spine

Problems with the **lumbosacral spine,** or low back, are some of the most common complaints that clients present to the massage therapist. **Low back pain (LBP)** is the second leading symptom for which patients consult their physicians.[1] Disorders of the low back are the leading cause of disability in people younger than 45 years of age.[2] Every year 50% of the adult population in the United States experiences at least a day of back pain, and yet 80% of LBP is nonspecific, meaning the cause is unknown.[3] It has been estimated that mechanical disorders of the spine, that is, problems of function and not pathology, represent at least 98% of LBP.[4]

Anatomy, Function, and Dysfunction of the Lumbosacral Spine

GENERAL OVERVIEW

- The spine consists of 33 bones divided into five regions: **cervical, thoracic, lumbar, sacral,** and **coccygeal** (Fig. 3-1).
- There are 24 distinct vertebrae: seven cervical, twelve thoracic, and five lumbar.
- Five vertebrae are fused to form the **sacrum,** and four are fused to form the **coccyx.**
- The lumbopelvic region consists of five lumbar vertebrae, the right and left innominate **bones,** which function as lower-extremity bones, and the sacrum, which functions as part of the spine. The pelvis has three joints: a **symphysis pubis** and two **sacroiliac joints.**

Primary and Secondary Curves

When the body is viewed from the side, there are three visible curves: the lumbar, the thoracic, and the cervical. The sacrum and the coccyx, which is not visible, form a fourth curve. The thoracic and coccygeal curves are called **primary curves** because the vertebral column at birth has one curve that is convex posteriorly. The cervical and lumbar curves are convex anteriorly and are called **secondary curves** because they develop after birth in response to the infant's lifting his or her head and standing upright, respectively.

The degree of curve in the healthy spine represents the balance between stability and mobility. With too little curve, the spine is stiffer. With too much curve,

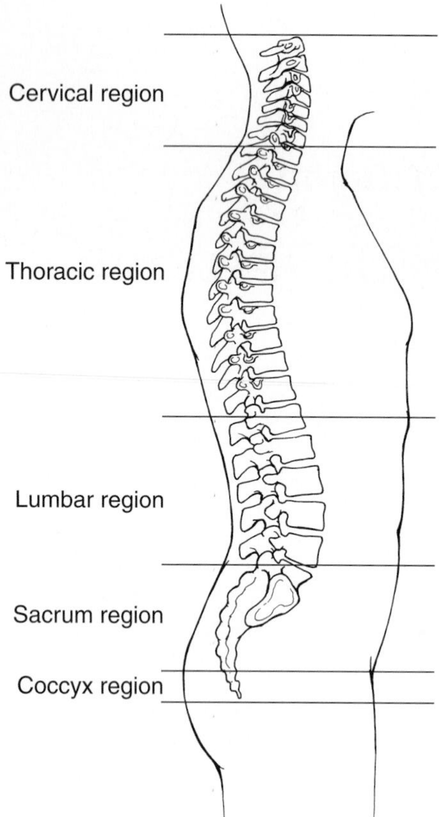

Figure 3-1. Lateral view of the spine showing the five regions and the four curves.

General Anatomy of the Vertebrae

Each vertebra consists of an anterior and a posterior portion (Fig. 3-3).

- The anterior portion is composed of the **vertebral body** and **intervertebral disc,** which forms a **fibrocartilaginous** or **amphiarthrodial joint.**
- The posterior portion is composed of two vertebral arches formed by a pedicle and lamina; two transverse processes; a central spinous process; and paired articulations, the **inferior** and **superior facets,** which form **synovial joints.**

There are five vertebrae in the lumbar spine, and each vertebra forms three joints with the vertebra above and three joints with the vertebra below (or the sacrum). This three-joint complex includes an intervertebral disc and two facet joints. The intervertebral foramen is an opening between two vertebrae through

the spine is often hypermobile and unstable. However, an increase in the thoracic curve, which is often caused by bony changes such as osteoporosis, represents bony degeneration.

Pelvic rotation determines the amount of curve in the spine (Fig. 3-2). Anterior rotation of the pelvis creates an increase in the lumbar curve, and all other curves are increased to keep the body in gravitational balance. Posterior rotation of the pelvis creates a flattening of the lumbar curve and a decrease of the thoracic and cervical curves. As is discussed in this chapter, many muscular factors contribute to the amount of pelvic rotation.

Posture

Posture is determined by many factors, including genetics, structural abnormalities caused by disease, habits of work and play, mimicking parents and peers, compensations resulting from injury, emotional and psychological factors, and gravity.[5]

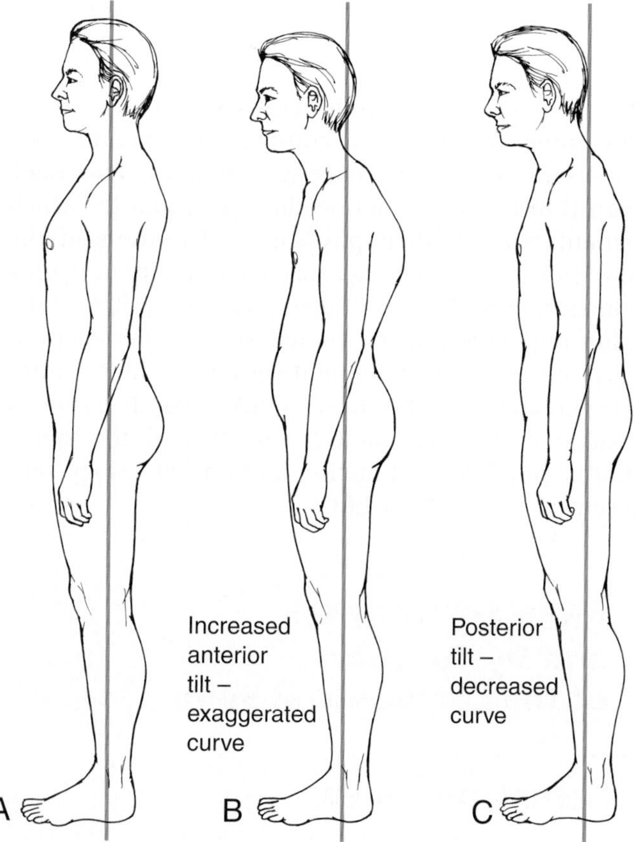

Figure 3-2. A. Normal spinal curves. B. Increased anterior pelvic tilt and exaggerated curve. C. Decreased curve due to a posterior pelvic tilt.

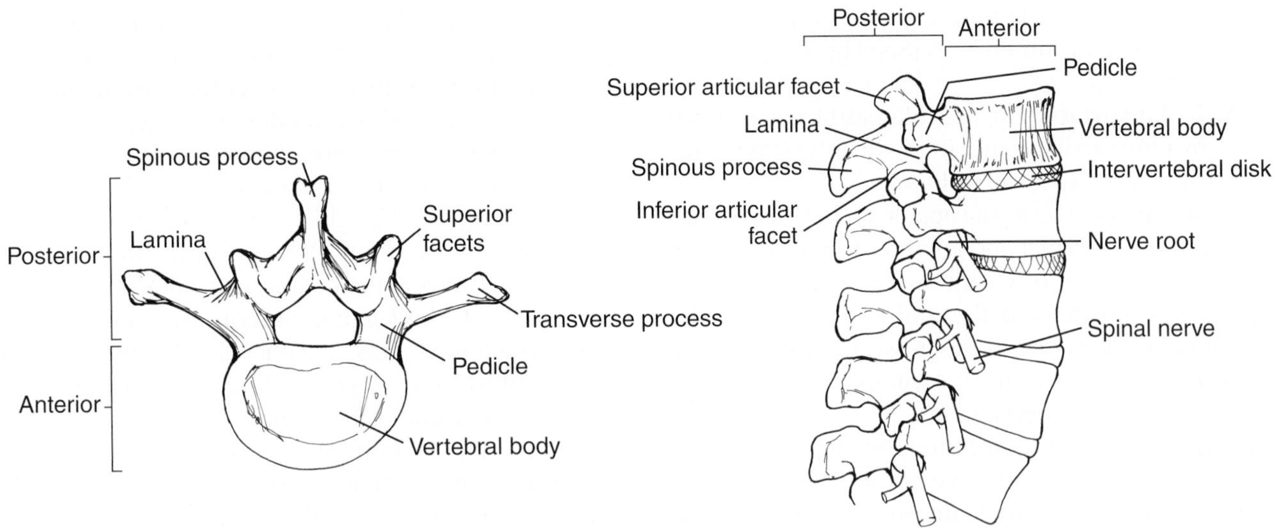

Figure 3-3. Vertebral anatomy. The anterior portion of the vertebrae consists of the vertebral body and the intervertebral disc. The posterior portion consists of a pedicle and lamina, two transverse processes, a central spinous process, and the inferior and superior facets.

which the ventral and dorsal nerve roots travel along the spine.

Intervertebral Disc

- *Definition:* The **intervertebral disc (IVD)** is a fibrocartilage structure that binds two vertebral bodies together.
- *Structure:* The IVD is composed of a nucleus and an annulus.
  - **Nucleus:** The nucleus is a colloidal gel contained within a fibrous wall that is 80 to 90% water, which changes its shape, and releases and absorbs water. The nucleus obtains its nutrition by movement, and this water-binding capacity decreases with age.
  - **Annulus:** Concentric layers of interwoven fibrocartilaginous fibers form the annulus. In the young, the fibroelastic tissue is primarily elastic but becomes more fibrous with age, and therefore loses some shock-absorbing ability. The outer third of the annulus is innervated by mechanoreceptors and free nerve endings (pain receptors) that have automatic, unconscious (i.e., reflexive) communication with the surrounding muscles.[1]
- *Function:* Provides a shock-absorbing hydraulic system that permits a rocker-like movement of one vertebra upon the other because of a fluid shift in the nucleus and an elasticity of the annulus. The disc also provides proprioceptive and nociceptive functions. Disc nutrition into the annulus occurs by movement of the spine, which pumps fluids into the disc through compression and decompression.
- *Dysfunction and injury*: The IVD is prone to acute and chronic injuries and is a major source of LBP. It is susceptible to age-related degeneration that involves loss of fluid in the nucleus and loss of elasticity of the annulus.
  - Repetitive torsion forces (that is, repetitive bending and twisting) can cause: an internal derangement or tear of the annulus, also called a protrusion or bulge of the disc; or a prolapse, which is a leaking of disc material into the spinal canal.
  - When injured, the disc leaks inflammatory material that can be a source of LBP and referral of pain caused by irritation of the nerve root.
- *Treatment implications*: Orthopedic massage (OM) introduces a new method of treatment called *wave mobilization* that theoretically helps promote fluid exchange to the disc. Through rhythmic cycles of posterior to anterior (P–A) mobilization, the author postulates that this compression and decompression pumps the disc to help rehydrate a degenerated disc, and also helps disperse excess inflammatory fluids in an acute disc.

Facet Joint

- *Definition*: The **facet joint** is a diarthrodial or synovial joint, containing a synovial space surrounded by a connective tissue joint capsule, adipose tissue fat pads, and a fibromeniscus (See Fig. 3-3).

- *Structure*
  - **Articular surface:** The articular surface is covered by hyaline cartilage and, in the healthy state, is lubricated with synovial fluid.
  - **Joint capsule:** The joint capsule is composed of an inner synovial layer and an outer fibrous layer. It is reinforced anteriorly with the ligamentum flavum and posteriorly with the multifidus muscle. The joint capsule is one of the most richly innervated structures of the spine. It contains proprioceptive and nociceptive nerve fibers.
- *Function*: The facets determine the range and direction of movement and have some weight-bearing capacity. In the healthy state, they are designed to slide on each other. Extension closes the facets, and flexion opens them. Compression squeezes fluid out of the hyaline cartilage, and the cartilage is rehydrated as the fluid is reabsorbed with the release of the compression. Activities of daily life, such as walking, move the spine through these cycles of compression and decompression, thus promoting normal lubrication in the facets. Sitting, on the other hand, is only compressive, and dehydrates the facets.
- *Dysfunction and injury*
  - **Hypomobility:** Restricted motion at the lumbosacral facets implies a loss of the normal gliding motion on the cartilage surfaces. This is called a joint fixation. Restricted motion of the facet results in a reflex that typically creates hypertonicity of the muscles at the same vertebral level.
  - **Degeneration:** A sustained contraction of the paraspinal muscles (muscles on either side of the spine) increases the compression to the facets and accelerates their degeneration.
  - **Acute Facet Syndrome:** The cause of "locked back" is not well understood. One chiropractic theory proposes a fixation or microadhesion of the facet surfaces, and that manipulation introduces normal movement by releasing the fixation. There are other current theories that suggest that the cause is an entrapment of the fibromenisci between the facets.
  - **Joint Capsule Injury:** Because the capsule is highly innervated, sprains are painful, potentially giving local and referred pain into the leg. Injury also affects the mechanoreceptors, resulting in altered movement patterns, dysfunctions of coordination and balance, and altered reflexes to the muscles, creating either weakness or hypertonicity.
- *Treatment implications:* One of the intentions of OM is to induce P–A mobilization into the facets in rhythmic oscillations of compression and decompression. This stimulates the synovial lining of the capsule to increase lubrication and to rehydrate the facets. If the facets are swollen, the author theorizes that this same mobilization helps disperse excess fluids. Patients who have chronic LBP must have balance and coordination exercises as part of their rehabilitation to reeducate the proprioceptors. OM is especially effective with hypomobility and degeneration, whereas an acute facet syndrome often requires manipulation to correct the fixation. With a joint capsule injury, OM helps promote a healthy repair through mobilization and massage, thus reducing adhesions in the joint capsule.

Intervertebral Foramen

- *Definition:* The **intervertebral foramen (IVF)** is an opening (foramen) formed by:
  1. Two pedicles from the superior and the inferior vertebrae that form the roof and floor;
  2. The disc, posterior longitudinal ligament and vertebral body anteriorly;
  3. The facets, anterior capsule and ligamentum flavum posteriorly.
- *Function:* Provides an opening for the motor and sensory nerve roots that originate at the spinal cord.
- *Dysfunction:* Narrowing of the IVF can cause compression of the nerve roots creating pain, numbing, tingling, and weakness in the legs. The diameter of the IVF is narrowed by many factors: disc degeneration, disc protrusion, thickening and fibrosis of the ligamentum flavum and joint capsule, facet position, facet degeneration and calcification, and increased lordosis of the lumbar spine. If the narrowing is significant, it is called foraminal encroachment.

Nerves of the Lumbosacral Spine

Ventral (motor) and **dorsal (sensory)** nerve roots originate from the spinal cord and merge at the IVF. The union of these two roots is called a **spinal nerve.**

Dorsal Root Ganglion

The **dorsal root ganglion** (DRG) is a cluster of cell bodies of the sensory root and typically lies in the IVF near the disc. The DRG has been postulated to be a major site of pain, called radicular (which means root) pain.[5]

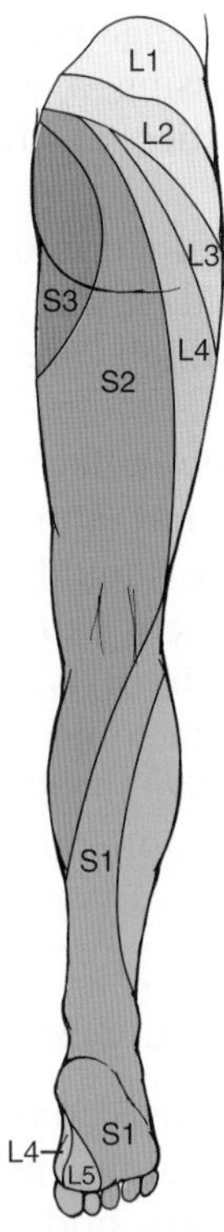

Figure 3-4. Dermatomes of the posterior lower limb.

It is also mechanically sensitive, so altered movement patterns may initiate reflex activity that results in sustained muscle contraction.

A **dermatome** is an area of skin supplied by the sensory (dorsal) root of a spinal nerve. Irritation of the DRG elicits a sharp pain in the dermatome corresponding to the root (Figs. 3-4 and 3-5).

Ventral Roots

- A **myotome** consists of the muscles that are supplied by the motor root(s) of the spinal nerve(s). Irritation of the motor (ventral) root elicits muscle weakness and potential atrophy.
- The corresponding myotomes of the lumbar nerve roots are L2-hip flexion (iliopsoas); L3-knee extension (quadriceps); L4-ankle dorsiflexion (anterior tibialis); L5-great toe extension (extensor hallucis longus); S1-foot eversion (peroneals); and S2-knee flexion (hamstrings). If weakness is detected in these muscles, one source of the weakness might be nerve root irritation. However, it takes a great deal of clinical experience to determine that the nerve root is the source of the weakness.
- Assessment of a nerve root involvement involves the straight–leg-raising (SLR) test to determine abnormal root tension (see p. 103, Assessment). The most common cause of increased root tension is a swollen or bulging disc.

Lumbar Plexus

Branches of nerves that communicate with other branches of nerves form a nerve plexus.

The **lumbar plexus** consists of nerves from L1–L4 and travels through the psoas muscle (Fig. 3-6). It innervates the anterior, medial, and lateral thigh, leg, and foot. It includes the femoral, lateral femoral cutaneous, obturator, and genitofemoral nerves.

Sacral Plexus

The **sacral plexus** consists of nerves from L4–L5 and S1–S3. It forms the sciatic nerve, which is actually two nerves within the same sheath, the common peroneal and tibial nerves. These nerves supply the posterior thigh, leg, and foot, as well as the anterior and lateral leg and the dorsum of the foot (See Figs. 3-6 and 3-8).

Sacroiliac Joint

- *Definition:* The **sacroiliac joint (SIJ)** is a synovial joint consisting of the articulation of the sacrum with the right and left iliac or innominate bones.

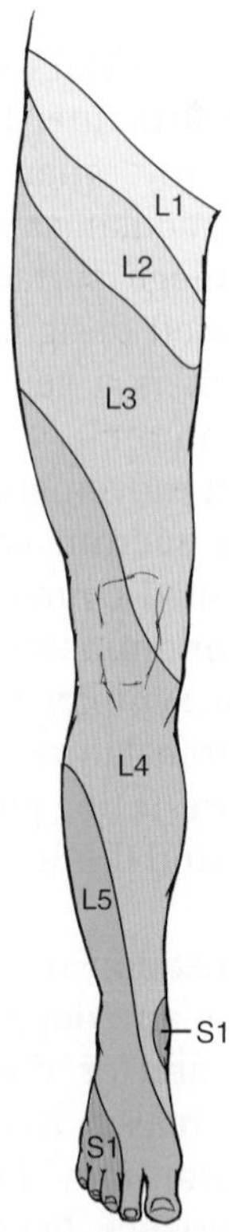

Figure 3-5. Dermatomes of the anterior lower limb.

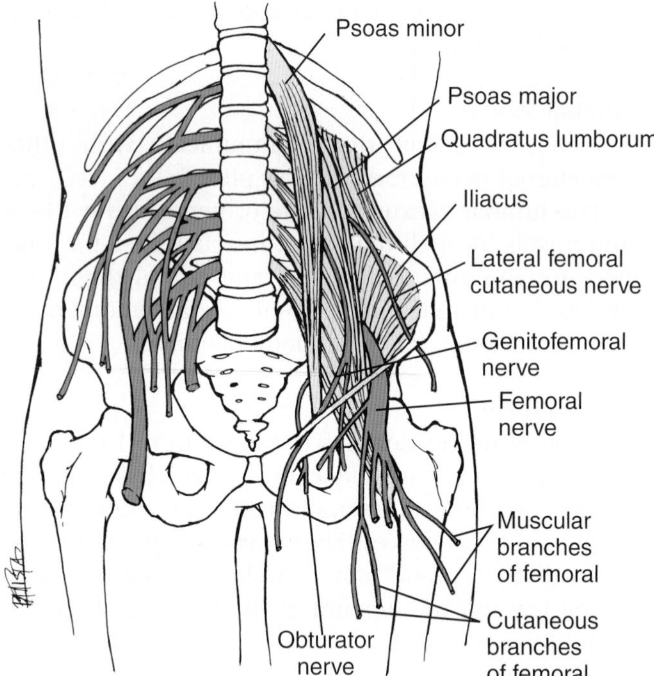

Figure 3-6. Muscles and nerves of the anterior pelvis. The lumbosacral plexus consists of nerves from L1–L4 and travels through the psoas muscles. It divides into many branches, including the femoral, lateral femoral cutaneous, obturator, and genitofemoral nerves.

- *Structure:* As in all synovial joints, its joint capsule is a pain-sensitive structure. The articular surfaces are different from any other joint in the body in that the hyaline articular cartilage of the sacrum faces the fibrocartilage surface of the ilium. The joint has a corrugated design, with ridges and depressions; that is, it is a self-locking mechanism, like a keystone of an arch.
- *Function:* The main movements of the SIJ are a forward tilting of the sacrum called nutation and a backward tilting called counternutation. The main movement of the innominates is rotation anteriorly and posteriorly. The symphysis pubis has a superior and an inferior translatory movement. Stability comes from the close-fitting joint surfaces, the muscles, the ligaments, and the fascia that cross the joint.
- *Dysfunction:*
  - Subluxation or fixation of the SIJ, in which the undulating ridges and depressions are no longer complimentary, and/or the normal movement of the SIJ is decreased (fixation) is a common dysfunction. There may be a loss of normal motion characteristics because of ligamentous shortening, irritation of the articular surfaces of the SIJ caused by ligamentous laxity, muscular hypertonicity causing a loss of normal movement characteristics at the SIJ, and articular dysfunction.
  - Pain from SIJ dysfunction or injury can be sharp, dull, or aching, and typically is in the buttock area, groin, posterior thigh, and, occasionally, below the knee.
- *Treatment implications:* Because the SIJ is stabilized with the muscles that attach to the pelvis and sacrum, assessment should consider the length, strength, and movement patterns of the major muscles of the SIJ. Since the SIJ is a synovial joint with lubricated surfaces with some movement, part of our intention is to mobilize the SIJ in posterior-anterior (P–A) glide to help restore motion and rehydrate the cartilage surfaces.

Lumbosacral Spine Ligaments

In addition to the dynamic stability provided by the musculature, a "continuous ligamentous stocking" wraps around the bones and interweaves with the muscles, providing essential passive stability to the lumbopelvic region.[6]

- **Anterior longitudinal ligament**: The anterior longitudinal ligament (ALL) is a dense band that runs along the anterior and lateral surfaces of the vertebral bodies and discs from the second cervical vertebra to the sacrum. The ALL serves as an attachment for the crura of the diaphragm and resists extension.
- **Posterior longitudinal ligament**: The posterior longitudinal ligament (PLL) runs within the vertebral canal along the posterior surfaces of the vertebral bodies from the second cervical vertebra to the sacrum. The PLL resists flexion.
- **Neural arch ligaments:** The ligamentum flavum, interspinous ligament, supraspinous ligament, and intertransverse ligament compose the neural arch ligaments. The interspinous ligament is continuous with the ligamentum flavum, which is a continuation of the joint capsule, which is continuous with the supraspinous ligament, which is attached to the thoracolumbar fascia (TLF).
- **Sacrotuberous ligament**: The sacrotuberous ligament is a triangular structure that extends from the posterior iliac spine, the SIJ capsule, the coccygeal vertebrae, and the ischial tuberosity. The biceps femoris, multifidus, and TLF all interweave with this ligament.

- **Sacrospinous ligament**: The sacrospinous ligament arises from the lateral margin of the sacral and coccygeal vertebrae and the inferior aspect of the SIJ capsule and attaches to the ischial spine.
- **Short and long dorsal (posterior) sacroiliac ligaments:** These sacroiliac ligaments are a complex array of multilevel, multidirectional ligaments. The long dorsal SIJ ligament travels under the sacrotuberous ligament, from the posterior superior iliac spine (PSIS) to the lateral sacral crest. This ligament resists counternutation.
- **Iliolumbar ligament**: The iliolumbar ligament arises from the transverse processes of L4–L5 and attaches to the iliac crest and adjacent region of the iliac tuberosity.
- **Inguinal ligament**: The inguinal ligament is formed by the inferior margin of the aponeurosis of the external abdominal oblique. It arises at the anterior superior iliac spine (ASIS) and inserts into the pubic tubercle.

- *Function:*
  - The ligaments of the lumbopelvic region provide passive stability to spine and pelvis. These ligaments and fascia serve as attachment sites to the major prime movers and to stabilizing muscles of the spine.
  - The ligaments and joint capsules have a neurosensory role. They have nociceptors and proprioceptors and play an important role in initiating reflex activity in the musculature.[2]
- *Dysfunction:*
  - Ligament injury decreases mechanoreceptor and proprioceptive functions, leading to reflexive muscle hypertonicity or weakness, altered movement patterns, altered coordination and balance, and instability.[7]
  - Ligament injury can also lead either to laxity and consequent joint instability or to shortening and thickening of the ligaments that lead to stiffness in the joint. Both outcomes alter joint mechanics and neurologic function.
- *Treatment implications:* Treatment of injured ligaments consists of four primary intentions:
  1. Rehydrate the tissue. This occurs through cycles of compression and decompression while performing the massage strokes.
  2. Reestablish normal neurologic communication between the muscle and the ligament with muscle energy technique (MET).
  3. Release adhesions with transverse massage and MET. As the fascia of the myotendon unit is attached to the ligaments, muscle contraction mobilizes the ligaments, helping to reduce adhesions.
  4. Exercise the ligament. If the ligaments have become weakened, exercise rehabilitation is the most effective therapy. In addition to strength training, balance and coordination exercises are essential.

Thoracolumbar Fascia

- *Definition*: The **TLF** is a sheet of dense connective tissue that covers the muscles of the back of the trunk.
- *Structure*: The TLF is divided into posterior, middle, and anterior layers.
  - The posterior layer is located under the skin and subcutaneous fat and begins as a continuation of the aponeurosis of the latissimus dorsi. It is thick and fibrous and is attached to the lumbar spinous processes and the supraspinous ligament and surrounds the erector spinae and multifidus.
  - The middle layer attaches to the transverse processes and intertransverse ligaments of the lumbar vertebrae.
  - The anterior layer surrounds the quadratus lumborum and attaches laterally to the transverse abdominus and the internal oblique. The TLF continues to the sacrum and ilium and blends with the fascia of the gluteus maximus (G. max.).
- *Function*: The TLF plays an important role in lumbopelvic function because it can be dynamically engaged through the muscles that attach to it. The latissimus dorsi, G. max., transverse abdominus, and internal oblique tighten the TLF and stabilize the lumbopelvic spine when they contract.
- *Dysfunction*: The fascia typically palpates as thickened and lacks resilience in the client who has chronic LBP. Theoretically, this thickening and lack of resilience is caused by the laying down of excessive collagen resulting from sustained hypertonicity in the latissimus dorsi and the pushing force on the fascia resulting from broadening of the erector spinae muscles when they contract. The TLF forms a container or septa for the muscles contained within it, and these muscles are designed to slide relative to their container. Fibrosis constricts these normal gliding characteristics.
- *Treatment implications*: Because the fascia often is thickened from sustained muscle contraction, MET and OM are used to reduce the hypertonicity in the muscles contained within the fascia, to lengthen the fascia, and to dissolve the adhesions between the muscles and the fascia.

Muscles of the Lumbopelvic Region

- *Function:* Muscles are not only the engines of voluntary and involuntary movement in the body, but they provide a dynamic stabilizing force to the joints. Muscles also unconsciously (reflexively) communicate with all of the other structures of the body, including the skin, nervous system, and connective tissue, including the ligaments and joint capsules. They express our emotions and reflect our comfort or distress. It is important to remember that muscles of the hip region, including the iliopsoas, gluteals, quadratus lumborum (QL), tensor fascia lata, rectus femoris, and hamstrings, as well as the abdominals, all have a profound influence on lumbopelvic function.
- *Dysfunction:* Muscle contraction is often a primary source of lumbopelvic dysfunction and pain.[8] In LBP or dysfunction, it is typical for the erector spinae to be held in a sustained contraction. The hypertonicity limits the movement in the joints, creating a fixation of the facets. This stimulates the joint mechanoreceptors, which have neurologic reflexes to the surrounding muscles. Some muscles increase their tension, and others become inhibited, such as the multifidus.

Jull and Janda[9] have discovered predictable patterns of muscle imbalance. These imbalances alter movement patterns and therefore add a continuing stress to the joint system. Hypertonicity is also a major source of pain itself. It is critical to understand these muscle imbalances because they may be a dominant factor in the cause of musculoskeletal pain and a major factor in the continuance of the pain. In the lumbopelvic region Jull and Janda[9] call this muscle imbalance **lower (pelvic) crossed syndrome,** because the tight iliopsoas and erector spinae and the weak abdominals and G. max. form a cross (Fig. 3-7).

Muscle Imbalances of the Lumbosacral Region or Lower (Pelvic) Crossed Syndrome

- **Muscles that tend to be tight and short:** The iliopsoas, the lumbar portion of erector spinae, the piriformis, the rectus femoris, the tensor fascia lata, the QL, the adductors, and the hamstrings are examples of tight, short muscles. (Although the lumbar erectors are usually tight and short, they often test weak. A muscle is weak in its shortened position, and sustained contraction weakens a muscle.)
- **Muscles that tend to be inhibited and weak:** The G. max., medius, and minimus and the abdominals are examples of inhibited, weak muscles.

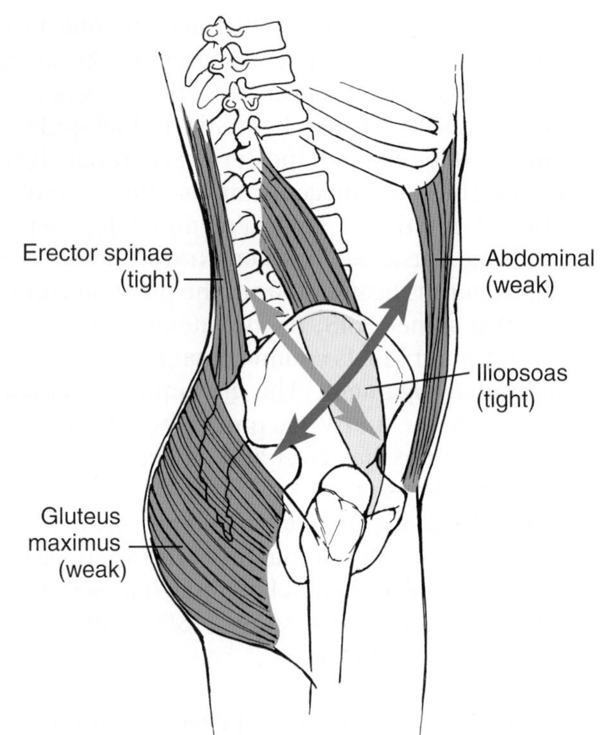

Figure 3-7. Pelvic crossed syndrome.

Postural Signs of the Lower Crossed Syndrome

- Lumbar hyperlordosis caused by short erector spinae.
- Anterior pelvic tilt and protruding abdomen caused by weak G. max., weak abdominals, and tight iliopsoas.
- Hypertonic muscles at thoracolumbar junction resulting from compensation for a hypermobile lumbosacral junction.
- Foot turned outward because of a tight piriformis.

Positional Dysfunction of the Lubopelvic Muscles

- The erector spinae roll into a medial torsion (i.e., toward the midline).
- The iliopsoas rolls into a medial torsion. One cause of this is the effect of a pronated foot, which shortens the leg and pulls the femur into an internal rotation and the pelvis forward, creating an internal or medial torsion to the iliopsoas.
- Gluteals and external rotators of the hip tend to roll into an inferior torsion.

- *Treatment implications*
  - Clinically, it is more effective to release the hypertonicity in a muscle and to lengthen a short muscle and its connective tissue before trying to strengthen a weak or inhibited muscle. As described by Sherrington's law of reciprocal inhibition (RI), a tight agonist inhibits its antagonist. For

example, a tight iliopsoas inhibits the G. max. Sometimes the muscle is weak because of this neurologic inhibition, and strength can be reestablished within a few contract-relax (CR) METs. If the muscle does not respond after a few sessions, then refer to a chiropractic or an osteopathic doctor for assessment of joint fixation, which is the next most likely cause of muscle weakness. A muscle may also be atrophied, in which case the client would be referred to a physical therapist.
- Use MET to help your client reestablish normal movement patterns through precise, controlled muscle contractions. If a muscle is weak, then other muscles will substitute for that muscle's action. For example, in hip abduction, if the G. medius is weak, the tensor fascia lata (TFL) will substitute. This creates an internal rotation of the hip with abduction, a dysfunctional pattern.
- Reestablish the normal position of the muscles by releasing their abnormal torsion.

Relation of Muscles to Lumbopelvic Balance
See Table 3-1.

Anatomy of the Muscles of the Lumbopelvic Region: The Seven Layers of the Back

The back muscles can be divided into seven layers (Fig. 3-8). See Table 3-2.

Muscular Actions of the Trunk

The trunk is capable of seven different movements: flexion, extension, lateral flexion to the right and left, rotation to the right and left, and circumduction. Flexion opens the lumbar facets, and extension is the close-packed position of the spine as it closes the facets.

The extent of motion in the nonacute spine is determined by many factors, including the tightness of the muscles, the extensibility of the ligaments, the elasticity of the articular capsule, the fluidity, and the elasticity of the disc. If a client is experiencing pain, the muscular guarding and swelling also limit movement.

- Flexion
  - Rectus abdominus: compresses the abdomen.
  - External abdominal oblique: causes lateral flexion to same side and rotation to the opposite side.
  - Internal abdominal oblique: causes lateral flexion and rotation to the same side.
  - Psoas major: flexes and rotates the hip laterally.

- Extension

Extension occurs mostly in the lumbar region of the spine.
  - Erector spinae (sacrospinalis), including the iliocostalis, longissimus, and spinalis: extend, rotate, and laterally flex the trunk on the side of the trunk to which they are attached.
  - Semispinalis thoracis: acts bilaterally to extend the trunk or acts unilaterally, laterally flexing the trunk and rotating it to the opposite side.
  - Multifidus: acts bilaterally to extend the trunk and neck or acts unilaterally, laterally flexing and rotating the trunk and the neck to the opposite side.
  - QL: causes lateral flexion.

Text continued on page 85.

TABLE 3-1 RELATION OF MUSCLES TO LUMBOPELVIC BALANCE

- Muscles that increase the lumbar curve and create an anterior pelvic tilt
  - Tight/short iliopsoas
  - Tight/short sartorius, rectus femoris, and TFL
  - Tight/short adductors—pectineus, adductor brevis, longus, magnus (anterior part), gracilis
  - Tight/short thoracic fibers of longissimus (bowstring effect)
  - Weak abdominals, weak or inhibited gluteals, especially gluteus maximus
- Muscles that decrease the lumbar curve
  - Tight/short gluteus maximus and posterior portion of the adductor magnus
  - Tight/short hamstrings
  - Tight/short abdominals
  - Weak paraspinal muscles
- Muscles that cause a lateral pelvic tilt (pelvic obliquity)
  - A lateral pelvic tilt typically is caused by tight adductors and weak/inhibited hip abductors, a tight quadratus lumborum (QL), tight tensor fascia lata (TFL) and tight iliotibial band (ITB)
  - Adductor hypertonicity can cause a high ilium on the side of contracture, an apparent short leg, and an abduction of the opposite hip
  - Abductor hypertonicity can cause a low ilium on the side of contracture, an apparent long leg, and adduction of the opposite hip
  - A tight TFL and ITB tilt the pelvis down on that side
  - Gluteus medius weakness causes the pelvis to be high on the corresponding side
  - Quadratus lumborum and lateral abdominal contracture elevates the ilium on the high side

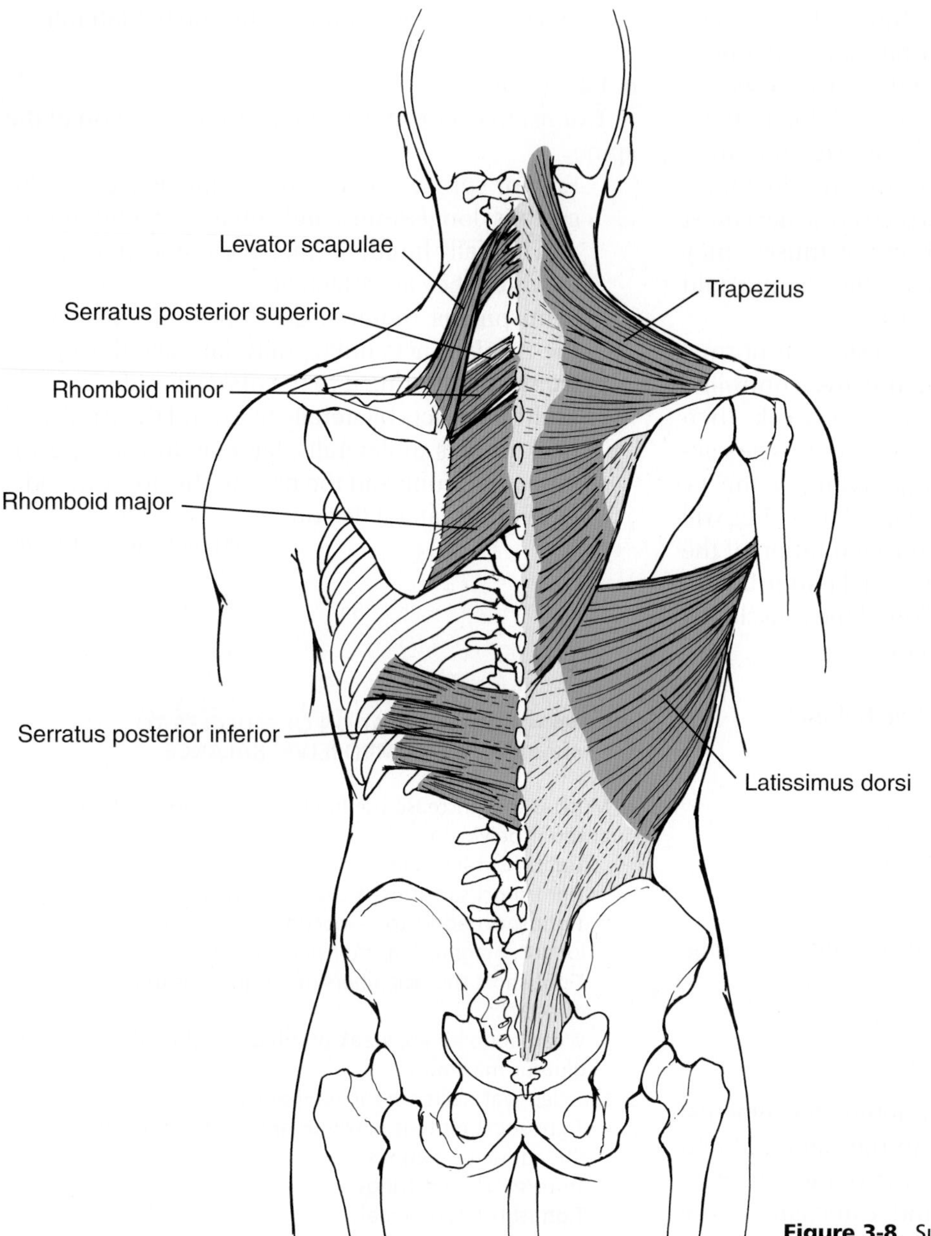

Figure 3-8. Superficial layer of back muscles.

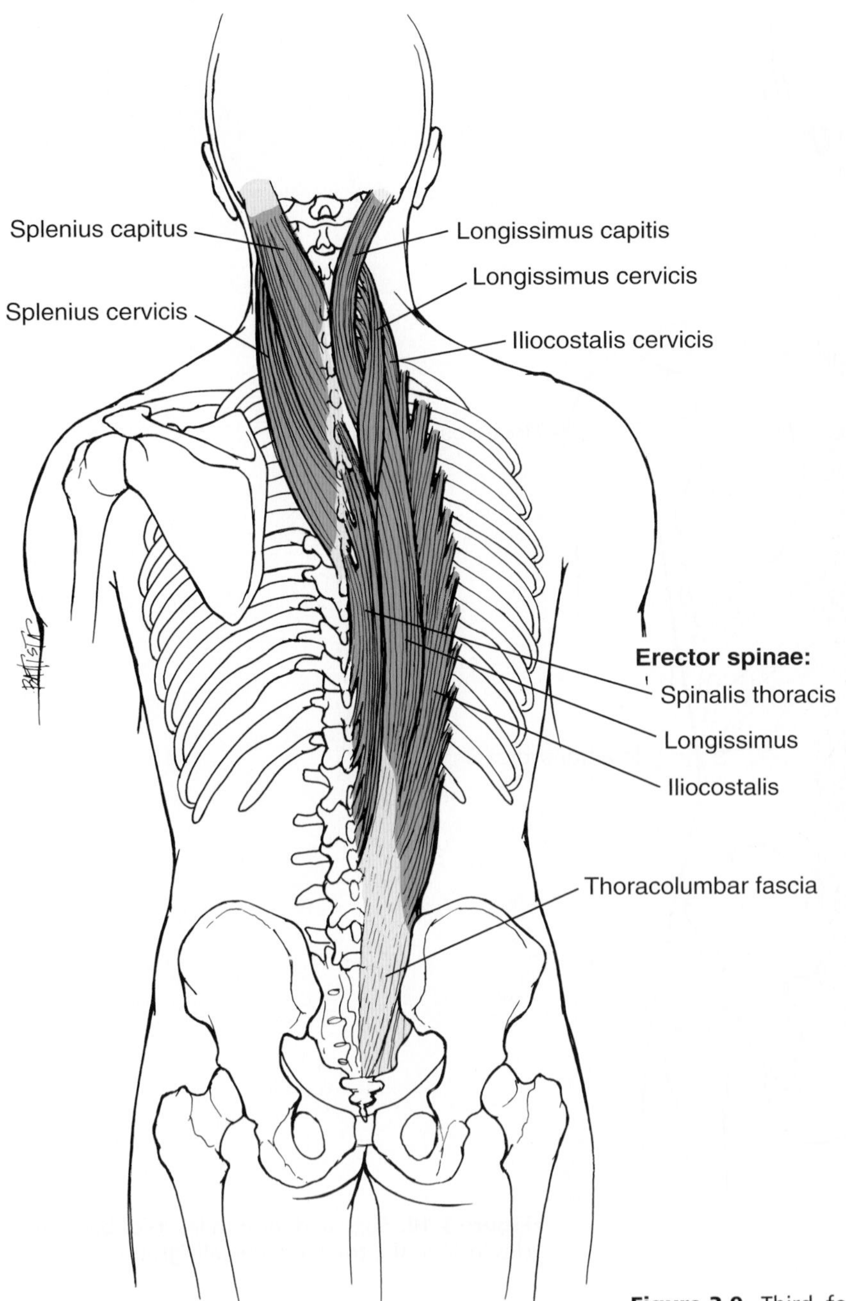

Figure 3-9. Third, fourth, and fifth layers of back muscles.

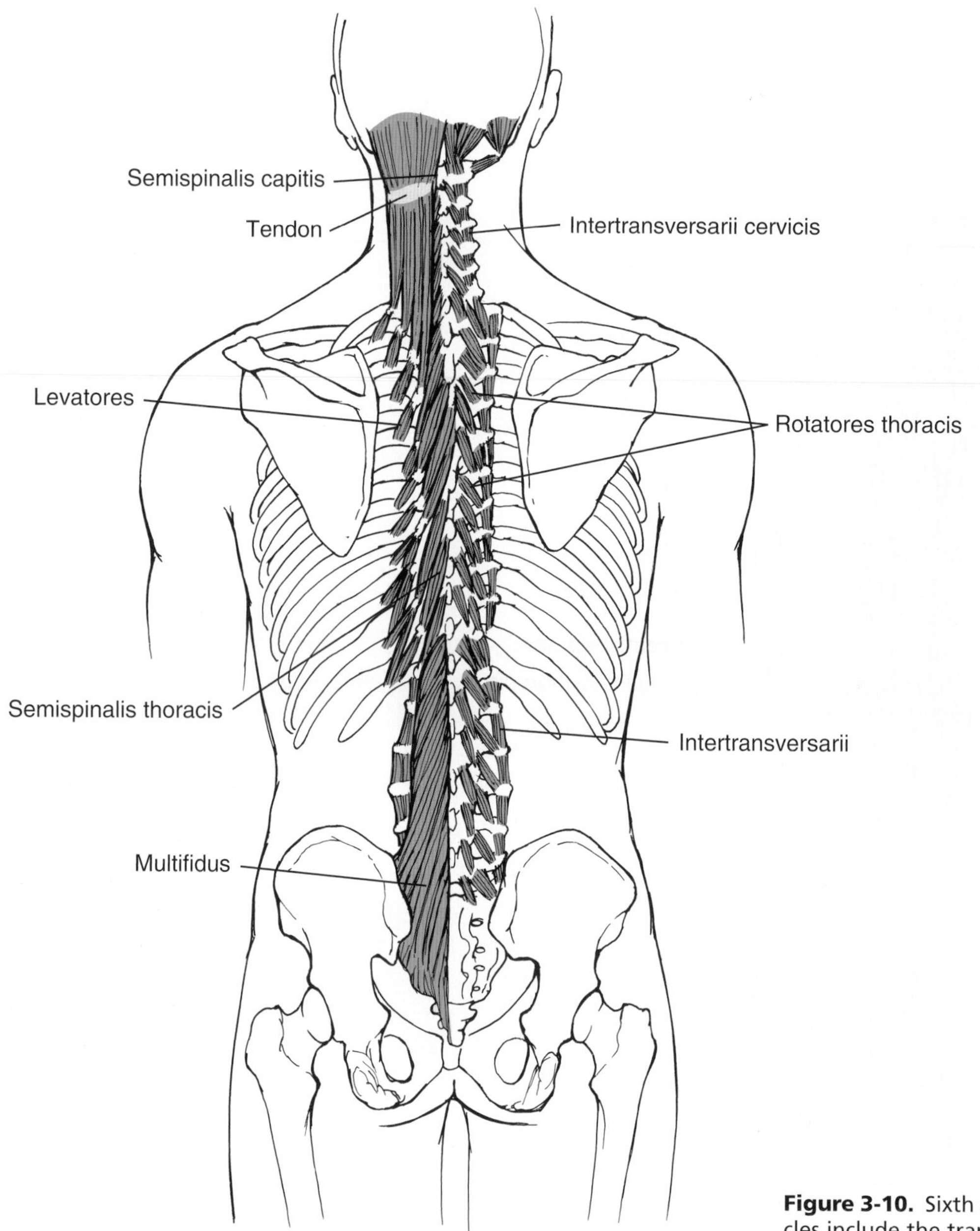

Figure 3-10. Sixth and seventh layers of back muscles include the transversospinalis group.

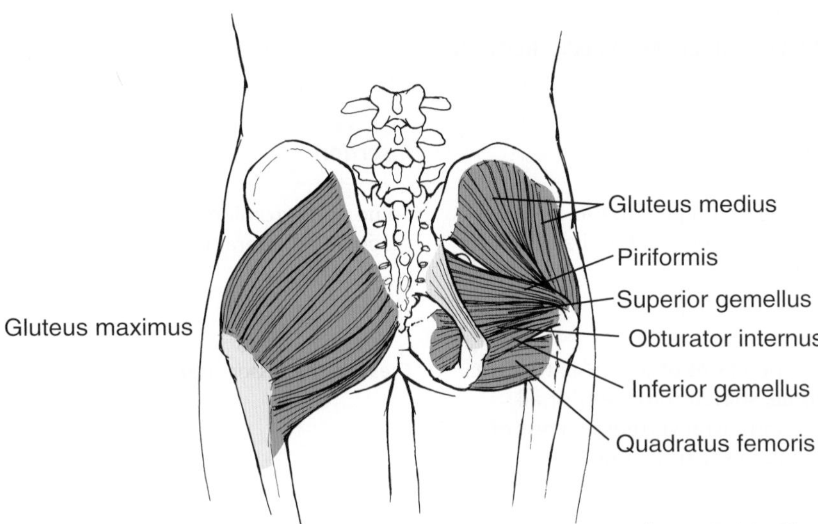

Figure 3-11. Gluteal muscles and deep rotators of the hip.

- Lateral Flexion

  Practically all trunk flexor and extensor muscles contribute to lateral flexion.

  - External and internal abdominal oblique
  - QL
- Rotation
  - External and internal abdominal oblique
  - Erector spinae
  - Semispinalis thoracis
  - Multifidus
  - Rotatores
- Circumduction

  Circumduction results from a sequential combination of flexion, lateral flexion, hyperextension, and lateral flexion to the opposite side.

Dysfunction and Injury of the Lower Back

PATHOGENESIS OF LOW BACK PAIN

The cause of LBP is controversial. A rational hypothesis, described by Kirkaldy-Willis and Bernard,[8] is outlined below.

- Three major factors predispose a client to an episode of LBP:
  1. Emotional upset, such as tension, stress, anxiety, fear, resentment, uncertainty, and depression. Emotional upset causes local areas of vasoconstriction and sustained muscle contraction that leads to muscle fatigue. These changes result in altered patterns of muscle contraction and movement.
  2. Abnormal function of the muscles of the lumbopelvic girdle creates abnormal movement patterns and excessive stresses on the facets and disc. The result of these changes is that movement becomes restricted and painful. These painful restrictions of movement lead to fibrosis around the joint.
  3. Facet joint hypomobility (fixation). As mentioned, this loss of the normal gliding characteristics has reflexive changes in the surrounding muscles, setting up a continuing cycle of muscle dysfunction and further joint dysfunction.
- Muscle dysfunction occurs in a predictable pattern in LBP. In the lower back, the paraspinal muscles tend to be tight. Sustained muscle contraction decreases the blood supply to the muscles, which leads to an accumulation of waste products, and eventual muscle fatigue.
- The multifidus is especially important in LBP. Its fibers interweave with the joint capsule. Sustained contraction adds a compressive load to the joint, and weakness decreases the stability of the lower back; both of these conditions accelerate the degeneration process.
- The client then reports a minor incident, such as gardening, or reaching for a light object, and experiences an episode of acute LBP either at the time, or within a day or two. There are two

Text continued on page 96.

TABLE 3-2 ANATOMY OF THE MUSCLES OF THE LUMBOPELVIC REGION

First Layer

Muscle	***Origin***	***Insertion***
Trapezius	External occipital protuberance, spinous processes of C7 and all thoracic vertebrae	Spine and acromion processes of scapula and lateral third of clavicle
Latissimus dorsi	Spinous processes of lower six thoracic vertebrae, spinous processes of all lumbar and sacral vertebrae, crest of ilium, and lower three ribs	Crest of the lesser tubercle of humerus

Second Layer

Muscle	***Origin***	***Insertion***
Rhomboid minor	Spine of C7 and T1	Vertebral border of scapula, superior to spine of scapula
Rhomboid major	Spines of T2–T5	Vertebral border of scapula below the spine of the scapula
Levator scapula	Posterior tubercles of the transverse processes of C1–C4. Significant attachment site as four major muscles blend into each other at this point: splenius cervicis, posterior scalene, longissimus capitis, and levator scapula	Superior angle of scapula and to the base of the spine of the scapula

Third Layer *(Fig. 3-9)*

Muscle	***Origin***	***Insertion***
Serratus posterior superior	Spinous processes of C7, T1 and T2	Second–fifth ribs
Serratus posterior inferior	Spinous processes of T11 and T12 and L1 and L2	Lower four ribs: T9–T12

Fourth Layer *(See Fig. 3-9.)*

Muscle	***Origin***	***Insertion***
Splenius capitis	A large, flat muscle from the spinous processes of C3–C7 and T1–T3	Lateral third of superior nuchal line and the mastoid process of the mastoid bone
Splenius cervicis	A large, flat muscle from the spinous processes of T4–T6	Posterior tubercles of transverse processes of upper three cervical vertebrae (C1–C3)

Action	Dysfunction
The upper fibers elevate the scapula, the lower fibers depress it, and the middle fibers retract the scapula. The trapezius is primarily a muscle of the shoulder girdle. For the scapula to be elevated, the anterior head and neck must be stabilized by way of the anchor of the longus capitis and longus colli on the front of the neck.	The upper fibers are tight and short, whereas the lower fibers are weak and long, allowing the scapula to migrate headward, decreasing its stability for movement of the arm.
Extends and adducts the humerus and rotates it medially, draws the arm and shoulder downward and backward, interweaves with the thoracolumbar fascia, and has a stabilizing effect on the lumbosacral spine by tensing the fascia.	Is tight and long (i.e., eccentrically loaded), especially with a rounded-shoulders posture.

Action	Dysfunction
Both major and minor: draws the scapula upward and medially, holds the scapula to the trunk along with the serratus anterior muscle, and retracts the scapula along with the fibers of the middle trapezius.	Rhomboids are weak, which contributes to a rounded-shoulder posture.
Pulls the scapula upward and medially (along with the trapezius); if the scapula is fixed, pulls the neck laterally; acts similar to the deep fibers of the erector spinae (see below) to prevent forward shear caused by cervical lordosis. Levator eccentrically contracts in the head-forward posture.	

Action	Dysfunction
Elevates second to fifth ribs.	
Draws lower four ribs downward and backward.	

Action	Dysfunction
Muscles of both sides acting together extend the head and neck; one side acting alone rotates the head to the same side.	
Muscles of both sides acting together extend the head and neck; muscle of one side rotates the neck and the head to the same side.	

TABLE 3-2 **ANATOMY OF THE MUSCLES OF THE LUMBOPELVIC REGION—cont'd**

Fifth Layer: Erector Spinae *(Fig. 3-9)*

Bogduk and Twomey[10] describes a deep and superficial layer to the iliocostalis and longissimus muscles.

Iliocostalis (Lateral Column): Ilium to Ribs

Muscle	*Origin*	*Insertion*
Lumbar fibers of iliocostalis (deep layer of iliocostalis)	Lumbar component consists of four to five overlying fascicles; attaches on iliac crest just lateral to the PSIS	Lateral aspect of the lumbar transverse process (t.p.) L1–L4
Thoracic fibers of iliocostalis (superficial layer of iliocostalis)	By a tendinous sheet of fascia referred to as the erector spinae aponeurosis to the PSIS, the dorsal surface of sacrum, the posterior sacroiliac ligament, and the sacrospinous ligament	Angle of the rib T12–T4
Iliocostalis cervicis	Angles of the ribs 3–6	Posterior tubercles of the transverse processes of C4–C6

Longissimus (Intermediate Column): Sacrum to Transverse Process

Muscle	*Origin*	*Insertion*
Lumbar fibers of longissimus (deep layer)	Composed of five fascicles, each attaching to the anterior-medial aspect of the PSIS, L5 fascicle is most medial	Transverse processes of all lumbar vertebrae
Thoracic component of longissimus (superficial layer)	Attaches to a broad tendinous sheet called the erector spinae aponeurosis, which attaches to the entire length of the medial sacral crest and the lateral sacral crest where it blends with the sacrotuberus and dorsal sacroiliac ligaments	Divided into two parts: the medial insertions reach the tips of the t.p.s of all thoracic vertebrae T1–T12, and the lateral insertions reach the ribs at the inferior margin, between the tubercle and the inferior angle
Longissimus cervicis	Lies under the splenius capitis, lateral to the semispinalis group and attaches to the t.p.s of upper four to six thoracic vertebrae (T1–T6)	Posterior tubercle of the transverse processes of C2–C6
Longissimus capitis	Transverse and articular processes of lower four cervical vertebrae	Posterior margin of mastoid process deep to the sternocleidomastoid (SCM) and splenius capitis

Spinalis (Central Column): Spinous Process to Spinous Process

Muscle	*Origin*	*Insertion*
Spinalis thoracis	Spines of T11 and T12 and L1 and L2	Spines of T1–T10
Spinalis cervicis (Not always present)	Spinous process of C7	Spinous process of C2
Spinalis capitis (Usually fused with semispinalis capitis)	C7 through T3 t.p.s	Attaches with the semispinalis capitis between the superior and the inferior nuchal lines of the occipital bone

Action	Dysfunction
Contracting unilaterally, acts as lateral flexors of the lumbar vertebrae. Acting bilaterally, extends the spine. The deep fibers help stabilize the lumbar vertebrae to the pelvis, and along with the psoas act as guy wires in the A–P plane. These fibers also decrease the lumbar curve, which is the opposite action as the psoas.	
As it does not attach to lumbar vertebrae, acting bilaterally can have bowstring effect, causing increased lumbar lordosis. Unilaterally, can laterally flex thoracic cage. They contract eccentrically when the trunk flexes forward. Through concentric contraction they extend the spine; isometrically, they control the position of the rib cage relative to the pelvis.[2]	
Acting bilaterally, extends the spine; unilaterally, causes lateral flexion.	

Action	Dysfunction
Same as lumbar fibers of iliocostalis described above.	
Same as thoracic fibers of iliocostalis described above.	
Acts as a significant stabilizer of the cervical spine along with the SCM and the posterior scalene. These muscles act as guy wires in three planes.[2] The longissimus capitis and cervicis also laterally flex and rotate the spine and head to the same side.	

Action	Dysfunction
Erector spinae muscles of both sides acting together extend the vertebral column and assist in maintaining erect posture; muscles on one side acting alone bend the vertebral column to the same side.	

TABLE 3-2 ANATOMY OF THE MUSCLES OF THE LUMBOPELVIC REGION—cont'd

Sixth Layer: Transversospinalis Muscles *(Fig. 3-10)*

The transversospinalis muscles consist of three groups that run from the t.p. to the spinous process.

Muscle	*Origin*	*Insertion*
Rotatores	Vertebra t.p.s	Base of spinous process of the first or second vertebra above
Multifidus	Largest and most medial of the lumbar back muscles; consists of a repeating series of fascicles, from the posterior sacrum, the aponeurosis of the erector spinae, the medial surface of the PSIS, and the posterior sacroiliac ligaments; fills the groove between the spinous process and the t.p. in the lumbar spine and forms the muscle mass over the sacrum, medial to the PSIS	Muscle runs superiorly and medially to attach to the spinous and mamillary process of L1 to L5; fibers also attach to capsule of lumbar facets and protect the capsule
Semispinalis group: Muscles run from transverse process to spinous process of the fourth to sixth vertebrae above.		
Semispinalis capitis (largest muscle in the back of the neck)	C7 through T6 t.p.s and C4 through C7 articular processes	Covered by the trapezius and splenius capitis in the cervical region, it inserts between the superior and the inferior nuchal lines of the occipital bone
Semispinalis cervicis	T1 through T6 t.p.s	Spinous processes of C2 through C5
Semispinalis thoracis	Transverse of T6–T12	Spines of T1–T6

Seventh Layer

Muscle	*Origin*	*Insertion*
Interspinales	Spinous processes of vertebrae	Adjacent spinous processes
Intertransversarii	Vertebrae t.p.s	Adjacent transverse processes

Gluteal Region *(Fig. 3-11)*

Muscle	*Origin*	*Insertion*
Gluteus maximus	Arises from posterior line of ilium, posterior aspect of the sacrum, coccyx, and sacrotuberous ligament	Ends in a thick tendinous lamina, passes lateral to the greater trochanter, and attaches to the iliotibial tract of the fascia lata; deeper fibers of the lower part attach to the gluteal tuberosity of the femur between vastus lateralis and the adductor magnus

Action	Dysfunction
Stabilizes the lumbar spine; helps control flexion and the shear force in the lower lumbar spine in forward flexion. Counters the action of the psoas.[2] Rotatores and multifidus, when acting bilaterally, extend the vertebral column; when acting unilaterally, bend the vertebral column to the same side and rotate the vertebrae to the opposite side.	
Extension of the cervical spine and head; increases cervical lordosis.	
Has a significant attachment to the spinous process of C-2 and an important stabilizing effect of C-2. Palpation: The semispinalis cervicis and capitis palpate as a rounded muscle bundle lateral to the cervical spinous processes. The trapezius and splenius muscles are flat by comparison.	
Semispinalis group, when acting bilaterally, extends the vertebral column, especially the cervical vertebrae and head, and rotates the head backwards; when acting unilaterally, draws the head to the opposite side.	

Action	Dysfunction
It has been suggested that these muscles may contribute to proprioceptive input.[2]	

Action	Dysfunction
Extensor and powerful lateral rotator of thigh. Inferior fibers assist in adduction; upper fibers are abductors. Balances trunk on femur; balances knee joint by means of the ITB; and is associated with bringing the trunk upright.	Is weak; inhibited by sustained contraction on the hip flexors, especially the iliopsoas, causing overuse of the hamstrings. Since it is often weak, hip extension may be initiated by the hamstrings, causing a dysfunctional gait pattern.
Principal muscle of abduction. Anterior fibers medially rotate and may assist in flexion; posterior fibers laterally rotate and may assist in extension of hip.	

TABLE 3-2 ANATOMY OF THE MUSCLES OF THE LUMBOPELVIC REGION—cont'd

Gluteal Region—*cont'd*

Gluteus medius	Broad, thick muscle arises from the outer surface of the ilium, between the anterior and the posterior gluteal lines, and the external aspect of ilium	Converges to a strong, flat tendon that is attached to the superior aspect of the lateral surface of greater trochanter
Gluteus minimus	Deep to the gluteus medius, smallest of three gluteals. Fan-shaped origin arises from outer surface of ilium between ASIS and greater sciatic notch	Attached to a ridge in the lateral surface of the anterior-superior portion of the greater trochanter and the hip joint capsule

Deep Lateral Rotators of the Hip

Muscle	*Origin*	*Insertion*
Piriformis	Anterior surface of sacrum among and lateral to sacral foramina one to four; margin of greater sciatic foramen and pelvic surface of sacrotuberous ligament	Passes out of the pelvis through the greater sciatic foramen and attaches by a rounded tendon to the superior-posterior border of greater trochanter; often blended with common tendon of obturator internus and gemelli
Quadratus femoris	Proximal part of lateral border of tuberosity of ischium	Attaches to posterior femur, extending down the intertrochanteric crest
Obturator internus	Internal or pelvic surface of obturator membrane and margin of obturator foramen, the inferior ramus of pubis and ischium	Travels from its origin toward the lesser sciatic foramen, making a right-angled bend over the surface of the ischium between the spine and the tuberosity; blends with the two gemelli, forming the "triceps coxae," inserting on the medial superior surface of the posterior greater trochanter
Gemellus superior	External surface of spine of ischium	Attaches with obturator internus on the medial surface of greater trochanter
Gemellus inferior	Upper part of tuberosity of ischium, below groove for obturator internus	Attaches with obturator internus (as above)
Obturator externus	Flat, triangular muscle covering the external surface of the anterior pelvic wall, arising from bone around the obturator foramen	Trochanteric fossa of femur

Lateral Pelvic Region *(See Fig. 3-6.)*

Muscle	*Origin*	*Insertion*
Quadratus lumborum (QL)	Internal lip of iliac crest and the iliolumbar ligament	Anterior surfaces of L1–L4 t.p.s and twelfth rib

Acting with gluteus medius, abducts the hip; the anterior fibers of the minimus rotate the hip medially. Both may also act as flexors of hip.	If weak, leads to lateral pelvic tilt; pelvis is high on the side of weakness; if contracted, pelvis is low on side of contracture.
	Tightness causes abduction and medial rotation of the thigh. In standing, there will be a lateral pelvic tilt, low on the side of shortness, accompanied by medial rotation of the femur.

Action	*Dysfunction*
Laterally rotates the extended thigh; abducts the hip when hip is flexed.	Sustained contraction in the piriformis may compress the sciatic nerve as it emerges through the sciatic notch, eliciting an ache, numbing, or tingling down the posterior thigh.
Laterally rotates and adducts the hip.	
The strongest lateral rotator of the hip with the gluteus maximus and the quadratus femoris. It acts as an abductor in the flexed position.	Lauren Berry, RPT, theorized that the obturator internus rolls into an inferior torsion with low back dysfunction, and this torsion could create a pulling force on the loose irregular connective tissue suspending the sciatic nerve, creating sciatica.
The two gemelli assist the obturator internus.	
Lateral rotation of the hip and assists in adduction.	

Action	*Dysfunction*
Concentric contraction causes lateral flexion of the trunk to the same side; eccentric contraction controls the rate of lateral bending to the opposite side; isometrically, helps to stabilize the trunk on the pelvis.[2] Palpation: Just lateral to the erector spinae at the top of the iliac crest.	Sustained contraction in the piriformis may compress the sciatic nerve as it emerges through the sciatic notch, eliciting an ache, numbing, or tingling down the posterior thigh.

TABLE 3-2 ANATOMY OF THE MUSCLES OF THE LUMBOPELVIC REGION—cont'd

Anterior Pelvic Region

Muscle	*Origin*	*Insertion*
Psoas major and minor	Divided into a superficial and a deep part—the deep part arises from the t.p.s, L1–L5 and the superficial part from the intervertebral discs of T12–L5 and the vertebral bodies T12–L5; lumbar plexus of nerves travels between the two parts and is susceptible to entrapment; psoas minor is an inconstant muscle from T12–L1 and inserts on the iliopubic eminence	Travels with the iliacus over the lateral pubic ramus to insert onto the lesser trochanter of the femur
Iliacus	Upper margin of iliac fossa and the inner lip of the iliac crest	Lesser trochanter

Abdominal Muscles

Muscle	*Origin*	*Insertion*
Rectus abdominus	Pubic crest and symphysis of pubic bone	Fifth to seventh cartilage of rib cage and xiphoid process
External oblique	Largest and most superficial of the abdominals, it attaches by fleshy digitations from the lower eight ribs, interdigitating with the serratus anterior	Attaches on the external lip of the iliac crest; on the inguinal ligament and the outer layer of the rectus sheath
Internal oblique	Intermediate lip of iliac crest; thoracolumbar fascia; lateral 2/3 of the inguinal ligament	Attaches on fleshy digitations to lower three ribs (9–12); the linea alba and aponeurosis help in formation of rectus sheath; also attaches with the transverse abdominus to the thoracolumbar fascia
Transverse abdominus	Costal—deep surfaces of costal cartilages of lower six ribs Vertebral—the thoracolumbar fascia from the t.p.s of the lumbar vertebrae Pelvic—internal lip of iliac crest, lateral third of inguinal ligament	Aponeurosis helps form the rectus sheath; attaches to xiphoid process and linea alba

Dysfunction of the abdominal muscles: The abdominal muscles are weak in a client with LBP, which causes an anterior pelvic tilt, increased lumbar lordosis, and a rounded-shoulder posture. Weak abdominals decrease the stability of the lumbopelvic region. They are often inhibited by tight extensors. Strengthening the abdominals decreases tension in the erector spinae, decreases the lumbar curve, and increases the stability of the lumbopelvic region. Shortness in the abdominals depresses the chest and contributes to thoracic kyphosis.

Action	Dysfunction
Because the psoas and the iliacus have the same insertion point and the same action, they are often described as one muscle, the iliopsoas; however, they are two distinct muscles. They are the main flexors of the hip; they also laterally rotate the hip; with the extremity fixed, the psoas flexes the trunk; unilateral contraction causes rotation of trunk to the opposite side. Acts to stabilize the lumbar spine on the pelvis, and as an anterior guy wire to balance the effect of the deep erectors.	Shortens, often owing to extensive sitting. This causes an increased lordosis, an anteriorly rotated pelvis, and an increased compressive load to the lumbar facets.
Has the same action as the psoas; they are the main flexors of the hip; also laterally rotates the hip; with the extremity fixed, the iliacus flexes the trunk; unilateral contraction causes rotation of the trunk to the opposite side. A sustained contraction causes an anterior torsion of the ilium, bringing the ASIS forward and down, and an extension of the lumbar facets, causing increased compression.[2]	

Action	Dysfunction
Flexes the vertebral column; pulls the sternum toward the pubis (antagonist of erector spinae); tenses the abdominal wall; all the abdominal muscles act to stabilize the trunk. They also eccentrically and isometrically contract to prevent excessive rotation and lateral flexion in the trunk.[2]	
Both sides acting together flex the vertebral column, rotate the trunk to the opposite side, and resist anterior torsion of the ilium.	
Same as for external oblique, except rotates toward same side, and bends the body laterally; also stabilizes the spine through the thoracolumbar fascia.	
Flattens abdominal wall.	

different mechanisms of injury: (1) a rotational strain that typically injures the facet joints, and (2) a compression force in flexion, which typically injures the disc. It is important to realize that in any given injury, the muscles, facets, and disc are all involved to some degree.

- This minor trauma leads to inflammation of the synovial lining of the capsule, called synovitis, and to sustained hypertonic contraction in the paraspinal muscles, usually on one side of the lower back. The inflammation releases enzymes that cause minimal degeneration of the articular cartilage.
- This phase of dysfunction is often followed by a phase of instability, which is demonstrated by abnormal, increased movement of the facets. There is laxity in the joint capsule and the annulus of the disc, and subluxation (partial dislocation) of the facets.
- The last phase of pathogenesis is the stable phase, in which the body responds to the continuing degeneration by laying down connective tissue and bone.
- Continuing degeneration leads to bony spurs under the periosteum, enlargements of the inferior and superior facets, periarticular fibrosis, and loss of motion.
- Changes in the disc begin in the dysfunctioning phase with small circumferential tears in the annulus that become larger and form a radial tear that passes from the annulus to the nucleus. These tears increase until there is internal disc disruption, which can lead to a disc herniation in which the nucleus shifts position.
- With further degeneration the normal disc height is reduced owing to the loss of proteoglycans and water.

FACTORS PREDISPOSING TO LOW BACK DYSFUNCTION AND PAIN

- *Functional factors:* Posture, joint dysfunction, muscle imbalances, deconditioning, fatigue, altered movement patterns, or emotional tension.
- *Structural factors:* rheumatologic, endocrine or metabolic, neoplastic (tumors), and vascular diseases; infection; congenital anomalies; referred pain from pelvic and abdominal disorders.

DIFFERENTIATION OF LOW BACK PAIN

LBP can be caused by many conditions in addition to functional problems, injury, or degeneration in the musculoskeletal system. These other causes are diverse but may be categorized as follows:

- Visceral diseases such as kidney stones or endometriosis
- Vascular diseases such as aneurysms
- Tumors, especially cancer that has metastasized from another site
- Stress-related disorders, such as adrenal exhaustion

The vast majority of LBP is caused by a mechanical disorder, a problem of function, and not pathology. The precise cause of the mechanical LBP can be difficult to determine. Sometimes it is a case of a frank injury, but more often there is an underlying chronic muscle imbalance, poor posture, or emotional stress. Assuming that the client's pain is caused by a mechanical disorder, there are two fundamental types of pain that refer into the leg(s): sclerotomal and radicular. The two types are differentiated by the quality of pain. These two types of referral are important to distinguish, because it helps you differentiate a simple mechanical disorder from a serious condition, such as a herniated disc.

Sclerotomal pain, the first type of referred pain, is caused by an injury to the paraspinal muscle, ligament, facet joint capsule, disc, or dura mater and can manifest locally and be referred to an extremity. For example, pain from a muscle strain in the lumbar region may be felt as a pain in the thigh in addition to the lower back. Usually, the sclerotomal referred pain is described as *deep, aching, and diffuse.*

Radicular pain, the second type of referred pain, is caused by an irritation of the spinal nerve root. If the sensory (dorsal) root is irritated, *sharp pain, numbing, or tingling that is well-localized* in dermatomes occurs. If there is compression of the motor (ventral) nerve root, in addition to the pain, numbing, and tingling, there may be a weakness in the muscles supplied by that nerve root (myotome) and a decrease in the response in the corresponding reflex. The most common cause of nerve root irritation is disc herniation. Nerve root pain is much more serious and requires an assessment by a doctor.

With these two categories in mind, we can enumerate nine common types of LBP. Note that these are artificial categories and that an injury or dysfunction usually has several of these causes of pain at the same time. For example, with a simple overuse injury of the lower back during gardening, muscles, ligaments (including joint capsule), and joint dysfunction would all typically be involved. These categories should be used as a guide to help differentiate simple from more complex problems.

COMMON TYPES OF DYSFUNCTION AND INJURY TO THE LOWER BACK

Muscle Strain

- *Cause:* Strains may be categorized as an acute episode, such as a sport injury; a cumulative stress, such as standing at work all day; or an acute episode overlaying a chronic problem. The causes are described in "Pathogenesis of Low Back Pain" on p. 85, and "Factors Predisposing to Low Back Dysfunction and Pain" on p. 96.
- *Symptoms:* Pain is usually described as diffuse and achy, either across the low back or on one side. Client reports being stiff and tight, especially with certain movements. Rest is relieving. An acute injury may present as a gripping spasm in the lower back that can be worse with active motion.
- *Signs:* Active motion localizes the area or line of pain. On palpation, muscles are tight and tender. Passive motion is not painful, except with full muscle stretch.
- *Treatment:* OM, CR-MET for weak muscles, and post-isometric relaxation (PIR) should be performed on short or tight muscles. Depending on the severity of the injury, the strain resolves in 1 to 4 weeks.

Ligament Sprain (Including Joint Capsule)

- *Cause:* The same causes described for "Muscle Strain" apply to ligaments.
- *Symptoms:* Pain is well localized and can be sharp in certain movements.
- *Signs:* Active and passive motion can be painful. Resisted motion usually is not painful. We assess the ligaments by movement characteristics in response to wave mobilization strokes. Ligamentous thickening in the lumbosacral region is either localized or diffuse. Localized thickening feels like a dense, leathery resistance to movement as P–A mobilization is introduced in that specific area. Diffuse thickening, such as that present in degenerative arthritis, reveals this same dense, leathery resistance to motion, but in a more diffuse area. We can palpate ligaments over the SIJ, and they feel thick and fibrous if they have shortened.
- *Treatment:* OM, passive motion in pain-free ranges and strengthening exercises should be performed. It often takes 6 weeks to 1 year to heal.

Fixation or Subluxation of the Vertebral Facets (Facet Syndrome)

- *Cause:* Poor posture, muscle imbalances, emotional or psychological tension leading to muscle hypertonicity, fatigue, and deconditioning all predispose to altered joint movement and potential fixation of the facets.
- *Symptoms:* Fixation or subluxation may be completely painless. They may present as either a sudden or an insidious onset of well-localized unilateral or bilateral paravertebral pain. It may radiate to the groin, buttock, or thigh.
- *Signs:* Active extension may cause a "catch" or abrupt restriction in area of the fixation. A decrease in lateral bending may occur, and flexion is cautious and limited. Hypertonicity and tenderness may be present in the paravertebral muscles. Motion palpation of the joint reveals loss of normal passive motion at the end range. SLR is normal.
- *Treatment:* OM and gentle mobilization of the joint are indicated. Refer to a chiropractic or osteopathic doctor for correction of fixation through manipulation.

Sacroiliac Joint Dysfunction

- *Cause:* Refer to cause of joint fixation described above.
- *Symptoms:* Pain in the buttock, groin, and posterior thigh pain can be sharp, dull, or aching; occasionally, pain below the knee occurs.
- *Signs:* Indicators of SIJ dysfunction are: an unlevelling of the pelvis measured at the PSISs or the ASISs, tenderness to palpation at the PSIS on one or both sides, a positive Kemp's test eliciting pain to the SIJ, and a diminished passive mobilization in P–A glide at the SIJ.
- Treatment: OM, especially gluteal work, including the sacrotuberous, sacrospinous, and interosseous ligaments of the SIJ, and balancing of the muscles attaching to the pelvis by means of MET, and mobilization of the SIJ are indicated treatments. To assess the need for an adjustment (manipulation), refer the client to a chiropractic or osteopathic doctor if he or she does not respond to treatment.

Piriformis Syndrome

- *Cause:* Piriformis syndrome is caused by a hypertonic piriformis muscle, often caused by SIJ dysfunction, or by overuse resulting from pelvic obliquity that leads to weakness of the G. medius of the ipsilateral side. The piriformis then overworks trying to substitute as an abductor.[1] In approximately 10% of the population, the sciatic nerve travels through the piriformis muscle, which causes a predisposition to sciatica when the muscle is in a sustained contraction. In the other 90%, the sciatic nerve travels under the muscle and is vulnerable to a sciatic irritation if the muscle is short and tight.

- ***Symptoms:*** Pain occurs in the middle of the buttock and can radiate down the posterior thigh, but rarely past the knee.
- ***Signs:*** Palpation reveals a tight and tender piriformis muscle; stretching the piriformis muscle by adducting the flexed hip over the supine client's extended leg increases buttock pain; straight leg raise (SLR) with internal rotation can increase the pain, which is relieved when the hip is externally rotated.
- ***Treatment:*** Perform MET and OM to relax, stretch, and reposition the piriformis; correct pelvic obliquities through MET; and facilitate weak G. medius.

Coccydynia

- ***Cause:*** Many patients report falling on the buttocks, or giving birth as the initial event. Often, articular and soft-tissue changes such as coccygeal ligamentous fibrosis, spasm in the muscles of the pelvic floor, and subluxation of the sacrococcygeal joint occur. Pain may be referred from the lumbar spine, SIJ, or pelvic viscera.
- ***Symptoms:*** Clients may experience coccyx pain, especially when sitting. It rarely refers to another location.
- ***Signs:*** Indicators of coccydynia are pain at the coccyx when sitting and the presence of thick, fibrotic ligaments about the coccyx.
- ***Treatment:*** Coccydynia treatment necessitates the release of the ligaments of the sacrococcygeal joint and the balancing of the musculature of the pelvic region. If patients do not respond to the soft-tissue therapy, refer them to a chiropractic or an osteopathic doctor to assess the need for manipulation of the subluxed or fixated joint.

Arthrosis (Arthritis): Degeneration of Vertebral Facets

- ***Cause:*** Arthrosis is caused by previous injury to the facets, chronic fixation of the facets, sustained muscle tension, muscle imbalances that create altered movement patterns through the joint, poor posture, deconditioning, and obesity.
- ***Symptoms:*** Clients experience a dull, achy pain that is worse in the morning, better with certain movements, and aggravated by others. Client feels diffuse stiffness in entire lower back.
- ***Signs:*** Arthrosis indicators are a chronic loss of lumbar extension with localized damage or a more complete loss of lumbar motion with diffuse changes in the affected joints. Another sign is a loss of passive motion ("joint play") at the involved facets.
- ***Treatment:*** Arthrosis clients need to move. Some pain accompanies increased movement, but it is a necessary pain to recover function in the joint. The general rule is that the client should be able to completely relax into the pain of moving the involved area. OM is helpful.

Spondylosis (Disc Degeneration)

- ***Cause:*** Spondylosis has the same factors described above under "Arthrosis."
- ***Symptoms:*** Clients report stiffness and a diffuse, dull ache across the lower back and gluteal region, relieved by short periods of rest. Long periods of rest increase stiffness. Stiffness and pain are worse in the morning.
- ***Signs:*** Decreased range of motion (ROM), especially extension, is an indicator of spondylosis. Disk degeneration is clear on x-rays.
- ***Treatment:*** OM and yoga are helpful. In addition, clients should walk briskly for 20 minutes or more per day. Traction on a slant board should be performed to promote fluid uptake in the disc.

Disc Herniation (Disc Bulge, Protrusion)

- ***Cause:*** Disc herniation is most common in young adults, between 30 and 40 years old. It is probably a result of repetitive stresses and eventual tearing of the annulus fibrosis, especially in rotation and forward flexion; however, some authors such as Kirkaldy-Willis and Bernard[8] suggest that the condition may start as a dysfunction caused by muscle imbalance. Sedentary lifestyle and obesity are risk factors.
- ***Symptoms:*** Clients report a sharp, nagging, or gripping pain in the gluteal region and the middle of the lower back. With disc herniation, pain, numbing, or tingling refers into the legs with irritation of the nerve root. Even at rest, pain is still present. Sitting usually worsens the symptoms.
- ***Signs:*** Often, the client presents to your office in slight forward flexion or in sustained lateral flexion (called antalgia). All active motion is painfully limited. Coughing, sneezing, and moving bowels may increase pain. The client usually has a positive SLR and well–leg-raising test, sensory changes in specific dermatomes, or weakness in the legs.
- ***Treatment:*** OM is done lightly, as deeper work could de-stabilize the spine. Work under the super-

vision of a doctor (chiropractic, osteopathic, or medical). Treatment should include strengthening, stabilizing, and proprioceptive reeducation.

Assessment

HISTORY QUESTIONS FOR CLIENTS WHO HAVE LOW BACK PAIN

Once you have ruled out the "red flags" (See Chapter 2, "Assessment & Technique") that may indicate a serious pathology and the need for an immediate referral to a doctor, you need to determine the "level of distress" in your client, that is, "how bad is the pain?" Questions such as "Did you sleep comfortably last night?" "Is the pain sharp or diffuse?" and "Do you have pain, numbing, or tingling in your legs?" will help you determine the following: (1) the appropriate depth of your massage strokes; (2) the appropirate amount of mobilization; (3) the necessity of referring your client to a doctor after your session; and (4) the recommendations for follow-up treatments. Refer to the section "Subjective Examination: Taking a History" in Chapter 2 for more information.

Did You Sleep Comfortably Last Night?

Pain that occurs when a client rolls over in bed is usually benign and caused by a mechanical problem. Pain that has decreased after a night's sleep usually indicates a mechanical problem, that is, muscle, ligament, or joint injury or dysfunction. Pain that is constant, even at rest is indicative of inflammation, such as a disc herniation, or a more serious pathology, such as a tumor, and needs referral to a doctor.

Is the Pain Sharp or Diffuse?

A sharp pain in the lower back or SIJ area usually indicates a joint problem. If there is a referral of sharp and gripping pain into the legs, then it indicates a nerve-root problem. A diffuse LBP can be muscle, ligament, or joint dysfunction or injury. Your active ROM assessment helps differentiate these various conditions (see "Summary of Possible Findings of Active ROM," p. 102).

Do You Have Pain, Numbing, Or Tingling in Your Legs?

If the client answers yes, you need to perform the SLR test before you begin your massage (see p. 103). If the SLR test creates intense, sharp pain in the legs, it typically indicates a nerve-root problem, and you need to refer your client to a doctor. If your client can lie on the table comfortably in the fetal position, you may perform gentle massage. The intention is to relax the client and not attempt to perform deep release of the muscles as that could be destabilizing. If the SLR creates a diffuse pain, numbing, or tingling in the legs, it is usually a sclerotomal pain (see "Differentiation of Low Back Pain"), and OM is indicated. As mentioned, a constant, gripping pain in the legs needs an immediate referral, and massage on the lower back is contraindicated.

OBSERVATION: CLIENT STANDING

Note any redness or swelling of the skin that may indicate inflammation and the need for much lighter pressure in your strokes. Also, notice any scars that may indicate a previous serious injury or previous surgery.

Observe any asymmetry in your client's posture from the posterior and the side views. A detailed postural assessment is for clients with chronic pain. If the client is experiencing acute pain, perform a postural assessment to determine if the sustained position, usually lateral bending (antalgia) or forward flexion, is a result of muscle spasms. If these postures are associated with acute pain, it usually indicates a facet syndrome or a disc protrusion. Postural assessment for acute pain is brief.

Posterior View

- **Is the client listing to the side?** It may be a result of chronic muscle and joint imbalance. If the client cannot straighten because of the pain, it usually indicates a disc protrusion or muscle strain in the QL or the iliopsoas.
- **Is the spine vertical?**
  - ☐ ***Position:*** Have your client stand in front of you.
  - ☐ ***Action:*** Place your index and middle finger on either side of the C7 spinous process, and slowly move your fingers down the spine to L5.
  - ☐ ***Observation:*** Does your client have a lateral curvature, called scoliosis, in the thoracic or lumbar spine? Lumbar scoliosis may be caused by sciatic neuritis, joint dysfunction, muscle spasm, irritation of the disc, or degenerative joint disease (DJD) (see Chapter 4 for further assessment of scoliosis).

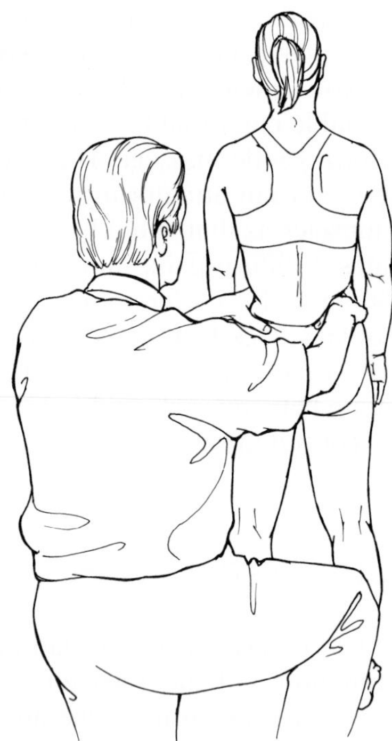

Figure 3-12. Assessment of iliac crests. To assess whether the iliac crests are level, place your fingertips on the top of the iliac crests.

- **Are the iliac crests level?** (Fig. 3-12)
  - *Action:* Place your fingertips on the iliac crests.
  - *Observation:* If they are uneven, then make a note of the high side in your chart. Compare this finding with a seated assessment. If the iliac crests are uneven in standing and level sitting, there may be a leg-length difference or pronation in the ankle on the short side. If they remain uneven in standing and sitting, it indicates a muscle and joint dysfunction in the lumbopelvic region.
- **Is the head tilted to one side or balanced in the midline?**
- **Are the shoulder heights equal?** Place your index fingers horizontally under the inferior angles of the scapulae.

Side View

- The earlobe should be in line with the upright acromion process. The most common dysfunction is the forward-head posture.
- **Observe the lumbar curve from the side to see if it is increased or decreased.**
  - *Action:* Place your index fingers on the ASIS and the PSIS on the side the closest to you.
  - *Observation:* The ASIS and the PSIS should be approximately level with a normal curve.
- **Correct the client's standing posture.**
  - *Action:* Adjust the lumbar spine so that the ASIS and the PSIS on the same side are level. Next, bring the head back if necessary so that the opening of the ear is over an upright acromion.

MOTION ASSESSMENT

Start by asking your client if any particular motion brings up the pain. Have your client perform that motion last. While the client performs the movements, note the ROM and whether the movement is painful. If it is painful, ask the client about the quality of the pain and its location.

Forward Flexion

- *Position:* Have your client stand in front of you, feet placed shoulder-width apart.
- *Action:* Ask the client to bend forward as far as comfortable, with knees kept straight (Fig. 3-13).

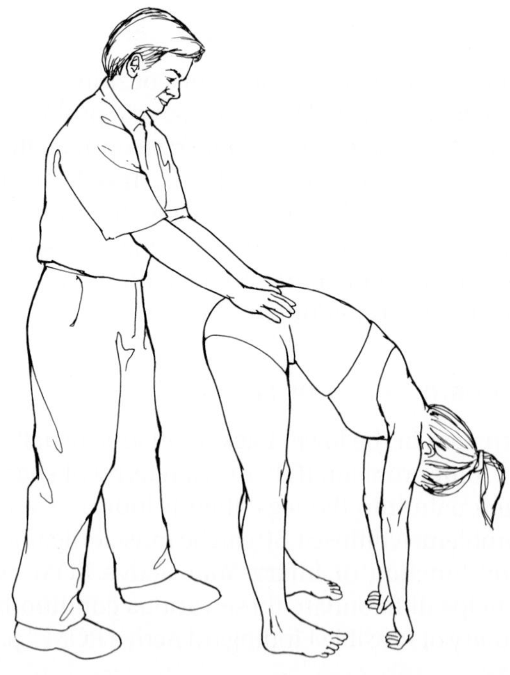

Figure 3-13. Assessment of active flexion. To assess active flexion in the lumbopelvic region, ask the client to bend forward as if she is going to touch her toes. Tell her to stop if it becomes painful. Have her bend her knees when coming back to standing.

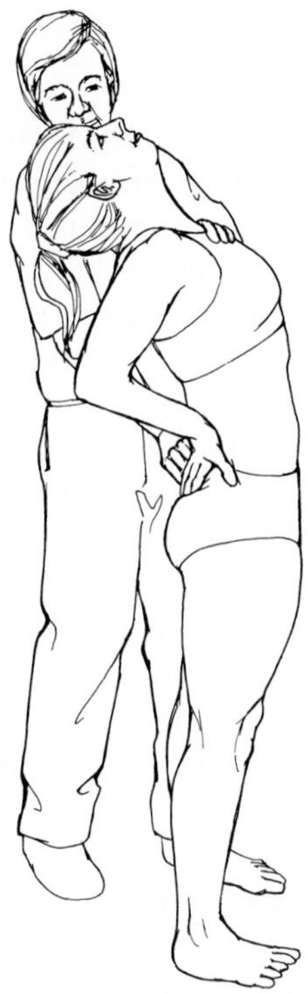

Figure 3-14. Assessment of extension. To assess extension, have the client place her hands on her lower back and bend backwards to her comfortable limit.

- *Observation:* Flexion is a combination of hip, lumbar, and thoracic motion. The trunk should flex at least to 90°, that is, parallel to the floor. You can measure the distance from the fingertips to the floor. Observe the spine from the side. The lumbar curve should flatten in bending forward. If the lumbar lordosis is maintained, it indicates erector spinae muscle spasms or hypomobility of the joints. Diffuse soreness or pain in the lower back indicates an injury to the muscle, ligament, or joint. A sharp pain in the lower back indicates joint involvement. A dramatic limitation of motion indicates inflammation and swelling and a more serious injury.

Extension

- *Position:* The therapist stands at the client's side and asks the client to stand with feet shoulder-width apart and palms on the lower back (Fig. 3-14).
- *Action:* Have the client bend backward to a comfortable limit, keeping the knees straight.
- *Observation:* The ROM of lumbar extension is approximately 30°. Does lumbar spine curve? Or is the client bending only at the hips? Active extension is the best test for joint dysfunction and injury since extension compresses the facets. A sharp local pain in extension indicates a facet syndrome. With a facet syndrome, diffuse pain, numbing, or tingling may refer into the gluteal region, thigh, and leg. A sharp, dermatomal pain in extension often indicates a nerve-root problem, as extension also closes down the IVF slightly.

For clients who have chronic pain or dysfunction, a more accurate assessment of pure lumbar extension may be done with your client lying prone on the massage table, resting on his or her elbows, with the pelvis remaining on the table. Is there a round curve in the lumbar spine? If there is limitation of this motion, it indicates a chronic degenerative condition or hypomobility of the joints. A loss of motion and stiffness indicates muscle and connective tissue shortening, including ligaments.

Side Flexion

- *Position:* The client stands with feet shoulder-width apart and arms at sides. The therapist stands behind the client and places both hands on the client's hips to stabilize the pelvis so that it does not sway or rotate (Fig. 3-15).

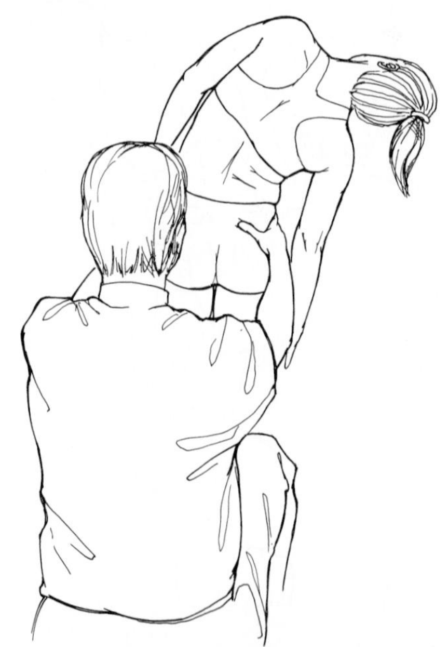

Figure 3-15. Assessment of lateral flexion. To assess lateral (side) flexion, stand behind your client and hold her pelvis to prevent any rotation or swaying. Ask her to slide her hand down the side of her leg to her comfortable limit.

- *Action:* Ask the client to slide one hand down the side of his or her leg without rotating the trunk.
- *Observation:* The client should be able to slide his or her hand down equally on both sides, almost to knee level (approximately 30°). The lumbar spine should form a smooth curve in side bending. If there is a sharp angle, then it indicates hypomobility at the facet joints. Pain on the bending side indicates a joint problem because the facet is being compressed. Pain, stiffness or tightness on the opposite side often indicates QL irritability.

Kemps Test (Quadrant Test)

- *Intention:* To help differentiate narrowing of the IVF caused by degeneration or SIJ problems.
- *Position:* Assume the same position as the side-bending test.
- *Action:* Have the client slide his or her hand down the back of the leg, one leg at a time, to a comfortable limit.
- *Observation:* Kemps test compresses the IVF and SIJ slightly and elicits referral of sharp pain into the leg with disc problems, diffuse referred pain with SIJ problems, or LBP with sacroiliac or lumbar joint dysfunctions and injuries (Fig. 3-16).

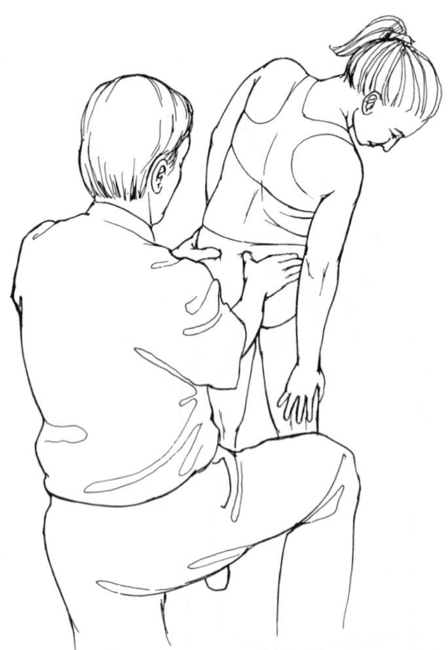

Figure 3-16. Kemps test. Kemps test is used to help differentiate sacroiliac problems and compression of a nerve caused by narrowing of the IVF. Have your client slide her hand down the back of her leg. This combines rotation and extension of the spine and compresses the IVF on the side of turning.

Summary of Possible Findings of Active Range of Motion

A dramatic limitation of the ROM is indicative of a facet syndrome, a disc injury, or a moderate to severe strain or sprain of the musculoligamentous tissues. If the ROM is normal, and the movement elicits diffuse LBP, then it is usually a muscle problem. If active motion is slightly decreased, and the motion elicits a sharp back pain, then it often indicates a joint or ligament problem. If there is a generalized loss of all motions without pain, just stiffness, there is often a diffuse arthrosis or spondylosis in the lumbosacral spine. Diffuse loss of motion, joint stiffness, and referral of pain into the legs with extension and Kemps test may indicate foraminal encroachment, a degenerative condition in which the IVF is narrowed and the nerve root is being compressed. This requires a referral to a chiropractic or osteopathic doctor.

BALANCE ASSESSMENT

- *Intention:* To assess chronic LBP. Chronic LBP often leads to balance problems from instability and dysfunction of the proprioceptors.
- *Position:* Have your client stand next to the wall so that he or she can place a hand on the wall for support while performing this test. The therapist stands facing client.
- *Action:* Ask your client to lift one foot off the ground a few inches and attempt to balance on the other leg for 10 seconds. Repeat on the other side.
- *Observation:* Chronic LBP patients and geriatric patients often have problems with balance. If your client cannot balance comfortably on each leg, then have him or her do this as an exercise at home for 30 seconds to 1 minute on each leg, once a day.

SEATED ASSESSMENT

- **Place your thumbs under the PSISs to see if they are level.** An unlevelling is called a pelvic obliquity. This may be a result of muscle spasms, DJD, sciatic neuritis, disc herniation, or joint fixation in the SIJs or lumbar spine.
- **Assess sitting posture.** Is the client's posture slumped? Correct a slumped posture by introducing a slight lumbar curve and placing the client's head so that the opening of the ear is over the upright acromion (see Fig. 5-12).

PALPATION

Client Seated

- Most of the palpation is done in the context of performing the strokes. A scanning palpation is done in a few areas to rule out a serious lower back problem. Severe pain with medium pressure to the bone is a red flag for serious pathology.
- Press with a medium amount of pressure on the following structures: the sacrum, both PSISs, each spinous process in the lumbar spine, the gluteal muscles, and the paraspinal muscles.

Client in the Side-Lying Position

- *Intention:* Perform palpation to assess the condition of the soft tissue and joints of the lumbosacral region; palpation is best accomplished with the client in the side-lying position.
- *Position:* Ask the client to lie in the fetal position, with a pillow between the knees. This is the most relaxed position for the soft tissue of the spine.
- *Action:* Begin by rocking the client gently. This rocking movement introduces a wave into the body, and like sonar, returns information to the therapist regarding the level of relaxation in the client. A guarded, tense person is rigid to this motion, and a relaxed, open person is pliable and resilient. Next, use the supported-thumb position to perform a series of slow P–A wave mobilization strokes along the SIJ and the lumbar spine (Fig. 3-17).

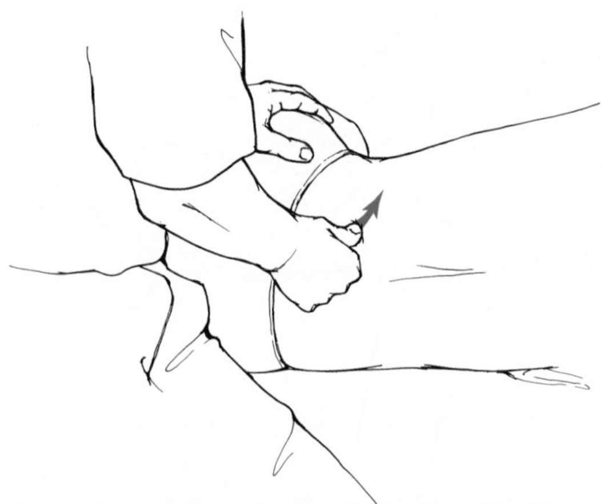

Figure 3-17. Palpation in the side-lying position. Assess the soft tissue and the motion of the spine.

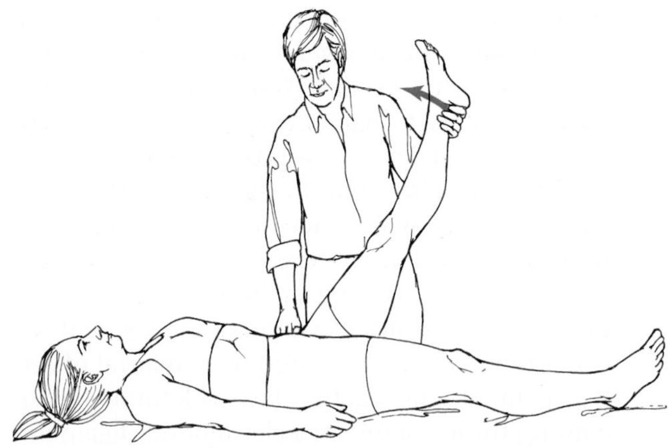

Figure 3-18. SLR test. The SLR test is performed if there is pain, numbing, or tingling into the leg. The therapist slowly lifts the client's leg off the table until there is pain in the leg or until there is tissue tension, usually occurs at approximately 70°.

- *Observation*
  - A healthy lumbosacral spine is resilient and bends with your pressure. The strokes are relaxing and completely pain-free.
  - Inflamed tissue is painful. The degree of pain indicates the level of inflammation.
  - Hypertonic muscles have a tight, springy resistance to movement.
  - Thickened soft tissue in the ligaments and capsule has a thick resistance to your movement.
  - A localized degeneration has a hard resistance to movement, whereas more diffuse degeneration has a similar hard resistance in a broader area.

OTHER TESTS

Straight–Leg-Raising Test

- *Intention:* Perform the SLR test if the client has pain radiating to the leg (Fig. 3-18). The test helps differentiate a nerve root lesion from sclerotomal pain.
- *Position:* The client is supine. The therapist stands at the side of the table by the leg with the referred pain.
- *Action:* The therapist grasps the client's leg just proximal to the ankle and slowly lifts it up, keeping the knee straight, until there is pain or until an elevation of 70° is attained.
- *Observation:* The test is positive if lifting the leg increases or initiates leg pain, numbing, or tingling below the knee before 70° of elevation. Note the

quality and location of the pain. Intense, sharp pain usually indicates nerve-root tension, probably an injury to the disc. Pain that is only in the back indicates a ligament sprain or facet syndrome. If the client has a positive SLR test, then perform the SLR test on the "good leg." If the test elicits pain below the knee on the involved leg, it indicates a much more severe disc problem. If the SLR test is negative, that is, there was no aggravation of leg pain with elevation of the leg, and the client reports that they often have referral of diffuse pain into the leg, they have sclerotomal pain coming from a joint, muscle, tendon, ligament, etc. (see "Differentiation of Low Back Pain").

Techniques

MUSCLE ENERGY TECHNIQUE

Remember that clients should never perform MET if it is painful.

- In this chapter, MET variations for the piriformis and iliopsoas are shown within the context of the strokes.
- Refer to Chapter 7 for evaluation of the hip joint and for information on MET for the hip abductors, adductors, TFL, and iliotibial band (ITB).

Muscle Energy Technique for Acute Low Back Pain

1. Contract-Relax for the Lumbar Erector Spinae

- ☐ ***Intention:*** An acute low back can be irritated if the facet joints are moved too much. A safe and effective way to reduce muscle hypertonicity in the lumbosacral region is isometric contraction of the lumbar extensors. If this motion is painful, then begin with an RI MET, illustrated below.
- ☐ ***Position:*** Client is side lying in the fetal position, with a pillow between the knees and hips flexed to 90°. To prevent trunk rotation, make sure the client lines up the top shoulder over the lower shoulder and the top hip over the lower hip. The therapist places one hand on the sacrum and one hand on the midthoracic region.
- ☐ ***Action:*** Instruct the client to resist as you press P–A on the spine for approximately 5 seconds. Cue the client by saying, "Don't let me move you." Press for 5 seconds, and then have the client relax. Remember, the client's body should not move as he or she resists your pressure. These are isometric contractions. I often alternate the CR and RI techniques several times, which reduces the hypertonicity in the lumbar erectors and decreases the pain in the lower back.

2. Reciprocal Inhibition for the Lumbar Erector Spinae

- ☐ ***Intention:*** An acute low back may be irritated if the extensor muscles are contracted. A safe and effective way to reduce muscle hypertonicity in the lumbosacral region is isometric contraction of the flexors of the trunk, the iliopsoas. When the iliopsoas contracts, the lumbar extensors relax by means of RI (Fig. 3-19).
- ☐ ***Position:*** Client is side lying in the fetal position, with a pillow between the knees and hips flexed to 90°. The therapist places one hand on the anterior thigh just above the knee and the other hand on the lower back.
- ☐ ***Action:*** Have the client resist your attempt to lightly pull the thigh into extension, that is, toward the foot of the table. Cue the client by saying, "Don't let me move you." Hold for 5 seconds. Alternate the CR and RI techniques several times, which reduces the hypertonicity in the lumbar erectors and decreases the pain in the lower back.
- ☐ ***Observation:*** The lumbar spine should not arch during the RI. Place your hand on the client's back and have him keep the spine against your hand as he resists.

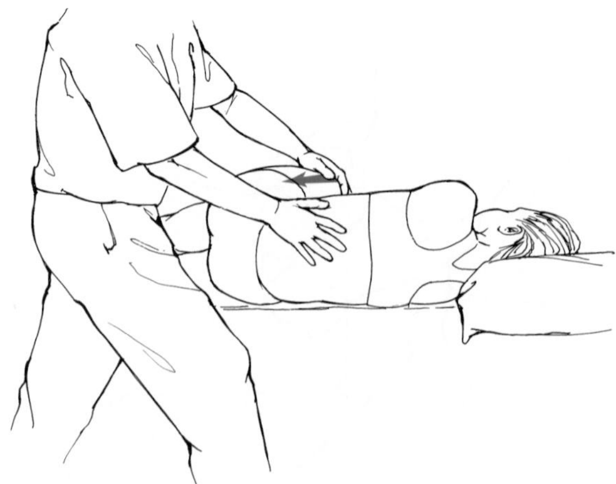

Figure 3-19. RI MET for the lumbar erector spinae. To perform RI on the extensors of the spine, have your client resist as you gently try to pull her thigh into extension.

Muscle Energy Technique to Release Hypertonic Muscles of the Lumbopelvic Region

3. Contract-Relax Muscle Energy Technique for the Lumbar Erector Muscles in the Subacute or Chronic Phase

- *Intention:* To reduce muscle hypertonicity by performing CR MET. Hip extension engages the lumbar erectors. If the erectors palpate as hypertonic, then CR MET is a safe and effective way to reduce their hypertonicity (Fig. 3-20).
- *Position:* Client is side lying. Have the client straighten the top leg, making sure the knee is fully extended, and lift it off the pillow and into a few degrees of extension.
- *Action:* Instruct the client to resist as you attempt to press the client's extended leg forward for approximately 5 seconds. It is often helpful to tap lightly on the lumbar extensors to give a sensory cue to the muscles. You might say, "Feel these muscles working," as they contract. Have the client put the leg back on the pillow and lie in the fetal position. Next, place your hand on the top of the client's thigh just above the knee and have the client resist as you attempt to pull the thigh into extension, as was described in the section "Reciprocal Inhibition for the Lumbar Erector Spinae." Repeat this cycle three to five times.

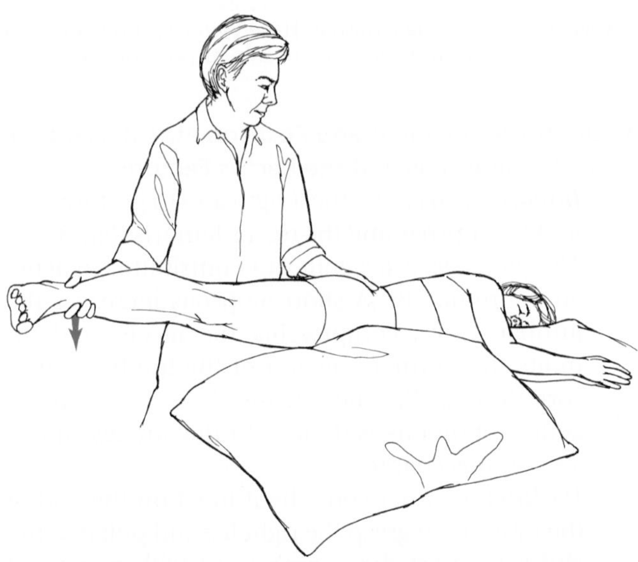

Figure 3-20. CR MET for the lumbar erector muscles in the subacute or chronic phases. To release hypertonicity in the extensors in the client who is not in acute pain, have her straighten her leg and gently lift it off the pillow. Have her resist as you lean your body into her leg, attempting to push it forward.

4. Contract-Relax and Reciprocal Inhibition Muscle Energy Technique for the Piriformis

- *Intention:* To perform CR MET to release the hypertonicity of the piriformis.
- *Position:* Client is side lying in the fetal position with a pillow between the knees.
- *Action:* Have the client lift his or her leg off the pillow and resist as you gently attempt to press it back down to the pillow for approximately 5 seconds (Fig. 3-21). To perform RI on the piriformis, have your client squeeze his or her knees together. This contracts the adductors and reciprocally inhibits the piriformis. You can give a sensory cue by lightly attempting to pull the client's knees apart.

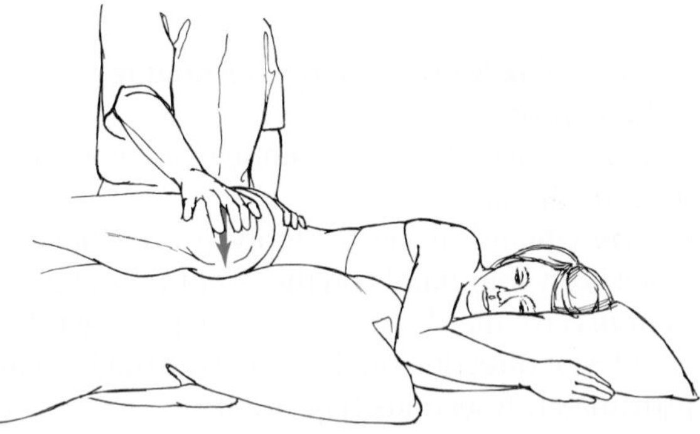

Figure 3-21. CR MET for the piriformis. Have your client lift her leg off the pillow a few inches, parallel to the floor, and resist as you gently attempt to press it back down to the pillow for approximately 5 seconds.

5. Postisometric Relaxation of the Piriformis

- *Intention:* The intention is to lengthen the piriformis. The piriformis is typically short and tight, so it compresses not only the SIJ but also the sciatic nerve. PIR of the piriformis should be performed on chronic clients only.
- *Position:* The client is supine. To lengthen the right piriformis, have the client cross the right leg over the left, placing the right foot on the table on the outside of the left knee (Fig. 3-22). You may stand on either side, facing the table (although I prefer to stand on the client's left side). Use your superior hand to hold the client's right ASIS to stabilize the pelvis, and place your left hand on the lateral aspect of the client's right distal thigh.
- *Action:* Have the client resist as you attempt to pull the leg across the body and push the knee toward the table for approximately 5 seconds. Relax, and as the client relaxes, pull the leg further across the body and press the knee further toward the table, until there is pain or you feel

the resistance barrier. Repeat this CR–lengthen cycle several times.

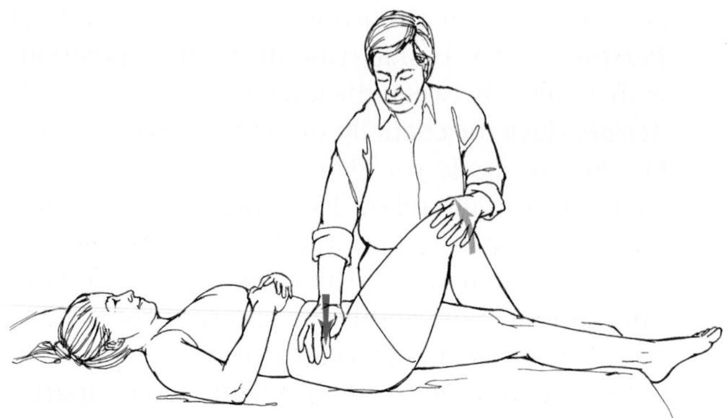

Figure 3-22. PIR of the piriformis.

6. Contract-Relax Muscle Energy Technique for the Iliopsoas

- *Intention:* Use CR MET to reduce the hypertonicity of the iliopsoas.
- *Position:* Stand in the 45° footward position and place both your hands on the client's distal thigh.
- *Action:* Have the client resist as you press gently in an inferior direction on the top of the thigh for approximately 5 seconds (Fig. 3-23).

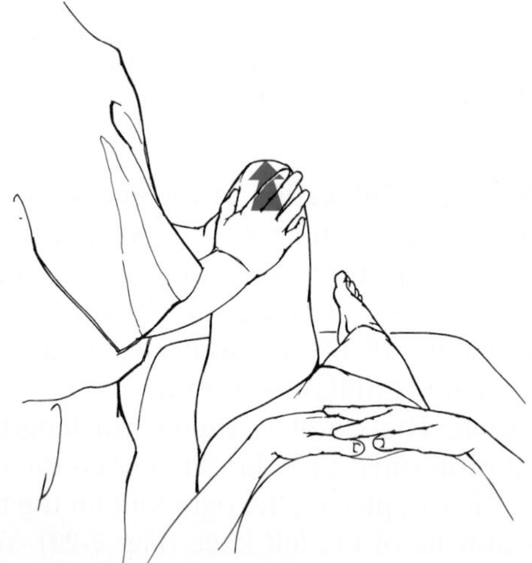

Figure 3-23. CR MET of the iliopsoas. Therapist stands in the 45° footward position and places both hands on the client's distal thigh. Have the client resist as you press gently in an inferior direction on the top of her thigh for approximately 5 seconds.

7. Reciprocal Inhibition Muscle Energy Technique for the Iliopsoas

- *Intention:* To perform RI to reduce the pain and hypertonicity of the iliopsoas by contracting the hip extensors, antagonists of the iliopsoas.
- *Position:* Stand in a 45° headward direction and place both your hands on the client's shin or posterior thigh.
- *Action:* Have your client resist as you press gently in a headward direction for approximately 5 seconds. This engages the hip extensors, and reciprocally inhibits the iliopsoas, the main hip flexors (Fig. 3-24).

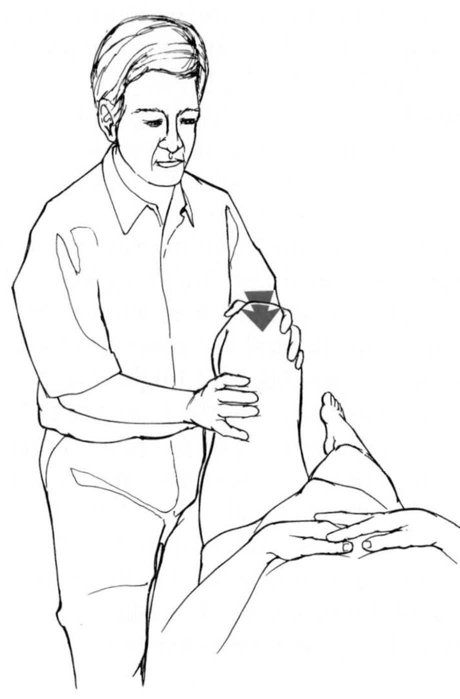

Figure 3-24. RI of the iliopsoas. Have your client resist as you press in a superior direction on her shin or posterior thigh.

8. Length Assessment and Postisometric Relaxation for the Iliopsoas and the Rectus Femoris

- *Intention:* To assess the length and to perform PIR for the iliopsoas and the rectus femoris (Fig. 3-25). The iliopsoas is a significant contributor to acute and chronic LBP. A short iliopsoas increases the lumbar curve, compressing the facets, and inhibits the normal function of the lumbar extensors through RI. The release of the iliopsoas for acute conditions is done with the strokes shown later in this chapter.
- *Position:* Instruct your client to sit on the end of the table, then grasp the right leg and pull it to the chest. Support the client's head with one hand and place the other hand on the flexed leg. Ask your client to tuck his or her chin, and then rock the client back onto the table, resting the head on a pillow. The left leg will hang over the edge of the

table. The knee should be pulled to the chest just enough to keep the lower back flat on the table.

- ☐ ***Observation:*** If the length of the iliopsoas is normal, then the left thigh will be parallel to the floor or lower. If the length of the rectus is normal, the lower leg will be perpendicular to the floor. If the TFL is short, the leg will be abducted slightly.
- ☐ ***Action:***
  - ☐ To lengthen the iliopsoas, perform PIR. Have the client resist as you press down on his or her left thigh. Press for 5 seconds, and after the client has relaxed for a few seconds, press down on the distal thigh to a new resistance barrier, stretching the iliopsoas and anterior hip joint capsule.
  - ☐ To lengthen the rectus femoris, have the client resist as you use your leg to press into the client's leg, attempting to press the leg into further flexion. Press for 5 seconds, have the client relax, then press again into a new resistance barrier.
  - ☐ Repeat the CR–lengthen cycle several times.

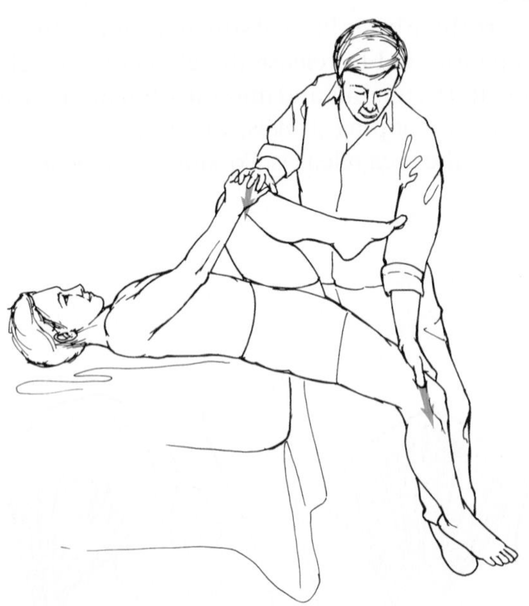

Figure 3-25. Length assessment and postisometric release of the iliopsoas.

9. Postisometric Relaxation of the Quadratus Lumborum

- ☐ ***Intention:*** To lengthen the QL (Fig. 3-26). The QL is typically tight in chronic LBP, and performance of PIR is a safe and effective way to lengthen it.
- ☐ ***Position:*** Client is side lying, with the top leg straightened, the bottom leg flexed. You may need to cue the client by asking him or her to hike the hip to resist you as you pull the leg. Explain that you want him or her to use the muscles on the top of the hip (crest of the ilium) to resist your pull, holding the hip toward the shoulder.
- ☐ ***Action:***
  - ☐ Hold the client's leg above the ankle and abduct the leg approximately 20° from the midline. Instruct the client to resist, saying, "Don't let me move you," as he or she pulls the leg for approximately 5 seconds. Make sure the client's body is neutral and not rotated forward or backward. If the leg is too heavy or creates discomfort in this position, then place pillows under the top leg to support it, or tuck the leg under your armpit. After the client holds for 5 seconds, have him or her relax, and as the client relaxes, pull the leg and stretch the quadratus. Then repeat the CR–lengthen cycle a few times. At the end of the PIR cycle, use PIR to help "set" the QL in its new lengthened position. Place your fist on the heel of the client's straightened leg and have the client resist as you push headward for approximately 5 seconds.
  - ☐ If the QL is acute, flex the client's hips in the fetal position. Face footward, place your hands on the iliac crest, and ask client to resist as you gently push the ilium inferiorly.

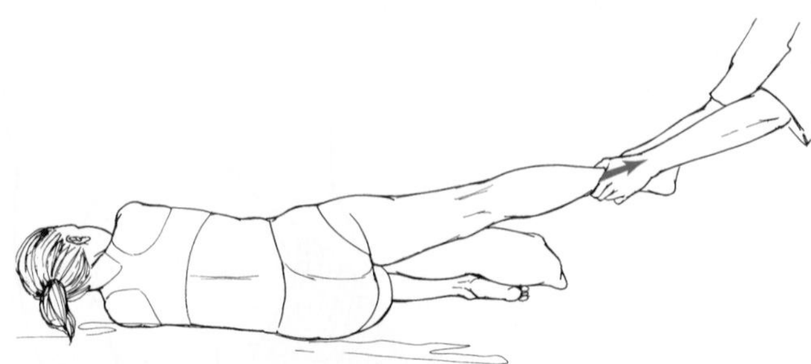

Figure 3-26. PIR of the QL.

Isotonic Muscle Energy Technique for the Gluteus Maximus

- ☐ ***Intention:*** Hip extension is primarily accomplished by the hamstrings and G. max. and secondarily by the erector spinae (Fig. 3-27). Weakness in the G. max. is common and may cause the lumbar erectors to initiate hip extension, which hyperextends the lumbar spine and compresses the facets. MET helps facilitate (strengthen) the G. max.

- *Position:* Have your client lie face down on the table and bend one knee to 90°. Place one hand on the G. max. and the other hand on the back of the thigh.
- *Action:* Instruct the client to lift his or her thigh slowly off the table a few inches and to hold it for 5 seconds. This movement is accomplished primarily by the G. max. Tap the muscle lightly with your fingertips and say, "Feel this muscle working," as the client is contracting. Repeat this five times. Perform this action on both sides.
- *Observation:* Note the trunk position. Make sure your client does not rotate his or her trunk to perform this motion.

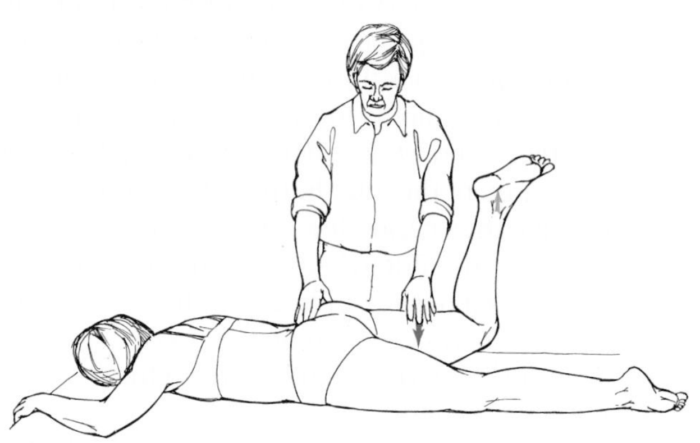

Figure 3-27. Isotonic-MET for the gluteus maximus. With her knee flexed, have the client slowly lift her thigh off the table. It is important to perform the movement slowly to isolate the gluteus maximus.

ORTHOPEDIC MASSAGE

Level I-Lumbosacral

1. Release of Gluteus Medius and Minimus

- *Anatomy:* Gluteal fascia; G. max., medius, and minimus; and superior cluneal nerves (Fig. 3-28)
- *Dysfunction:* The G. medius is a strong abductor of the hip, and its dysfunction contributes to pelvic unlevelling, and LBP. Although the G. medius and minimus tend to be weak, they may also be hypertonic, known as *tightness weakness,* or weak because of RI of hypertonic adductors. The superior cluneal nerves may become entrapped in the gluteal fascia just below the crest of the ilium.

Position

- Therapist Position (TP)—standing, facing the line of the stroke
- Client Position (CP)—side-lying, in the fetal position, with a pillow under the head and between the knees, with the hands resting on each other in a "prayer position"

Strokes

There are three basic lines of strokes to assess the region by palpation and to release the gluteal fascia, cluneal nerves, and G. medius and minimus. Begin superficially with broad, scooping strokes, and proceed with deeper strokes as the area releases. Possible hand positions in-

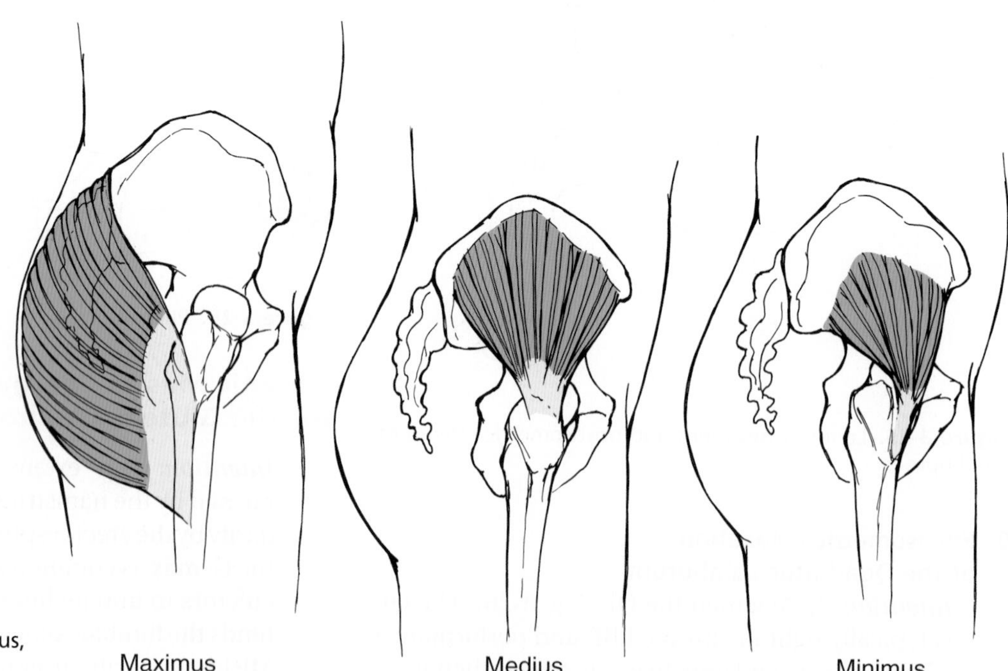

Figure 3-28. Gluteus maximus, medius, and minimus.

clude double thumb, braced thumb using the pisiform of the opposite hand, the fifth metacarpophalangeal (MCP) area of a soft fist, or the forearm and elbow area, which can be angled to be rounded, flat, or fleshy.

1. Begin your spinal sessions by placing both hands on the gluteal region and gently rocking the client's entire body with a rhythm of approximately one cycle per second. This rocking creates a wave in the client's body that is like sonar and that reflects the client's level of relaxation or guarding. It is also a way to make nurturing contact with the client.
2. The first line of strokes begins midway between the greater trochanter and the iliac crest in the belly of the G. medius (Fig. 3-29). Perform a series of 1-inch scooping strokes, perpendicular to the line of the G. medius. Begin another series of strokes approximately 1 inch below your previous stroke, and continue this line of strokes to the area between the PSIS and the greater trochanter.
3. A second line of strokes begins approximately 1 to 3 inches from the greater trochanter at the myotendinous junctions of G. medius and minimus. Start at the superior aspect of this area and work inferiorly in 1-inch scooping strokes around the greater trochanter.
4. The third line is along the superior portion of the iliac fossa to release the gluteal fascia, superior cluneal nerves, and superior portion of the G. medius and minimus. Begin at the most lateral-superior aspect of the ilium, using 1-inch scooping strokes and move your hands more medially and inferiorly as you work down the iliac fossa.

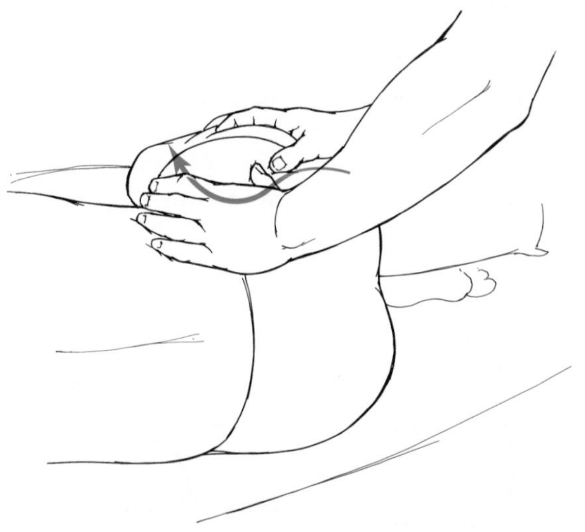

Figure 3-29. Double-thumb technique to release the gluteal fascia, cluneal nerves, and the gluteus medius and minimus.

2. Release of Gluteus Maximus and Sacrospinous and Sacrotuberous Ligaments

- *Anatomy*: G. max. and the sacrospinous and sacrotuberous ligaments. Work the G. max. superficially; work the sacrotuberous and sacrospinous ligaments deeply (Fig. 3-30).
- *Dysfunction:* In dysfunction, the G. max. is weak. It may be hypertonic, especially with hypertonic hamstrings, and a loss of the lumbar curve might occur. The ligaments tend to develop fibrotic change because of excessive tension caused by pelvic obliquity (unlevelling), hyperlordosis, inflammation from trauma, etc. Microscopically, the sacrotuberous ligament tends to develop an inferior torsion and needs to be repositioned superiorly. Fibrosis of the ligaments of the coccyx is a common cause of coccydynia (coccyx pain).

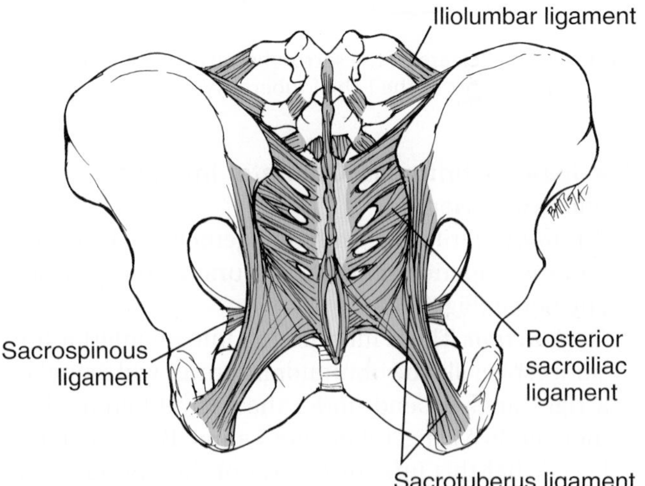

Figure 3-30. Sacrotuberous and sacrospinous ligaments.

Position

- TP—standing
- CP—side-lying, fetal position, with the top part of the client's body angled diagonally forward on the table, and the pelvic area at the edge of the table, the ischial tuberosity facing toward you

Strokes

Work three lines of strokes from the sacrum and coccyx to the ischial tuberosity.

1. Lift the G. max. muscle in short, scooping, inferior to superior (I–S) strokes from below the PSIS to the ischial tuberosity. Begin another series of I–S strokes just below the first line, from the lateral portion of the sacrum and coccyx, and again continue to the ischial tuberosity.

2. Release the sacrotuberous ligament by penetrating underneath the G. max. in the same areas as described in the previous stroke. Perform a series of deep, scooping I–S strokes, lifting this ligament superiorly (Fig. 3-31). Begin at the sacrum and coccyx and work to the ischial tuberosity.
3. Release the sacrospinous ligament from the area of the sacrococcygeal joint to the ischial spine. Perform a series of strokes, lifting the ligament superiorly.

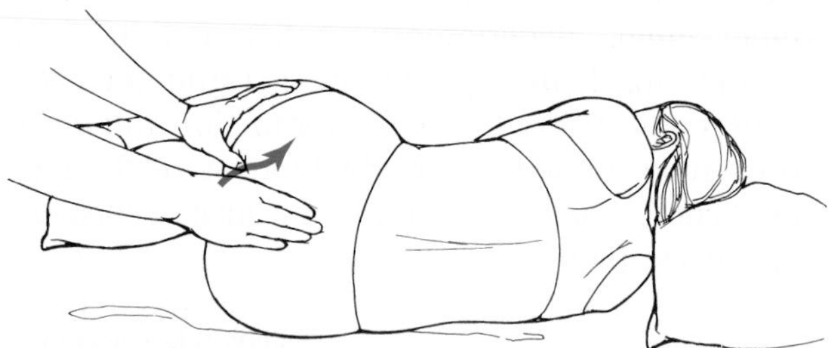

Figure 3-31. Release of the sacrotuberous ligament from the sacrum and coccyx to the ischial tuberosity.

3. Release of Piriformis, Obturator Internus, and Sciatic Nerve

- *Anatomy*: Piriformis, inferior gemellus, quadratus femoris, superior gemellus, obturator internus, sciatic nerve (Fig. 3-32).
- *Dysfunction*: These muscles roll into an inferior torsion, especially the obturator internus, which makes a right-angled bend under the sacrotuberous ligament at the ischial tuberosity. Lauren Berry, RPT, believed that this inferior torsion of the obturator internus and its fascia could have a tethering effect on the sciatic nerve, creating sciatica. The sciatic nerve can become entrapped under a hypertonic piriformis, which is a condition called the *piriformis syndrome*. It can also become entrapped in the space between the ischial tuberosity and the greater trochanter.

Position

- TP—standing
- CP—side lying, fetal position

Strokes

1. Palpate the piriformis and perform a CR and RI MET for this muscle. This is the same technique described in the MET section on p. 105.
2. Perform a series of lifting, scooping strokes perpendicular to the line of the fiber of the piriformis (Fig. 3-33). Begin just inferior to the PSIS and continue to the greater trochanter.

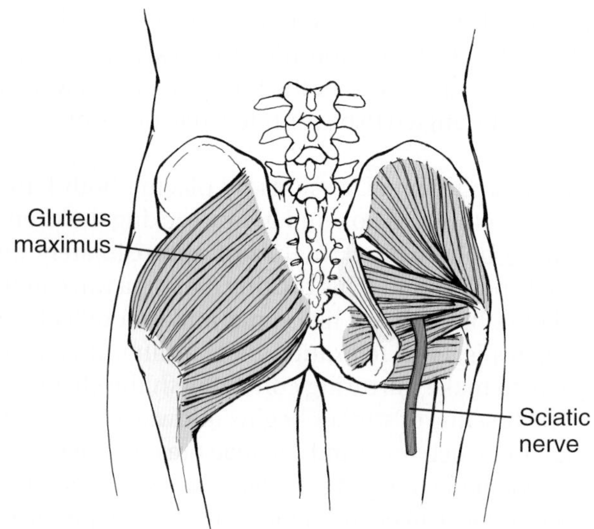

Figure 3-32. Deep rotators of the hip and the sciatic nerve.

3. Perform a series of strokes on the obturator internus along the superior and lateral border of the ischial tuberosity. Lift the soft tissue in a circular motion, scooping laterally to medially, following the contour of the bone (Fig. 3-34).
4. If your client has some mild numbing and tingling down the leg and does not have a positive SLR test, then perform a series of 1-inch scooping strokes with the thumbs, in the M–L plane, going from the lateral surface of the ischial tuberosity to the greater trochanter perpendicular to the sciatic nerve (Fig. 3-35). An entrapped sciatic nerve normally manifests some mild numbing and tingling down the leg as it is being released. *Perform this stroke no more than six times and only if it is needed.*

***CAUTION:* Do not repeat this stroke if pain radiates toward the spine, as it usually indicates a nerve-root lesion, in which case crossing the nerve only aggravates the condition.**

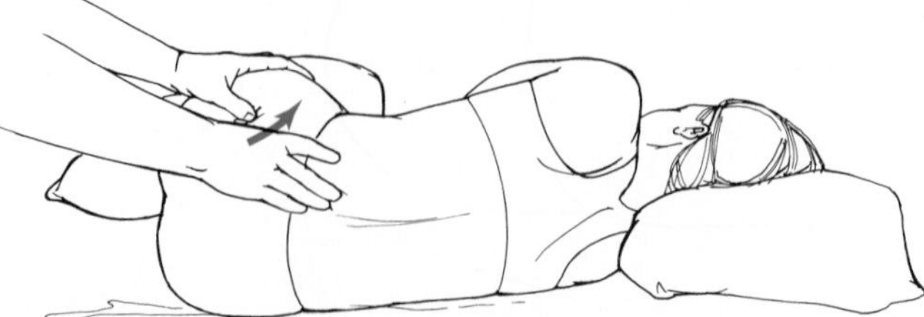

Figure 3-33. Double-thumb release of the piriformis. Begin your strokes just below the PSIS and continue to the greater trochanter.

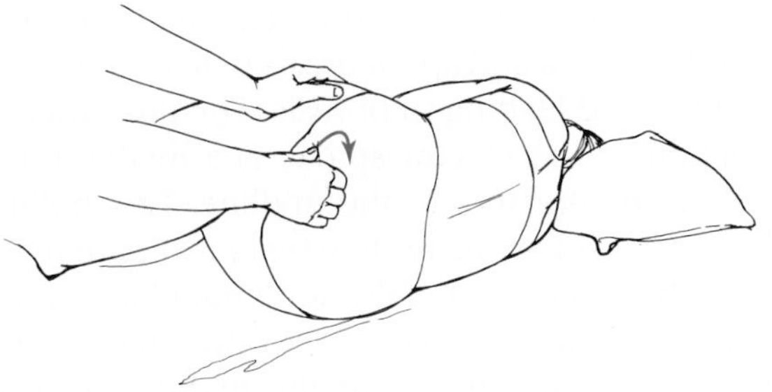

Figure 3-34. Supported thumb technique to release the obturator internus. Lift the soft tissue in a circular motion, scooping laterally to medially along the superior and lateral border of the ischial tuberosity.

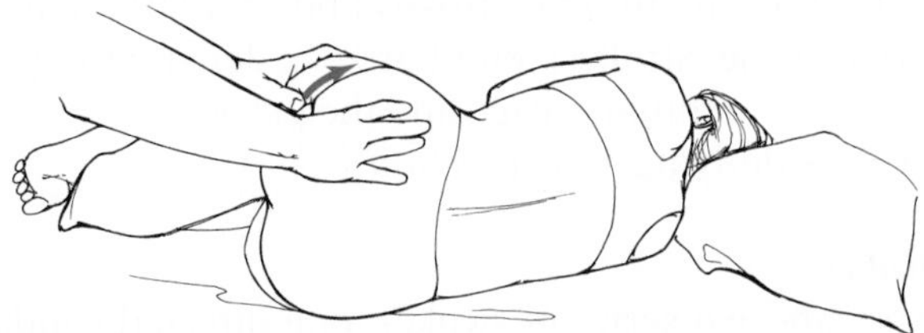

Figure 3-35. Release of a peripheral entrapment of the sciatic nerve from the trough formed between the ischial tuberosity and the greater trochanter.

4. Transverse Release of the Quadratus Lumborum

- *Anatomy*: QL (Fig. 3-36)
- *Dysfunction*: The quadratus tends to shorten with both acute and chronic lower back dysfunction. If it is in a sustained contracture on one side only, due to trauma, postural faults, etc., it will laterally flex the lumbar spine to that side, called antalgia. Antalgia may be caused by many factors, including a protruding disc.

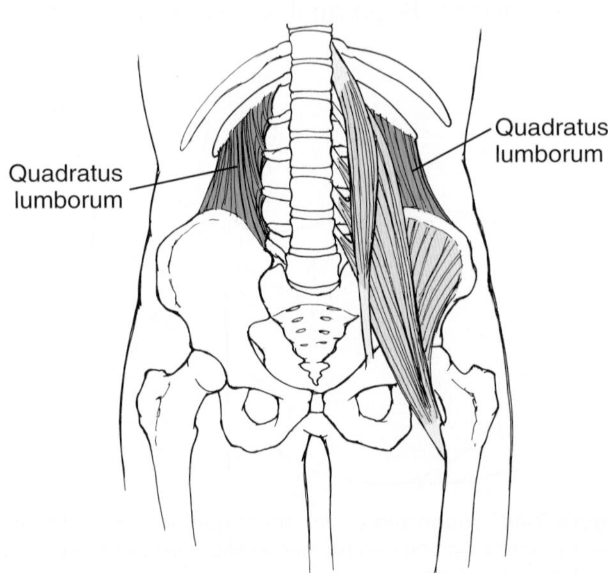

Figure 3-36. Quadratus lumborum.

Position

- TP—standing, 45° headward or 45° caudally
- CP—side lying, fetal position, with back close to edge of table

Strokes

1. Facing 45° headward, use fingertips (Fig. 3-37) or a supported thumb and place your hand just above the iliac crest lateral to the erector spinae. Perform a series of 1-inch scooping strokes on the QL in an M–L direction. The series begins at the most lateral aspect of the QL, and each new stroke begins 1 inch more medially. The supporting hand compresses the ilium headward slightly with each stroke, bringing the origin and insertion of the QL together, helping to relax the QL by turning off the muscle spindles.
2. An alternate position is to face 45° caudally and use a double-thumb technique to perform the same strokes described previously (Fig. 3-38).

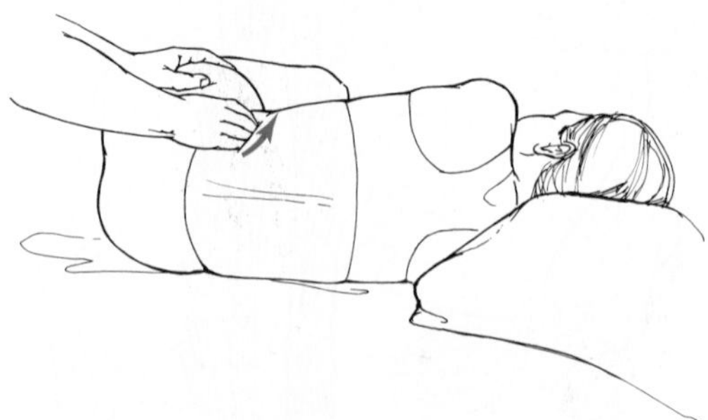

Figure 3-37. Fingertip release of the QL.

3. Begin another series of strokes approximately 1 inch superior to the last series, working into the belly of the QL. Release the entire muscle from the iliac crest to the twelfth rib.

CAUTION: **Do not use strong pressure under the last rib, as the kidneys lie in this region and could be irritated by too much pressure.**

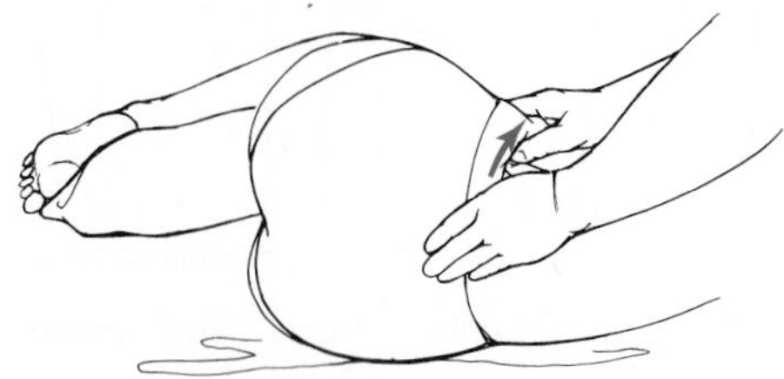

Figure 3-38. Double-thumb technique to release the QL.

5. Release of the Thoracolumbar Fascia and Erector Spinae Aponeurosis

- *Anatomy*: TLF (Fig. 3-39), erector spinae aponeurosis (tendinous sheet of attachment)
- *Dysfunction:* The most common form of chronic lumbosacral dysfunction is hypomobility or lack of movement. The erectors tend to be tight, compressing the facets and the intervertebral discs. This tightness dehydrates these tissues, leading to degeneration. The fascia and aponeurosis tend to shorten, dehydrate, and leading to fibrosis. The positional dysfunction of the erector spinae is a medial torsion, pulling the erectors to the midline. This pulling is demonstrated by the finding that most patients who have LBP—and most of the adult population for that matter—are in some sustained trunk flexion. Since the erectors attach toward the midline, a forward trunk increases this pulling to the midline.

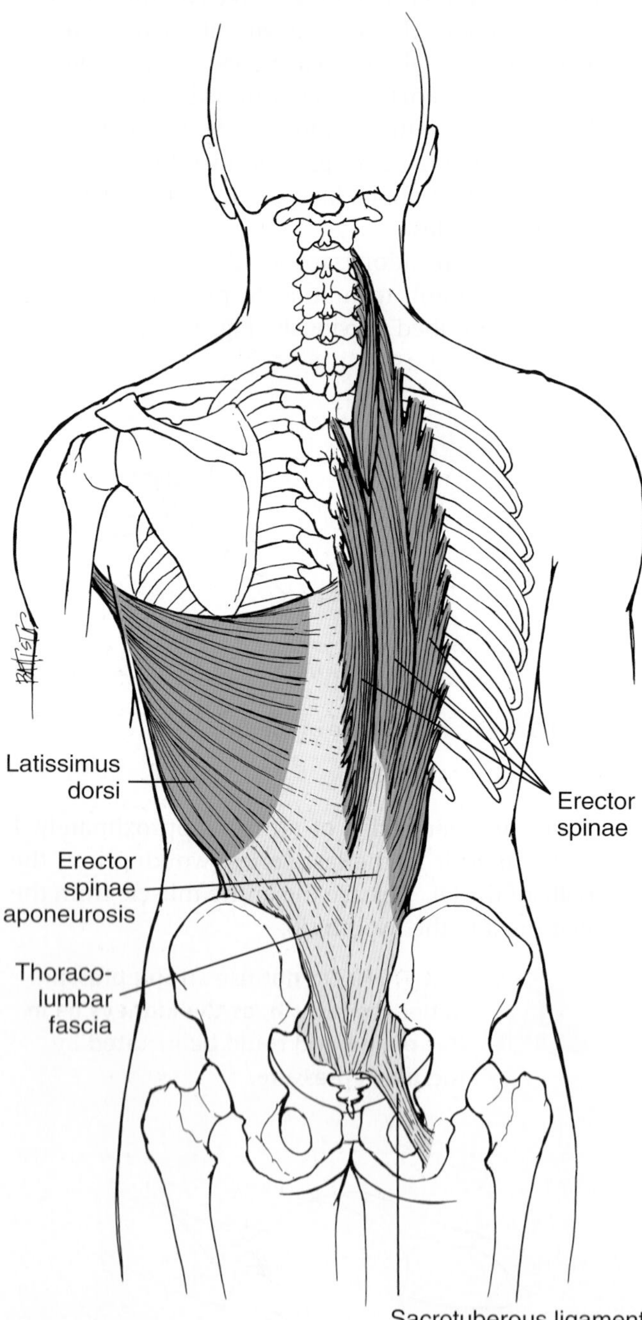

Figure 3-39. Thoracolumbar fascia and erector spinae aponeurosis.

Position

- TP—standing, facing the table at a 45° angle inferiorly for longitudinal strokes and at a 90° angle for transverse strokes; emphasize a lengthening between the thoracic cage and the pelvis
- CP—side-lying, fetal position

Strokes

There are two series of strokes, one directed caudally and the other laterally. These strokes also introduce a P–A glide into the spine. This mobilization technique promotes hydration of the facet joints, the intervertebral discs, the ligaments, and the muscles that have dehydrated due to fibrosis from previous inflammation or hypertonicity. This mobilization "resuscitates" the spine. Use gentle rocking if the client is in acute pain and deeper rocking if the client is chronic.

1. Using a supported-thumb technique, perform a series of strokes approximately 1 inch long that are directed caudally (Fig. 3-40). Begin immediately next to the spinous processes near L4, that is, near the top of the ilium, and work down to the apex of the sacrum. Begin another series approximately

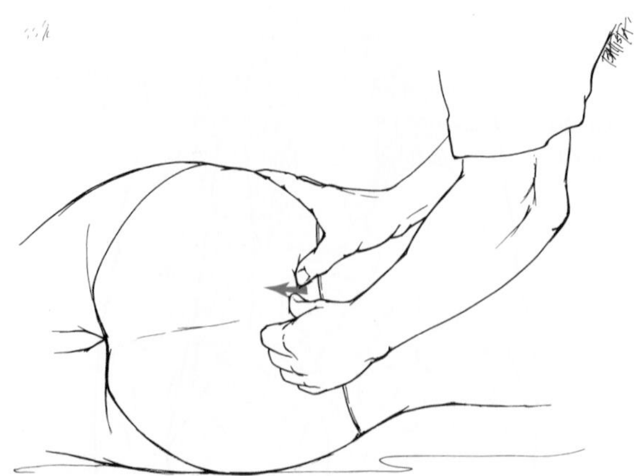

Figure 3-40. Supported-thumb technique to release the thoracolumbar fascia and erector spinae aponeurosis in a superior to inferior direction.

1 inch laterally and include the entire area between the lumbar spinous processes and the ilium. The more superficial strokes release the fascia and the aponeurosis of the erector spinae muscles. The deeper strokes affect the multifidi, ligaments, joints, and discs.

2. Using a supported-thumb technique, perform a series of transverse strokes to release the TLF and erector spinae aponeurosis, working medially to laterally (Fig. 3-41). Begin at the lumbar spinous processes, scooping laterally. Release the entire soft tissue between the lumbosacral spine and the ilium, working from L4 down to the sacral apex.

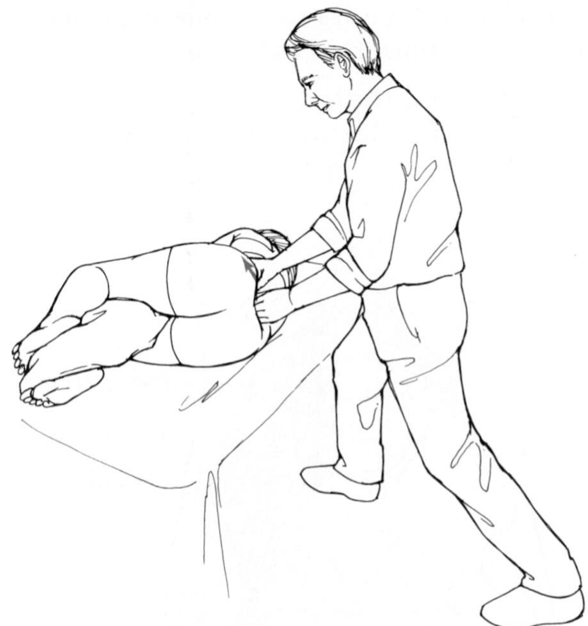

Figure 3-41. Supported-thumb technique to release the thoracolumbar fascia and erector spinae aponeurosis in an M–L direction.

6. Transverse and Longitudinal Release of Soft Tissue of Lumbar Spine from L4 to T12

- *Anatomy:* Latissimus dorsi, TLF, erector spinae (Fig. 3-42)
- *Dysfunction:* The latissimus dorsi is eccentrically loaded in chronic LBP; that is, it is long and tight. With the trunk typically in some sustained flexion, the latissimus contracts to assist the extensors and the TLF to which it attaches. The aponeurosis of the latissimus blends with the fascia and palpates as thickened if there is a history of LBP. A sustained contraction in the latissimus internally rotates the humerus, contributing to the position of dysfunction of the glenohumeral joint.

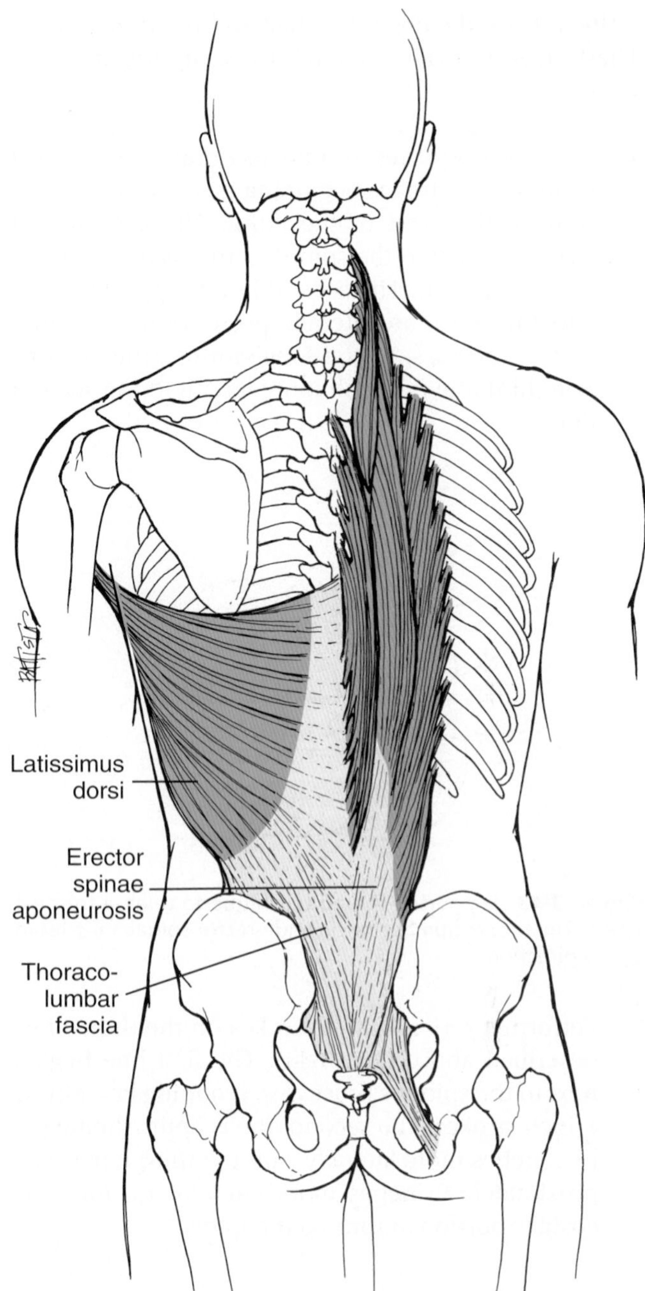

Figure 3-42. Latissimus dorsi, thoracolumbar fascia, and erector spinae.

Position

- TP—standing, facing the table at a 45° angle headward for the longitudinal strokes and at a 90° angle for transverse strokes on the erectors
- CP—side-lying, fetal position

Strokes

There are two types of strokes in three lines. Release the TLF, latissimus, and trapezius (at T-12) superficially; release the erector spinae and multifidi deeply. These strokes are all scooping strokes approximately 1 inch long.

1. Using a supported-thumb technique, perform a series of I–S strokes beginning near L4, that is, the level of the crest of the ilium. The first line of strokes is next to the spinous process of the vertebrae (Fig. 3-43). The second line is approximately 1 to 2 inches more laterally, posterior to the transverse processes, at the longissimus attachments. The third line is 1 inch more lateral to the second line.

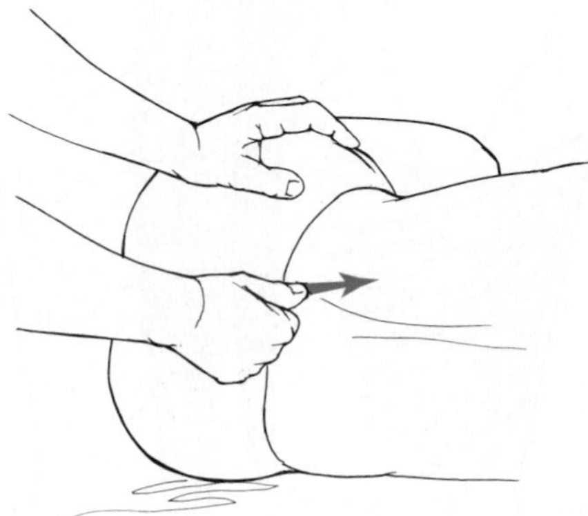

Figure 3-43. Supported-thumb technique to release the first line of the thoracolumbar fascia and erector spinae muscles in an I–S direction.

2. Perform a series of M–L strokes on the three lines described above (Fig. 3-44). The first line begins next to the spinous processes, scooping laterally in 1-inch strokes. The second line is approximately 1 to 2 inches more laterally, and the third line is approximately 2 inches more laterally, on the iliocostalis portion of the erector spinae.

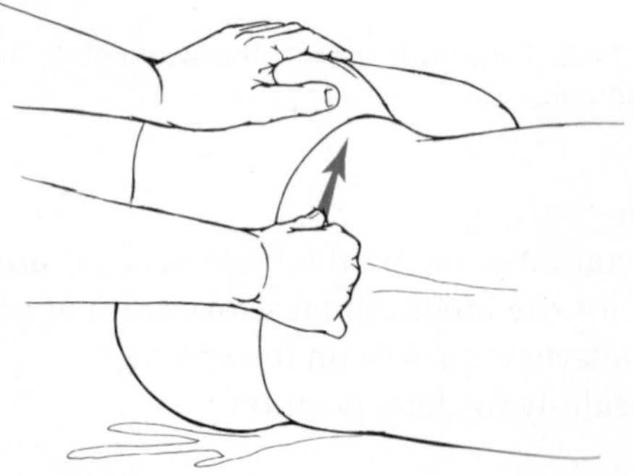

Figure 3-44. Supported-thumb technique to release the thoracolumbar fascia and erector spinae muscles in an M–L direction.

Remember: Pull the skin back 1 inch as you move onto your back leg; scoop into the tissue as you shift your body forward onto your front leg. Stay relaxed. Move your hands with each new stroke, and get into a gentle, calm rhythm as you work. These strokes are deeply relaxing when performed correctly.

7. Transverse Release of the Psoas and Iliacus

- ***Anatomy:*** Psoas major and iliacus (Fig. 3-45)
- ***Dysfunction:*** The iliopsoas tends to roll into a medial torsion, which is often demonstrated as a genu valgum (knock-knees) and pronated ankles, a common weight-distribution dysfunction. The iliopsoas tends to be tight, increasing the lordosis of the lumbar spine, which causes a compression of the lumbar facets. Sitting shortens the iliopsoas.

CAUTION: **Do not perform deep iliopsoas work on a pregnant woman.**

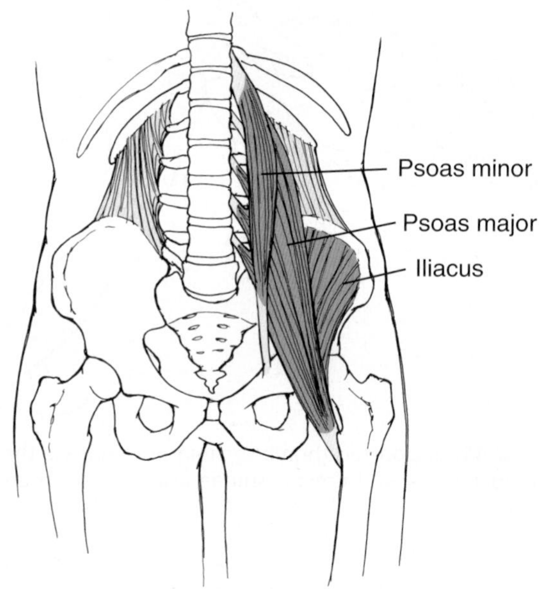

Figure 3-45. Psoas major and iliacus muscles.

Position

- TP—standing, facing the direction of your stroke
- CP—supine

Strokes

1. Palpate the psoas (Fig. 3-46) and perform CR and RI MET on the iliopsoas with the hip at 90° flexion. This MET is described in the "Muscle Energy Technique" section.
2. To release the psoas, assume a 45° headward position, flex the client's hip and knee, and stabilize the

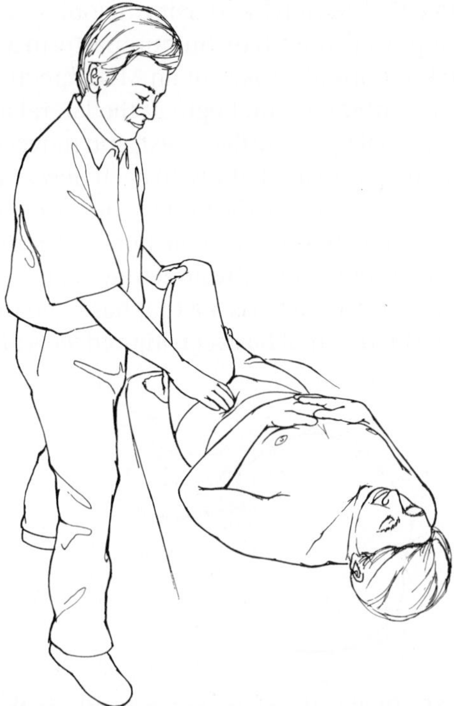

Figure 3-46. Palpation of the psoas. Find the psoas by first placing your fingertips on the ASIS. Move medially approximately 2 to 3 inches, along the inguinal ligament. Gently roll your fingertips slowly into the abdominal tissue just over the superior surface of the ligament. Have your client begin the motion of lifting his thigh toward his chest. You will feel the psoas contract under your fingertips. If the client is ticklish or sensitive to being touched in this area, have him place his hand on top of your hand. This reduces the sensitivity.

client's lower leg against your body (Fig. 3-47). Place the fingertips of both hands on the iliopsoas; rock your body and your client's body rhythmically back and forth as you stroke back and forth on the iliopsoas, parallel to the inguinal ligament. You can also place your flexed knee on the table to stabilize the client's leg.

3. Using the same hand position described in the second stroke, palpate the iliacus by first placing your fingertips on the ASIS. Gently roll your fingertips over the bone and into the iliac fossa. Maintain contact with the iliacus covering the bone by flexing your fingertips, so as not to compress the viscera. Release the iliacus with gentle, lateral to medial, scooping strokes, following the contour of the bone, as if you are cleaning the inside of a bowl. Begin at the ASIS, and then perform another series of strokes 1 inch superiorly and continue in 1-inch segments, covering the entire iliac fossa.
4. Bring the client's hip into approximately 90° flexion. Using fingertips, scoop the iliopsoas laterally in 1-inch strokes as you move the client's hip in circles of abduction and external rotation (Fig. 3-48). This resets the muscle fasciculi. You sink into the tissue as the hip is being flexed, and scoop laterally as the hip is abducted. Then release your fingers as the thigh is being brought to the midline, and repeat the scooping stroke in a slightly new area.

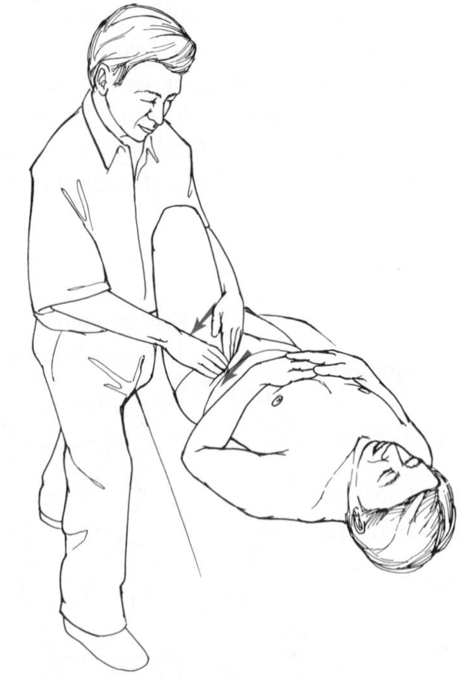

Figure 3-47. Release of the iliopsoas. Place the fingertips of both hands on the iliopsoas and move the client's entire leg with your strokes.

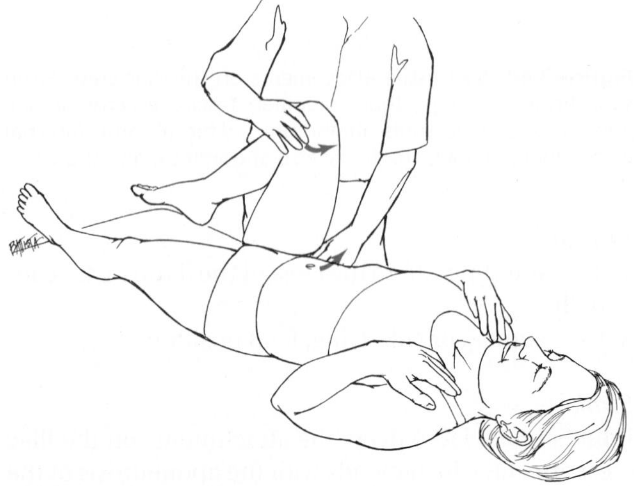

Figure 3-48. Fingertip release of the torsion of the iliopsoas. Move the hip in circles of abduction and external rotation as you roll the fibers of the iliopsoas laterally.

Level II–Lumbosacral

1. Transverse Release of Soft-Tissue Attachments to the Crest of the Ilium

- *Anatomy*: TLF, internal and external abdominal obliques, erector spinae aponeurosis, transverse abdominus, iliocostalis lumborum, QL (Fig. 3-49).
- *Dysfunction*: The iliac crest is a significant attachment site for fascia and muscles, and acts as a stabilizer for the pelvis and the lumbar spine. The soft tissue here thickens with chronic irritation associated with injuries and dysfunctions of the lumbosacral spine. The abdominal muscles can be strained at their attachments to the lateral iliac crest, called a "hip-pointer" injury. This area also thickens due to chronic muscle imbalance.

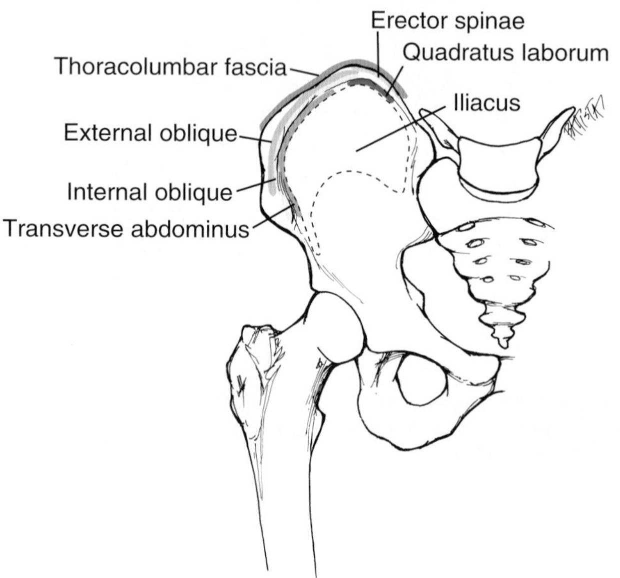

Figure 3-49. Soft-tissue attachments on the iliac crest. From superficial to deep: thoracolumbar fascia, erector spinae aponeurosis, iliocostalis lumborum, external and internal abdominal obliques, the transverse abdominus, and the QL.

Position

- TP—standing, 90° to the crest of the ilium or 45° caudally
- CP—supine; or side-lying, fetal position

Strokes

From superficial to deep, the attachments on the iliac crest are TLF, which blends with the aponeurosis of the latissimus dorsi, iliocostalis lumborum, external abdominal oblique, internal abdominal oblique, transverse abdominus, the QL, and the iliolumbar ligament.

1. Facing 45° inferiorly and using a double (Fig. 3-50) or supported-thumb technique, perform a series of 1-inch scooping strokes in an M–L direction along the crest of the ilium. Begin at the lateral aspect of the external lip of the iliac crest, and move in 1-inch segments more medially with each new stroke. The intention is to "clean the bone." Your strokes should move along the surface of the bone without digging into the bone. A healthy attachment site feels glistening and smooth. Tissue that has been under excessive load or that has been injured feels fibrotic.

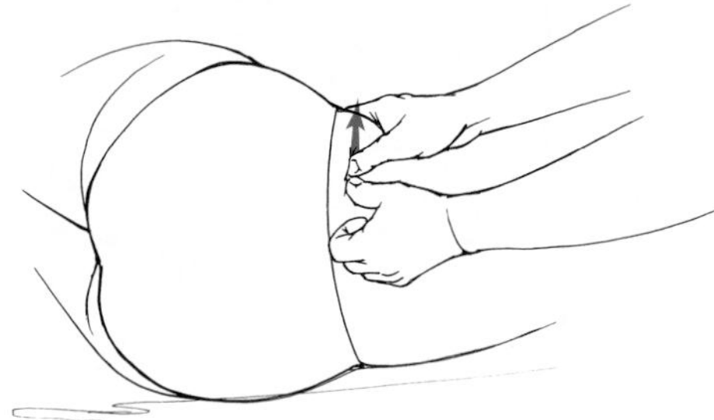

Figure 3-50. Double-thumb technique to release the crest of the ilium.

2. Repeat the same stroke in two more lines on the intermediate and internal lip of the iliac crest. Your body faces more caudally with these strokes. As you perform these strokes, move the entire pelvis into an inferior traction.
3. To release the abdominal attachments from the lateral portion of the iliac crest, ask your client to lie on his or her back, with legs extended. You may place a pillow under the client's knees. Using fingertips over thumb technique, perform scooping strokes from anterior to posterior on the iliac crest (Fig. 3-51). Begin the strokes on the most posterior portion of this area, and move more anteriorly with your strokes.

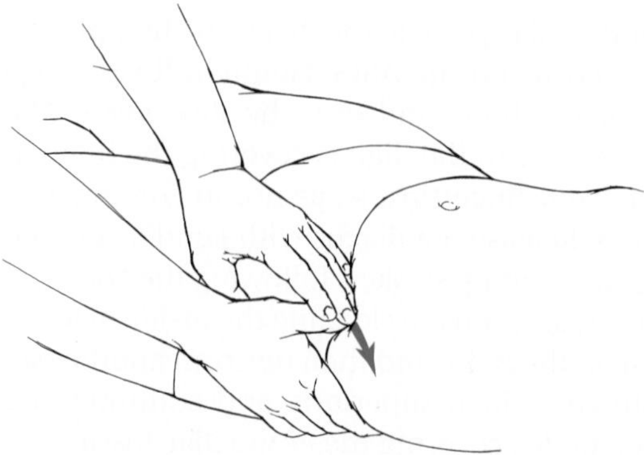

Figure 3-51. Release of the abdominal attachments to the lateral aspect of the ilium.

2. Transverse Release of the Soft-Tissue Attachments to the Posterior Superior Iliac Spine

- *Anatomy:* Thoracic fibers of iliocostalis lumborum, lumbar fibers of the iliocostalis, lumbar fibers of longissimus (Fig. 3-52).
- *Dysfunction:* As mentioned in the anatomy section, Bogduk and Twomey[10] has described a superficial and deep portion of the erector spinae. Now the attachments of the deep portion are addressed. These muscles stabilize the lumbar spine and act to prevent anterior shear of the vertebrae relative to the sacrum and ilium.[2] Injury or dysfunction shortens and thickens soft tissue. Attachment points dry out, becoming ischemic and eventually fibrous. The intention is to dissolve the fibrosis, broadening and rehydrating the tissue.

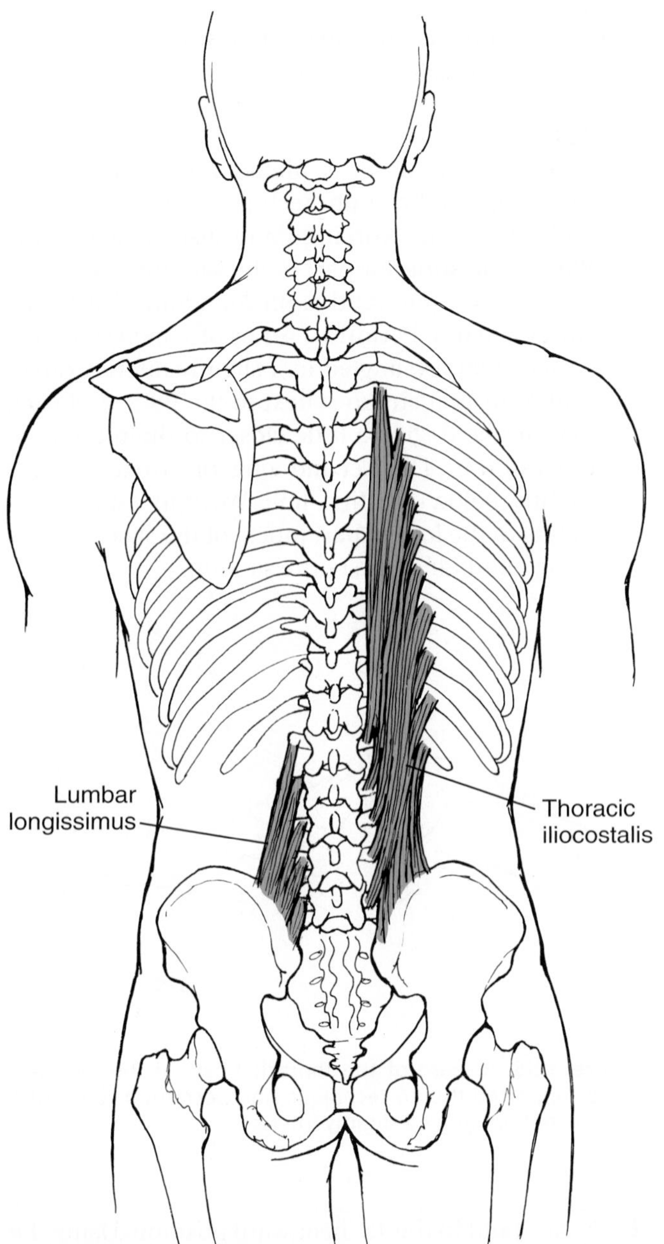

Figure 3-52. Deep portion of the erector spinae muscles. Shown here are the thoracic fibers of the iliocostalis lumborum, the lumbar fibers of the iliocostalis, and the lumbar fibers of the longissimus.

Position

- TP—standing, facing the direction of your stroke
- CP—side-lying, fetal position

Strokes

We use a double- or supported-thumb technique and follow the contour of the bone with our strokes. We are working on the tenoperiosteal attachments of the above muscles to the PSIS. The following strokes are from superficial to deep.

1. Facing slightly headward, perform a series of M–L scooping strokes on the lateral portion of the PSIS and the adjoining portion of the iliac crest (Fig. 3-53). This releases the thoracic fibers of the iliocostalis.
2. To release the lumbar fibers of the iliocostalis, perform a series of 1-inch scooping strokes in an I–S direction on the superior, medial, and inferior aspect of the PSIS. Follow the contour of the bone.
3. Working in the same area as the previous stroke, but more deeply, perform a series of scooping strokes on the deepest portion of the medial aspect of the PSIS. These strokes release the lumbar fibers of the longissimus, which are the deepest muscle fibers attaching to the PSIS.

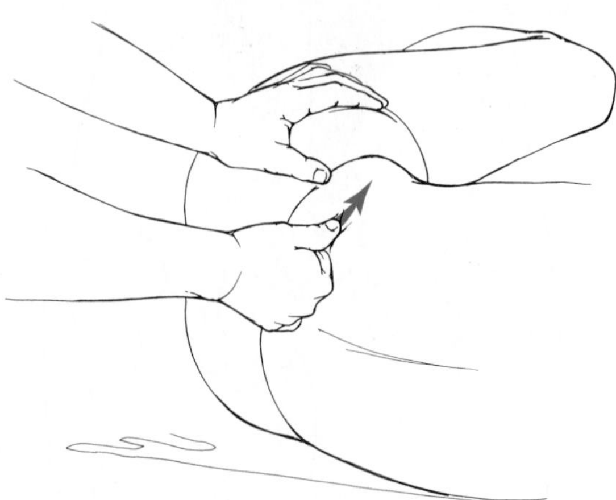

Figure 3-53. Supported-thumb technique to release the lateral portion of the iliac crest and the lateral portion of the PSIS.

3. Release of the Soft-Tissue Attachments to the Sacrum

- *Anatomy*: From superficial to deep, the attachments on the sacral base are TLF, thoracic fibers of longissimus, multifidus, posterior sacroiliac ligaments which are next to the bone (Fig. 3-54).

As the thoracic fibers of longissimus run headward, they angle approximately 10° to 15° laterally. Deep to the fibers of the longissimus is the multifidus. The muscle mass you palpate medial to the PSIS is the multifidus.

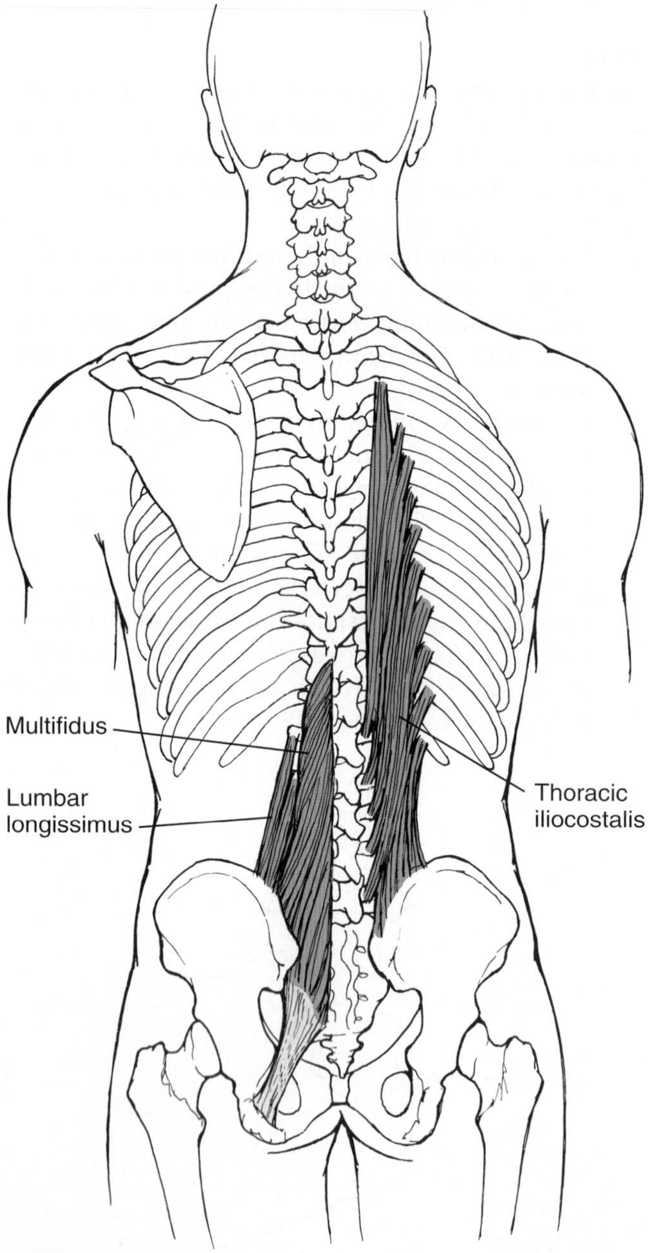

Figure 3-54. From superficial to deep, the attachments to the sacrum are the thoracolumbar fascia, the thoracic fibers of longissimus, the multifidi, and the posterior sacroiliac ligaments.

- *Dysfunction*: Soft tissue tends to shorten and become fibrotic with overuse or injury. The multifidus attaches to the joint capsules of the vertebral facets, and releasing the multifidus at the sacrum assists in the release of the lumbar facets.

Position

- TP—standing, facing direction of stroke
- CP—side lying, fetal position

Strokes

1. To release the thoracic fibers of longissimus, use the supported-thumb technique. Face caudally and place your working hand just medial to the PSIS at the superior part of the sacrum (Fig. 3-55). Your supporting hand is on the ilium next to the working hand. Perform a series of 1-inch scooping strokes that are angled in a slightly inferior direction. Your first stroke is next to the PSIS, and each new stroke begins a little closer to the midline of the sacrum. The second line of strokes begins slightly below the first line. Work in 1-inch segments to the lowest part (apex) of the sacrum, covering one-half of the entire sacrum.

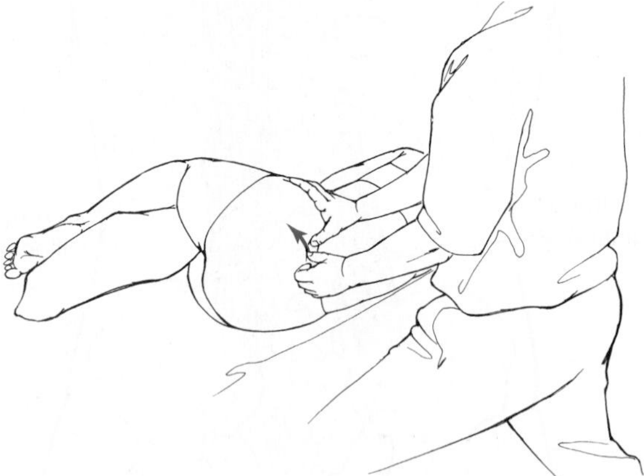

Figure 3-55. Release of the thoracic fibers of the longissimus. Use a supported-thumb technique and perform a series of M–L strokes that are angled slightly inferior.

2. Next, stand in the 45° headward position. Using the supported-thumb technique, perform a series of 1-inch, scooping strokes in an approximately 45° headward direction (Fig. 3-56). To release the multifidi attachments on the sacral base, work at a

deeper level than the previous stroke. Begin just medial to the PSIS, scoop M–L in 1-inch strokes, and work to the midline of the sacrum. Cover one-half of the entire sacrum.

3. Using the same hand technique, perform short, back and forth strokes at various angles for the posterior sacroiliac ligaments. Place your supporting hand on the ilium, and rock the client's body in short oscillations with each stroke. Use your palpation skills to feel for thickened, fibrous tissue. The thicker the tissue, the deeper the transverse strokes to broaden and rehydrate the tissue. These deep strokes on the ligaments are used only as needed to release fibrotic tissue.

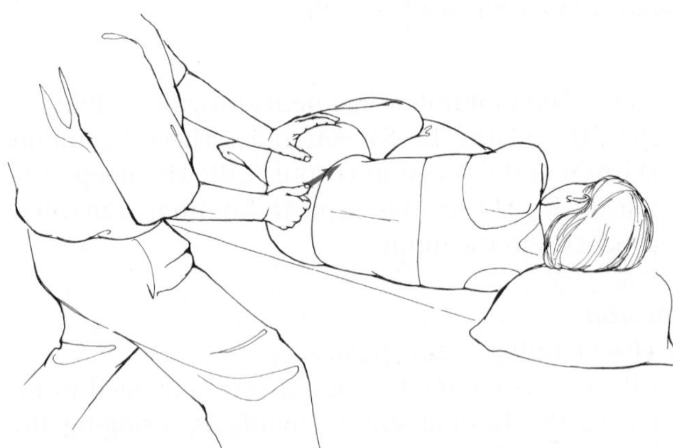

Figure 3-56. Release of the multifidi. Standing in a 45° headward stance, scoop in an M–L direction.

4. Release of Multifidi and Rotatores from L5 to L1

- *Anatomy:* multifidus, rotatores (Fig. 3-57)
- *Dysfunction:* The multifidi and rotatores attach to the joint capsule and are often strained in back injuries. They either develop a sustained contraction, leading to dehydration and fibrosis, or become inhibited, leading to atrophy and destabilization of the lumbar spine. You must be able to palpate the difference, as it is contraindicated to work deeply on atrophied tissue.

Position

- TP—standing, facing headward
- CP—side-lying, fetal position

Strokes

1. To release the multifidus and rotatores from the area between L5 and L1, use a supported- or double-thumb technique (Fig. 3-58). Stand in the 45° headward stance. Begin near the spinous process of L5, and perform a series of strokes in a 45° headward direction. Scoop under the erector spinae, working transverse to the line of the fiber of the multifidi and rotatores.

CAUTION: **These next strokes are for chronic conditions only.**

2. To release the soft tissue attachments on the lateral aspect of the lumbar spinous processes, stand facing the table or in a 45° headward stance. In the

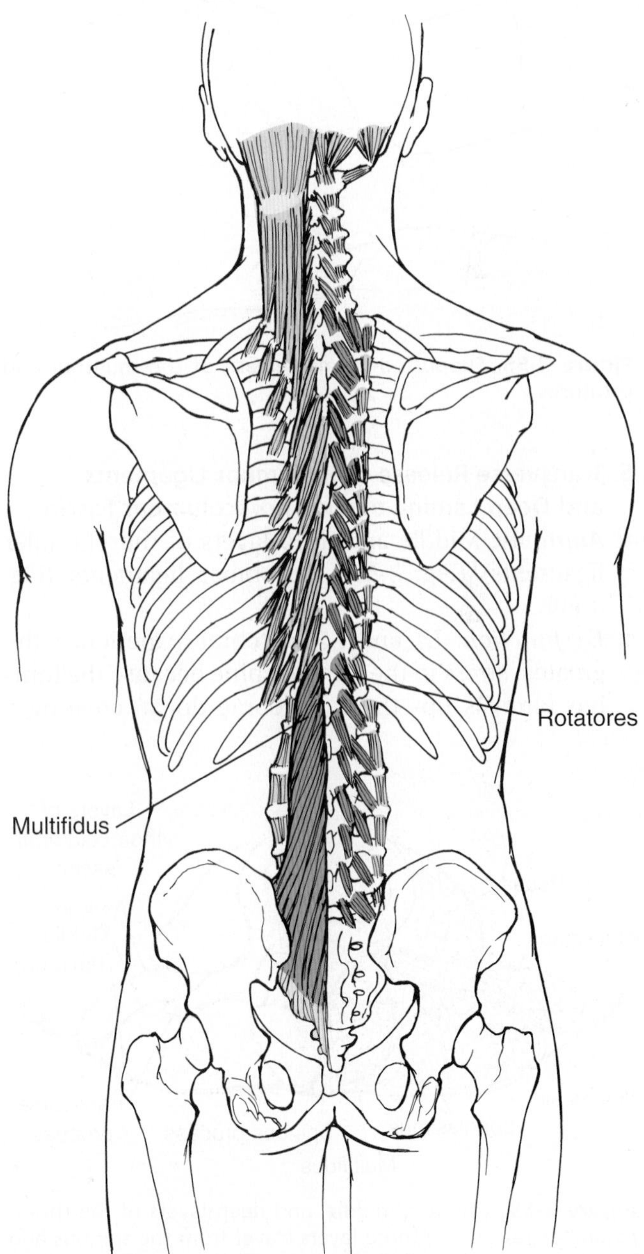

Figure 3-57. Multifidi and rotatores.

lumbar spine the spinous processes are angles almost straight posteriorly. Using a supported-thumb position, perform a series of 1-inch back and forth strokes in the I–S plane on the spinous processes. The bone is cleaned with strokes that scoop across the bone. Do not press into the bone. Work on each spinous process, from L5 to L1.

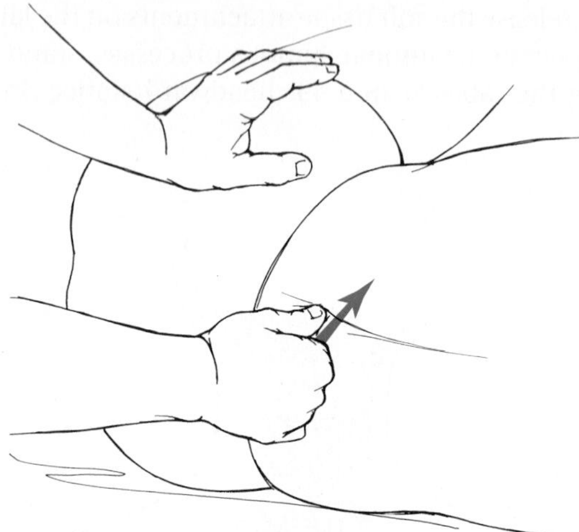

Figure 3-58. Supported-thumb release of the multifidi and rotatores.

5. Transverse Release of Iliolumbar Ligaments and Deep Lamina of the Thoracolumbar Fascia

- *Anatomy:* Middle and deep layers of the TLF (alar ligaments) (Fig. 3-59), iliolumbar ligaments (Fig. 3-60).
- *Dysfunction*: L4 and L5 vertebrae experience the greatest stress in the lumbar spine because the lumbar lordosis tips these vertebrae down, creating a

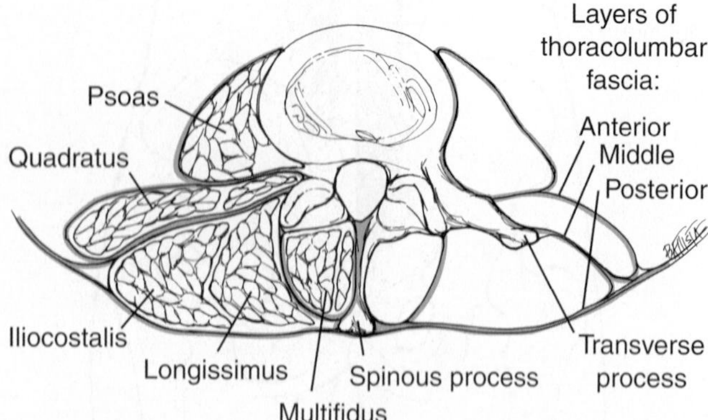

Figure 3-59. Anterior, middle, and deep layers of the thoracolumbar fascia. The three layers travel from the spinous and transverse processes of the lumbar vertebrae to the ilium.

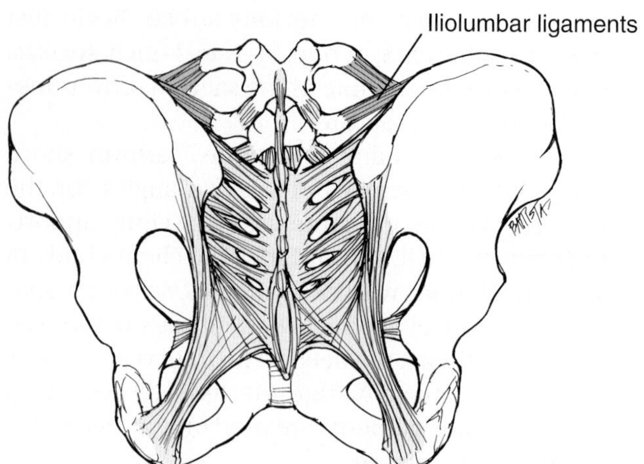

Figure 3-60. Iliolumbar ligaments.

shear. The iliolumbar ligaments provide stability to the SIJ and the L5–S1 vertebrae. These ligaments shorten and thicken in chronic LBP. The deep lamina of the TLF travels from the lumbar transverse processes to the ilium.

Position

- TP—standing, facing headward
- CP—side-lying, fetal position; you may need to increase the lumbar curve slightly by bringing the knees away from the client's chest slightly to put the erector muscles in more slack.

Strokes

Now you are working the deepest layers of soft tissue between the medial aspect of the ilium and the spinous and transverse processes on the lowest lumbar vertebrae. The intention is to scoop transverse to the line of the fiber, broadening these fibers to release any fibrosis. It takes a great deal of preparation to work this deeply. These strokes are for chronic conditions only.

1. Using the supported-thumb position (Fig. 3-61), place your working hand next to the spinous process of L4, which is at the level of the iliac crest. Your supporting hand rests on the ilium. Perform a series of 1-inch scooping strokes in a superior direction between the L4 vertebra and the sacrum, transverse on the deep lamina of the TLF and iliolumbar ligaments. As you move onto your back leg gathering your chi, pull the client's ilium back with you slightly. As you scoop into the tissue, push the client's ilium toward your working hand. This brings the erectors into slack and allows for deeper work.

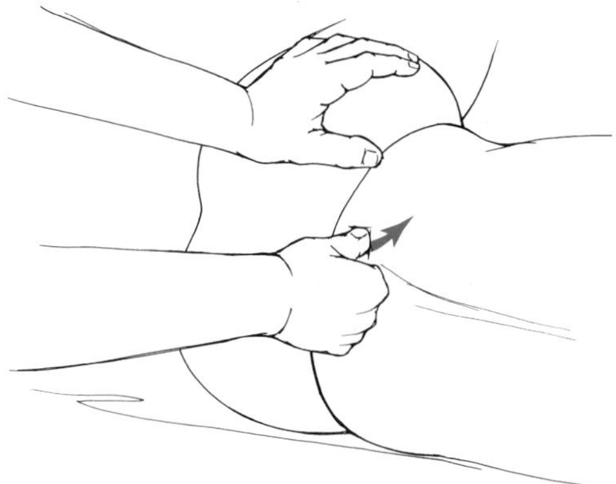

Figure 3-61. Supported-thumb release in three lines for the middle and deep layers of the thoracolumbar fascia and the iliolumbar ligaments.

2. The second line of strokes begins at the L4 area again, but approximately 1 inch lateral to the first line. Perform another series of 1-inch scooping strokes in the superior direction. Continue your series of strokes to the top of the sacrum (sacral base).
3. The third line of strokes is along the medial aspect of the ilium, at the level of L4 and L5. You are now cleaning the bone to release any fibrosis. Scoop next to the bone, not into the bone. Rock your entire body and your client's body as you perform your strokes. If you find fibrotic tissue, your strokes may become more brisk, but always maintain the rocking movement.

CASE STUDY

MB is a 45-year-old, 5'6", 210 lb female accounting supervisor who presented with pain, numbing, and tingling in the left lateral thigh and calf. She reported that the pain began approximately 3 months previously, without any incident. She stated that she had one previous episode approximately 18 months prior to our visit. Again, there was no incident, and it resolved in a few weeks. She said that the pain was worse in the morning, that sitting made it worse, and lying on her back was relieving. She had x-rays taken after the first episode, but the alignment and disc spaces were normal. Prior to our visit, she had received a series of acupuncture and physical therapy treatments, but they were only temporarily relieving.

Examination revealed an elevated ilium on the right side in standing. The spinal curves were normal in the posterior and lateral views. The lumbar ranges of motion were normal, without any pain. The Kemps test was normal. Motor strength testing revealed a moderate weakness in the left hip flexors (iliopsoas), but no pain. The SLR test was normal. Length testing showed that she had a short iliopsoas and piriformis on the left, and the piriformis test elicited symptoms into the left thigh and leg.

A diagnosis was made of piriformis syndrome. Treatment began on the noninvolved iliopsoas with the client supine. Both knees were flexed, her feet on the table. A CR MET was performed for five cycles on the iliopsoas and hip extensors, with the hip in 90° of flexion. Manual work to release the iliopsoas was performed for a few minutes. The same work on the symptomatic iliopsoas was performed. She was asked to move into the fetal position, with the noninvolved side up. CR MET was then performed on the piriformis by having her lift her leg off the pillow for 5 seconds and RI on the adductors by having her squeeze her knees together for 5 seconds. This cycle was repeated for five times. Then, she was asked to roll onto her other side, and the same CR technique was performed on the involved piriformis. Next, she was asked to roll onto her back again, knees up, feet on the table. PIR MET was performed on the involved piriformis to lengthen it. She was shown a simple piriformis-stretching exercise that she could do at home.

MB returned to the office 1 week later for a follow-up and said that she had only slight, occasional symptoms, even after a long drive. She was treated again with the same protocol as described above, and in a follow-up 1 week later, she was asymptomatic. She was encouraged to begin an exercise program, and recommendations for future treatment were on an as-needed basis.

STUDY GUIDE

Lumbosacral Spine, Level I

1. List the names of the muscles in the seven layers of the back, from superficial to deep.
2. Describe the basic origins and insertions of the erector spinae, the psoas, and the QL.
3. Describe the difference between the signs and the symptoms of muscle strain, facet syndrome, disc degeneration, and disc herniation.
4. Describe the MET used for acute LBP.
5. Describe the positional dysfunction of the erector spinae and psoas, and the directions of a therapist's strokes.
6. What is the stroke direction for the sacrotuberous and sacrospinous ligaments?
7. Explain the intention of MET and how to perform MET to release the hypertonic lumbar extensors, piriformis, and QL.
8. What muscles are tight and what muscles are weak in the lower-crossed syndrome?
9. List three major factors that predispose a person to an episode of acute low back pain.
10. List what functional factors predispose to LBP.

Lumbosacral Spine, Level II

1. Describe the basic origins and insertions of the piriformis, gluteals, and multifidus muscle.
2. Describe the main muscles responsible for an increased lumbar curve, and a decreased lumbar curve.
3. Describe the length assessment test and PIR MET for the iliopsoas.
4. List the attachments on the crest of the ilium, from superficial to deep.
5. List three factors that affect the diameter of the IVF.
6. List what attaches to the sacral base, from superficial to deep.
7. Describe the direction of our stroke to release the multifidi and rotatores.
8. Explain how abnormal muscle function can predispose a person to an episode of LBP.
9. Describe the two types of referral of pain and their causes.
10. Describe the SLR test. What are the implications of a positive test?

REFERENCES

1. Kaul M, Herring SA. Rehabilitation of lumbar spine injuries. In: Kibler WB, Herring SA, Press JM, eds. Functional Rehabilitation of Sports and Musculoskeletal Injuries. Gaithersburg, MD: Aspen, 1998:188–215.
2. Porterfield JA, DeRosa C. Mechanical Low Back Pain. Philadelphia: WB Saunders, 1991.
3. Mooney V. Sacroiliac joint dysfunction. In: Vleeming A, Mooney V, Dorman T, Snijders CJ, Stoeckart R, eds. Movement, Stability, and Low Back Pain. New York: Churchill Livingstone, 1997:37–52.
4. Swenson R. A medical approach to the differential diagnosis of low back pain. Journal of the Neuromusculoskeletal System 1998;6:100–113.
5. Cailliet R. Low Back Pain Syndrome. Philadelphia: FA Davis, 1995.
6. Willard FH. The muscular, ligamentous and neural structure of the low back and its relation to low back pain. In: Vleeming A, Mooney V, Dorman T, Snijders CJ, Stoeckart R, eds. Movement, Stability, and Low Back Pain. New York: Churchill Livingstone, 1997:3–35.
7. Freeman MA, Dean MR, Hanham IW. The etiology and prevention of functional instability of the foot. J Bone Joint Surg Br 1965;47:678–685.
8. Kirkaldy-Willis WH, Bernard TN Jr. Managing Low Back Pain, 4th Ed. New York: Churchill Livingstone, 1999.
9. Jull GA, Janda V. Muscles and motor control in low back pain: assessment and management. In: Twomey L, Taylor JR, eds. Physical Therapy of the Low Back. New York: Churchill Livingstone, 1987:253–278.
10. Bogduk N, Twomey L. Clinical Anatomy of the Lumbar Spine, 3rd Ed. London: Churchill Livingstone, 1998.

SUGGESTED READINGS

Calais-Germain B. Anatomy of Movement. Seattle: Eastland Press, 1991.

Chaitow L. Muscle Energy Techniques. New York: Churchill Livingstone, 1996.

Clemente C. Anatomy: A Regional Atlas of the Human Body, 4th Ed. Baltimore: Williams & Wilkins, 1997.

Corrigan B, Maitland GD. Practical Orthopaedic Medicine. London: Butterworths, 1983.

Greenman PE. Principles of Manual Medicine, 2nd Ed. Baltimore: Williams & Wilkins, 1996.

Kendall F, McCreary E, Provance P. Muscles: Testing and Function, 4th Ed. Baltimore: Williams & Wilkins, 1993.

Kessler R, Hertling D. Management of Common Musculoskeletal Disorders, 3rd Ed. Baltimore: Williams & Wilkins, 1993.

Lewit K. Manipulative Therapy in Rehabilitation on the Locomotor System, 3rd Ed. Oxford: Butterworth Heinemann, 1999.

Liebenson C. Rehabilitation of the Spine. Baltimore: Williams & Wilkins, 1996.

Magee D. Orthopedic Physical Assessment, 3rd Ed. Philadelphia: WB Saunders, 1997.

Norkin C, Levangie P. Joint Structure and Function, 2nd Ed. Philadelphia: FA Davis, 1992.

Platzer W. Locomotor System, vol 1, 4th Ed. New York: Thieme Medical, 1992.

Reid DC. Sports Injury and Assessment. New York: Churchill Livingstone, 1992.

Thoracic Spine

The thoracic region has been the subject of few studies or clinical trials compared with the cervical and lumbar regions, as disability is rarely associated with this region.[1] Disc lesions in the **thoracic spine** are rare and represent approximately 2% of disc problems.[2] Degenerative joint disease occurs as frequently in the thoracic spine as in the cervical and lumbar regions, but symptoms are uncommon.[2] However, occupational factors, including heavy lifting, bending and twisting, vibration, and static work posture, are also known to affect this area.[1] Excessive sitting, especially with poor posture, commonly leads to thoracic pain. The most common disease affecting the thoracic spine is **osteoporosis,** a thinning of the bone leading to microfractures, principally in postmenopausal women.

Anatomy, Function, and Dysfunction of the Thoracic Spine

GENERAL OVERVIEW

- The thoracic region consists of intervertebral discs, 12 vertebrae, 12 ribs and their associated cartilage, sternum, and scapula; it is also composed of nerves, ligaments, muscles, and associated soft tissues (Fig. 4-1). The scapula is considered in more detail in Chapter 6, "The Shoulder."
- The thoracic region is the longest part of the spine with the least mobility and the most stability. The stability is caused by the rib cage and the thinness of the discs.
- Flexion, extension, lateral bending, and rotation are possible in the thoracic spine but are extremely limited, owing to the rib cage and the thinness of the discs. Because of the orientation of the facets, rotation produces the greatest movement.
- The resting position of the thoracic spine is midway between flexion and extension. The close-packed position is extension.

Thoracic Curve

The thoracic spine normally has a mild, smooth posterior curve. However, as Grieve[2] points out, the degree of thoracic curve can vary greatly. The interscapular region may be flat with a normal x-ray.

Posture

- The curve in the thoracic spine is affected by the position of the pelvis and the lower back, just as the position of the head and neck are influenced

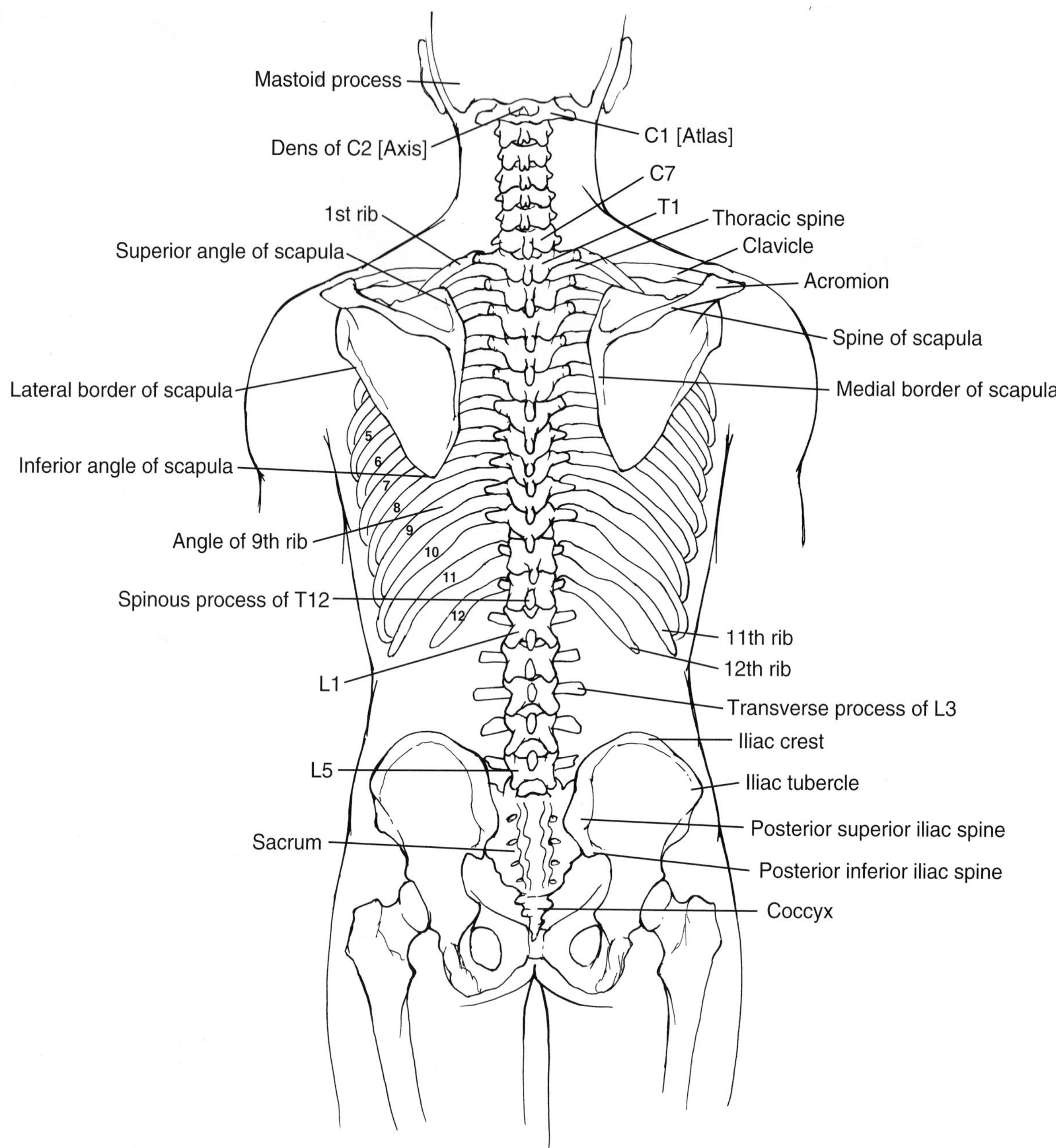

Figure 4-1. Posterior view of the thoracic region showing the 12 vertebra, 12 ribs, and the scapulae overlying the rib cage.

by the thoracic spine. An increased lumbar curve causes an increase in the thoracic and cervical curves. A common postural fault is a rounded-shoulder, forward-head posture (FHP), which also creates an increase in the thoracic curve, further contributing to an increase in the cervical curve.

- *Dysfunction and injury:* With a rounded-shoulder, FHP, the thoracic spine goes into flexion, compressing the discs, potentially leading to early degeneration (Fig. 4-2). The facets are held in a flexed position, losing their ability to move into extension. The joint capsules have an increased load in the flexed position and develop abnormal crosslinks and adhesions, leading to loss of normal joint motion. The tension in the extensor muscles of the upper thoracic spine must increase dramatically to prevent the head and upper back from falling forward because of gravity. This increased tension is not only

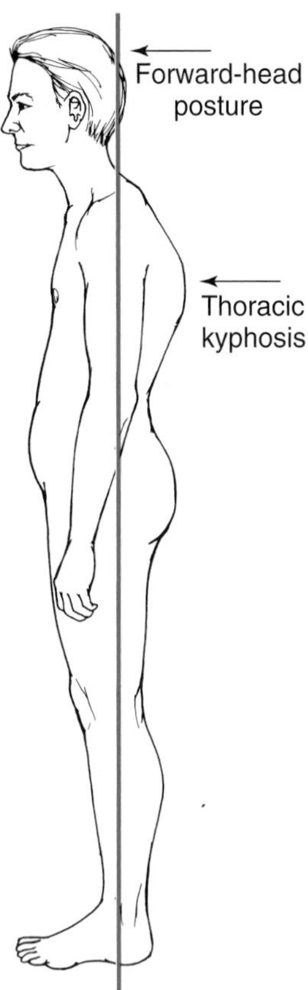

Figure 4-2. Thoracic kyphosis is an exaggeration of the normal thoracic curve and contributes to a forward-head posture.

fatiguing but also adds a compressive force to the facets. Compression can also occur in the space above and below the clavicle, called the thoracic outlet, which can compress the nerves and blood supply into the arm. Slumped posture decreases vital lung capacity and creates excessive tension in the temporomandibular joint (TMJ).

Thoracic Vertebrae Anatomy

- The thoracic spine includes 12 vertebrae, and each vertebra forms 3 joints with the vertebra above and 3 joints with the vertebra below. This three-joint complex includes an **intervertebral disc (IVD)** and two **facet joints.** The **intervertebral foramen** is an opening between two vertebrae through which the motor (ventral) and sensory (dorsal) nerve roots travel along the spine.
- As in the lumbar spine, each vertebra has an anterior and a posterior portion. Many structural and functional similarities as well as some important differences exist.
  - The **anterior portion** consists of a vertebral **body** and an **IVD,** which forms a fibrocartilaginous joint with the vertebral body (Fig. 4-3).
  - The **posterior portion** consists of two vertebral arches formed by a pedicle and lamina, a central spinous process, two transverse processes, and paired articulations, called the **inferior** and the **superior facets,** which form synovial joints.
- A unique feature of the thoracic vertebrae is that the body and transverse processes have synovial joints for articulation with the ribs. These joints are called **costovertebral joints** and are discussed in the section, "Costovertebral Joints."

Vertebral Body

- Unlike the cervical and the lumbar spine, the vertebral body in the thoracic spine is shorter anteriorly than posteriorly, giving this area its normal thoracic kyphosis. As in the lumbar and cervical regions, a fibrocartilage joint is located between the two vertebral bodies and the disc.
- ***Dysfunction and injury:*** The vertebral body is the site of pathologic fractures secondary to osteoporosis; these are most common in the midthoracic region.[1]

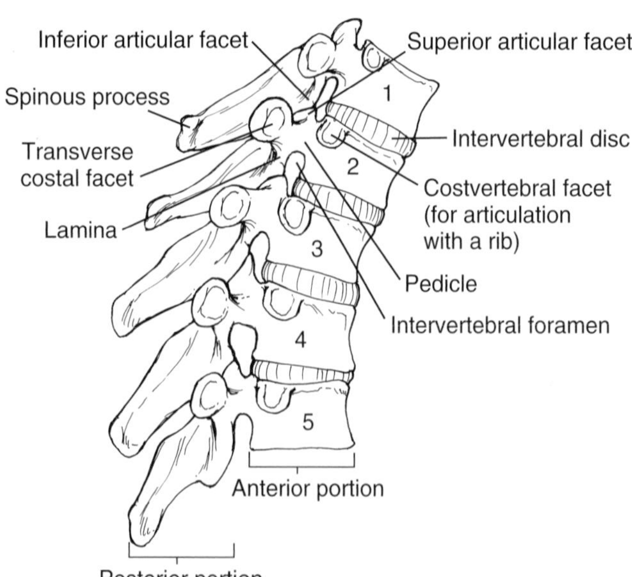

Figure 4-3. Anterior and posterior portions of the thoracic vertebra.

Intervertebral Disc

- *Structure:* The IVD is composed of a **nucleus** and **annulus.** The nucleus is a colloidal gel contained within a fibrous wall that is 80 to 90% water. Concentric layers of interwoven fibrocartilaginous fibers form the annulus. The thoracic discs are proportionally smaller than the cervical or lumbar discs, and the disc height is symmetric, rather than wedge-shaped as in the other two regions. Therefore, discs give the cervical and lumbar regions their curves and the vertebral body shape defines the thoracic curve.
- *Function:* The discs provide a shock-absorbing hydraulic system that permits a rockerlike movement of one vertebra upon the other owing to a fluid shift in the nucleus and an elasticity of the annulus. The disc also provides proprioceptive and nociceptive functions. Disc nutrition into the annulus occurs by movement of the spine, which pumps fluid into the disc through compression and decompression.
- *Dysfunction and injury:* The IVD is susceptible to age-related degeneration that involves loss of fluid in the nucleus and loss of elasticity of the annulus. Disc degeneration is common in the thoracic region, but it rarely becomes symptomatic, other than the stiffness associated with decreased mobility.[2] Disc herniation is rare in the thoracic spine because of the protection and stability afforded by the rib cage. Compression injuries fracture the vertebra before they injure the disc.[1]
- *Treatment implications:* Orthopedic massage (OM) introduces a new method of treatment called *wave mobilization* that theoretically helps promote fluid exchange to the disc. Through rhythmic cycles of posterior to anterior (P–A) mobilization, the author postulates that this compression and decompression pumps the disc to keep the disc well hydrated and potentially help rehydrate a degenerated disc.

Intervertebral Facets

- *Structure:* The **superior and inferior vertebral facets** are synovial joints between two vertebrae (See Fig. 4-3). As in the lumbar and cervical regions, joint capsules that are highly innervated with mechanoreceptors and pain receptors surround these facet joints. They also contain fibrocartilage meniscoid structures.[2]
- *Function:* The facets determine the range and direction of movement and have reflexive (automatic) communication to the surrounding muscles. They are designed to slide on each other in the healthy state. Extension closes the facets, and flexion opens them. For facets to maintain a healthy state, it is necessary for them to be moved through their full range of motion (ROM) regularly. Stretching programs, such as yoga, are extremely beneficial to the spinal facets.
- *Dysfunction and injury*
  - *Hypomobility:* Restricted motion at the thoracic facets implies a loss of the normal gliding motion on the cartilage surfaces. This restriction is called a **fixation** and may be caused by poor posture, injury, sustained muscle tension, entrapment of the articular meniscoid, or roughened articular surfaces because of degeneration. Restricted motion of the facets result in a reflex that typically creates hypertonicity of the muscles at the same vertebral level.
  - *Degeneration:* Degenerative changes are common in the thoracic spine and cause stiffening, called **hypomobility syndrome.** In the thoracic spine the most hypomobile areas are C7 to T1 and T12 to L1. High stress occurs in these two areas where the curves change direction. Hypertonicity in the muscles compresses the facets, reducing their mobility and, therefore, reducing their nutritional exchange, which depends on movement. This compression and decreased lubrication of the facets accelerates their degeneration.
  - *Irritation and injury:* When the thoracic joints are irritated as a result of acute injury or cumulative stress, they produce local pain and may refer pain into the anterior chest.[3] The pain is described as a deep, dull ache.
- *Treatment implications*: Dysfunction and injury to the facets are best treated with muscle energy technique (MET), manual release of the hypertonic thoracic extensor muscles, and P–A mobilization of the joints. Unlike the cervical and lumbar spine, the thoracic spine is rarely unstable. Rather, it typically becomes too stiff and requires increased movement, especially extension.

Costovertebral Joints

- *Structure:* The **costovertebral joints** are synovial joints on the body and transverse processes of the thoracic vertebrae that articulate with the ribs (Fig. 4-4). The articulation between the body and the transverse process is also called the **costotransverse joint.**
  - Except for T-1, which has only one joint at the body, each vertebra has two joints on its body for

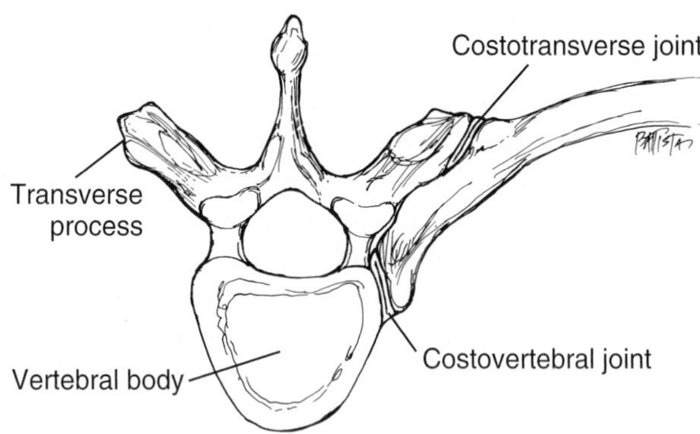

Figure 4-4. Costovertebral joints. Each rib forms a joint with the thoracic vertebra at two places, the vertebral body and the transverse process.

articulation with the rib. Each articulation is a synovial joint with a joint capsule and articular meniscoid, supported by numerous ligaments. The center of the head of the rib is attached to the intervertebral disc by interarticular ligaments.

- The costovertebral joints are highly innervated with pain fibers and mechanoreceptors. A powerful reflex creating hypertonicity in the muscles overlying the joint can be caused by irritation of these nerves.[2]

- ***Function:*** In the healthy state, the ribs have considerable movement at their articulation with the transverse processes and vertebral body.[4] Respiration, bending and twisting of the thoracic cage, and reaching with the arm all generate movement at the costovertebral joints.
- ***Dysfunction and injury:*** The costovertebral joints are susceptible to loss of their normal gliding characteristics due to injury, muscle spasm, meniscoid entrapment, and degeneration. Fixation of the costovertebral or costotransverse joints alters respiratory function and potentially causes a "catch," or sharp pain, on inspiration. This catch may be felt a few inches lateral to the spinous process, along the lateral portion of the chest wall, or in the anterior chest.[4]
- ***Treatment implications***: MET helps reduce muscle hypertonicity in the intercostal muscles and diaphragm and increases movement to the joints. P–A mobilization of the costovertebral joints stimulates the secretion of synovial fluid and helps reintroduce normal gliding characteristics. If your client has a catch in the thoracic spine with inspiration and your treatment does not resolve it, refer the client to a chiropractor or an osteopath for manipulation.

Spinous Process

The spinous processes (SPs) slope inferiorly and overlap the SP of the inferior vertebra. They are frequently asymmetric. It is fruitless to try to determine dysfunction merely by the position of the SP.

Sternum

The sternum is divided into three parts, the **manubrium, body,** and **xiphoid** (Fig. 4-5). The manubrium articulates with the clavicle and first rib at its superior-lateral aspect and with the second rib at the inferior-lateral aspect. The sternum protects the heart and lungs and other vital structures in the thoracic cavity.

Sternocostal and Costochondral Joints

- ***Structure:*** The **sternocostal joints** are synovial articulations between the costal (rib) cartilages and the sternum (see Fig. 4-5). At the first rib the articulation is cartilaginous, not synovial.
- The **costochondral joints** are the articulations of the bony portion of the T1 to T7 ribs with cartilage. They are located 1 to 2 inches lateral to the sternocostal joints. Costochondral joints are cartilaginous joints (synchondrosis) in which cartilage and bone are bound together by periosteum.
- ***Dysfunction and injury:*** Excessive weight training of the pectoral muscles or repetitive pushing or pulling can irritate or injure these joints. Acute trauma, such as falling on an outstretched arm; a blunt sports injury; or the impact of the shoulder harness during a car accident can create an acute inflammation that typically manifests as a localized, painful swelling.

Rib Cage

- ***Structure:*** There are 12 ribs on each side (see Fig. 4-5). The first seven are called "true ribs" because they attach directly to the sternum. Ribs 8 to 10 articulate below the sternum through cartilage, and the last two ribs, 11 and 12, are called "floating ribs" because they have no attachment to the sternum.
  - Twenty muscles that attach to the rib cage provide stability and movement to the trunk, pelvis, head, neck, and arms and assist in respiration.
  - An intercostal nerve travels between the ribs and can be irritated with injury to the ribs or from the synovial joints of the spine and ribs (Fig. 4-6).

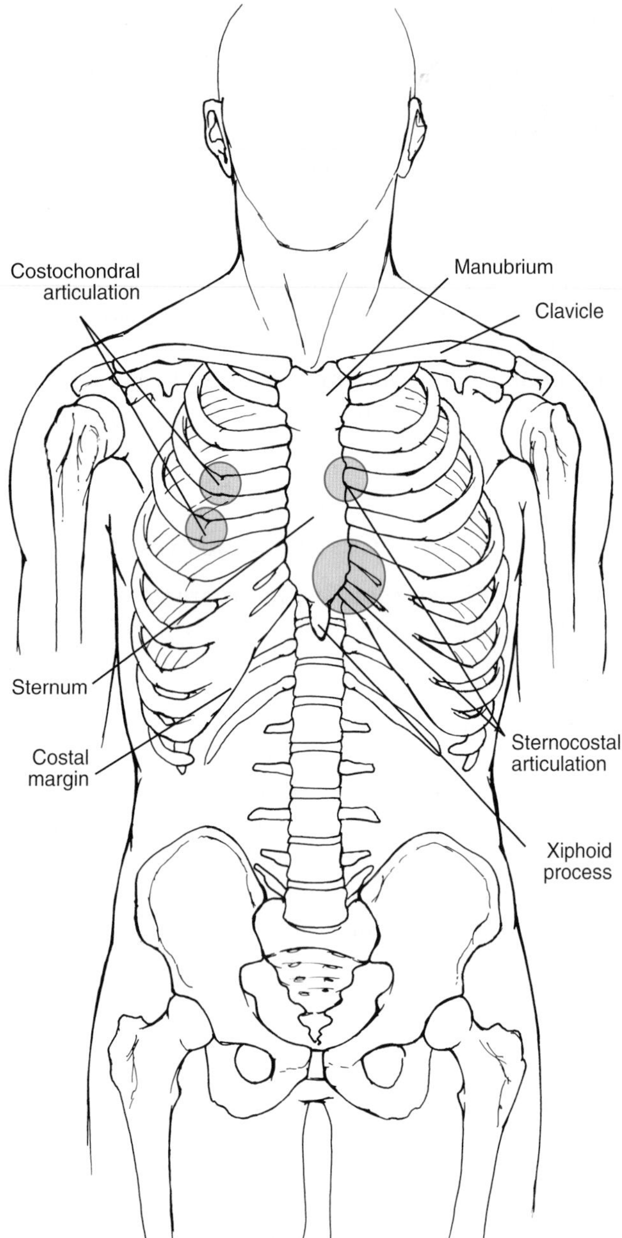

Figure 4-5. Anterior view of the rib cage, showing the costochondral and sternocostal joints.

- ***Function:*** The rib cage serves as protection to the heart and lungs, as attachment sites for the muscles, and its movement increases thoracic volume for respiration. The rib cage is resilient in the normal state; this springing quality is essential to maintain full respiratory capacity.
  - Movement of the rib cage is primarily concerned with respiration. The chest can expand in three directions: vertically, owing to the contraction of the diaphragm; and in the transverse and anterior to posterior directions due to the movement of the ribs.[1] The lateral aspect of the ribs elevates during inspiration, then lowers on expiration.
- ***Dysfunction and injury:*** The most common dysfunction of the rib cage is hypomobility that leads to stiffness and rigidity. This loss of movement contributes to hypomobility of the facet joints of the thoracic spine and to the costovertebral joints, decreasing respiratory function. Causes include adhesions as the result of trauma, respiratory diseases such as emphysema or asthma, chronic shallow breathing from emotional depression, or from the depression of the anterior rib cage caused by rounded shoulders.
  - Weakness of the extensors of the upper thoracic spine and the middle and lower trapezii prevents straightening of the upper back and decreases the ability of the chest to expand.[5]
  - Using the arms influences the rib cage because of the attachments of the powerful arm muscles. Polishing or scrubbing; repetitive reaching, especially overhead; or reaching with a twisting motion, such as reaching into the backseat of a car, can create irritation to the costovertebral joints.

Intervertebral Foramen

- ***Structure:*** The IVF is an opening (foramen) formed by:
  1. two pedicles from the superior and inferior vertebrae that form the roof and floor;
  2. the disc, posterior longitudinal ligament, and vertebral body anteriorly;
  3. the facets, anterior capsule, and ligamentum flavum posteriorly.
- ***Function:*** The IVF provides an opening for the motor and sensory nerve roots that originate at the spinal cord.
- ***Dysfunction and injury:*** The IVF of the thoracic spine is large; bone spurs seldom decrease the opening. Unlike in the lumbar spine, the IVF is posterior to the vertebral body rather than the disc, and therefore thoracic disc lesions do not affect the IVF. Also, because of restriction from the ribcage, the movements of the thoracic spine are much smaller than those of the cervical and lumbar regions. Therefore, the nerve roots, which lie in the IVF, have much less movement, and consequently the risk of irritation is not as great.[6]

Thoracic Region Nerves

- ***Structure:*** As in the other areas of the spine, the **thoracic nerves** are mixed nerves formed from the union of **motor (ventral)** and **sensory (dorsal) roots** that have emerged from the spinal cord. The roots merge to become the **spinal nerve.**

- *Sclerotomes:* No sclerotomes are in the thoracic spine
- *Myotomes:* There are no myotomes in the thoracic region, except T1, which innervates the intrinsic muscles of the hand and controls abduction and adduction of the fingers.
- *Dermatomes:* Dermatomes are segmentally arranged, correspond to the level of the vertebrae, and follow the ribs. Note that the T1 dermatome covers the inner arm to the medial wrist and that the T2 covers the pectoral, scapular, and axillary regions.

■ ***Dysfunction and injury:*** Except for T-1 and T-2, the thoracic spine is not generally involved in radicular (nerve root) pain, which would refer sharp, well-localized pain into the arm.[1] However, when the upper half of the thoracic spine is involved, diffuse, achy pain in the upper arm and axillary region may be greater than thoracic pain.[6]

- The irritation of the thoracic spinal nerve roots may also simulate visceral disease. For example, pain over the stomach or pancreas can be produced by T6 to T7; pain over the gallbladder, from T7 to T8; and pain in the kidney, from T-9.

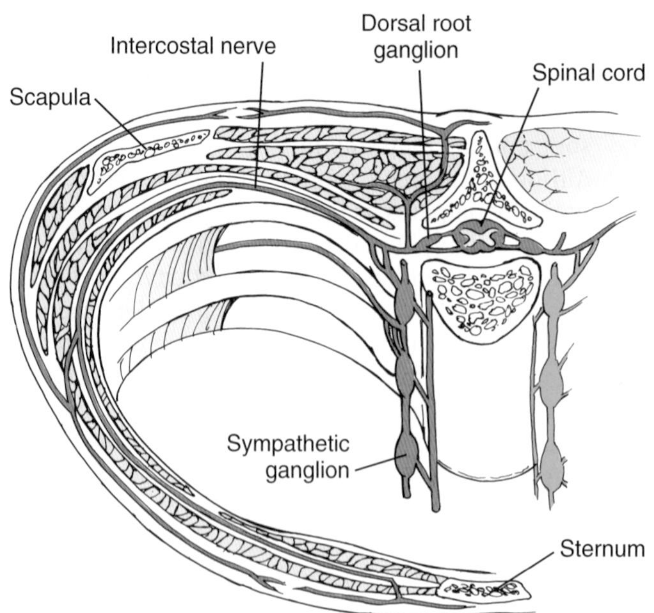

Figure 4-6. Nerves of the thoracic region, showing the intercostal nerves, the spinal cord, dorsal root ganglion, and sympathic ganglion.

Sympathetic Nervous System

■ ***Structure and function:*** Fibers from the **sympathetic nervous system** emerge from the spinal cord from T1 to L2 and innervate the cardiac, respiratory, and digestive systems. Sympathetic nerves mediate neurological reflexes, called *viscerosomatic* and *somatovisceral reflexes,* between the internal organs and the somatic structures such as the muscles, ligaments, and joint capsules.

■ ***Dysfunction and injury:*** Pain may be referred into the thoracic region from irritation of the abdominal organs (Fig. 4-7). For example, gallbladder irritation can refer pain to the right scapular region. The pain can vary from mild to severe and is not well-localized. Pain in the thoracic somatic structures may create increased sympathetic nerve impulses to the internal organs, creating pain and decreased function.[2]

Thoracic Region Muscles

■ ***Function:*** Muscles not only provide a dynamic stabilizing force to the thoracic region for posture and movement of the arms, the diaphragm creates the movement of the breath. Muscles also unconsciously (reflexively) communicate with the ligaments and joint capsule. Remember that muscles of the shoulder complex have a profound influence on thoracic function. Muscle contraction is often a primary source of thoracic stiffness, and restoration of proper muscle function is essential to an upright posture and normal mobility of the spine.

■ ***Dysfunction***

- Muscular imbalance in the thoracic spine is most commonly caused by poor posture. The client typically has a forward head, rounded shoulders, and increased thoracic curve (kyphosis).
- As the connective tissue of the fascia, muscle coverings, ligaments, and joint capsules adapt to faulty posture, shortening occurs in the upper chest, the thoracic outlet regions of the supraclavicular and infraclavicular spaces, the anterior shoulder, and the posterior cervical region. A reciprocal lengthening and weakening occurs in the scapular muscles, erector spinae, and lower trapezius.

As mentioned, Janda[5] has identified predictable patterns of muscle imbalance. The thoracic region participates in **upper-crossed syndrome,** because the tight pectoralis and upper trapezius and the weak deep-neck flexors, rhomboids, and middle and lower trapezius form a cross (Fig. 4-8).

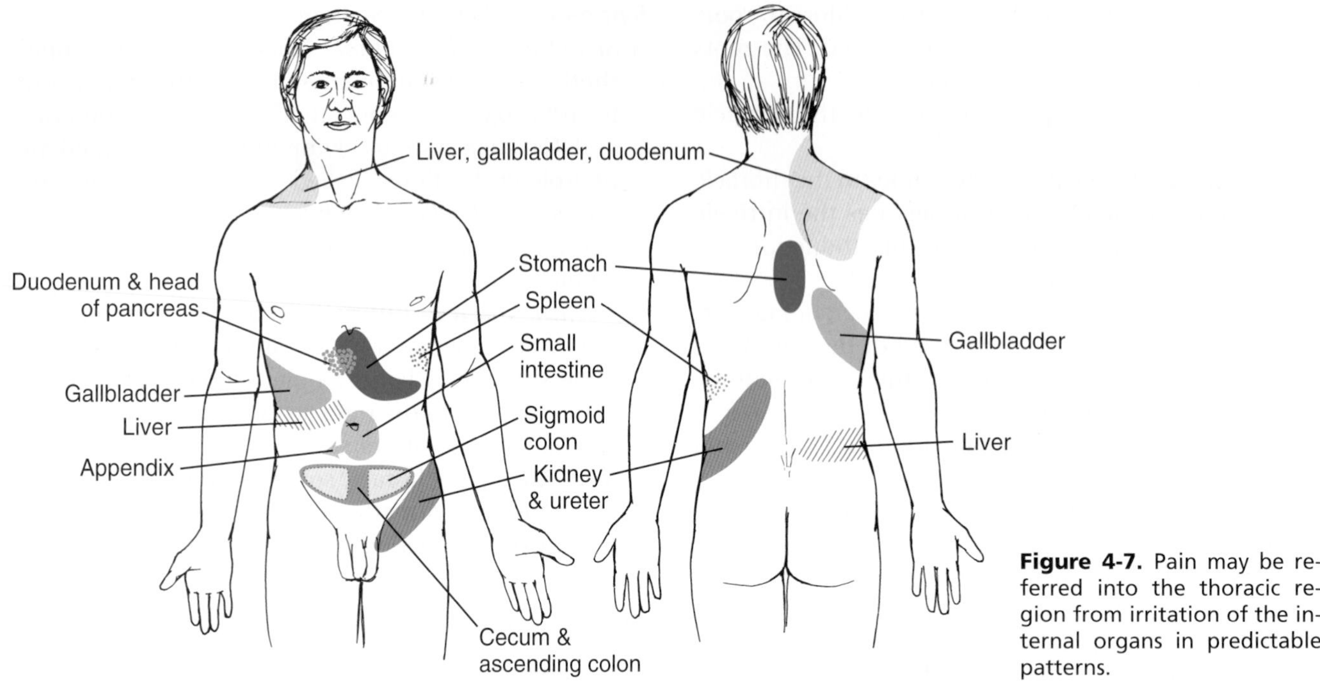

Figure 4-7. Pain may be referred into the thoracic region from irritation of the internal organs in predictable patterns.

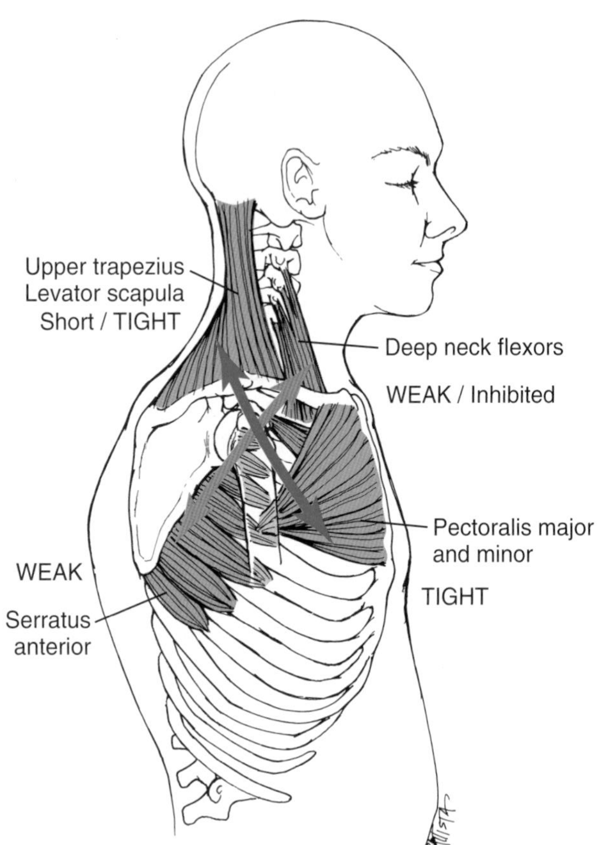

Figure 4-8. Upper crossed syndrome, a typical pattern of muscle imbalance. The upper trapezius and levator scapula are usually short and tight, and the deep neck flexors and the serratus anterior are typically weak and inhibited.

Muscle Imbalances of the Thoracic Region

- Muscle imbalances in the thoracic region can be caused by muscles that are weak and inhibited or muscles that are tight and short.
  - **Muscles that tend to be weak and inhibited:** are the middle and lower trapezius, rhomboids, serratus anterior, deep neck flexors, and scalenes.
  - **Muscles that tend to be tight and short:** are the upper trapezius and levator scapula, thoracic extensors, pectoralis major and minor, neck extensors, and the diaphragm.
  - Although the erector spinae of the thoracic region typically palpates as tight, these muscles are usually in a lengthened contraction and often test weak. This weakness is called a *stretch weakness,* as a muscle loses strength in its most lengthened position. Although the rhomboids are weak in the rounded-shoulder posture, they are often short and tight in the client with retracted and elevated shoulders. The scalenes may be either weak and long, or short and tight. With a decreased cervical curve, the deep neck flexors are short and tight.

Positional Dysfunction of the Thoracic Spine Muscles

- Thoracic spine muscles can have the following dysfunctions of position:
  - The thoracic and cervical extensors are pulled toward the midline into a medial torsion.

- The levator scapula rolls into an inferior torsion as the scapula protracts and rotates upward.
- The diaphragm is pulled toward the midline.
- The pectorals and anterior deltoid roll into an anterior and medial torsion.

- ***Treatment implications:*** When treating muscle imbalances anywhere in the body, it is important to release the short and tight muscles first, then strengthen the weak and inhibited muscles. This release may be accomplished with MET or manual techniques. For example, first release the thoracic and cervical extensors, levator, pectorals, upper trapezius, and diaphragm. Next, facilitate and strengthen the lower and middle trapezii, rhomboids, abdominals, and deep neck flexors. A typical session may involve postural assessment and correction before table work as well as after the session.

Anatomy of the Thoracic Region Muscles

The following are muscles of the thoracic spine (Table 4-1) that are not listed in Chapter 3 ("The Lumbosacral Spine").

Thoracic Region Dysfunction and Injury

FACTORS PREDISPOSING TO DYSFUNCTION AND PAIN IN THE THORACIC REGION

- Poor posture
- Excessive sitting
- Joint dysfunction
- Muscle imbalances
- Deconditioning
- Fatigue
- Altered movement patterns
- Emotional tension

TYPICAL REGIONS OF DYSFUNCTION IN THE THORACIC SPINE

The junctions between the cervical and the thoracic spine and between the thoracic and the lumbar spine are two common areas of increased functional disturbances and are areas of high incidence of degenerative changes in the facet joints. This increased vulnerability has several causes.

- **Cervicothoracic junction**
  - A change occurs in the orientation of the facets between C-7 and T-1, creating increased mechanical stress.
  - This junction represents the point in the curves where the highly mobile cervical spine meets the relatively immobile thoracic spine.
  - It is an area of attachment for many scapular muscles and muscles that support the weight of the head. The FHP causes a drastic increase in tension to the muscles attaching in this area.
- **Thoracolumbar junction:** Dysfunction and injury occur in this region for the following reasons:
  - The orientation of the facets changes in this area from the coronal-facing facets of T-12 to the mostly sagittal-facing facets at L1.
  - This area often becomes hypertonic and hypomobile to compensate for a hypermobile and unstable lumbosacral junction.
  - It is a high-stress area because it is where the curves change direction.
  - It is prone to rotational injury.[1]

TYPICAL POSTURAL FAULTS IN THE THORACIC SPINE

Kyphosis

- A **kyphotic thoracic spine** is an increase in the normal posterior curve. A common cause is slouching (poor posture), which presents as the forward-head, rounded-shoulder appearance. Congenital factors, a localized healed fracture, osteoporosis, or degeneration of the vertebrae may cause a kyphotic thoracic spine.
- If the increased curve is a result of postural changes, the following muscle imbalances typically occur:
  - Elevation and protraction of the shoulders caused by a short upper trapezius and levator scapula and a weak middle and lower trapezius.
  - FHP, tight thoracic erector spinae, and weak lower trapezius.
  - Rounded shoulders as a result of a short and tight pectorals, especially pectoralis minor, and an internally rotated humerus with a short anterior joint capsule.
  - Winging of the scapula caused by a weak serratus anterior.
- **A flat upper thoracic spine** may be a normal variant, with completely normal x-rays and good motion characteristics, as determined by motion palpation. However, a flattened thoracic curve is often

TABLE 4-1 MUSCLES OF THE THORACIC SPINE THAT ARE NOT LISTED IN CHAPTER 3

Muscle	*Origin*	*Insertion*
Diaphragm	From the dorsum of the xiphoid process, inner surfaces of the lower six costal cartilages and lower six ribs and the bodies of the upper lumbar vertebrae	Into a central tendon in the middle of the muscle
External and internal intercostals	The external intercostal arises from the lower border of the ribs, and the internal intercostal arises from the inner surface of the ribs	The external and internal intercostals insert into the superior border of the ribs
Levator costarum	The transverse processes of C7 and the upper 11 thoracic vertebrae	
Serratus Anterior: See Chapter 6, "The Shoulders."		Onto the rib immediately below each vertebra

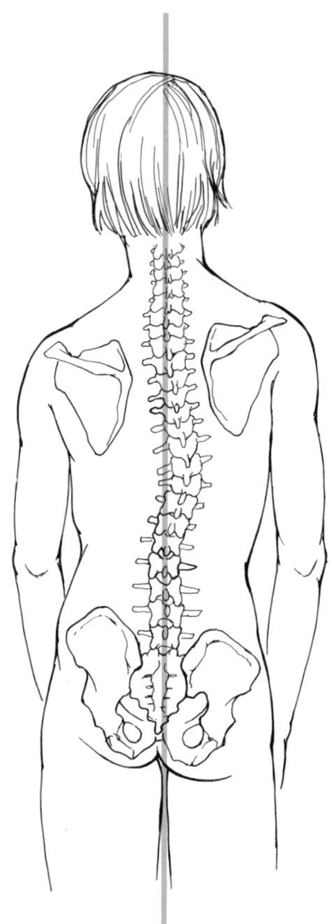

Figure 4-9. Scoliosis is a lateral deviation of the spine. View of a right thoracic scoliosis as the convexity of the curve is to the right.

an area of painful stiffness. Postural changes and muscle imbalances with a flat thoracic spine are as follows:

- Decreased thoracic curve, depressed scapula and clavicle, and decreased curve in the cervical spine (military spine).
- Muscle imbalances, for example, tight erector spinae, tight scapula retractors (rhomboids and middle and lower trapezii), and decreased scapulothoracic mobility.

Scoliosis

- *Definition:* **Scoliosis** is defined as one or more lateral curves in the spine (Fig. 4-9). The curve is described to the side of convexity. For example, a left thoracic scoliosis has the convex part of the curve to the left.
- *Causes:* There are many known causes of scoliosis that are the result of disease or injury. However, 70 to 80% are classified as idiopathic; that is, there is no known cause.[7] Although there is a genetic predisposition, with 25 to 33% occurring among relatives, Lauren Berry, RPT, believed that scoliosis often begins as a mechanical disorder. The situation begins when a young child has a hard fall, which creates muscle hypertonicity and a vertebral fixation or subluxation. When left untreated, this muscle hypertonicity and fixation or subluxation

Action	Dysfunction
The principal muscle of respiration. During inspiration, the diaphragm contracts and descends. During expiration, the muscle relaxes, and the elastic recoil of the lungs moves the air out. The diaphragm is often held in a sustained tension, shortening its fibers, and pulling the anterior-inferior portion of the rib cage toward the spine. This tension reduces full inhalation.	In the author's clinical experience, the sustained tension in the diaphragm is also an underlying cause of many conditions that have been diagnosed as hiatal hernia. The tension pulls the stomach up slightly.
These muscles elevate the ribs and expand the chest. They play an important role in respiration and posture, as they stabilize and maintain the shape of the rib cage.	When the chest is depressed as in the rounded-shoulders posture (a kyphotic spine) or because of adhesions after injury, there is a decreased ability to expand the chest.
Elevates and abducts the ribs and assists in inspiration.	

causes an unlevelling of the pelvis and the spine grows unevenly. This situation is based on the Heuter-Volkman theory that states that increased pressure across an epiphyseal (growth) plate inhibits growth, whereas decreased pressure accelerates growth.[8]

- The paraspinal muscles have been implicated as a major causative factor in the production and progression of adolescent idiopathic scoliosis.[9] Paradoxically, some studies show greater electrical activity in the muscles at the apex of the convex side, suggesting that a deep muscle contracture of the multifidus on the convex side can create scoliosis.[9]
- Scoliosis has two types: functional and structural.
  - ***Functional:*** Functional scoliosis disappears with forward flexion of the trunk. It is caused by muscle imbalances, postural imbalances, or leg-length differences. The functional curve is believed to be the precursor of the structural curve.[9]
  - ***Structural:*** The lateral curve does not straighten with forward or lateral flexion of the spine. The vertebrae have a fixed rotation of the body toward the convexity. Since the ribs rotate with the vertebrae, there is a prominence of the ribs posteriorly on the side of vertebral body rotation. This prominence is the result of bony deformity or soft-tissue changes in the discs, ligaments, joint capsules, and muscles. Structural scoliosis is classified into two major types: irreversible and reversible.[8]
  - ***Irreversible:*** Structural scoliosis that is irreversible is caused by structural deformity within, between, or around the vertebrae. The soft-tissue changes are the same as described below under reversible.
  - ***Reversible:*** Structural scoliosis that is reversible is caused by structural changes that are the result of possible reversible ligament shortening or chronic muscular hypertonicity.[8] The joint capsules shorten on the concave side. The intertransversarii, erector spinae, quadratus lumborum, psoas major, and oblique abdominals all shorten on the concave side, limiting lateral flexion toward the convex side.[7]
- ***Muscle imbalances related to scoliosis:*** A complex pattern of imbalance affects the pelvis. The erectors are typically short on the concave side and weak on the convex side. In addition, there is sustained contraction in the multifidi at the apex of the convex curve.
- ***Treatment implications:*** As Kendall et al[10] point out, scoliosis is a problem of asymmetry. As muscle imbalances play an important role in the development of scoliosis, assess the length of the iliopsoas, adductors, quadratus lumborum, hamstrings, thoracolumbar fascia (TFL), iliotibial band (ITB), and latissimus. Assess the strength of the back extensors, abdominals, hip extensors, hip abductors, and lower trapezius. Also release the diaphragm, as it is typi-

cally short and tight. OM and contract-relax (CR) MET on the tight muscles and MET to help facilitate the weak muscles provide a valuable contribution. It is essential that the client receives proper exercise instruction and maintain a home program that involves stretching the tight areas and strengthening the weak areas.

DIFFERENTIATION OF THORACIC PAIN

- The thoracic spine and chest wall are common sites of referral from conditions other than the neuromusculoskeletal system, including inflammation and diseases of the heart, lungs, and abdominal organs. Dysfunction and injury to the thoracic spine and costovertebral joints can also mimic symptoms of diseases from these organs. These symptoms can generate a lot of anxiety because of the concern about heart disease. Refer to the section titled "Contraindications to Massage Therapy: Red Flags" in Chapter 2 for information on when a massage therapist should refer a client to a doctor. Here it is assumed that your client is under the care of a doctor for any persistent pain in the thoracic region.
- The vast majority of midback pain is caused by a mechanical disorder. The most common disorders include sustained muscle tension, hypomobility of the thoracic intervertebral and costovertebral facets, and acute fixation of those facets.
- Hypertonicity of the thoracic muscles is typically caused by poor posture or emotional tension, which can create a diffuse, dull ache in the midback and stiffness in the upper trapezius region. It is worse at the end of the day and better with rest.
- Corrigan and Maitland[3] state that the most common cause of chest pain is a referral from irritation of the thoracic or lower cervical facet joints. The thoracic vertebral facets produce both local and referred pain.[11] The pain is typically described as a deep, dull ache, worse with extension and rotation toward the side of pain and better with rest. With an acute episode of joint fixation and capsular inflammation, the symptoms can be sharp and well-localized. If the client does not gain symptom resolution after a brief trial of therapy, refer him or her to a chiropractor or an osteopath for a trial of manipulation.
- Except for T-1 and T-2, generally, the thoracic spine is not involved in radicular (nerve root) pain that would refer sharp well-localized pain into the arm.[1] However, when the upper half of the thoracic spine is involved, pain in the upper arm and axillary region may be greater than that of the thoracic region.[12]
- Fixation of the costovertebral or costotransverse joints often causes a "catch," or sharp pain, on inspiration that may be felt posteriorly along the lateral portion of the chest wall, in the anterior chest, or through the chest.[1]
- Degeneration of the intervertebral facets (osteoarthrosis) or degeneration of the intervertebral disc (spondylosis) create a dull, achy stiffness in the midback region. The symptoms are typically worse in the morning and at the end of the day.
- A cervical disc lesion or injury to the lower cervical spine is a common cause of pain in the upper thoracic spine.[6] The scapular region is innervated primarily by cervical nerves and is often a referral site for cervical injury.
- The pain from pathologic fractures of the vertebral body, secondary to osteoporosis, is most common in the mid-thoracic region and is described as a persistent ache, even at rest. Remember that osteoporosis may be asymptomatic.[1]

COMMON TYPES OF DYSFUNCTION AND INJURY OF THE THORACIC REGION

Thoracic Muscle Strain (Upper Trapezius Most Common)

- *Causes:* Forward head, rounded-shoulders posture; emotional or psychological stress; prolonged sitting; or injury, such as a whiplash.
- *Symptoms:* Dull, diffuse, achy pain or stiffness—typically located in the posterior neck and upper scapular region with trapezius involvement, and in the upper back and midback with rhomboid hypertonicity—or sustained contraction of the lower attachments of the cervical erectors. Pain is made worse with neck movements, especially cervical flexion, or sitting, and it is relieved with rest. The suboccipital nerves are often entrapped in the fascia and muscle of the trapezius attachment to the occiput, creating an occipital headache.
- *Signs:* Upper trapezius, rhomboids, levator scapula, and cervical extensors are taut and tender to palpation; postural slumping; and weakness in the deep neck flexors.
- *Treatment:* The entire OM series of Level I thoracic and cervical strokes, strengthening exercise for the lower trapezius and scapular stabilizers, postural training, and stress management.

Arthrosis (Arthritis) or Spondylosis

- *Causes:* Degeneration of the facet joints, often caused by adaptive shortening from poor postural habits or prior trauma, that leads to fibrosis of the joint capsules. Spondylosis is a degeneration of the intervertebral disc. In the early stages this condition begins as hypomobility of the vertebral facets.
- *Symptoms:* Dull, diffuse, achy pain located in the middle of the back; usually feels stiff, but can get sharp with certain movements. Pain is worse in the morning and at the end of the day.
- *Signs:* Client often presents with forward-head and rounded-shoulder posture, with increased kyphosis. Active ROM is limited, especially extension, and lateral flexion and rotation to painful side. Passive motion of the spine reveals a stiffened or hardened spine, with a capsular or bony-end-feel. Palpation reveals thick, fibrous soft tissue.
- *Treatment:* OM strokes that emphasize mobilization of the joints by means of compression and decompression to hydrate the soft tissue and joints; stretching exercises that emphasize extension and rotation. Yoga is recommended.

Fixation or Subluxation of the Vertebral Facets

- *Cause:* Poor posture, muscle imbalances, emotional or psychological tension leading to muscle hypertonicity, fatigue, deconditioning all predispose to altered joint movement and potential fixation of the facets.
- *Symptoms:* An acute episode involves sharp, local pain, often radiating laterally. The upper thoracic spine can cause arm pain, and the lower thoracic spine can refer pain to the lumbar spine, iliac crest, buttock, and anterior groin.
- *Signs:* Loss of joint play at the involved joint; hypertonic and tender muscles at the fixated segment.
- *Treatment:* The thoracic series of OM strokes and an adjustment or manipulation by a chiropractic or an osteopathic doctor.

Scoliosis

- *Cause:* Idiopathic, no known cause. See p. 132 for further discussion.
- *Symptoms:* Stiff, achy back, often localized to one side. May be asymptomatic, but if the curve is noticeable, it often creates embarrassment and emotional distress.
- *Signs:* Adam's test is positive. Client stands with feet together and with palms together, then bends over as if to place his fingertips between his feet. A positive test reveals a rib hump on the side of spinal rotation, indicating a structural scoliosis. In functional scoliosis, the curve is evident in standing and straightens in forward bending.
- *Treatment:* The thoracic, cervical, lumbar, and hip series of OM strokes; proper exercise instruction, and manipulation by a chiropractic or an osteopathic doctor. Curves are classified by x-ray as mild, moderate, or severe. Mild curves in children should be evaluated every 3 to 4 months. Moderate curves are treated with massage, manipulation, exercise, and bracing. For severe curves, conservative treatment should be tried before surgery is considered.

Costovertebral Joint Fixation

- *Cause:* The costovertebral joints are susceptible to loss of their normal gliding characteristics due to injury, muscle spasm, meniscoid entrapment, and degeneration.
- *Symptoms:* Localized pain, typically a few inches lateral to the SP, and when the upper ribs are involved, a dull ache in the scapular area. Often refers pain to the lateral and anterior chest. Pain can be sharp, stabbing, burning, or aching. Client may report a pain through the chest.[4] The first rib is commonly involved; symptoms include a dull, nagging ache in the lower neck, with occasional burning pain in the upper trapezius.[2]
- *Signs:* Increase in pain on deep inspiration; localized areas of extreme sensitivity to pressure at the transverse processes and rib angles; muscular spasm in the interscapular area. With first rib involvement, decreased cervical rotation to the side of fixation occurs, and cervical extension increases the pain.
- *Treatment:* OM and MET to the rhomboids, erectors, and serratus posterior superior for the upper ribs. As the scalenes, serratus anterior, and subclavius all attach to the first rib, manual release and MET to those areas often help release the fixation.

Osteoporosis

- *Cause:* Calcium deficiency, estrogen loss, and lack of weight-bearing exercise cause a thinning of the bone and wedge-shaped vertebrae due to microfractures. Because the weight is placed on the anterior part of the vertebrae, a round back called *senile kyphosis* may occur.

- ***Symptoms:*** Osteoporosis can be asymptomatic even with a pronounced kyphotic spine. Typically, a persistent ache in the thoracic spine and a lower backache are present.
- ***Signs:*** Observation reveals either a rounded kyphosis or a sharp angulation if there is a localized collapse of a vertebra.
- ***Treatment:*** OM can be temporarily relieving, but these clients need extension exercises, postural education, and encouragement to walk. As diet and hormone levels play a significant role, these areas must be addressed.

Assessment

HISTORY QUESTIONS FOR CLIENT'S WHO HAVE THORACIC PAIN

Client typically uses words such as tightness, stiffness, or aching when describing their complaints in the thoracic region. It is important to differentiate between muscle tension problems that arise during periods of high stress and an acute episode of pain that results from chronic conditions in this area. The thoracic spine is a classic area where chronic poor posture, underlying degeneration, or hypomobility in the spine or a combination of the foregoing may be underlying causes. It can be frustrating for both therapist and client to have the client return week after week with the same tension, even after a great massage therapy treatment. A few simple questions will help differentiate complaints arising from poor posture and degeneration from simple muscle tension.

- How long has this area been troubling you?
  - Obviously, the longer the area has been problematic, the more you suspect an underlying postural or degenerative condition. The assessment can differentiate between these two causes.
- Is your discomfort (pain, stiffness) better or worse in the morning?
  - Muscle tension is typically better after a night's rest. Clients who have degenerative arthritis and hypomobility syndromes are stiffer or ache more in the morning and at the end of the day.
- Is the pain sharp and well-localized or dull and achy?
  - Sharp pain in the thoracic spine typically indicates a joint fixation, either at the vertebrae or at the articulation of the rib to the vertebrae. A fixation of the rib and vertebrae is often painful with breathing. Sharp pain in the spine in the elderly may also be an indication of microfractures from osteoporosis. If the client can lie comfortably on the table without pain, proceed with the massage. After the massage, refer the client who has sharp local pain to a chiropractor or an osteopath for further assessment and treatment.

OBSERVATION: CLIENT STANDING

Posterior View

- Observe the skin for any redness or swelling that may indicate inflammation and the need for much lighter pressure in your strokes. Also, notice any scars that may indicate a previous serious injury or surgery.
- Observe any asymmetry in the level of the client's shoulders and iliac crests (see lumbar assessment).

Adam's Test

- The Adam's test is performed to detect whether the client has scoliosis (Fig.4-10).
  - ***Position:*** Have the client stand, with feet and palms together, in front of you.

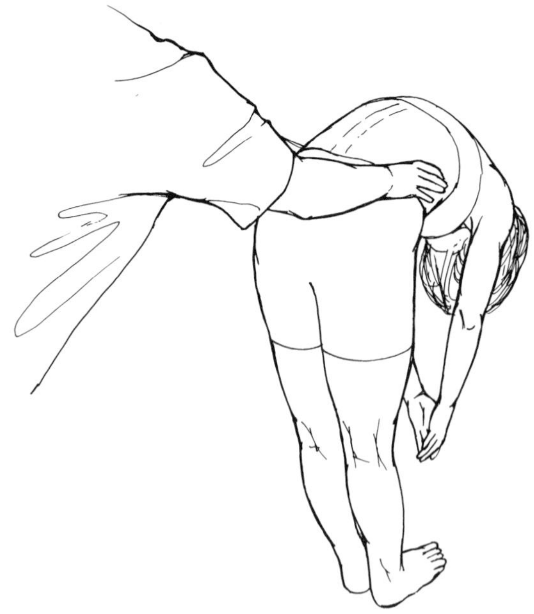

Figure 4-10. Adam's test. Therapist observes the thoracic spine to see if the ribs deviate or form a hump to one side, a sign of structural scoliosis.

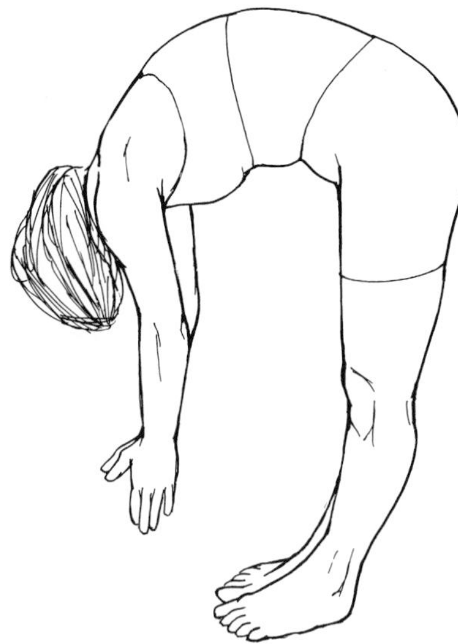

Figure 4-11. Side view of normal thoracic curve. Notice the smooth bend to the spine, rather than a sharp angle that would indicate a kyphotic spine.

- *Action:* Instruct the client to bend forward until his or her spine is parallel to the floor. Have the client relax his or her arms and head, pointing the fingertips midway between the feet.
- *Observation:* Bend down so that your eyes are level with the spine. This is called the "skyline view." Note the presence of a rib hump on one side of the rib cage. The rib hump indicates that the bodies of the vertebrae have rotated to the side of the hump and that the client has structural scoliosis. If you noticed a curvature in the spine when the client was standing and the curve straightens out with performance of Adam's test, the client has functional scoliosis.
- *Structural scoliosis:* Client has a rib hump when performing Adam's test. This indicates a dysfunction or growth deformity in the spinal body, joint structure, or both.
- *Functional scoliosis:* Lateral curve in the spine noted in standing, but there is no rib hump with Adam's test. This finding indicates that muscle hypertonicity or fascial shortening has caused the curvature. This curvature can be a result of work or postural habits.

Side View

- Observe whether the client has an increased thoracic curve (kyphosis), a decreased curve (flat thoracic spine), or a normal curve.

Test to Differentiate Between a Structural and a Functional Kyphosis

- *Position:* Have the client stand, with feet shoulder-width apart. Stand to the client's side (Fig.4-11).
- *Action:* Instruct the client to bend forward, arms hanging, until the spine is approximately parallel to the floor.
- *Observation:* Note whether the spine has a smooth, even curve to it or whether it has a sharp bend in the thoracic region. A sharp bend in the thoracic spine is indicative of structural kyphosis.

MOTION ASSESSMENT

Active Motion

- Active motion assessment of the thoracic spine is considered part of the "Motion Assessment Lumbosacral Spine" (see p. 100).

Test to Confirm a Structural Kyphosis

- *Position:* Have the client lie prone on the massage table, with arms at the sides. Stand at the side of the table.
- *Action:* Have the client slowly lift his or her head and chest off the table to the comfortable limit.
- *Observation:* Note whether the kyphosis changes as the client lifts into extension. Structural kyphosis remains on active extension. A structural kyphosis is caused by bone distortion, fixation in the joints, or ligamentous shortening. A functional kyphosis is caused by sustained muscular imbalances, most commonly in the erector spinae, iliopsoas, quadratus lumborum, and diaphragm.

PALPATION

- *Intention:* To assess the condition of the joints and soft tissue of the thoracic region, perform P-A glide into the joints and medial to lateral scooping strokes into the soft tissue.
- *Position:* Have the client lie in the fetal position, with a pillow between the knees and the arms and hands folded together in the "prayer position."

- *Action:* Using the supported-thumb position, first perform a series of slow, medial to lateral scooping strokes into the medial portion of the erector spinae muscles, from approximately T-12 to C-7. Next, using a soft fist, press into the thoracic spine in a P–A direction, performing a series of P–A mobilizations on the joints.
- *Observation:* The mobilization and palpation strokes should feel relaxing and completely pain-free in the healthy spine. Healthy muscles are relaxed, pliable, and resilient. Inflamed tissue is painful. The degree of pain indicates the level of inflammation. Hypertonic muscles have a tight, springy resistance to pressure. Fibrous, chronic tension in the muscles feels thick and gristly.

Healthy facet joints of the thoracic spine and costovertebral joints are resilient and bend with your pressure. Thickened soft tissue of the ligaments and capsule have a thick resistance to your P–A mobilization. A localized degeneration has a hard resistance to movement, while more diffuse degeneration also has this hard resistance but in a broader area.

Specific Muscle Palpation

Specific muscle palpation is performed in the context of doing the strokes. Through OM you can assess not only the quality of the soft tissue but also the mobility of the joints (see Chapter 2, "Assessment & Technique").

Techniques

MUSCLE ENERGY TECHNIQUES

- Remember, METs should never be painful.
- Typically, the thoracic erector spinae muscles are tight and long, held in an eccentric contraction because of FHP. In this lengthened position, they often are weak, a phenomenon called *stretch weakness.*
- METs are typically given within the context of performing the strokes.

Muscle Energy Technique for Acute Thoracic Pain

1. Contract-Relax Muscle Energy Technique for the Thoracic Extensors

- *Intention:* To help reduce hypertonicity in the thoracic extensors. This MET is particularly indicated for clients in acute pain (Fig. 4-12).

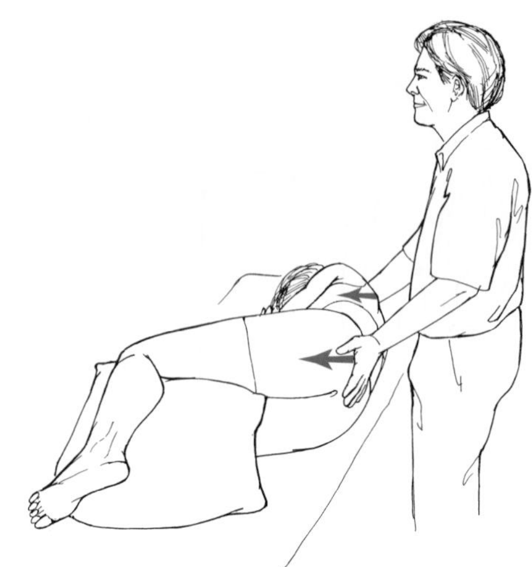

Figure 4-12. CR MET for acute thoracic pain.

- *Position:* Client is in the side-lying position, with the chin tucked slightly to lengthen the cervical extensors. Place your hand on the occiput and your other hand on the sacrum.
- *Action:* Have your client resist as you press P–A with both hands. This resistance engages the client's extensors. To reciprocally inhibit, place one hand on the anterior humerus and one hand on the anterior superior iliac spine (ASIS) and have the client resist as you attempt to pull posteriorly.

Muscle Energy Techniques to Release Hypertonic Muscles in the Thoracic Region

2. Postisometric Relaxation Muscle Energy Technique for the Latissimus Dorsi and Thoracolumbar Fascia

- *Intention:* To reduce muscle hypertonicity, lengthen the latissimus dorsi, and reduce tension in the TLF (Fig. 4-13).
- *Position:* The client is in the side-lying position, and the top arm is overhead. The knees are tucked to flatten the lower back, which stretches the latissimus. Hold the distal forearm with both hands.
- *Action:* Have the client resist from the pelvic attachment of the latissimus as you attempt to pull the arm further overhead. Have the client relax, and as he or she is relaxing, pull the arm until you reach a new resistance barrier. Have the client resist as you attempt to pull again, and repeat this CR–lengthen cycle several times. Reciprocally inhibit the muscle by having the client make a fist and resist as you push on the fist toward his or her body.

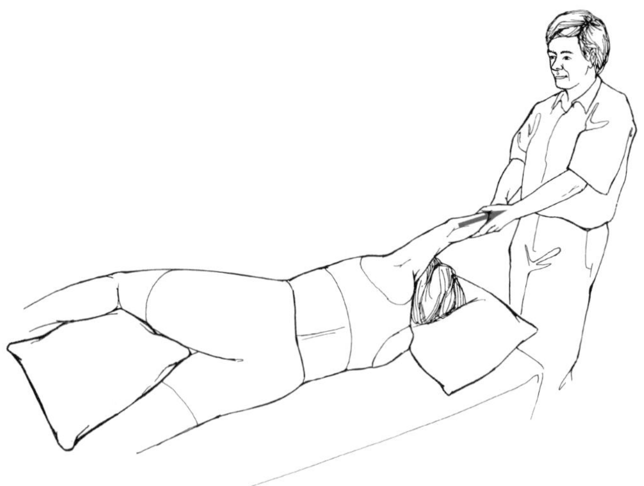

Figure 4-13. PIR MET for the latissimus dorsi and TLF.

3. Contract-Relax Muscle Energy Technique and Sensory Awareness for the Middle and Lower Trapezius

- ***Intention:*** To increase sensory awareness and strengthen the middle and the lower trapezius. The lower trapezius is typically weak, which allows the scapula to migrate headward, losing essential stability in the shoulder complex. This MET helps the client learn to use this muscle effectively, bringing strength and sensory awareness to the muscle (Fig. 4-14).

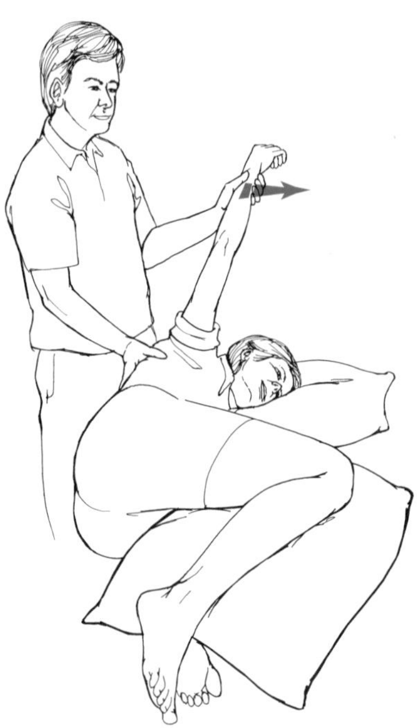

Figure 4-14. CR MET for the lower trapezius.

- ***Position:*** The client is side-lying. Client lifts his or her arm into two different positions, one at a time. First, have the client lift his or her arm in a "T" position, that is, reaching toward the ceiling, for the middle trapezius. After you perform MET on the middle trapezius, have the client lift his or her arm in the "Y" position, that is, approximately 135° of abduction, with the palm facing overhead. Place one hand on the client's distal forearm and the other hand on the middle border of the scapula for the middle trapezius and the lower border of the scapula for the lower trapezius.
- ***Action:*** Have the client resist as you attempt to press the arm anteriorly for approximately 5 seconds. Tap on the muscle fibers and say, "Feel this muscle working" to bring sensory awareness to the muscle. Perform the "T" and "Y" positions. Reciprocal inhibition (RI) is having the client resist as you attempt to pull the arm back toward you for approximately 5 seconds.

4. Contract-Relax Muscle Energy Technique to Reduce Hypertonicity in the Thoracic Erector Spinae

- ***Intention:*** To reduce the hypertonicity of the thoracic erector spinae and release tension in the TLF.
- ***Position:*** The client is in the side-lying position, and the top arm is overhead in the "I" position, with palms facing the head (Fig 4-15). The knees are tucked to flatten the lower back, which stretches the erector spinae and TLF. Place one hand on the distal forearm and the other hand on the erector spinae.
- ***Action:*** Instruct the client to resist as you attempt to press the arm forward for approximately 5 seconds. Do not allow the client to arch the lower back as he or she resists you.

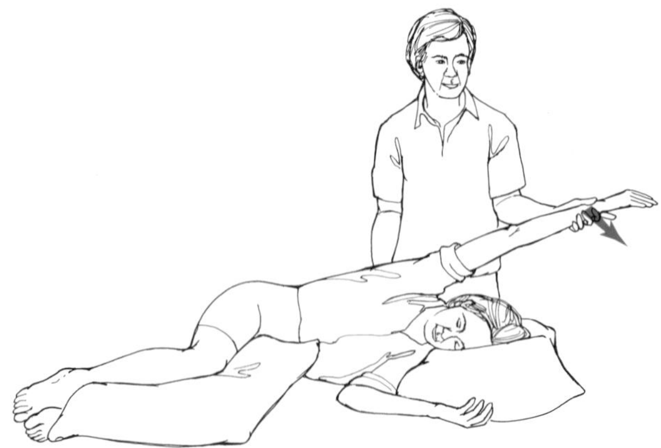

Figure 4-15. CR-MET to reduce the hypertonicity in the thoracic extensor muscles.

5. **Contract-Relax and Postisometric Muscle Energy Technique for the Rhomboids**
   - ☐ ***Intention:*** To reduce hypertonicity and lengthen the rhomboids. (Fig 4-16)

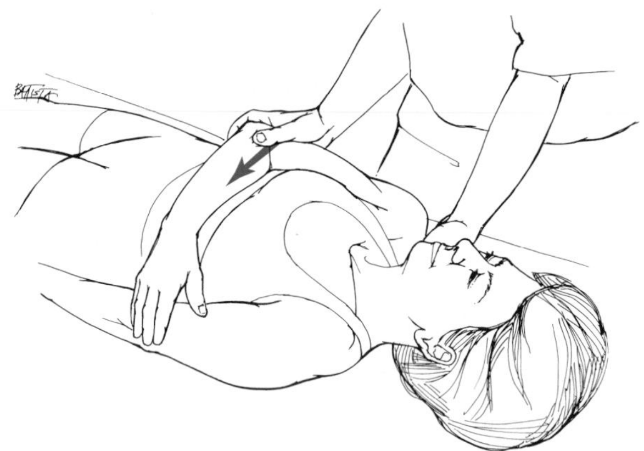

Figure 4-16. CR and PIR-MET for the rhomboids.

   - ☐ ***Position:*** Client is supine, with arm resting on the chest. Place one hand on the elbow, and the other hand on the rhomboids.
   - ☐ ***Action:*** Instruct the client to resist as you attempt to push the arm across his or her chest. Push for 5 seconds, have the client relax, and either repeat in the same position, or while the client is relaxing, stretch the rhomboids by moving the arm further across the chest, protracting the scapula. After the client relaxes, use your fingertips to scoop the rhomboids headward, as you push the elbow toward the pelvis, approximately 1 inch.

6. **Contract-Relax Muscle Energy Technique for the Muscles Attaching to the Scapula**
   - ☐ ***Intention:*** To reduce the hypertonicity of the muscles attaching to the scapula (Fig 4-17).
   - ☐ ***Position:*** Client is in the side-lying fetal position. Place both hands on the scapula.
   - ☐ ***Action:*** Have the client resist for approximately 5 seconds in four directions: (1) client resists as you attempt to push the scapula headward to reduce lower trapezius hypertonicity; (2) client resists as you attempt to pull the scapula inferiorly to help release the upper trapezius, rhomboids, and levator scapula; (3) client resists as you push the scapula anteriorly, to release the middle trapezius and rhomboids; and (4) client resists as you attempt to pull the scapula posteriorly for the pectoralis minor and major. After performing the MET, mobilize the scapula in a circular motion.

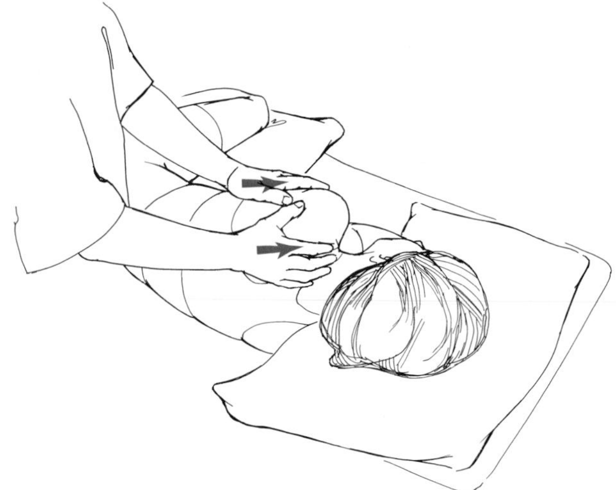

Figure 4-17. CR MET for muscles attaching to the scapula.

7. **Postisometric Relaxation Muscle Energy Technique for the Levator Scapula**
   - ☐ ***Intention:*** To reduce hypertonicity and lengthen the levator scapula (Fig 4-18).
   - ☐ ***Position:*** Client is in the side-lying fetal position. Place one hand over the acromion and one hand on the mastoid process.
   - ☐ ***Action:*** Ask your client to rotate his or her head slightly toward the pillow. Next, pull the shoulder caudally until the slack in the tissue is taken out. Then, ask the client to resist as you attempt to push his or her head into the pillow. Have the client hold for 5 seconds and then relax, and after the client relaxes for a few seconds, pull the scapula away from the head. Repeat the CR–stretch cycle several times.

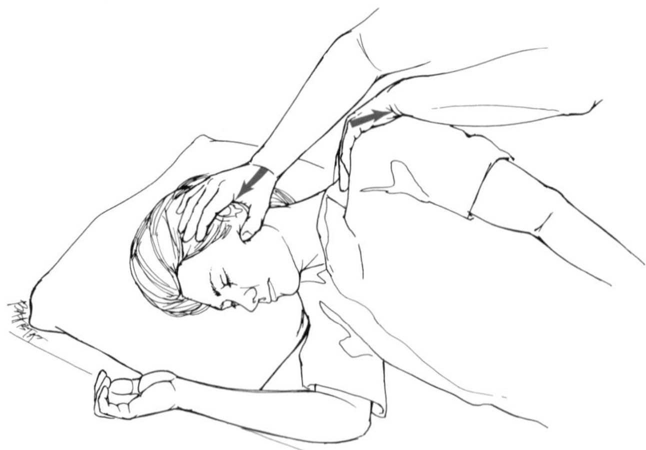

Figure 4-18. PIR MET for the levator scapula in the side-lying position.

8. Contract-Relax Muscle Energy Technique for the Diaphragm and Intercostals and Mobilization of the Rib Cage

- *Intention:* To reduce hypertonicity in the diaphragm and intercostals and increase respiratory capacity (Fig 4-19).

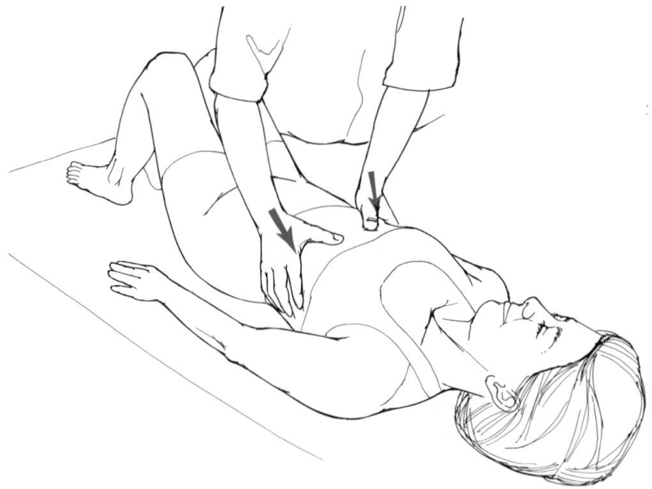

Figure 4-19. CR MET for the diaphragm and intercostal muscles and mobilization of the rib cage.

- *Position:* Place the client in the supine position, with knees up, feet on the table. Facing 45° headward position, place both hands on the lateral aspect of the lower ribs, with your fingers in the intercostal spaces.
- *Action:* Gently compress the rib cage and offer slight resistance as you ask the client to inhale slowly and fully, expanding the rib cage. As the client is inhaling, cock your wrists into ulnar deviation to elevate the anterior portion of the ribs. Tell the client to relax, and as he or she exhales, gently compress the rib cage to squeeze the air out and mobilize the ribs. Repeat this several times.

9. Contract-Relax Muscle Energy Technique for the Transversospinalis Group

- *Intention:* To reduce hypertonicity in the transversospinalis group.
- *Position:* The client is in the fetal side-lying position. Place one hand on the upper back and one hand on the lower back (Fig 4-20).
- *Action:* Have the client rotate his or her trunk posteriorly and then resist as you attempt to rotate the trunk forward. Press for approximately 5 seconds, relax, and repeat several times. To reciprocally inhibit these muscles, place one hand on the anterior portion of the head of the humerus and the other hand on the ASIS. Have the client roll forward slightly and resist as you attempt to rotate him or her posteriorly.

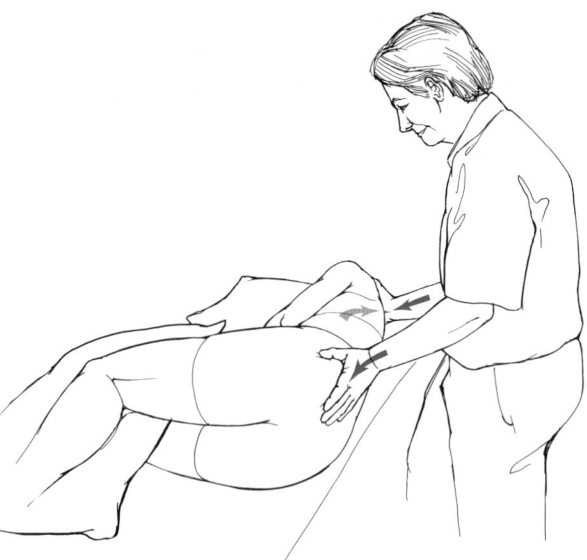

Figure 4-20. CR MET for the transversospinalis group.

10. Assessment of the Length of the Latissimus Dorsi

- *Intention:* To assess the length of the latissimus dorsi. The latissimus is often short, contributing to a rounded-shoulder posture, which also contributes to the humerus being internally rotated.
- *Position:* The client is supine, with arms at sides, with hips and knees flexed, and with feet on the table (Fig 4-21).
- *Action:* Have the client do a pelvic tilt to bring the lower back flat on the table. Then have the client raise his or her arms overhead, keeping them as close to the head as possible. Tightness in the latissimus prevents the arms from lying flat on the table when they are in an elevated position. A tight pectoralis minor pulls the scapula down and forward and also prevents the arms from lying flat on the table.

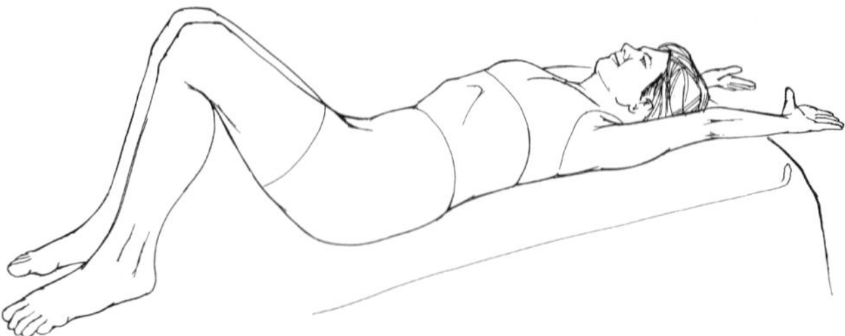

Figure 4-21. Assessment of the length of the latissimus dorsi.

11. Supine Contract-Relax-Antagonist-Contract Muscle Energy Technique for the Latissimus Dorsi

- *Intention:* To lengthen the latissimus dorsi. If the assessment of the latissimus shows that the arms cannot lie comfortably on the table next to the head, either on one or on both sides, CRAC MET is an effective technique to lengthen this muscle. A normal length in the latissimus contributes to a person's ability to assume an upright posture.
- *Position:* The client is supine, with the hips and knees flexed, feet on the table, and arms overhead to their comfortable limit. Hold the distal forearm with one hand and stabilize the arm with the other hand (Fig 4-22).
- *Action:* Instruct the client to tighten the abdominals, which flattens the lower back and thus lengthens the lower attachment of the latissimus. Next, have the client resist as you attempt to lift the client's distal forearm away from the table. Pull for 5 seconds. Have the client relax, then have him or her pull the distal arm back toward the table to the new limit. Relax, and have the client resist as you again pull the distal forearm away from the table. Repeat this CRAC cycle several times. CRAC may be performed simultaneously on both arms.

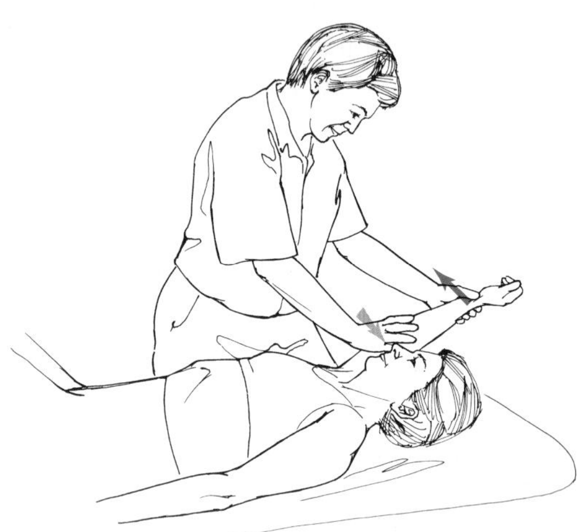

Figure 4-22. Supine CRAC MET for the latissimus dorsi.

ORTHOPEDIC MASSAGE

Level I-Thoracic

1. Release of the Thoracolumbar Fascia (TLF), Latissimus, Trapezius, and Erector Spinae

- *Anatomy:* TLF, latissimus, trapezius (Fig. 4-23), erector spinae (See Fig. 3-9).
- *Dysfunction:* The erector spinae tend to pull toward the midline and need to be moved in a medial to lateral direction. The fascia and ligaments thicken with chronic tension, a common cause of hypomobility in the thoracic spine.

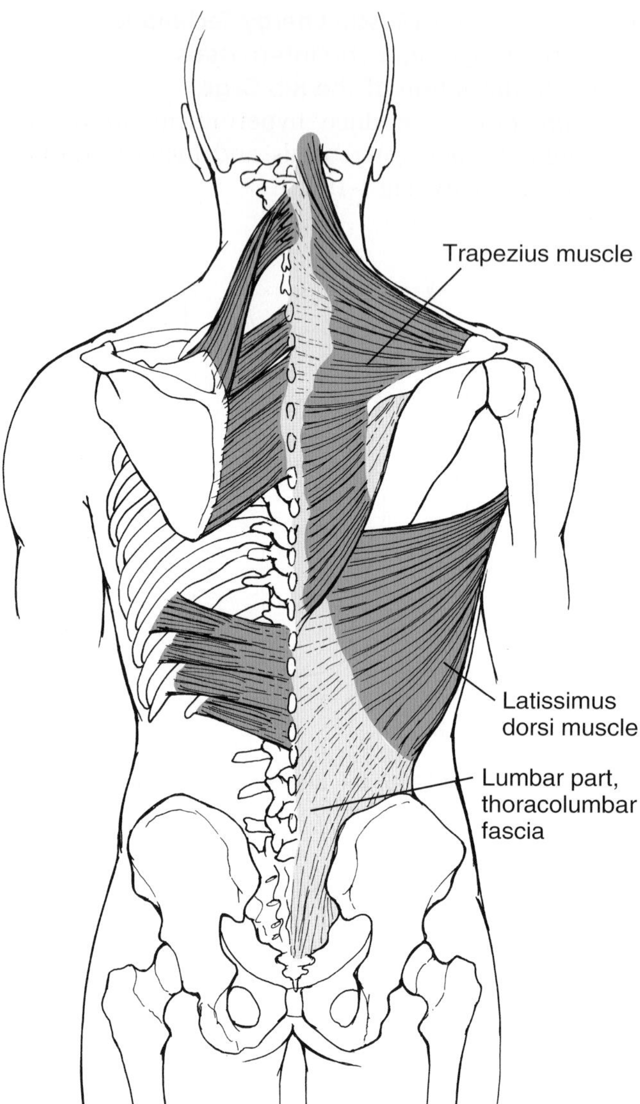

Figure 4-23. Thoracolumbar fascia, latissimus dorsi, and trapezius.

Position

- Therapist Position (TP)—standing, facing 45° headward for longitudinal strokes and 90° towards the client for transverse strokes.
- Client Position (CP)—side-lying.

Strokes

The strokes have two directions in three lines. The first line is along the SP, the second line is approximately 1 to 2 inches laterally over the area of the costotransverse joint, and the third is on the ribs approximately 2 to 4 inches laterally. These strokes also promote hydration of the joints through gentle mobilization in P–A glide.

1. Perform MET for the trapezius, latissimus, TLF, and erector spinae (see Figs. 4-13 to 4-15).
2. Using the supported-thumb technique, perform a series of short, scooping strokes, in an inferior to superior direction, approximately 1 inch in length, beginning at L4 and continuing to C7 on the areas outlined above, covering all three lines (Fig. 4-24). Superficially, these strokes release the TLF, the latissimus dorsi, and the trapezius. More deeply, these strokes release the erector spinae.

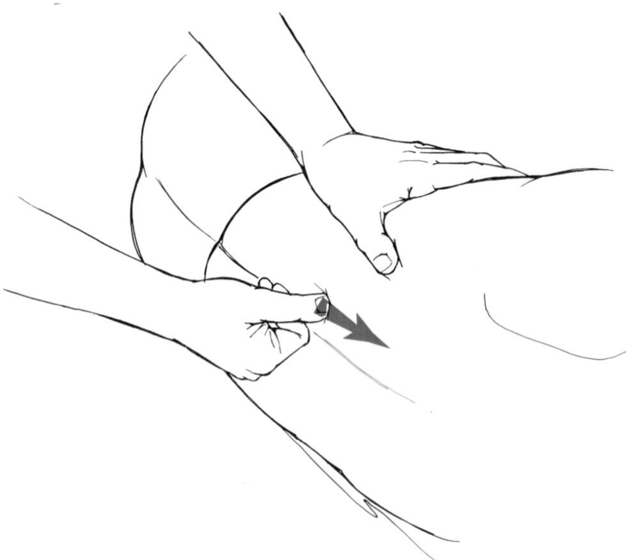

Figure 4-24. Supported-thumb technique for inferior to superior release of the thoracolumbar fascia, latissimus dorsi, trapezius, and erector spinae.

3. Perform a series of strokes, in a medial to lateral direction, approximately 1 inch in length. Begin at L4, just lateral to the spinous process (Fig. 4-25). Inch by inch move to the C7 area. Begin a second line approximately 1 inch laterally, from L4 to C7. Repeat a third series on the soft tissue over the ribs from T-12 to C-7.

Note: To assist in the effectiveness of these strokes, gently compress the rib cage with the supporting hand as you are sinking into the tissue with the working hand. This brings the tissue into slack, helps turn off the muscle spindle cells, and mobilizes the ribs and the vertebral facets. Pull the rib cage back as you are moving onto your back leg, then gently compress the rib cage as you move onto your front leg with the stroke. If a client is particularly tense, it is important to slow your strokes down and work on the client's exhale, as this also enhances relaxation.

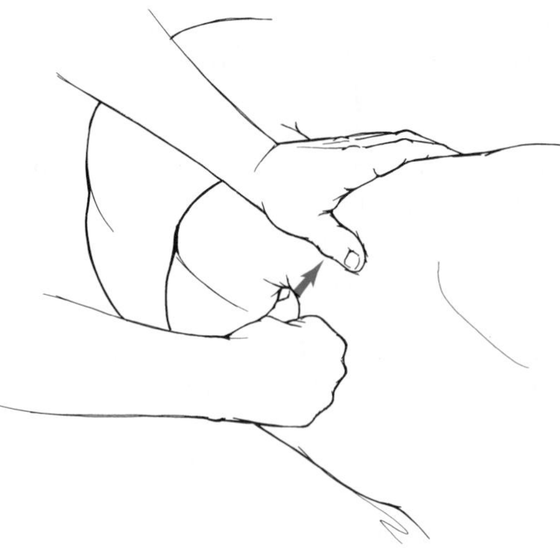

Figure 4-25. Supported-thumb technique for medial to lateral release of the medial line of soft tissue next to the spinous process.

2. Transverse Release of Rhomboids

- ***Anatomy:*** Rhomboid major and minor (Fig. 4-26).
- ***Dysfunction:*** These muscles tend to shorten, from chronic stress, or become weak, allowing the scapula to protract away from the spine. In the weakened position, there is a decreased scapular stabilization and an increased likelihood of glenohumeral impingement, as the acromion overhangs the head of the humerus.

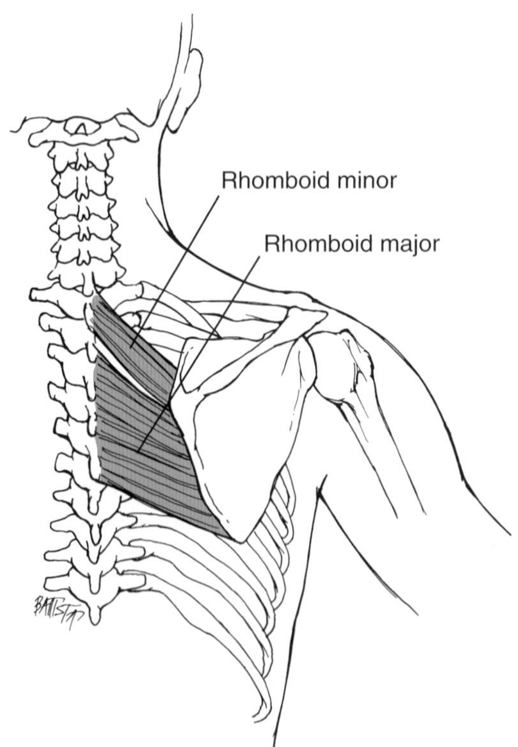

Figure 4-26. Rhomboid major and minor.

Position

- TP—standing, facing 45° headward.
- CP—supine and side-lying.

Strokes

1. With the client supine, perform MET on the rhomboids (see Figs.4-16, p. 140).
2. Perform CR MET on the muscles that attach to the scapula (see Fig. 4-17, p. 140).
3. Using a supported-thumb, double-thumb, or fingertips technique, perform 1-inch, inferior to superior, scooping strokes on the rhomboids (Fig. 4-27). The strokes are performed as rhythmic oscillations. Your supporting hand is on the scapula and moves it headward, coordinated with the movement of each stroke. Work the entire area from the T5 to C7 SPs to the vertebral border of the scapula.

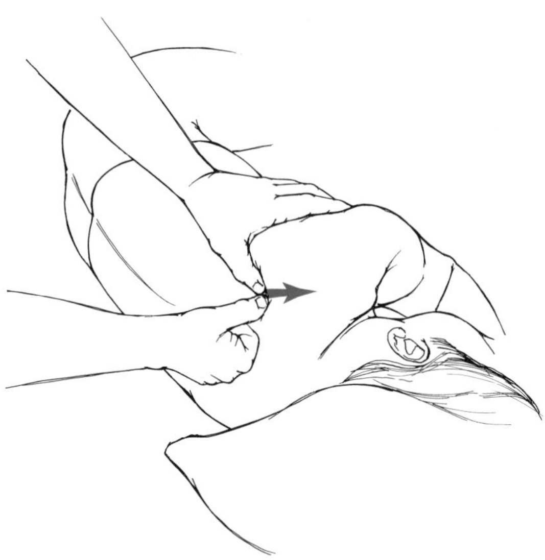

Figure 4-27. Double-thumb release of the rhomboids.

4. Beginning on the vertebral border at the superior angle of the scapula, use the supported thumb or fingertips of your superior hand to perform short, lifting, headward strokes on the rhomboids as your inferior hand cups the head of the humerus and pulls the scapula in an inferior direction (Fig. 4-28). Continue to the inferior angle. These strokes are more staccato, quicker paced. Rotate your entire body from the waist as you perform the strokes.

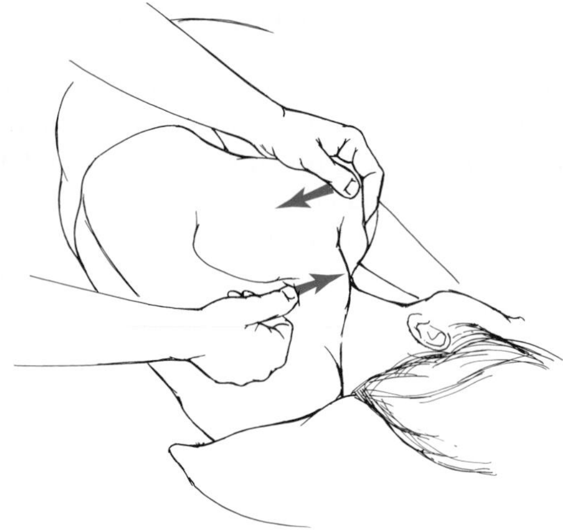

Figure 4-28. Shearing stroke to release the rhomboids.

3. Release of the Levator Scapula at the Superior Angle of the Scapula

- *Anatomy:* Levator scapula (Fig. 4-29).
- *Dysfunction:* The superior angle of the scapula is a critical stress point due to the strain on the levator as it holds the head in an upright position. The levator tends to drop into an inferior-medial torsion relative

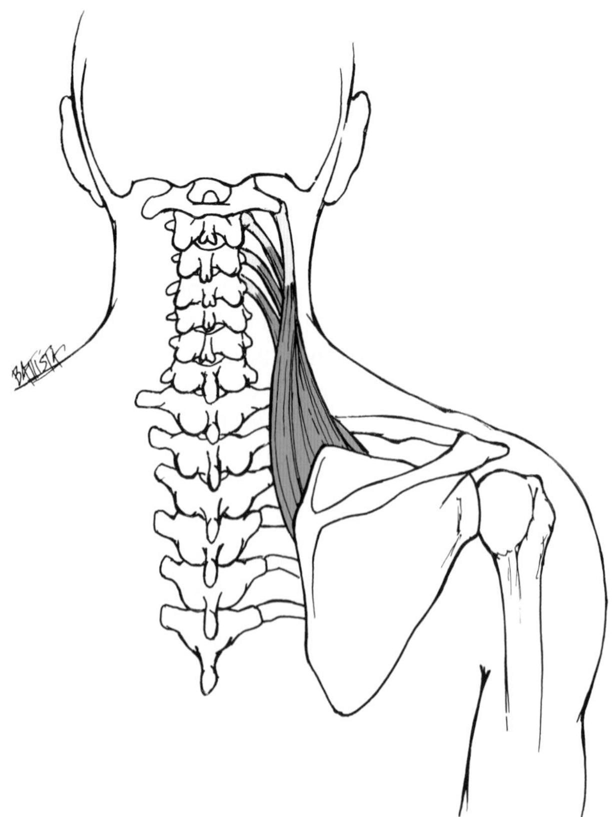

Figure 4-29. Levator scapula.

to the superior angle of the scapula and must be lifted in a 45° headward direction. This may seem paradoxical, but Lauren Berry, RPT, taught that the typical pattern of dysfunction is for the scapula to rotate anterolaterally around the rib cage in the forward-head, rounded-shoulder posture and for the levator to roll in an inferior direction relative to the upward scapula. Therefore, finish the work in this area by moving the scapula down.

Position

- TP—standing, 45° headward.
- CP—side-lying. If the shoulder is painful or especially tight, place a pillow under the client's arm.

Strokes

1. To help release a short and tight levator scapula, perform PIR MET (see Fig. 4-18, p. 140).
2. Perform 1-inch, scooping strokes on the levator scapula in a 45° headward direction, using fingertips, single-thumb, or supported-thumb technique with your superior hand (Fig. 4-30). Begin at the superior angle of the scapula, and continue your strokes to the cervical spine. The strokes are performed as rhythmic oscillations. Your supporting hand is on the scapula and moves it headward, coordinated with the movement of each stroke.

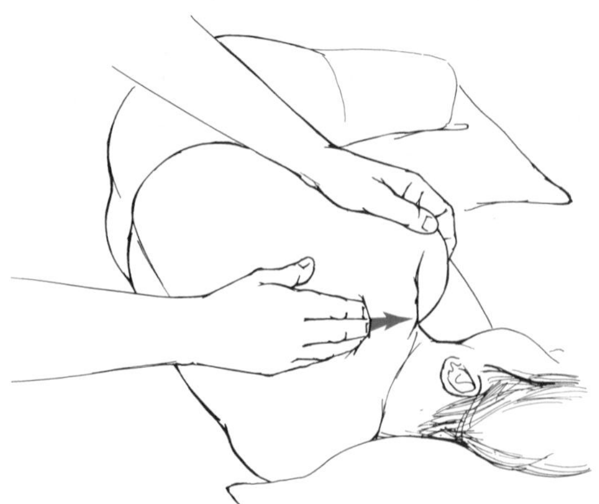

Figure 4-30. Fingertip release of the levator scapula.

3. Perform shearing strokes on the levator scapula (Fig. 4-31). Using the thumb or fingertips of your superior hand, perform short, scooping strokes in a 45° headward direction. Your supporting hand cups the head of the humerus and draws it toward you, moving the scapula inferiorly. Coordinate the movement of the two hands in a rhythmic oscillation.

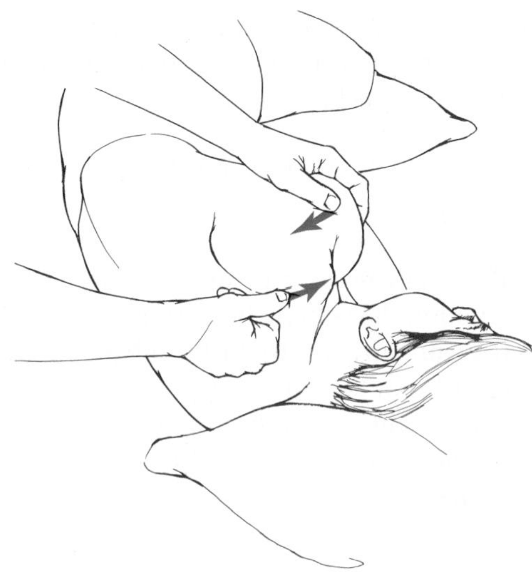

Figure 4-31. Supported-thumb shearing stroke for the levator scapula. Pull the scapula back with one hand as you scoop the levator 45° headward.

4. Release of the Lateral Rib Cage and the Anterior Surface of the Scapula

- *Anatomy:* Latissimus dorsi, pectoralis minor, serratus anterior (Fig. 4-32).
- *Dysfunction:* The scapulothoracic joint can become hypomobile due to chronic tension or adhesions at the inferior angle caused by tension in the latissimus or a short serratus anterior. It can also become hypermobile owing to a weak serratus, rhomboid, and

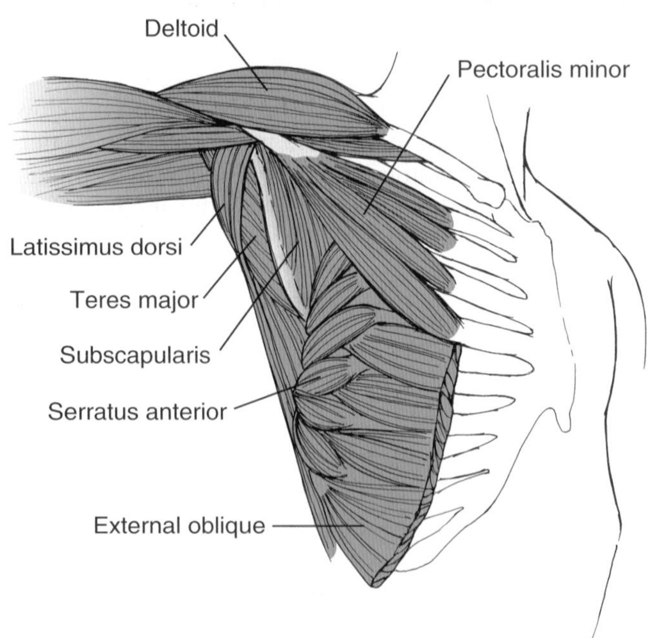

Figure 4-32. Latissimus dorsi, external abdominal oblique, serratus anterior, and the pectoralis minor.

trapezius; when strong, these muscles provide scapular stabilization. These strokes are for hypomobility and adhesions.

Position

- TP—standing, 45° or 90° to the client.
- CP—side-lying.

Strokes

1. Have the client rest his or her arm on a pillow in 90° abduction, 90° elbow flexion. Facing 45° headward, use a fingertips-next-to-thumb technique, and perform anterior to posterior (A–P) scooping strokes on the lateral rib cage, following the contour of the bone, to release the latissimus dorsi and serratus anterior. Proceed to the hairline of the axilla (Fig. 4-33).

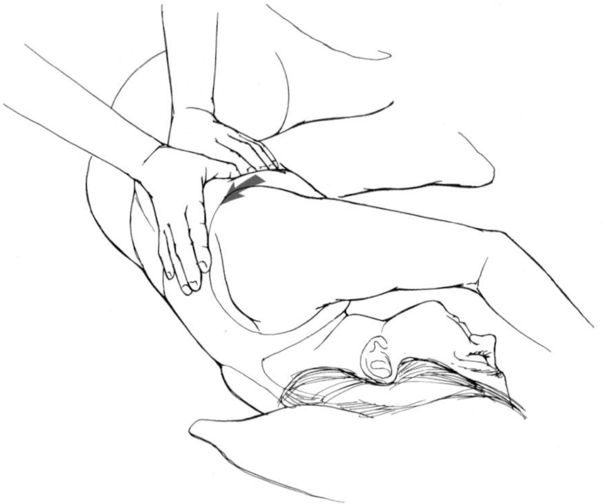

Figure 4-33. Release of the lateral and anterior rib cage using fingertips and thumb.

2. With the client resting his or her arm on a pillow, face 45° headward and use your fingertips to perform short, scooping strokes in a lateral to medial direction on the anterior rib cage for the pectoralis minor (Fig. 4-34).

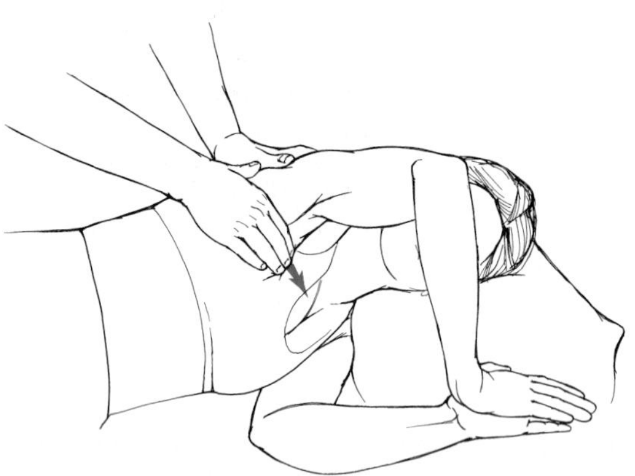

Figure 4-34. Fingertip release of the pectoralis minor.

3. Facing 90° to the table, release the latissimus from the inferior angle of the scapula by using the thumb of the inferior hand to push the latissimus anteriorly, while using the superior hand to cup the humerus and pull the scapula posteriorly (Fig. 4-35). This is a back-and-forth shearing stroke to dissolve the adhesions.

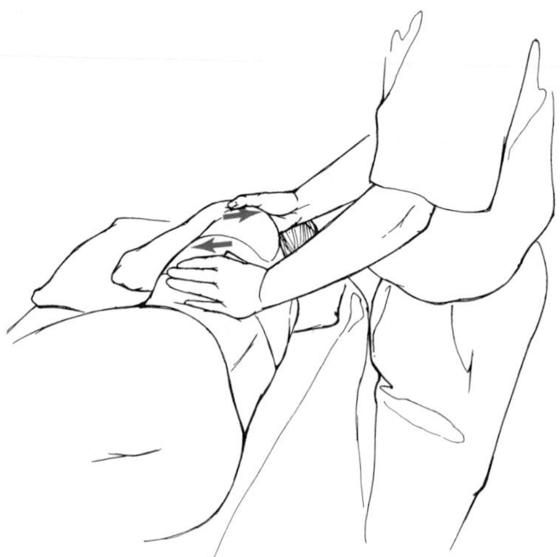

Figure 4-35. Thumb release of the inferior angle of the scapula.

4. Facing 45° headward, place the client's arm on the lateral aspect of his or her rib cage. Stabilize the client's arm by placing your forearm next to his or her arm, cupping the head of the humerus. Cup the fingertips of your superior hand under the vertebral border of the scapula to touch the attachments of the serratus anterior. Scoop headward with your fingertips in 1-inch strokes as you mobilize the client's arm and scapula headward (Fig. 4-36). If you cannot

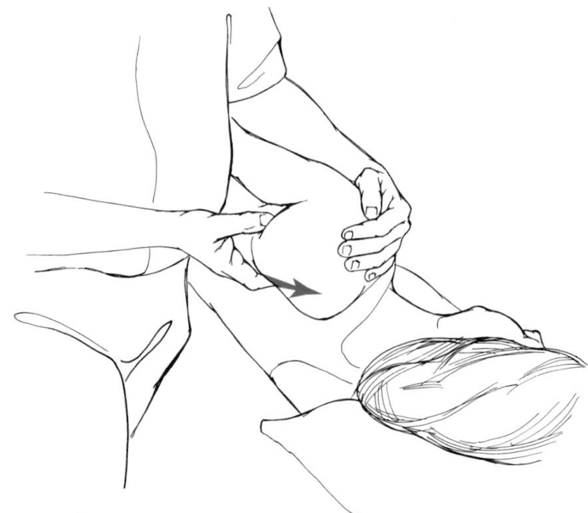

Figure 4-36. Fingertip release of the attachments of the serratus anterior on the anterior surface of the scapula.

place your fingertips under the scapula, have the client roll backwards slightly and place his or her arm behind the back, as this position wings the scapula and exposes the undersurface.

5. Release of the Diaphragm

- *Anatomy:* Diaphragm (Fig. 4-37).
- *Dysfunction:* The diaphragm attachments tend to thicken with chronic tension, which is often due to rounded-shoulders posture, lack of aerobic exercise, shallow breathing from emotional tension, lung problems such as asthma, or chronic hypomobility of the costovertebral joints. Chronic tension in the diaphragm adds significantly to the hypomobility of the spine and to thoracic kyphosis. Tension in the diaphragm pulls the muscle fibers toward the midline and pulls the thoracic cage forward. The diaphragm attaches to the lumbar vertebrae by means of a powerful tendon called the crus. Persistent coughing or even a sneeze can severely irritate the lumbar discs.

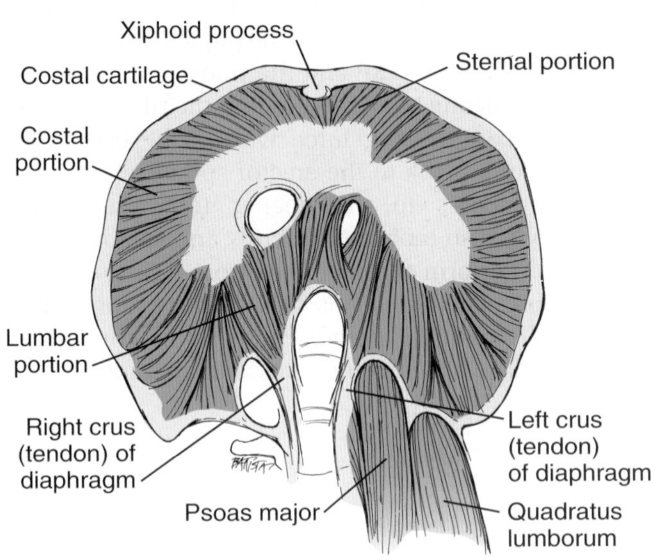

Figure 4-37. The diaphragm, showing its attachments to the inner surface of the rib cage.

Position

- TP—standing.
- CP—supine, with knees up, or side-lying position.

Strokes

1. Perform MET for the diaphragm (see Fig. 4-19, p. 141).
2. With the client supine, stand in the 45° headward position, opposite the side being worked on (Fig. 4-38). Beginning on the most lateral aspect of the anterior rib cage, place your thumb or braced thumb approximately 1 inch below the ribs. This hand placement allows some slack in the tissue. On

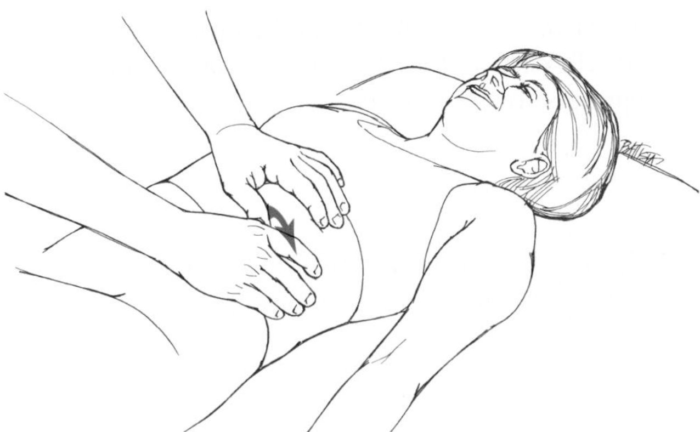

Figure 4-38. Supine release of the diaphragm

the client's exhale, gently press under the ribs and flex your thumb onto the posterior surface of the ribs, then scoop in a medial to lateral direction. Perform a series of slow, gentle, scooping strokes on the inner surface of the ribs in 1-inch segments, continuing to almost 1-inch lateral to the xiphoid process at the midline. Tell the client that there may be some sensitivity in this area if there are adhesions of the diaphragm to the rib cage, including a burning or biting pain. Remember to mention to the client that he or she should be able to completely relax. Releasing this area may elicit an emotional response. Proceed slowly and with sensitivity.
3. Another position that is used more frequently than no. 2 above is to place your client in the side-lying position (Fig. 4-39). Place your working hand on the lateral aspect of the rib cage such that your flexed fingertips are approximately 1 inch inferior to the ribs. As the client exhales, use your stabilizing hand to compress the lateral rib cage gently into your working hand to give some slack to the tissue. Tuck your fingertips under the rib cage,

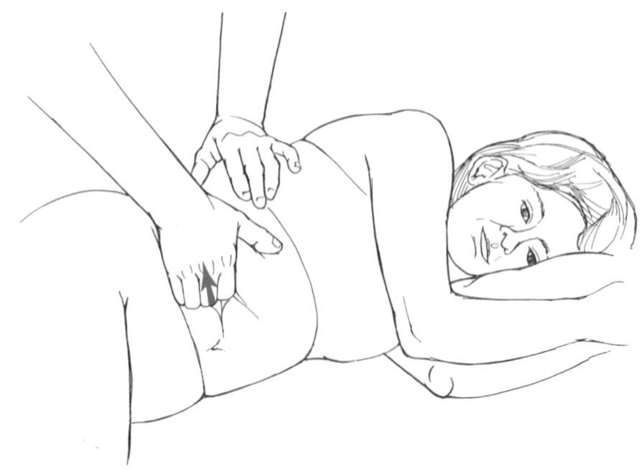

Figure 4-39. Side-lying release of the diaphragm.

then stroke on the posterior surface of the ribs in a medial to lateral direction. Proceed in 1-inch segments to the midline.

Level II–Thoracic

1. Release of the Transversospinalis Group

- *Anatomy*: Semispinalis thoracis, cervicis, multifidus (Fig. 4-40).

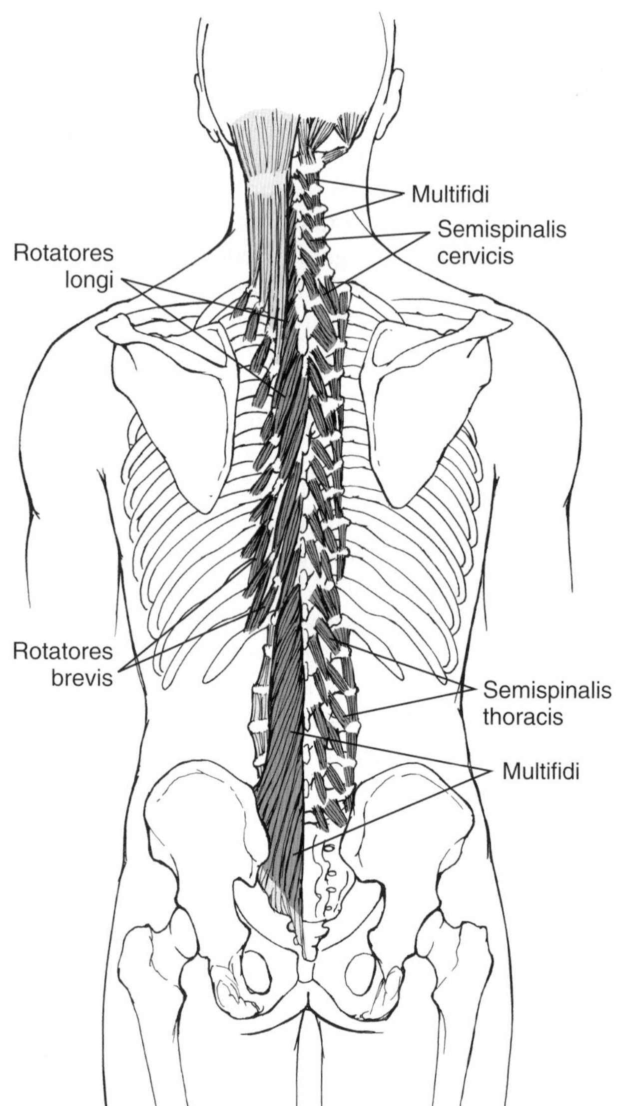

Figure 4-40. Transversospinalis muscle group.

- *Dysfunction:* The transversospinalis group of muscles help stabilize the spine. With lack of movement, such as occurs during prolonged sitting, they tend to shorten and develop fibrosis through chronic tension, especially if there is hypomobility in the joints. Since the multifidi attach to the joint capsules, chronic tension contributes significantly to the lack of glide in the facet joints. The multifidi may also be in a sustained contraction in scoliosis, at the apex of the curve on the convex side. Pay particular attention to the T12 to L1 and the C7 to T1 junctions, as these are the most common areas of facet degeneration.

Position

- TP—standing, facing 45° headward.
- CP—side-lying.

Strokes

1. Perform CR MET on the transversospinalis group (see Fig. 4-20, p. 141).
2. Using a supported-thumb or a braced-thumb technique, perform a series of scooping strokes in a 45° headward direction (Fig. 4-41). Place your thumb next to the SP, and slide it along the spinous process, tucking your thumb under the erector spinae to release the multifidi and semispinalis group in the area between the SP and the transverse processes. The stabilizing hand presses into the rib cage with a gentle compressing force with each stroke. This gives some slack to the erector spinae, allowing an easier access to the deeper transversospinalis group. It also mobilizes the ribs and costovertebral joints. Perform these strokes from T12 to C7, one vertebra at a time. This series can be done many times to dissolve the adhesions in the connective-tissue layers of the muscles and to mobilize the spine.

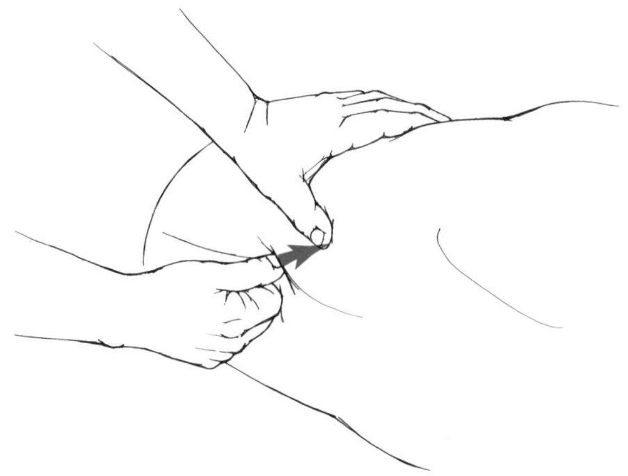

Figure 4-41. Supported-thumb release of the transversospinalis group.

2. Release of the Attachments to the Spinous Processes

- *Anatomy:* Trapezius, TLF, supraspinous ligament, rhomboid major, splenius cervicis, spinalis, multifidus, and rotatores (Fig. 4-42).
- *Dysfunction:* The tenoperiosteal junctions on the SPs are an interweaving of the fascia, the supraspinous ligament, and the fascial expansions of the muscles. Attachments thicken as the result of previous injury or chronic dysfunction, such as poor posture. Extended periods of sitting, especially in a slumped posture, create a tethering or pulling force on the SPs. Over time, the tissue thickens and becomes ischemic and tender. This treatment is for chronic conditions only.

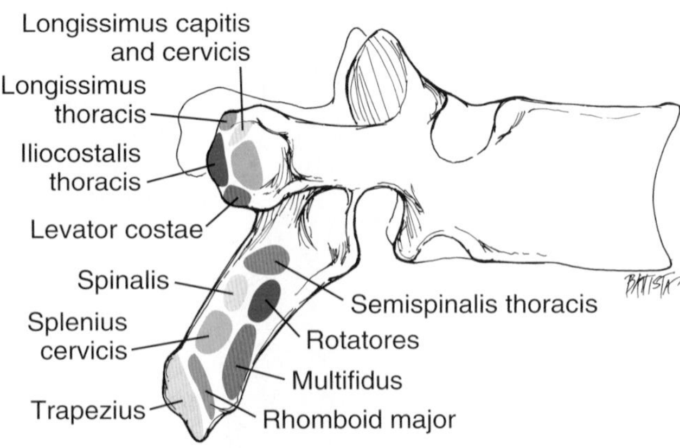

Figure 4-42. Muscle attachments to thoracic spinous processes.

Position

- TP—standing, facing 45° headward.
- CP—side-lying.

Strokes

Note that the mid-thoracic SPs are angled steeply in an inferior direction, whereas the upper thoracic spinous are almost straight posterior. Your intention is to clean the bone, as a healthy bone has a smooth and glistening feel to it.

1. Beginning at the SP of T12, use a supported-thumb technique to perform short, back-and-forth strokes in the inferior to superior plane on the SP of each of the thoracic vertebrae (Fig. 4-43). Your flexed index finger rests on the other side of the SP. You may use a slight pinching grasp of the SP to stabilize your thumb. Use your supporting hand to compress the rib cage gently as you are working, thus bringing the overlying soft tissue into slack. Rock the entire body as you work. If the soft-tissue attachments to the SP feel fibrous, you may use brisk, transverse-friction strokes.

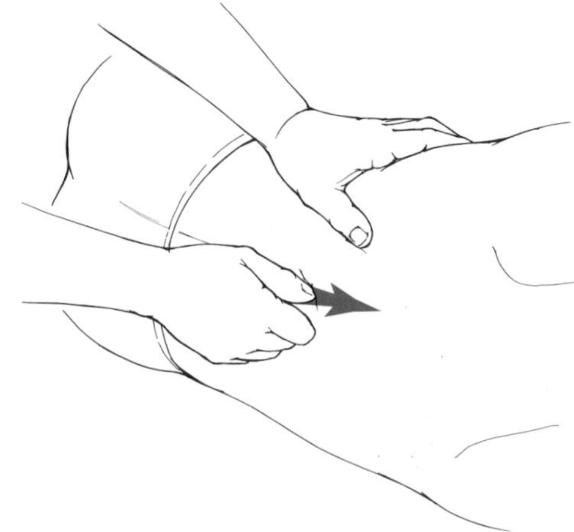

Figure 4-43. Supported-thumb technique to release attachments to the thoracic spinous processes.

3. Release of the Soft Tissue at the Transverse Processes

- *Anatomy:* Longissimus thoracis, cervicis, and capitis; semispinalis thoracis, cervicis, and capitis; iliocostalis thoracis and intertransverse; multifidus; and levator costarum (Fig. 4-44).
- *Dysfunction:* The area in the region of the transverse process is clinically significant for two main reasons. One, there are significant muscle attachments on the transverse processes between the midback and the neck and head. These muscles become chronically taut in a FHP. Second, hypertonicity in the muscles attaching to the transverse process can cre-

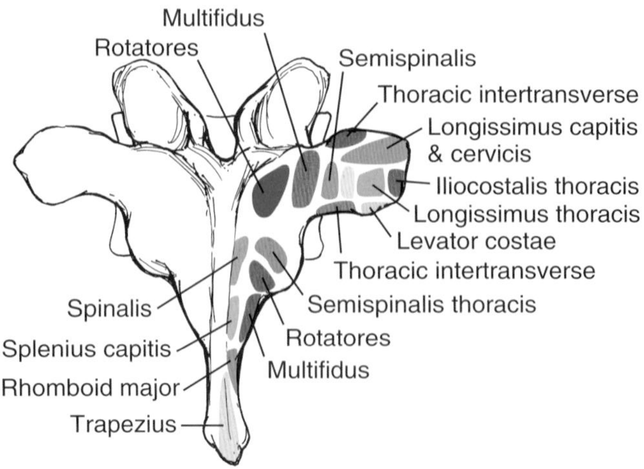

Figure 4-44. Muscle attachments to thoracic transverse processes.

ate compression in the rib joints owing to the interweaving of the muscles, fascia, and ligaments. This would decrease the mobility of the ribs. Hypertonicity may also be caused by a rib fixation, which can create greater hypertonicity caused by irritation of the joint, called an arthrokinetic reflex.

Position

- TP—standing, 90° to the line of the fiber.
- CP—side-lying.

Strokes

1. Using a supported-thumb or a braced thumb technique, begin a series of strokes on the muscle attachments to the transverse processes and on the muscle attachments to the ribs at the area of the T12 vertebra approximately 1 to 2 inches lateral to the SP (Fig. 4-45).

   First, perform short, slow, scooping strokes, and then brisk transverse strokes where you find areas of fibrosis. You are "looking" with your hands for a feeling of hypertonicity or thickening and fibrosis. The direction of the strokes may be slightly inferior, slightly superior, 45° headward, or 90° to the midline. As you perform the slow, scooping strokes, you are pressing P–A into the area of the costotransverse joint. Identify areas of hypomobility, and repeat the strokes many times in that area. Emphasize the P–A mobilization in your strokes to help restore normal mobility to these joints.

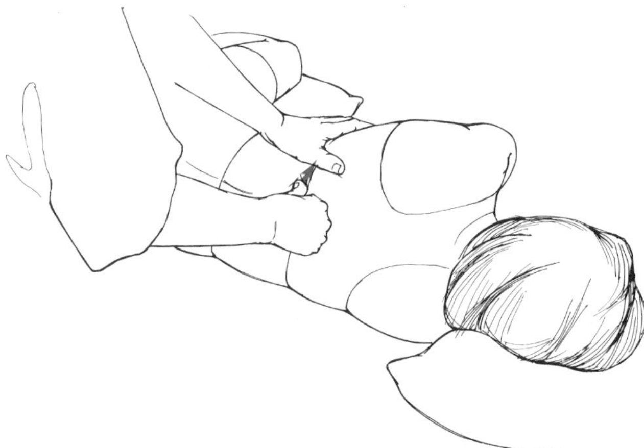

Figure 4-45. Supported-thumb release of attachments to the thoracic transverse processes and mobilization of the costotransverse joints.

2. Continue this series of strokes to the C7 vertebra. Perform several strokes in the area of one vertebra, then move approximately 1 inch higher and perform another series of strokes.

4. Release of the Iliocostalis Thoracis, Cervicis, Serratus Posterior Superior

- ***Anatomy:*** Iliocostalis thoracis, cervicis, serratus posterior superior (Fig. 4-46).
- ***Dysfunction:*** The iliocostalis thoracis and cervicis are often hypertonic as a result of FHP or an injury to the neck. The iliocostalis develops an eccentric contraction with a FHP that leads to tenderness under the scapulae. These muscles tend to develop fibrosis under chronic tension. The serratus posterior superior acts like a retinaculum holding down the erector

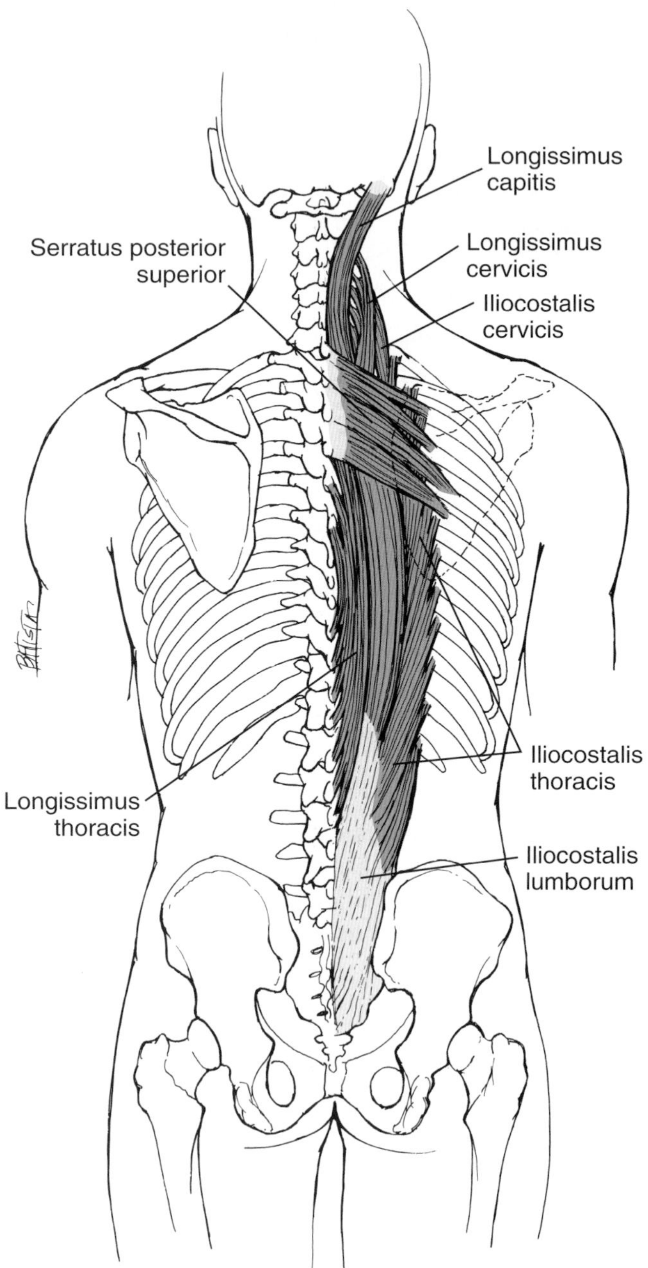

Figure 4-46. Iliocostalis thoracis and cervicis and serratus posterior superior.

spinae and can also assist in elevating the ribs. As this muscle is attached to ribs 2 to 5, it is often hypertonic and can develop a tender thickening, especially with fixation of the upper ribs.

Position

- TP—standing, 90° to the line of fiber.
- CP—side-lying and supine.

Strokes

Locate the serratus posterior superior under the rhomboids and the trapezius. The serratus feels flat and fibrous, like a tuck in a sheet over the ribs, not fleshy like the rhomboids. To palpate the difference, move the scapula toward the spine. As the rhomboids attach to the scapula, they slacken and feel fleshy at the vertebral border of the scapula. The serratus remains flat against the ribs. If you press deeply over the ribs in a 45° headward direction, you feel the serratus.

1. Using a supported-thumb or fingertips technique, perform a series of 45° headward, scooping strokes through the rhomboids on the serratus posterior superior. Cover the entire muscle from its attachments at the SPs of C7 and upper two or three thoracic vertebrae to its attachments to ribs 2 to 5 under the scapula. (Fig. 4-47).

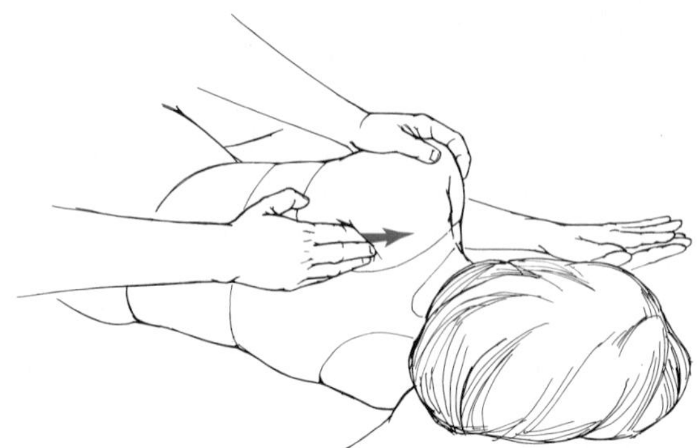

Figure 4-47. Fingertip release of serratus posterior superior.

2. Using a supported-thumb, fingertips, or double-thumb technique, perform short, scooping strokes in a medial to lateral direction to release the iliocostalis thoracis and cervicis (Fig. 4-48). They are running underneath the vertebral border of the scapula. With your supporting hand, move the scapula laterally as you stroke, coordinating the two hands in a rhythmic oscillation. Cover the entire area under the scapula.
3. Use the supine technique, which is an alternative technique for releasing the iliocostalis. Place the client's forearm on his or her chest, and grasp the elbow with your inferior hand. Place the fingertips of your superior hand on the iliocostalis, and perform a series of medial to lateral scooping strokes, as you move the client's arm across the chest.

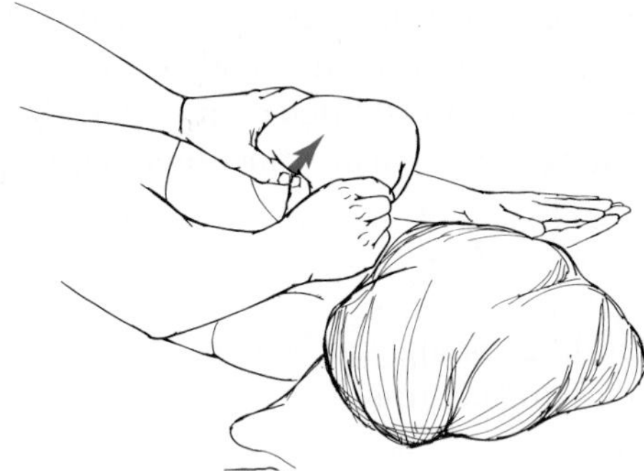

Figure 4-48. Double-thumb release of the iliocostalis thoracis and cervicis.

5. Release of the Posterior Scalene and Iliocostalis Cervicis at the Upper Ribs

- ***Anatomy:*** Posterior scalene, iliocostalis cervicis (Fig. 4-49).

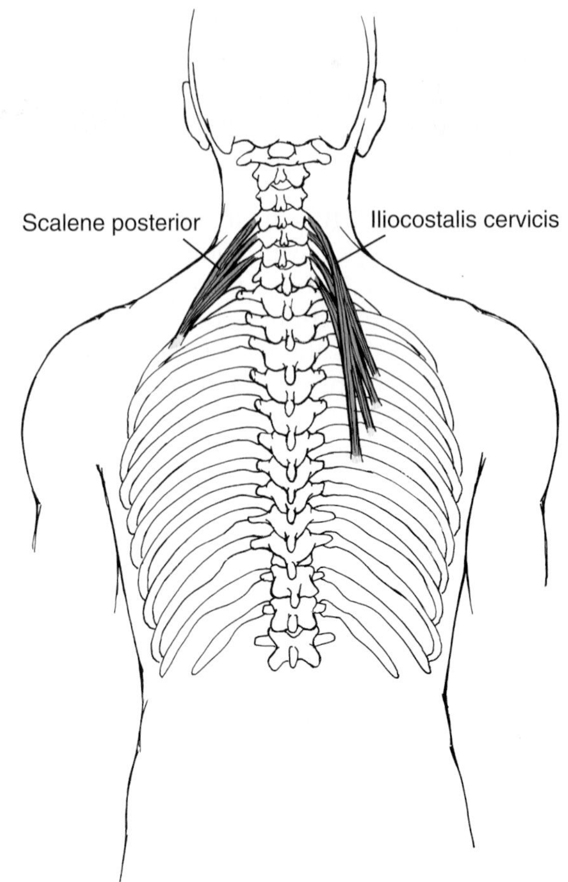

Figure 4-49. Posterior scalene and iliocostalis cervicis.

- *Dysfunction:* These muscles are eccentrically contracted under an excessive load from a FHP. They can also develop a sustained contraction after a neck injury such as a whiplash. Attachment points tend to thicken.

Position

- TP—standing, facing your stroke.
- CP—side-lying or supine.

Strokes

Use short, scooping strokes in the P–A plane or brisk transverse friction strokes at the attachment points if fibrosis is found.

1. Place the fingertips of your superior hand above the superior angle of the scapula on the upper ribs. Place your supporting hand on the scapula. Perform a series of short, scooping strokes following the contour of the ribs. You are working on the posterior scalene, and iliocostalis cervicis attachments on the T1 to T3 ribs (Fig. 4-50). As you are working, gently move the scapula in the direction of your stroke. This brings the superficial tissue into slack and allows for deeper work on the attachments to the ribs. Since the direction of the strokes follows the contour of the upper ribs, the strokes begin in an inferior to superior direction and then change to a medial to lateral direction. Move your stance to face the direction of the strokes. Your series of strokes should cover the entire posterior and superior area of the upper ribs.

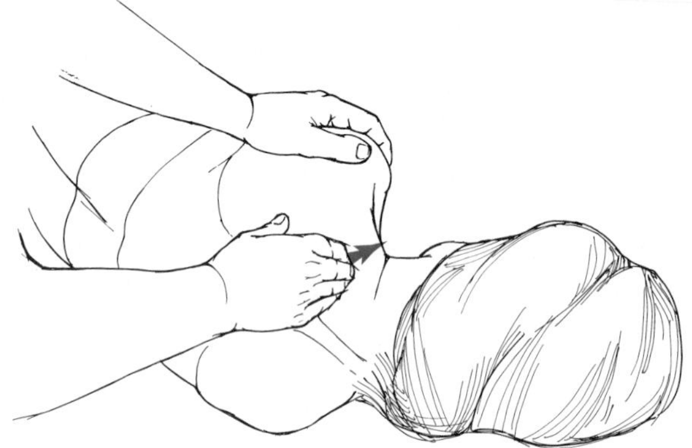

Figure 4-50. Fingertip release of posterior scalene and iliocostalis attachments T1 to T3. ribs.

CASE STUDY

JK is a 67-year-old, 5'10", 169-lb, male professor who presented to my office with complaints of stiffness and an occasional jabbing pain in the midback. He reported that the stiffness began approximately 15 years ago and that the occasional jabbing began approximately 1 month previously. There was no particular incident that preceded the jabbing pain. He consulted with an orthopedist, and was given an anti-inflammatory drug, but it did not resolve his complaints.

Examination revealed that the iliac crests were level in standing. The left shoulder was elevated (the patient is right-handed). There were decreased curves in the thoracic and the lumbar spines, a FHP, and an increased cervical curve. Active lumbar and cervical ROMs were moderately decreased, and he felt stiffness at the end range. Passive motion of the thoracic spine revealed a drastic loss of the normal P–A glide in the entire thoracic region. The SPs of T3 to T10 were mildly tender to palpation. The paraspinal musculature was hypertonic and fibrous.

A diagnosis was made of thoracic hypomobility syndrome and a costovertebral fixation. Treatment began by instructing the patient in the correct posture of the head. The patient was then asked to lie in a side-lying fetal position. CR and RI MET were performed for the hypertonic thoracic, cervical, and lumbar extensors. Level I OM strokes were performed, beginning with the lumbar series for the gluteal region, quadratus lumborum, and lumbar erectors. Then, slow, deep transverse strokes were performed on the thoracic extensors, emphasizing the P–A glide mobilization of the spinal facets and costovertebral joints. Transverse release was performed on the cervical muscles, followed by the diaphragm. He was asked to lie on his other side, and the same treatment was repeated.

A series of four treatments was recommended for the acute jabbing pain and to help increase the mobility in the thoracic spine. Recommendations were made for a home program of stretching and postural reeducation.

JK returned to my office 1 week later with no real change. The same treatment was repeated. At his third visit he reported that the jabbing pain was gone and that he felt looser and more relaxed. Motion palpation of the spine revealed a slight increase in mobility. Two treatments a month for a 3-month period and monthly treatments for a year for his chronic hypomobility, with a reevaluation at that time, were recommended. Because of the chronicity of his condition and the severity of the hypomobility, monthly OM treatments were recommended to help improve function and to prevent future degeneration. The importance of a daily exercise and stretching program were also emphasized.

STUDY GUIDE

Thoracic Spine, Level I

1. Describe the signs and symptoms of thoracic muscle strain, arthrosis, and facet joint fixation.
2. Describe the upper-crossed syndrome. List the muscles that tend to be weak and the muscles that tend to be tight.
3. Name three factors predisposing to dysfunction and pain in the thoracic region.
4. Describe how the first series of massage strokes promotes hydration of the joints of the thoracic spine.
5. Describe a kyphotic spine, and describe the typical muscle dysfunctions in the pectoralis minor, lower trapezius, and upper trapezius.
6. Name the three lines of strokes, and the two basic directions of strokes in the thoracic erector spinae muscles.
7. Describe the direction of positional dysfunction of the levator scapula and the direction of our stroke to correct it.
8. Describe the direction of our stroke to release the diaphragm.
9. Describe what scoliosis is, and describe Lauren Berry's theory of its origin.
10. List the three most common mechanical disorders that cause midback pain.

Thoracic Spine, Level II

1. Describe the MET for acute thoracic pain and for the lower trapezius.
2. Describe the signs and symptoms of osteoporosis and a costovertebral fixation.
3. Describe the muscular imbalances of a kyphotic spine.
4. How do we palpate the serratus posterior superior and differentiate it from the rhomboids?
5. Describe the palpation findings in a healthy thoracic spine and in a degenerated spine.
6. List the stroke direction for the multifidus and iliocostalis cervicis.
7. Describe the Adam's test, and describe how you differentiate between a structural and a functional scoliosis.
8. Describe how you would differentiate between a functional and a structural kyphosis.
9. Describe the MET to release the rhomboids and to increase respiratory function.
10. Describe why the area of C7 to T1 is often thick and fibrotic to palpation.

REFERENCES

1. Hayek R, Henderson C, Hayek A. Unique features of the thoracic spine: impact on chiropractic management. Top Clin Chiro 1999; 6:69–78.
2. Grieve G. Common Vertebral Joint Problems. Edinburgh: Churchill Livingstone, 1981.
3. Corrigan B, Maitland GD. Practical Orthopaedic Medicine. London: Butterworths, 1983.
4. Triano J, Erwin M, Hansen D. Costovertebral and costotransverse joint pain: a commonly overlooked pain generator. Top Clin Chiro 1999;6:79–92.
5. Janda V. Evaluation of muscular imbalance. In: Liebenson C, ed. Rehabilitation of the Spine. Baltimore: Williams & Wilkins, 1996:97–112.
6. Kessler R, Hertling D. Management of Common Musculoskeletal Disorders, 3rd Ed. Baltimore: Lippincott, Williams & Wilkins, 1993.
7. Faraday JA. Current principles in the nonoperative management of structural adolescent idiopathic scoliosis. Phys Ther 1983;66:512–523.
8. Schafer RC. Clinical Biomechanics. Baltimore: Williams & Wilkins, 1983.
9. Ford DM, Bagnall KM, McFadden KD, et al. Paraspinal muscle imbalance in adolescent idiopathic scoliosis. Spine 1984;9:373–376.
10. Kendall F, McCreary E, Provance P. Muscles: Testing and Function, 4th Ed. Baltimore: Williams & Wilkins, 1993.
11. Dreyfuss P, Tibiletti C, Dreyer S. Thoracic zygapophyseal joint patterns. Spine 1994;19:807–811.
12. Blair JM. Examination of the thoracic spine. In: Grieve GP, ed. Modern Manual Therapy of the Vertebral Column. New York: Churchill Livingstone, 1986:536–546.

SUGGESTED READINGS

Calais-Germain B. Anatomy of Movement. Seattle: Eastland Press, 1991.

Chaitow L. Muscle Energy Techniques. New York: Churchill Livingstone, 1996.

Clemente C. Anatomy: A Regional Atlas of the Human Body, 4th Ed. Baltimore: Williams & Wilkins, 1997.

Corrigan B, Maitland GD. Practical Orthopaedic Medicine. London: Butterworths, 1983.

Greenman PE. Principles of Manual Medicine, 2nd Ed. Baltimore: Williams & Wilkins, 1996.

Janda V. Evaluation of muscular imbalance. In: Liebenson C, ed. Rehabilitation of the Spine. Baltimore: Williams & Wilkins, 1996:97–112.

Kendall F, McCreary E, Provance P. Muscles: Testing and Function, 4th Ed. Baltimore: Williams & Wilkins, 1993.

Kessler R, Hertling D. Management of Common Musculoskeletal Disorders, 3rd Ed. Baltimore: Lippincott, Williams & Wilkins, 1993.

Lewit K. Manipulative Therapy in Rehabilitation on the Locomotor System, 3rd Ed. Oxford: Butterworth Heinemann, 1999.

Liebenson C. Rehabilitation of the Spine. Baltimore: Williams & Wilkins, 1996.

Magee D. Orthopedic Physical Assessment, 3rd Ed. Philadelphia: WB Saunders, 1997.

Norkin C, Levangie P. Joint Structure and Function, 2nd Ed. Philadelphia: FA Davis, 1992.

Platzer W. Locomotor System, vol 1, 4th Ed. New York: Thieme Medical, 1992.

Reid DC. Sports Injury and Assessment. New York: Churchill Livingstone, 1992.

5

Cervical Spine

Neck pain is one of the most common complaints presented to a massage therapist. The causes of neck pain are diverse, but include injuries from sports or motor vehicle accidents, cumulative stress from poor posture, or emotional and psychological tension. Approximately one-third of the population has experienced neck pain within the past year, and nearly 14% of the population experiences chronic neck pain.[1] Outside of injury, the most common cause of neck ache is postural strain. Studies suggest that the soft tissue is the source of the neck pain in 87% of patients who have neck pain from injuries.[2]

Anatomy, Function, and Dysfunction of the Cervical Spine

GENERAL OVERVIEW

- **Seven vertebrae** form the cervical spine (Fig. 5-1). They are numbered from the vertebra under the skull, called C1, or the atlas, to C7, also called the vertebra prominens, because the spinous process (SP) is significantly longer than the SPs of the other cervical vertebrae. C2 is also called the axis. The occipital portion of the skull is included in the cervical spine, because it forms a joint with the atlas, the occipitoatlantal joint (Occ-C1).
- These seven vertebrae may be divided into two segments based on their anatomy.
  - The lower segment includes C3 to C7 and consists of typical vertebrae.
  - The upper segment includes C1 to C2 and the occiput, as they are atypical.

Cervical Curve

- The cervical spine has a normal lordotic curve (i.e., the curve is convex anteriorly). Lordosis is a position of stability, maintained by the ligaments, muscles, facets, and shape of the discs.
- The apex of the forward cervical curve occurs at C5 to C6. The greatest amount of flexion, extension, and rotation in the lower cervical spine occurs here. This great mobility makes this area susceptible to injury.

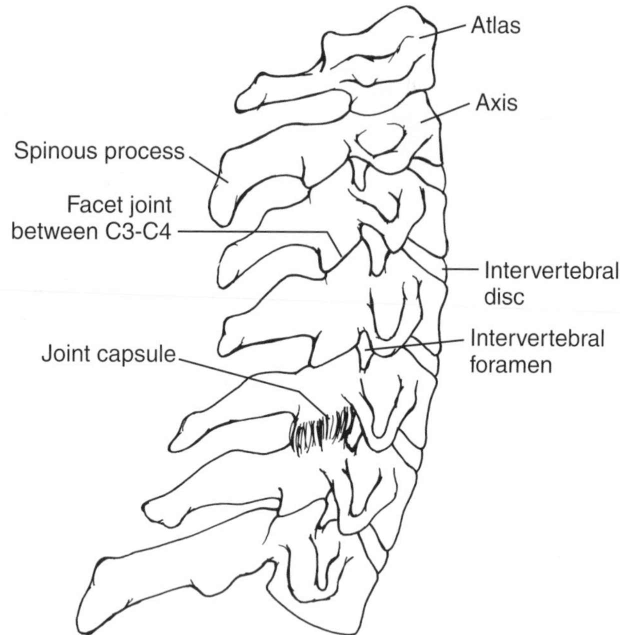

Figure 5-1. Lateral view of the anterior and the posterior portions of the cervical spine showing the vertebral body, intervertebral disc, facet, intervertebral foramen, transverse process, and transverse foramen.

- The curve may be increased or decreased by many factors. Essentially, muscle tone is the primary factor in determining the degree of spinal curves.[3]
- With an increase in the curve, as in a forward-head posture (FHP), the facets are excessively compressed.
- A decrease of the curve places an excessive compressive force on the intervertebral discs.[4] This loss of the curve may be caused by previous trauma and consequent shortening of the anterior ligaments or by sustained muscle contraction of the deep cervical flexors.

Posture

- Grieve[5] states that "Head posture governs body posture." This is an important insight because it emphasizes the critical importance of the position of the head. How a person carries their head is also an expression of their self-image and self-esteem.
- There are three major factors that influence posture: heredity, disease, and acquired habit.[3] As Cailliet[3] points out, since postural habits develop in childhood, slumped posture may be the result of family or peer pressure, or the result of anxiety, insecurity, fear, anger, or depression.
- The upper cervical connective tissue, including the joint capsules and ligaments, contain an extremely dense concentration of proprioceptive nerves that serve as an important sense organ for posture.[6] The muscles of the suboccipital triangle are some of the most finely controlled muscles in the body. They have approximately one motor nerve per 4 to 5 muscle fibers, the same ratio as the muscle moving the eyes, compared with one motor nerve for every 500 muscle fibers in the quadriceps. The proper function of the upper cervical area is critical to our sense of balance, coordination, and finely tuned movements of the head in response to visual and auditory cues.
- ***Dysfunction and injury***: With a rounded-shoulder, FHP, the cervical spine goes into extension, closing the intervertebral foramen (IVF) slightly, potentially leading to nerve-root pressure. The facets are compressed, which creates increased weight bearing on the cartilage and leads to early degeneration. The joint capsules shorten and develop abnormal crosslinks, leading to loss of normal joint motion. The tension in the extensor muscles of the cervical spine and upper thoracic spine must increase dramatically to hold the weight of the head. This is not only fatiguing but also adds a compressive force on the facets and the disc and further closes the IVF. There is also compression of the space above and below the clavicle, called the *thoracic outlet,* which can compress the nerves and blood supply into the arm. Slumped posture decreases vital lung capacity and creates excessive tension in the temporomandibular joint (TMJ).
- FHP also compromises the blood flow through the vertebral artery, which is deep within the suboccipital triangle. The artery travels over the superior surface of the atlas and under the occiput before it enters the foramen magnum and travels to the brain. Lauren Berry, RPT, theorized that sustained FHP could compress the vertebral artery and could be a major contributing factor to early senility. This compression is caused by the narrowing of the space between the occiput and the atlas due to the posterior rotation of the occiput and extension of the cervical spine that occurs during FHP.

General Anatomy of Cervical Vertebrae

- As in the lumbar and thoracic spine, there is an anterior and posterior portion to each of the vertebra. There are many similar structural and functional similarities and some important differences.
- The anterior portion consists of a vertebral body and an intervertebral disc that forms a fibrocartilaginous joint with the vertebral body (Fig. 5-1). The two up-

per joints, Occ-C1 and C1 to C2, do not have discs, and C1 does not have a body.

- The posterior portion consists of two vertebral arches formed by a pedicle and lamina; two transverse processes; a central SP; and paired articulations, the inferior and superior facets, which form synovial joints. The atlas does not have an SP. Instead it has a posterior tubercle that is generally not palpable.

Unique Anatomy of Cervical Vertebrae

- *Transverse processes* are bony processes that project from both sides of the body of each vertebra. They are unique in the cervical spine (Fig. 5-2). Transverse processes have two distinct portions, the anterior and posterior portions, with an opening in the middle for the vertebral artery, called the **transverse foramen.** The most lateral projections of the transverse process are the anterior and posterior tubercles, which serve as attachment points for nine muscles in the lower segment and six muscles in the upper segment. The transverse process also has a groove or sulcus in its superior surface on which the spinal nerve travels.

Unique Anatomy of Lower Cervical Vertebrae

- The *vertebral bodies* are much smaller than the thoracic or the lumbar bodies. The increased size that would have afforded stability has been exchanged for the increased mobility allowed by the smaller size.[2] The vertebral bodies are also unique in that the anterior portion has a lip that projects downward slightly in front of the intervertebral disc, which contributes greater protection to the disc.
- *The spinous processes* are the bony prominences that project posteriorly and can be palpated on the back of the neck. They increase in length from C3 to C7. The axis (C2) has the first SP that you can palpate under the skull. C4 to C6 have bifid, or two parts to the SPs, that may be asymmetric.
- The *uncinate processes* are elevated edges on the posterolateral rim of the superior surfaces of the body of C3 to C7 (see Fig. 5-2). They articulate with a bevelled edge of the lower border of the vertebra above. These articulations are called uncovertebral joints or joints of von Luschka. Grieve[5] describes them as synovial joints, lined with hyaline cartilage and surrounded by a joint capsule. They are bordered by the intervertebral disc (IVD). These joints add stability to the region by limiting lateral flexion and protecting the posterolateral disc. Like other synovial joints they have a rich supply of proprioceptors and nociceptors.[7]
- ***Dysfunction and injury:*** It is important to realize that you cannot assess the function of the vertebrae by the position of the SPs. The SPs should not be tender to palpation. Pain with digital pressure on the SPs should alert the therapist to a dysfunction or injury to the vertebrae. The uncovertebral joints are especially susceptible to degenerative changes, as shearing occurs at these joints with flexion and extension. There often develop thickened soft-tissue and bony outgrowths that may irritate the neighboring nerve root and vertebral artery.[5] Because of their location, these processes minimize lateral bending. As they are the first areas to degenerate in the cervical spine, a chronic loss of lateral flexion is a clinical sign of cervical degeneration.

Unique Anatomy of Upper Cervical Vertebrae

- The *atlas (C1)* is the first cervical vertebra. The superior aspect of the atlas forms a synovial joint with the occipital portion of the skull, called the Occ-C1. The atlas is shaped like a ring and does not have a body or an SP. It is like a "washer" between the skull and axis.[8]
- The *axis (C2)* is the second cervical vertebrae. It has a unique vertical projection from the anterior body

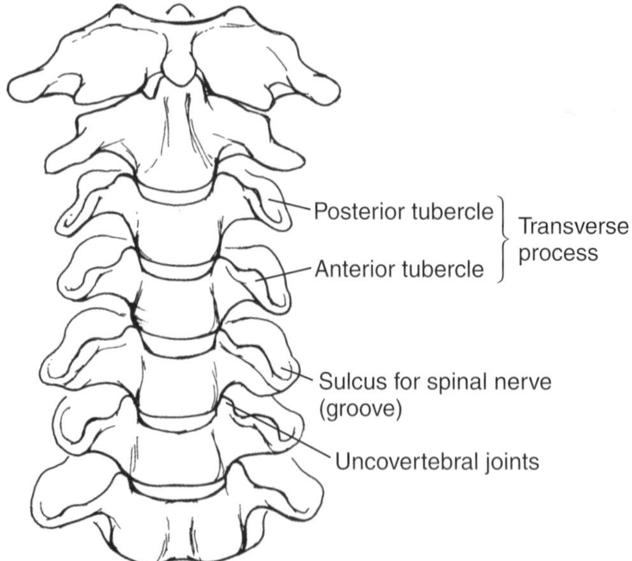

Figure 5-2. Anterior view of the cervical vertebrae showing the uncinate process, the anterior and the posterior tubercle of the transverse process, and the groove or sulcus for the spinal nerve.

called the dens, or odontoid process. The anterior portion of the dens forms a synovial joint with the posterior portion of the arch of the atlas, forming the atlantoaxial joint. The posterior tip of the dens abuts the anterior aspect of the brainstem and upper spinal cord.

- *Function:* Fifty-percent of flexion and extension of the entire cervical spine occurs at the Occ-C1 joint, and 50% of cervical rotation occurs at the atlantoaxial (C1–C2) joint. C1 to C2 is the most mobile joint in the spine.[8] Both of these joints do not have discs between them, and therefore lack the tight fit offered by the IVDs. These joints are consequently less stable. Their stability relies on a dense network of ligaments and the surrounding muscles and fascia.
- *Dysfunction and injury*: The upper segment of the cervical spine is one of the most common sources of dysfunction and injury in the body. Because of the lack of stability in this region it is susceptible to strains from falls, whether from sports or daily life, or car accidents. It is also commonly strained due to postural stresses in the common FHP. When the head is held in this forward posture, it has to rotate posteriorly on the atlas to keep the eyes on the horizon, thus shortening the suboccipital muscles. This can lead to tension headaches from the entrapment of the first and second cervical nerves. Diseases that weaken the connective tissue, such as rheumatoid arthritis (RA), can create further instability and require extreme caution from the therapist. It is **contraindicated** to introduce vigorous movement in the upper cervical spine.

Intervertebral Disc

As mentioned, there are IVDs between each of the vertebrae except the occiput and the atlas and the atlas and the axis.

- *Structure:* A nucleus and an annulus compose the IVD.
  - *Nucleus:* The nucleus is a colloidal gel that is 80 to 90% water contained within a fibrous wall. In the cervical spine it is located in the anterior portion of the disc, compared with the central location in the lumbar spine. The disc is wedge shaped, with its anterior height two times greater than its posterior height, and contributes to the normal cervical lordosis. In the lumbar spine the discs are parallel.
  - *Annulus:* Concentric layers of interwoven fibrocartilaginous fibers form the annulus.
- *Function:* The IVD provides a shock absorbing hydraulic system that permits a rocker-like movement of one vertebrae upon the other due to a fluid shift in the nucleus and the elasticity of the annulus. The disc also provides proprioceptive and nociceptive functions. Disc nutrition into the annulus occurs by movement of the spine, which pumps fluids into the disc through compression and decompression.
- *Dysfunction and injury:* Two major lesions occur in the IVD: degeneration and herniation. Disc herniation is not as common in the neck as in the lumbar spine because of the protection afforded by the uncovertebral joints, the more anterior location of the nucleus, and the much stronger posterior longitudinal ligament (PLL). The PLL is double-layered in the neck and completely surrounds the disc, whereas in the lower back it is thin and narrow.
  - Disc herniations can compress the nerve roots in the IVF, creating ischemia. Most nerve root irritations occur at C5 to C6 and at C6 to C7.
  - Disc injuries can create local neck pain and referral of pain. If the lesion is internal to the disc, it creates neck pain and referral of pain to the interscapular area. If the disc has herniated and is irritating the nerve roots, pain is referred into the arm in specific myotomes (muscles supplied by motor roots of spinal nerves) and dermatomes (areas of skin supplied by the spinal nerve sensory root) described in the section "Cervical Spine Nerves."
  - Sustained muscular contraction creates compressive forces that can lead to disc degeneration, and according to Cailliet,[3] may cause disc herniation.
- *Treatment implications*: Clients who have a disc herniation are approached with special precaution. Some of the muscle tension in the neck is providing stability to the disc, and deep massage is **contraindicated.** Disc herniations are treated with contract-relax (CR) muscle energy technique (MET) with a neutral spine. Gentle massage work is performed, but mobilization of the spine is minimized. The purpose of using these techniques is disc decompression, by reducing muscle hypertonicity. The chronic, degenerated disc is treated with CR-MET, mobilization, and manual release to help rehydrate the disc.

Facet Joints

- *Definition*: The facet (see Fig. 5-1) or apophyseal joint is a synovial joint, surrounded by a connective tissue joint capsule, fat tissue pads, and a fibromeniscus. As in the lumbar and thoracic spine, the vertebrae articulate at two superior and two inferior facet joints.

- ***Structure***
  - *Articular surface:* In the healthy state, the articular surface of the facets is covered by hyaline cartilage that is lubricated with synovial fluid. As in the other regions of the body, the nutrition to the articular cartilage depends on cycles of compression and decompression that arise from movement.
  - *Joint capsule:* An inner synovial layer and a thick and dense outer fibrous layer compose the joint capsule. In the cervical spine the capsule is loose and elastic, which allows the cervical spine to have the greatest mobility of all the regions in the spine. The capsule also has fibromenisci infoldings, which allows the joint to bear a greater load.
- ***Function***
  - The facets determine the range and direction of movement and have some weight-bearing capacity. In the healthy state, they are designed to slide on each other. The closed-packed position of the cervical facets is extension and lateral flexion, and the open position is flexion.
  - The joint capsule (capsular ligament) functions to passively stabilize the facet joints. The capsules are highly innervated and serve as receptors for proprioception or position sense, movement and pressure through mechanoreceptors, and pain through pain fibers (nociceptors). Proprioception in the cervical spine is more refined than in the lumbar spine, as a higher concentration of proprioceptors exists in the facet joint capsules.[4]
- ***Dysfunction and injury:*** The facets are susceptible to cumulative stresses and acute injury. The most common causes are as follows:
  - *FHP:* This posture places the facets in a sustained extension, the closed-packed position, compressing the joints, decreasing the joint lubrication, and leading to early degeneration.
  - *Hypomobility:* The facets can lose their normal gliding characteristics due to muscular tension, FHP, ligamentous and capsular thickening, joint fixation, degeneration or herniation of the disc, or arthritic changes.
  - *Degeneration:* Many factors cause facet degeneration. Muscle imbalances generate abnormal stresses to the cartilage, creating instability in the joint. Sustained muscle contraction decreases joint motion, creating hypomobility, and adds a compressive load to the cartilage.
    - Degeneration of the cartilage of the facets is a source of local and referred pain. Clients describe it as a dull, achy pain that can be felt in the neck, shoulder, or interscapular area. Eventually the cartilage can form osteophytes that can encroach into the IVF and lead to nerve-root irritation, which would manifest as pain, numbing, tingling, or weakness in the arm, in the hand, or in both.
  - *Injury:* The cartilage is susceptible to acute injury (e.g., a sports injury, a fall, a blow to the head or neck), to the cumulative stresses of sustained muscular contraction or FHP.
  - *Acute facet syndrome:* A common complaint is a "crick" in the neck, in which the client in unable to turn his or her neck. As mentioned, theoretically, this is caused by a fixation of the articular cartilage surfaces or an entrapment of the fibromenisci between the facets.
  - *Joint capsule injury:* Because the capsule is highly innervated, a sprain is painful, potentially giving local and referred pain into the arm. Injury also affects the mechanoreceptors, resulting in dysfunctions of coordination and balance, altered movement patterns, and altered reflexes to the muscles, creating either weakness or hypertonicity.
  - Pain in the neck is often caused by limited joint movement and capsular thickening.[5] Restricted motion of the facets results in a reflex that typically creates hypertonicity of the muscles at the same vertebral level.
- ***Treatment implications***
  - Examination reveals hypertonic muscles; muscle length and strength imbalances; thickened, fibrous tissue, especially in the multifidi and capsular ligaments; and loss of normal joint play at the facets. As motion in the joint creates lubrication, decreased motion means decreased lubrication and, consequently, increased friction and wear and tear of the joint surfaces.
  - Many clients tell the therapist that "the doctor says I have arthritis in my neck, and that I just have to live with the pain." They are afraid to move their necks, or worse, have been instructed not to move their necks if it is uncomfortable. It is important to realize, as Cailliet[3] notes, "There is little or no correlation found between the degree of pain felt in the neck and the degree of arthritic changes found on X-ray." In the author's clinical experience, most of these patients can have a dramatic reduction in pain and improvement of function with orthopedic massage (OM) and MET and instruction in proper posture and exercise.

- The basic treatment protocol is to release the hypertonicity in the short and tight muscles, broaden the fibers in the capsular ligaments, facilitate the weak muscles through CR MET, rehydrate the cartilage through compression and decompression, and reintroduce the normal gliding characteristics in the facets with gentle mobilization.
- It is important to instruct the client in proper posture. Postural strain is one of the major sources of neck pain.
- Some clients, on the other hand, are unstable and weak in their cervical muscles because of previous injury. They need proper instruction in strengthening exercises to help stabilize the cervical spine. This typically requires a referral to a physical therapist. And finally, because of the high concentration of proprioceptors in the neck, balance exercises are important to rehabilitate the function of these nerves.
- Acute facet syndrome requires a referral to a chiropractor or an osteopath for manipulation.

Intervertebral Foramen

- *Structure:* The IVF is narrow in the cervical spine, and relatively wide in the thoracic and lumbar regions (see Fig. 5-1). The IVDs form a much smaller part of the boundary of the IVF than in the lumbar region. Most cases of narrowing of the IVF caused by bony spurs are in the cervical spine, but more than 90% of the disc protrusions in the spine are in the lumbar region.[3]
- *Function:* The IVF provides an opening for the sensory and motor nerve roots and for the blood vessels. The IVF opens on flexion and closes slightly on extension.
- *Dysfunction and injury:* Narrowing of the IVF can cause compression of the nerve roots creating pain, numbing and tingling, and weakness in the arms or hands. The IVF can be narrowed because of disc degeneration, disc herniation, osteophytes or spurs, facet inflammation, sustained muscle contraction, thickening and fibrosis of the ligamentum flavum and joint capsule, malposition of the facets, osteoarthritis (OA) of the facets or uncovertebral joints, or increased lordosis caused by FHP. Significant narrowing of the IVF is called **foraminal encroachment** and can lead to nerve root irritation.

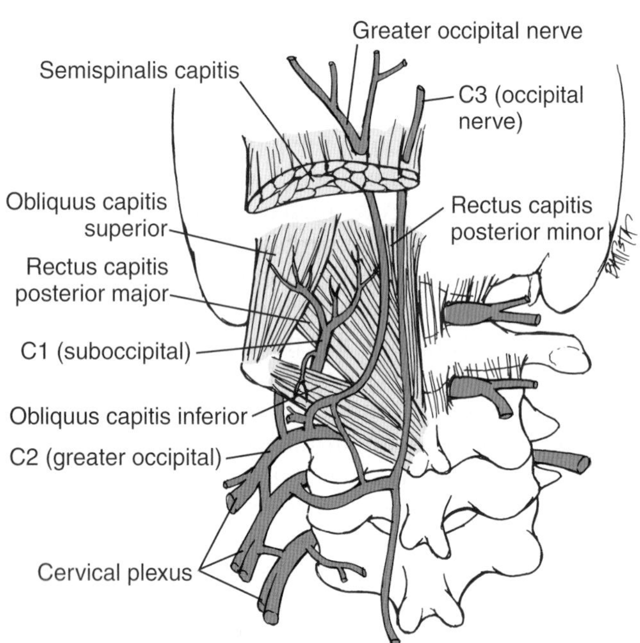

Figure 5-3. Suboccipital muscles and the nerves of the suboccipital region showing the C1 to C3 nerves.

Cervical Spine Nerves

- As in the other areas of the spine, the cervical nerves are mixed nerves from the union of **motor (ventral)** and **sensory (dorsal)** roots that have emerged from the spinal cord. The roots merge to become the spinal nerve. The motor nerve has intimate contact with the uncovertebral joints, and the sensory root lies close to the facet joint and capsule.
- The C1, C2, and C3 nerves innervate the head and face. These first three cervical nerves travel through the muscles at the base of the skull and are sensitive to irritation from sustained muscle contraction (Fig. 5-3). The medial branch of C2 is also called the greater occipital nerve and travels through the semispinalis capitis and pierces the scalp as it travels onto the back of the skull. C3 extends forward to the area above the eye, and if irritated, can feel like sinus pain.[3]
- The **spinal cord** occupies four-fifths of the spinal canal, and as the neck flexes, the nerve roots are pulled taut and have a pulling or tethering effect on the spinal cord. Normally, there is enough slack in the roots and the cord, but many factors can compromise their free movement.

Dorsal Root Ganglion

- **The dorsal root ganglion** (**DRG**) is a cluster of cell bodies of the sensory nerves and has been postulated to be a major site of pain, called radicular

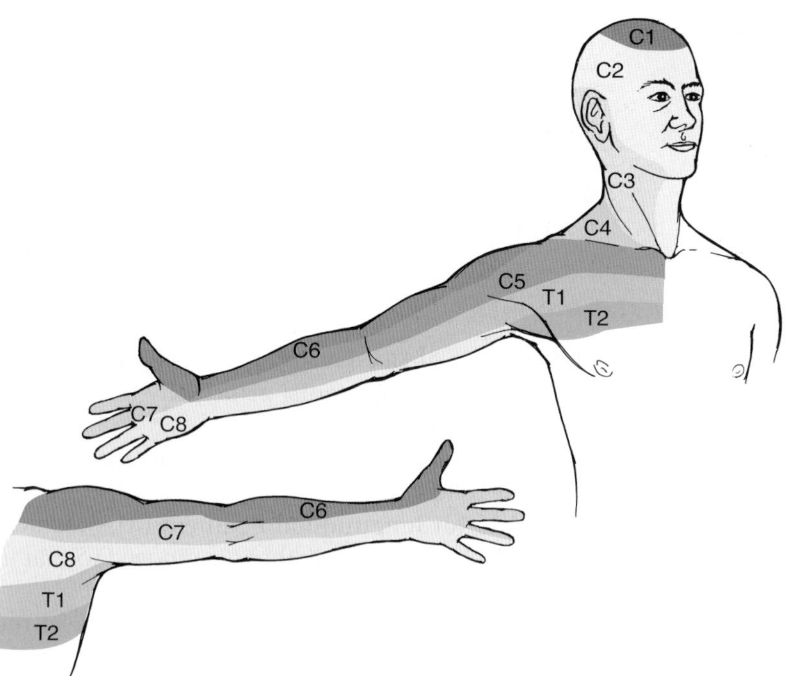

Figure 5-4. Dermatomes of the cervical spine, which cover the head, neck, shoulder, arm, and hand.

(which means root) pain. DRG irritation elicits a sharp pain, numbing, and tingling in the dermatome corresponding to the root. A **dermatome** is an area of skin supplied by the sensory root of a spinal nerve (Fig. 5-4).

Ventral (Motor) Root

- The ventral (motor) root is a cluster of cell bodies of the motor nerves. A **myotome** is the muscles supplied by the motor (ventral) root(s) of the spinal nerve(s). Irritation of the motor root elicits muscle weakness and potential atrophy. The corresponding myotomes of the cervical nerve roots are C1 to C2, neck flexion; C3, side flexion of the neck; C4, shoulder elevation; C5, shoulder abduction; C6, elbow flexion and wrist extension; C7, elbow and finger extension and wrist flexion; C8, thumb extension; and T1, abduction of the fingers.

Brachial Plexus

- The anterior portion of C5 to C8 and T1 nerves forms the brachial plexus (Fig. 5-5) that becomes the ulnar, median, and radial nerves of the arm. They emerge from the transverse processes and travel between the anterior and the middle scalenes, under the clavicle and subclavius, under the pectoralis minor, and then into the arm. The covering of the nerve, called the epineurium, of C4 to C6 is partially anchored to the scalene muscle group, and sustained contraction of these muscles could irritate these nerves.
- ***Dysfunction and Injury***
  - The nerve roots and spinal cord can become compressed or stretched near the IVF due to disc herniations, thickening of the ligamentum flavum, osteophytes (bone spurs), or degeneration and hypertrophy (bone deposits) of the facets.
  - Three types of referred pain, numbing, or tingling into the extremities occur: spinal cord irritation, nerve root irritation, or brachial plexus peripheral irritation.
    - Irritation from the spinal cord is a condition called **cervical myelopathy.** This cord compression often affects the elderly and causes gait disturbances, impaired fine-hand movements, lower-extremity weakness, and numbness in the trunk.[3] Passive neck flexion causing lower-extremity numbness is a sign of cord compression.
    - Nerve root pain is also called **radicular pain** and results from irritation of the cervical nerve roots in the region of the IVF. If the sensory root is irritated, it creates pain, numbing, and tingling, localized to a specific area, called the dermatome, rather than to a diffuse region. The pain varies from a deep aching to sharp. If the motor root is irritated, it causes deep and bor-

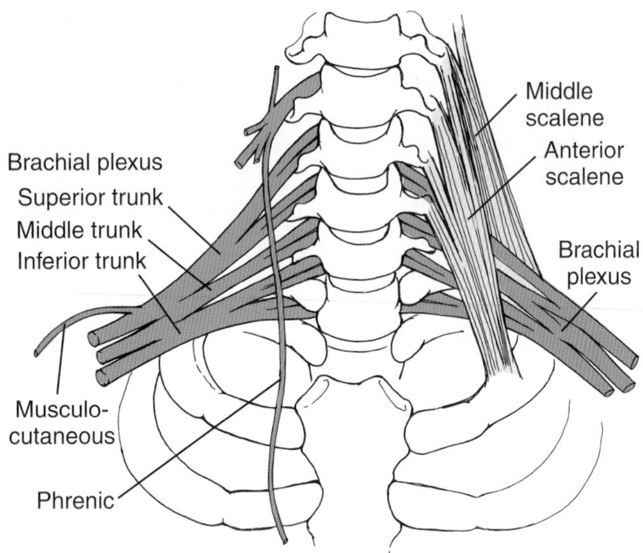

Figure 5-5. Brachial plexus and the scalenes muscle. The brachial plexus travels in between the anterior and the middle scalenes, under the clavicle, under the pectoralis minor, and into the arm.

ing pain in the muscles supplied by that root and weakness. The cause of the pain is often hard to differentiate.

- The third source of referred pain comes from the brachial plexus, which may also become compressed by sustained contraction in the anterior and the middle scalenes or under the pectoralis minor or subclavius or by thickened fascia in the area above or below the clavicle. These conditions are broadly defined as thoracic outlet syndrome (TOS). TOS is often caused by slumped posture but may be the consequence of injury or overuse from work or recreational habits.

Sympathetic Nerves

- Major components of the sympathetic nervous system are located in the neck. The sympathetic nerves travel through the longus colli and are susceptible to irritation with sustained muscle contracture or may be irritated from an excessive stretch caused by a hyperextension injury.
- *Dysfunction and injury:* Whiplash injuries can damage the cervical sympathetic nerves.[9] Irritation of these nerves can lead to the following symptoms: headache, vertigo, tinnitus, nasal disturbance, facial pain, facial flushing, and pharyngeal paresthesias, nausea, and blurred vision.[3]
- *Treatment implications:* OM has been found to be clinically effective in many cases to reduce or relieve symptoms of sympathetic irritation with MET and manual release of the deep cervical flexors. All clients who have these symptoms should also be under the care of a chiropractor or an osteopath to evaluate and treat potential joint fixations.

Ligaments

- The stability of Occ-C1 and C1-C2 is provided primarily by dense ligaments, principally the cruciate, alar, and apical ligaments.
- The principal ligaments of the lower segment include the following:
  - An **anterior longitudinal ligament (ALL),** which, in the cervical spine, is thin as opposed to that in the lumbar spine, where it is thick.
  - A **PLL,** which, however, is wide and thick in the neck and narrow in the lumbar spine. PLL thickness offers protection from a posterior protrusion of the disc.
  - A **ligamentum flavum,** which blends with the joint capsule.
  - A **supraspinous ligament** and its broad expansion called the ligamentum nuchae, which extends from C7 to T1 to the external occipital protuberance (EOP). As the center of the mass of the head lies anterior to the center of gravity, the ligamentum nuchae and extensor muscles are designed to resist this forward pull.
  - A **capsular ligament** of the facet joints (see joint capsule above).
- *Dysfunction and injury:* Cervical spine degeneration has the potential to cause folds in the ligamentum flavum, which can buckle during extension, and to contribute to narrowing of the spinal canal.[2] Because the ligamentum flavum blends with the joint capsule, sprains of the joint can create hypertrophy to the capsule and ligamentum flavum, decreasing the space of the IVF, causing encroachment of the nerve roots. Diseases that weaken the connective tissue, such as RA, can severely affect the stability of the upper cervical spine.
- *Treatment implications*
  - Because many clients who have chronic neck pain have fibrotic capsular ligaments, the intention of massage therapy is to gently and gradually broaden these fibers and rehydrate these tissues through manual techniques. Thick and dense capsular ligaments prevent the normal gliding of the vertebral facets and contribute to joint degeneration.

- Clients who have a history of RA or acute neck injury need protection from vigorous mobilization. If a client tests weak in their cervical muscles, then treatment is geared toward stabilization through CR MET with the client in a neutral position. These clients are referred to a physical therapist for rehabilitation exercises to strengthen the muscles and to increase the density of the ligaments.

Cervical Fascia

- ***Structure:*** Fascia is a sheet of dense connective tissue. In addition to the fascia that surrounds each muscle, there are six layers of fascia in the cervical spine. The **prevertebral fascia,** which completely surrounds each vertebra, is continuous with the thoracolumbar fascia.[2]
- ***Function:*** Fascia plays an important role in transmitting the forces generated by the muscles and in giving shape to the body. The fascia forms muscle compartments that allow for the precise direction of muscle contraction.
- ***Dysfunction and injury:*** Injury or irritation thickens the fascia through abnormal crosslinks and collagen deposition (adhesions). This fascial thickening restricts the normal muscle movement within the fascial compartments and decreases the range of motion (ROM) of the joints.

Cervical Region Muscles

- ***Function:*** Muscles of the cervical spine provide dynamic stabilization, mobility, and proprioceptive feedback essential to our balance and fine postural control. In the lumbopelvic region, the essential function of the muscles and associated fascia is to promote stability for lifting and carrying activities. In the cervical spine, mobility is more essential, so as to be able to move the eyes and ears quickly and efficiently. There are vast reflex connections between the organs of balance, called the vestibular apparatus, the muscles of the eyes, and the musculature of the head and neck.[2]
- The muscles of the cervical spine may be divided into four functional groups: superficial posterior, deep posterior, superficial anterior, and deep anterior.[7] The superficial posterior includes the trapezius, levator scapula, and splenius cervicis and capitis. They serve to hold the head up against gravity and extend the head and neck. The deep posterior includes the longissimus cervicis and capitis, iliocostalis cervicis, semispinalis cervicis and capitis, multifidi, and suboccipital muscles. The superficial anterior muscles include the sternocleidomastoid (SCM), scalenes, and hyoid muscles. The deep flexors are the longus colli and capitis.
- A further division may be made between muscles that move the head, what Cailliet[3] calls the capital muscles, and those that move the cervical spine. In addition to the suboccipital group, the muscles that move the head are the longissimus capitis; semispinalis capitis; splenius capitis; the deep flexors of the cranium, including the rectus capitis anterior and lateralis; and the suprahyoid muscles, which because of their attachment to the mandible, assist in flexing the head. These two categories also describe a functional differentiation in that the occiput, atlas, and axis can be moved independently of the lower cervical spine.[2] This independent movement allows for stability in the lower segment, whereas the upper segment is fine-tuning its movement for sight and hearing.
- An intimate relationship exits between the jaw and the muscles of the cervical spine. Swallowing, chewing, and vocalization all involve the hyoid muscles. For the jaw to open, the occiput must be stabilized.
- ***Dysfunction and injury***
  - *Muscle tightness*: Muscle tightness usually develops from postural faults or psychological and emotional stress. As in the lumbar spine, it is typical for the extensor muscles of the cervical spine to be held in a sustained contraction. With a FHP, the extensors shorten, increasing the lordosis of the cervical spine, placing the facets in the closed-packed position. These postural changes result in compression of the facet joints and disc, contributing to neck pain and headaches and to early degeneration of these structures.[4]
    - ***Anterior scalene syndrome:*** The brachial plexus and subclavian artery travel in between the anterior and the middle scalenes. With sustained contraction of these muscles, pain, numbing, and tingling can manifest, especially along the ulnar border of the hand. This is called anterior scalene syndrome (scalenus anticus syndrome). This condition is part of a constellation of similar lesions that fall under the broad category of TOS.
    - The hyoid muscles and muscles of the TMJ may also be held in a sustained contraction due to injury or FHP. As the head tilts posteriorly to keep the eyes level in FHP, the mandible is pulled down and posteriorly, which means that the masseter and temporalis must increase

their tension to bring the TMJ back into its resting position.[2,4]

- Headaches caused by muscle tension: According to Kendall et al.,[4] two types of headaches are associated with muscle tension: the occipital headache and the tension headache. The occipital headache develops from sustained contraction of the semispinalis capitis. The semispinalis capitis can entrap the greater occipital nerve, leading to pain, numbness, and burning from the occipital region to the top of the head. Tension headaches, on the other hand, are caused by faulty posture and emotional or psychological stress that lead to sustained tension in the posterior neck muscles. Periods of increased stress increase the tension. The rectus capitis posterior minor is also implicated in tension headaches, as it attaches to the covering of the brain called the dura, and sustained contraction creates a tethering or pulling force on the dura, creating a headache.
- *Muscle injury*: Muscle strain is often associated with an injury but may develop from minor repetitive strains. The SCM is the most commonly injured muscle in rear-end auto accidents, followed by the longus colli. If the SCM is held in a sustained contraction, it pulls the head forward. Typically, the longus colli, a deep flexor of the neck, is weak after injury, which allows an increase in the cervical curve. However, the longus colli may be short and tight as a result of injury, which would contribute to a decreased cervical curve.

- As mentioned previously, Janda describes predictable patterns of muscle dysfunction. In the upper body, this dysfunction is called the **upper crossed syndrome** (Fig. 5-6), because the muscles that are typically tight form one arm of the cross, and those that are typically weak form the other arm of the cross.

Cervical Region Muscle Imbalances

- *Muscles that tend to be tight and short:* Levator scapula; upper trapezius; SCM; suboccipitals; cervical extensors, including the splenius capitis and the semispinalis capitis; and pectoralis minor.
- *Muscles that tend to be weak and inhibited:* Deep neck flexors, including longus colli and capitis; scalenes; middle and lower trapezius; rhomboids; and serratus anterior.
- These patterns have common variations. For example, the scalenes may be either tight and short or weak and inhibited.

Positional Dysfunction of the Cervical Spine Muscles

- Cervical extensors develop a medial torsion.
- Scalenes and SCM tend to develop an anterior torsion.

Muscular Relations to the Balance of the Head and Neck

- Muscles that increase the cervical curve.
  - Semispinalis cervicis and capitis.
- Muscles that decrease the cervical curve.
  - Longus colli and capitis.

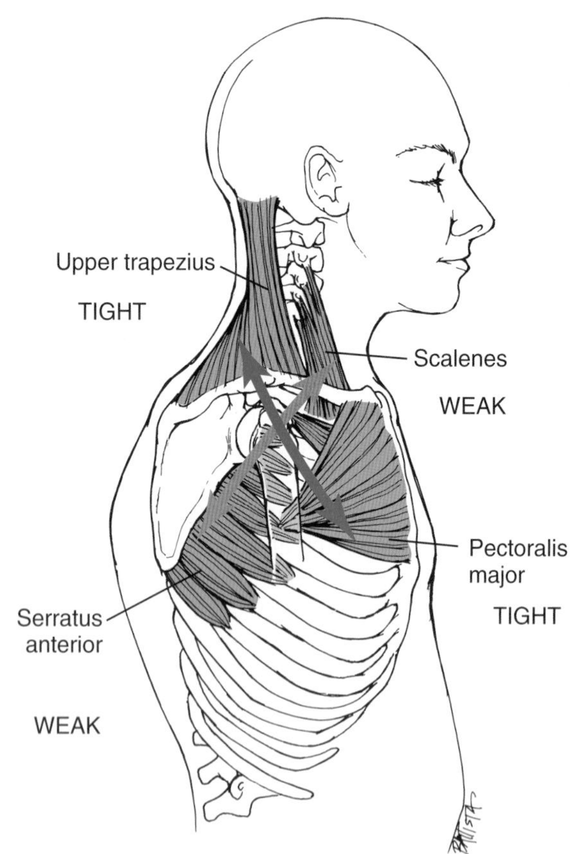

Figure 5-6. Upper crossed syndrome is characterized by short and tight suboccipitals, cervical extensors, upper trapezii, levator scapulae and pectoral muscles and by weak and inhibited deep cervical flexors, middle and lower trapezii, and serratus anterior. This syndrome is characterized by FHP, rounded shoulders, hyperextension of the head, elevated shoulders, and an increased cervical curve.

TABLE 5-1 POSTURAL SIGNS OF THE UPPER CROSSED SYNDROME

Postural Finding:	*Dysfunction:*
Rounded shoulders	Short pectoralis minor
Forward head	Kyphotic thoracic spine
Hyperextension of head	Short suboccipital muscles
Elevated shoulders	Short upper trapezius and levator
Winging of scapula	Weak serratus anterior
Increased cervical lordosis	Short cervical extensors, weak deep flexors

- Muscular imbalances that contribute to FHP.
  - Short and tight SCM.
  - Weak cervical extensors, lower trapezius, and abdominals.
- *Treatment implications*
  - The foundation of the treatment of the cervical spine is to correct faulty posture. The only exception is the client in acute pain, who will adopt compensatory postures due to the pain. As part of the correction of postural faults, exercises are recommended to strengthen the deep cervical flexors, lower trapezius, and latissimus. Kendall et al.[4] provide exercise guidelines.
  - *The primary intention in treating the acute client* is to apply gentle reciprocal inhibition (RI) MET or CR MET that helps disperse excess fluids, restore proper nutrition, and provide gentle stress to the collagen to promote healing of the fibers in their proper alignment. The muscles that have been strained will be swollen, boggy, and tight to palpation, with a thin-membraned rigidity caused by the swelling.
  - *The primary intention in treating the subacute or chronic client* is to reduce muscle hypertonicity, lengthen shortened muscles and their associated fascia, and promote mobility in the cervical spine. CR MET and postisometric relaxation (PIR) MET are used to promote strength and stability. And finally, balance exercises are recommended to restore proper function of the proprioceptors.
  - Treatment for clients who have a diagnosis of herniated discs involves CR MET and gentle manual release of the hypertonicity in the muscles, as this helps decompress the disc. However, it is **contraindicated** to perform deep-release techniques on these clients, as some of the tension in the muscle system is helping to stabilize the discs.

ANATOMY OF THE CERVICAL SPINE MUSCLES

Muscles cited in Table 5-2 are in addition to those listed in Chapter 3.

Muscular Actions of the Neck

See Table 5-3 for a comprehensive listing of the muscles responsible for neck movement, including flexion, extension, lateral flexion, rotation, and circumduction.

Anatomy, Function, and Dysfunction of the Temporomandibular Joint

The TMJ is part of what is called the stomatognathic system, which includes the muscles of chewing (the mandibular and cervical muscles); the tongue; the TMJ; the occlusion of the teeth; and the associated ligaments, muscles, nerves and vessels.[10] The TMJ is probably used more than any other joint in the body, as it is involved in eating, chewing, speaking, and swallowing.

TEMPOROMANDIBULAR JOINT ANATOMY

- ***Structure:*** The TMJ is a synovial joint formed by the articulation of the horseshoe-shaped mandible and the two temporal bones of the skull (Fig. 5-10). An intervening disc separates the two bones, essentially creating an upper and lower joint.[11] The mandible is composed of a body and a right and left rami. The articulating region of the mandible is called the mandibular condyle, which is a rounded projection of bone that sits in the concave portion of the temporal bone called the glenoid fossa. On the anterior portion of each ramus is another bony protuberance called the coronoid process, which serve as the attachment site for the temporalis and masseter muscles. The

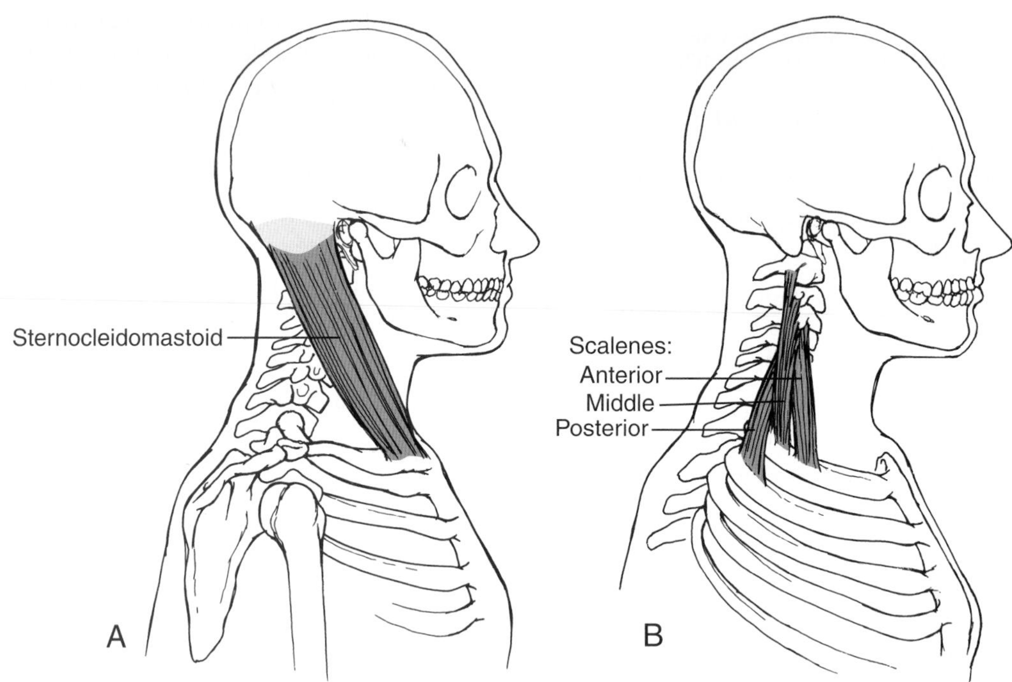

Figure 5-7. **A.** SCM. **B.** Anterior, middle, and posterior scalenes.

TMJ is located immediately anterior to the opening of the ear.

- *Function:* The TMJ functions during eating, chewing, speaking, and swallowing. The resting position of the mandible is when the teeth are held slightly apart, and in this position there is minimal muscular effort.[12] The resting position of the tongue is when the superior portion of the tongue is resting lightly against the palate and the anterior tip is lightly touching the back of the upper front teeth.[10]

  There is a functional relation among the cervical spine, the TMJ, and the occlusion or articulation of the teeth. A change in head position affects the way the mandible closes, the resting position of the mandible, and the way the teeth make contact.[12] The TMJ is capable of five motions: opening of the mouth, closing of the mouth, jutting the chin forward (protrusion), sliding the jaw backwards (retrusion), and lateral deviation of the mandible.

ARTICULAR DISC OR MENISCUS

- *Structure:* The meniscus is a fibrocartilage structure in the TMJ.
- *Function:* The meniscus functions to add congruency to the articulating surfaces throughout their ROM and to distribute the compressive forces.[11] The disc essentially follows the movement of the condyles of the mandible and moves forward during the opening of the mouth and moves posteriorly as it closes.[12] The lateral pterygoid muscle attaches to the disc and pulls the condyle and the disc forward.

LIGAMENTS

- The TMJ ligaments are the capsular ligaments, the stylomandibular ligament, the sphenomandibular ligament, and the lateral ligament (the temporomandibular ligament), which is a thickening of the joint capsule.

TEMPOROMANDIBULAR JOINT MUSCLES

- The mandible has eight muscles attached to it, and five of the eight muscles are essential to the movement of the TMJ: the digastric, temporalis, masseter, lateral pterygoid, and medial pterygoid muscles (Fig. 5-11 and see Fig. 3-10).
  - The primary muscles that open the jaw are the lateral pterygoids and the digastrics. The suprahyoid muscles assist in mandibular opening, as the hyoid bone is fixed by the infrahyoid muscles.[12]

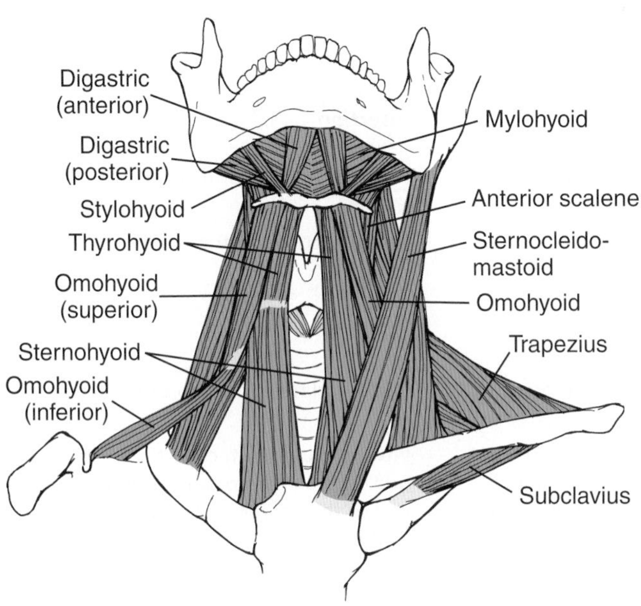

Figure 5-8. Superficial anterior muscles of the neck are the suprahyoid and infrahyoid muscles.

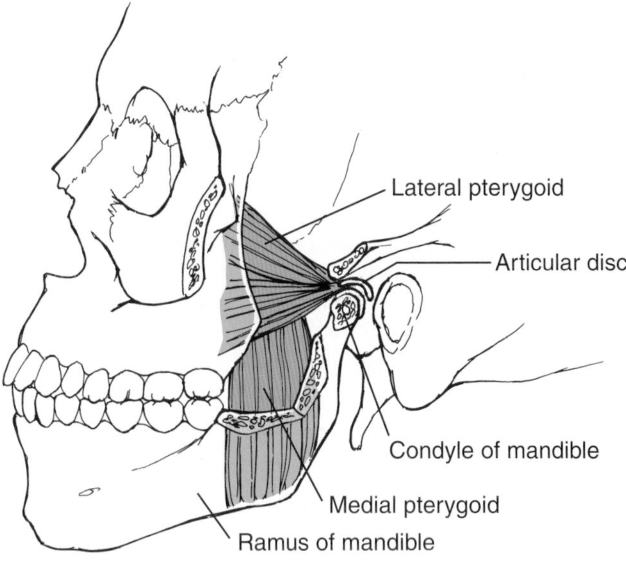

Figure 5-10. TMJ and the medial and lateral pterygoid muscles.

- The temporalis, masseter, and the medial pterygoid muscles close the jaw.
- The masseter and the medial and lateral pterygoids provide protrusion.
- The posterior fibers of the temporalis perform retrusion, which is also called retraction.
- The medial and lateral pterygoids on one side and the contralateral temporalis provide lateral move-

Text continued on page 172.

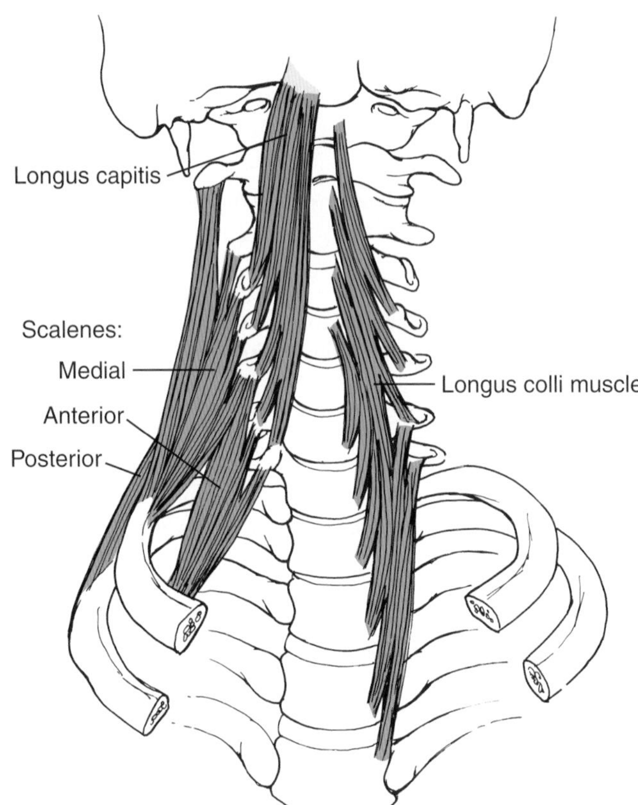

Figure 5-9. Muscles on the deepest aspect of the anterior neck are called the prevertebral muscles.

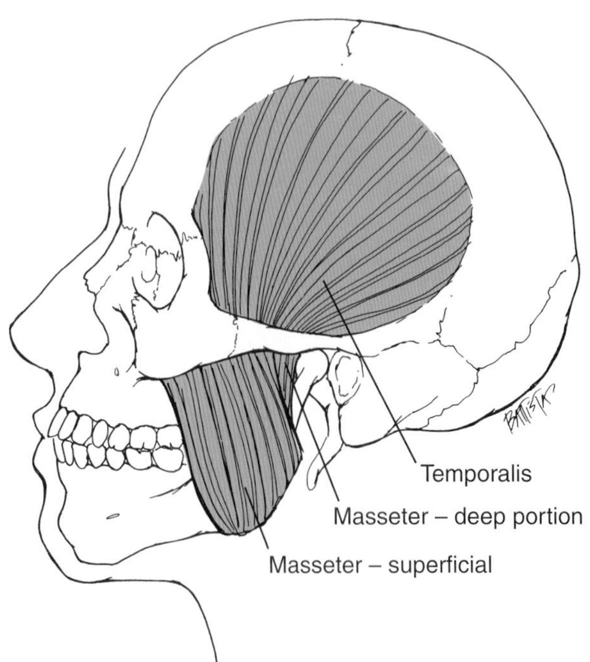

Figure 5-11. Temporalis and masseter muscles.

TABLE 5-2 ANATOMY OF THE MUSCLES OF THE CERVICAL SPINE[a]

Muscle	*Origin*	*Insertion*
Scalenus anterior (Anticus) (Fig. 5-7**A**)	Anterior tubercle of the transverse processes of C3–C6.	Anterior portion of first rib
Scalenus medius (Fig. 5-7**A**) ***Clinical Note:*** The brachial plexus travels between the anterior and the medial scalenes, under the clavicle, under the pectoralis minor, and into the arm.	Posterior tubercle of transverse processes C1–C7.	Lateral portion of the first rib
Scalenus posterior (Fig. 5-7**B**)	Posterior tubercle of transverse process of C5–C7.	Posterior-lateral portion of the second rib
Sternocleidomastoid (SCM) muscle (Fig. 5-7**C**)	This large, rounded muscle is twisted 90° like a screw about its longitudinal axis from the sides down toward the midline of the body.	Into the outer surface of the mastoid process from its tip to its superior border and to the center (or lateral two-thirds) of the superior nuchal line

Suboccipital Muscles *(See Fig. 5-3)*

Muscle	*Origin*	*Insertion*
Rectus capitis posterior major	Lateral and superior half of the spinous process of the axis. The thick muscle belly has a triangular shape, spreading toward the skull. The fibers are twisted so that the most anterior are inserted most medially.	Lateral half of the inferior nuchal line
Rectus capitis posterior minor	Tuberosity on posterior arch of atlas, interweaves with the dura of the brain, and therefore, implicated in tension-type headaches.	Medial one-third of the inferior nuchal line
Obliquus capitis superior	Thick tendinous fibers from the posterior corner and lateral segment of the transverse process of C1.	Superior to the lateral one-third of the inferior nuchal line
Obliquus capitis inferior	Anteriorly between the apex of the spinous process and the arch of the axis (C2).	Inferior and posterior surface of the transverse process of the atlas

Suprahyoid Muscles *(Fig. 5-8)*

Muscle	*Origin*	*Insertion*
Digastric	Two bellies united by a rounded tendon—extends from mastoid to chin. Posterior belly attaches in mastoid notch of temporal bone and passes downward and forward.	Anterior belly attaches to digastric fossa on the base of the mandible; the two bellies meet in an intermediate tendon, which perforates the stylohyoid muscle

Action	Sternal Position	Clavicular Position	Relation
Lateral flexion of the cervical spine			
Lateral flexion of the cervical spine			
Lateral flexion of the cervical spine			
Bilateral flexion of the head Unilateral lateral bending of the head to side of contraction and rotation to opposite side	Arises by a rounded, strong tendon from the anterior surface of the manubrium of the sternum, immediately medial and inferior to the sternoclavicular joint	Composed of muscular and aponeurotic (tendonous) fibers, arises from the superior surface and posterior border of the sternal end of the clavicle, and extends laterally to the first third of the clavicle. The flat muscle belly slides under the inferior surface of the sternal portion and enlarges superiorly.	

Action	Sternal Position	Clavicular Position	Relation
Bilateral extension of the head Unilateral lateral bending of the head to the same side			Under the trapezius and semispinalis capitis
Posture and stabilization of occipital-first cervical (OCC-C1) junction			Two-thumb widths below the external occipital protuberance (EOP)
Bilateral extension of the head Unilateral lateral bending of the head to the side of the contracting muscle Rotation of the head to the side of the contracted muscle			Approximately 1 inch lateral to the EOP, palpated below the most lateral insertion of semispinalis capitis

Action	Sternal Position	Clavicular Position	Relation
Depresses the mandible and can elevate the hyoid bone			

TABLE 5-2 ANATOMY OF THE MUSCLES OF THE CERVICAL SPINE*

Suprahyoid Muscles *(Fig. 5-8)*

Muscle	*Origin*	*Insertion*
Stylohyoid	Arises by a small tendon from the posterior surface of the styloid process	Into the body of the hyoid at its junction with the greater cornu
Mylohyoid	Forms the muscular floor of the mouth. It is a flat, triangular sheet attached to the entire length of the mylohyoid line of the mandible.	Passes medially and downward to the anterior medial body of the hyoid
Hyoglossus	Form the greater horn of the hyoid bone	Passes superiorly to the aponeurosis of the tongue

Infrahyoid Muscles *(See Fig. 5-8)*

Muscle	*Origin*	*Insertion*
Sternohyoid	Arises from the posterior surface of the medial end of the clavicle, the posterior sternoclavicular ligament, and the superior-posterior surface of the sternum.	Lower border of the most medial part of the body of the hyoid
Sternothyroid	Shorter and wider than above muscle and deep to it. Arises from the posterior surface of the manubrium below the origin of the sternohyoid.	Oblique line on lamina of thyroid cartilage
Thyrohyoid	Oblique line on lamina of thyroid cartilage.	Lower border of greater cornu and adjacent part of hyoid underneath the sternohyoid and omohyoid
Omohyoid	Arises from upper border of the scapula near the scapular notch. Consists of two fleshy bellies united by an intermediate tendon.	Lower border of hyoid bone body, lateral to insertion of sternohyoid

Prevertebral Neck Muscles *(Fig. 5-9)*

Muscle	*Origin*	*Insertion*
Rectus capitis lateralis	Upper surface of the transverse process of the atlas.	Inferior surface of the occipital bone lateral to the occipital condyle
Rectus capitis anterior	Anterior surface of the lateral mass of the atlas and the transverse process.	Inferior surface of the basilar part of the occipital bone in front of the occipital condyle
Longus capitis	Attached by tendinous slips to the anterior tubercles of the transverse processes of C3–C6.	Inferior surface of the basilar part of the occipital bone
Longus colli—Inferior oblique	Runs up and laterally from anterior bodies of T1–T3.	Anterior tubercles of transverse processes of C5 and C6.
Longus colli—Superior oblique	Anterior tubercles of C3 and C5.	Anterolateral surface of the anterior tubercle of atlas
Longus colli—Medial (intermediate) fibers	Anterior bodies of upper 3 thoracic and lower 3 cervical vertebrae	Anterior bodies of upper 3 cervical vertebrae

*In addition to those listed in Chapter 3, pp 86–90.

Action	Sternal Position	Clavicular Position	Relation
Elevates and draws back the hyoid			
Elevates the floor of the mouth in the first stage of swallowing; elevates the hyoid bone or depresses the mandible			
The hyoglossus moves the tongue in concert with the genioglossus and the styloglossus			

Action	Sternal Position	Clavicular Position	Relation
Depresses the hyoid after swallowing			
Draws larynx down after it has been elevated in swallowing or vocalization			
Depresses the hyoid or raises the larynx			
Depresses the hyoid after it has been elevated			

Action	Sternal Position	Clavicular Position	Relation
Bends the head to same side and stabilizes the head			
Flexes the head			
Flexes the head when acting bilaterally and straightens the upper cervical spine; side bends the head when acting unilaterally			
Flexes the head and straightens the upper cervical spine when acting bilaterally; unilaterally, it assists in side bending and rotation of the head to the same side			

TABLE 5-3 MUSCULAR ACTIONS OF THE NECK

The neck is capable of the same movements as the trunk (i.e., flexion, extension, right and left rotation, right and left lateral flexion, and circumduction).

- Flexion
  - SCM—contributes to neck flexion when acting bilaterally and to lateral flexion and rotation to the opposite side when acting unilaterally
  - Scalenes (anterior, medial, and posterior)—assist in forward flexion when acting bilaterally, and when acting unilaterally, assist in lateral flexion
  - Longus colli—bends the neck forward, and when acting unilaterally, assists in lateral flexion to the same side and rotation to the opposite side
  - Longus capitis—flexes the head forward
  - Rectus capitis anterior—flexes the head forward
- Extension
  - Erector spinae
  - Semispinalis capitis—extends the neck and head when acting bilaterally, bending the head backwards, and draws the head to the opposite side when acting unilaterally
  - Semispinalis cervicis—extension, lateral flexion, and rotation to the opposite side
  - Splenius capitis—extends the head and neck; lateral flexion and rotation of the head to the same side when acting unilaterally
  - Splenius cervicis—same as splenius capitis
  - Multifidus—extends the neck when acting bilaterally and provides lateral flexion and rotation of the neck to the opposite side when acting unilaterally
- Lateral Flexion
  - Splenius capitis
  - Splenius cervicis
  - SCM
  - Scalenes
  - Semispinalis capitis
  - Semispinalis cervicis
  - Erector spinae
  - Multifidus
  - Levator scapulae
- Rotation
  - SCM—rotates to opposite side
  - Semispinalis cervicis and capitis—rotate to opposite side
  - Multifidus—rotates to opposite side
  - Splenius cervicis and capitis—rotate to same side
  - Erector spinae—rotates to same side
- Circumduction

As with the trunk, neck circumduction is the combination of flexion, lateral flexion, and hyperextension in a sequential movement.

ment of the mandible. The muscles of the cervical spine stabilize the head, allowing for efficient mandible movements.

- ***Dysfunction and injury:*** Head posture has a significant and immediate affect on the resting position of the mandible.[11,12] In the FHP, as the cranium rotates posteriorly, the position of the tongue changes from the normal resting position of being up against the palate to the floor of the mouth. This contributes to tightness in the floor of the mouth and muscles in the anterior neck.[10] Sustained tension in the masseter muscles is often associated with emotional or psychological stress and contributes to grinding of the teeth (bruxism). TMJ injury is common and results from incidents such as a blow or fall or an acceleration force such as a car accident. OA of the TMJ is common and manifests as a painful reduction of the ability to open the mandible. OA develops from previous injury, the cumulative stress of chronic tension, or the imbalances of forces through the joint caused by malocclusion of the teeth or muscle imbalances.
- ***Treatment implications***: Postural correction is the first treatment goal. Second, if sustained muscle tension is palpated in the client who has chronic pain or dysfunction, encourage stress management, such as aerobic exercise, yoga, meditation, or biofeedback. The easiest way to reduce sustained hypertonicity and balance the muscles of the TMJ is by application of CR MET. These techniques are performed in the resting position of the mandible to help stabilize the joint in neutral. To increase the joint ROM, perform PIR MET.

Temporomandibular Joint Muscle Anatomy

See Figs. 5-10 and 5-11. See Table 5-4 for a comprehensive listing of TMJ muscles and their origin, insertion, and action.

Dysfunction and Injury of the Neck and Temporomandibular Joint

FACTORS PREDISPOSING TO NECK AND TEMPOROMANDIBULAR JOINT DYSFUNCTION AND PAIN

- ***Injury:*** An acceleration-deceleration strain of the neck, called whiplash, can result from a motor vehicle accident (MVA), sports injury, or fall. This whip-

TABLE 5-4 ANATOMY OF THE MUSCLES OF TEMPOROMANDIBULAR JOINT

Muscle	*Origin*	*Insertion*	*Action*
Temporalis	Entire temporal fossa; tendon passes through the gap between the zygomatic arch and the side of the skull	Medial surface, tip and front and back borders of coronoid process and front border of the ramus of the mandible	Elevates the mandible and so closes the mouth
Lateral pterygoid	■ Upper head from the infratemporal surface and crest of the greater wing of the sphenoid and lower head from the lateral pterygoid of the sphenoid ■ Fibers pass laterally and backwards	Into a depression on the front of the neck of the mandible and pterygoid fovea and the articular capsule and disc of the TMJ	Assists the mouth in opening by pulling forward the condyle and disc In closing the mouth, backward gliding of the disc and condyle are controlled by its slow relaxation
Medial pterygoid	Thick, quadrilateral muscle attached to the medial surface of the lateral pterygoid plate of the sphenoid and the palatine bone	Passes down, laterally and backwards and is attached to the inner surface of the mandibular ramus	Assists in elevating the mandible and with the lateral pterygoids, helps to protrude it
Masseter	Consists of three superimposed layers ■ The zygomatic process of the maxilla and the anterior two-thirds of the zygomatic arch ■ The deep surface of the front two-thirds of the zygomatic arch and the lower border of the posterior one-third of the arch ■ The deep surface of the zygomatic arch	■ The angle and lower half of the lateral surface of the mandibular ramus ■ The middle of the ramus of the mandible ■ The upper part of the ramus and into the coronoid process	Elevates the mandible to occlude the teeth in chewing

ping or jerking of the neck and jaw can damage ligaments, as well as the joint capsule, muscles, cartilage, and nervous system.

- ***Posture:*** The FHP compresses the facets of the cervical spine, irritating the joint capsule, and causes the extensor muscles to be tight and short. It also causes increased tension in the floor of the mouth and anterior neck muscles. This leads to fatigue in the soft tissue, which predisposes it to injury.
- ***Emotional and psychological stress:*** Tension, stress, anxiety, fear, resentment, uncertainty, and depression cause local areas of vasoconstriction and sustained contraction in the muscles of the neck and jaw, which leads to muscle fatigue. These changes result in altered patterns of muscle contraction and movement.
- ***Abnormal function of the muscles:*** Abnormal function of the muscles creates abnormal movement patterns and excessive stresses on the facets and disc. The result of these changes is that movement of the neck, jaw, or both becomes restricted and painful, leading to fibrosis around the joints.
- ***Joint dysfunction:*** Excessive mobility or loss of mobility in the joints of the cervical spine or TMJ predisposes the area to injury. The loss or the normal gliding characteristics has reflexive changes in the surrounding muscles, setting up a continuing cycle of muscle and joint dysfunction.

- ***Deconditioning or inactivity:*** As the muscles dynamically stabilize the spine, if there is generalized muscle weakness caused by immobilization, lack of exercise, or previous injury, the lack of stability creates excessive pressure on the joints, irritating the cartilage and capsular tissues.
- ***Fatigue:*** Factors that lead to fatigue include overuse, illness, and emotional and psychological stress, which leads to sustained muscle contraction. A muscle that is held in constant tension develops fatigue.
- ***Aging:*** The connective tissue becomes less resilient and less lubricated as a result of aging, and the soft tissues lose some of their shock-absorbing capacity.
- ***Structural factors:*** The most common structural factors are OA, RA, and congenital anomalies.

DIFFERENTIATION OF NECK AND ARM PAIN AND PAIN IN THE TEMPOROMANDIBULAR JOINT

- Neck pain and TMJ pain can be caused by many conditions, but we will assume that the following discussion applies to benign conditions (i.e., conditions that are not disease processes). Refer to Chapter 2, "Assessment & Technique"; see the section "Contraindications to Massage Therapy: Red Flags," for guidelines in ruling out pathologies.
- To help differentiate whether pain in the arm is a local problem or is referred from the neck, it is important to remember that there are two fundamental types of referred pain that are differentiated by the quality of pain. One type of referred pain is caused by a muscle, ligament, facet, joint capsule, disc, or dura mater. These tissues elicit what is called *sclerotomal pain* when they are injured. Sclerotomal pain can manifest locally and be referred to an extremity. For example, pain from a muscle strain in the neck may be felt as a pain in the arm in addition to the neck. Usually, the sclerotomal pain is described as deep, aching, and diffuse.
- A second type of referred pain, called *radicular pain,* is caused by an irritation of the spinal nerve root. If the sensory (dorsal) root is irritated, there is sharp pain, numbing, or tingling that is well-localized in dermatomes. If there is compression of the motor (ventral) nerve root, in addition to the pain, numbing, and tingling there may be weakness in the muscles supplied by that nerve root. The most common cause of nerve root irritation is disc herniation. Nerve root pain is much more serious and requires an assessment by a doctor.
- Muscle injury and dysfunction is clinically evaluated by the presence of swelling and heat, the degree of muscle hypertonicity, the tenderness to palpation, and the degree of pain elicited by isometric contraction. Muscle injuries are typically painful with isometric contraction and better with rest.
- Ligament injuries are extremely difficult to assess. The pain is sharper, more localized than muscle pain. There is pain with passive cervical rotation or passive opening of the jaw, but if the pain is at the end range, it may be a result of stretching an irritated muscle. It takes ligaments much longer to heal than muscles, and if recovery from a neck or TMJ injury has not been obtained in several weeks, one assumption is that there has been ligament damage, in addition to other structures that might be involved.
- Internal disc derangement in the cervical spine refers a deep, boring pain into the back of the neck and interscapular region. Disc protrusion typically affects the nerve roots.
- The facet joints (zygapophyseal joints) are also a source of neck pain and of referral of pain into the head, shoulder, scapular region, and anterior chest wall and arm. Active motion often elicits a sharp, local pain during the acute phase. The pain then becomes a more diffuse ache in the chronic phase. Assessment reveals loss of passive glide at the involved facet.

COMMON TYPES OF DYSFUNCTION AND INJURY TO THE CERVICAL SPINE AND TEMPOROMANDIBULAR JOINT

Muscle Strain

- ***Causes:*** FHP; emotional or psychological stress; repetitive strains, resulting from the dynamic movement of the neck in activities such as dance, gymnastics, martial arts, and sports; and injury from a specific trauma, such as a car accident.
- ***Symptoms:*** Muscle strains may be asymptomatic. They may also manifest as diffuse, dull, achy pain; or as tight areas or lines of stiffness and discomfort that worsen with certain movements. Moderate and severe muscle strain can manifest as sharp, local pain and is usually better with rest.
- ***Signs:*** Muscles involved palpate as tight and tender. There may be a thickened texture with chronicity. With an active inflammation, the muscles are painful with isometric testing. There may be loss of active ROM, eliciting discomfort in the muscles.

- *Treatment:* Correct the client's posture, perform CR MET, and perform the entire protocol of Level I massage strokes and mobilization described in this chapter.

Whiplash Syndrome (Cervical Acceleration or Deceleration Injury)

- *Causes:* A common cause of whiplash is a rear-end auto collision, but any jolt to the head and neck—from a fall off a bike or horse, a ski accident, or a fall down the stairs—can be considered a whiplash. A mild whiplash is essentially an injury of the soft tissue and would be diagnosed as a cervical sprain or strain injury. A moderate to severe whiplash may cause serious injuries to the muscles; ligaments; cartilage of the facets; disc; and nerves, including the brain. The main cause of the injury in a rear-end collision is the acceleration of the tissues, not necessarily the speed of the vehicles. When the car is hit, the head and neck accelerate at 250 milliseconds, overwhelming the integrity of the soft tissues.
- *Symptoms:* Whiplash may have a wide possibility of symptoms, and there is often a delay of symptoms due to the gradual swelling and accumulation of waste products.
  - *Neck pain and stiffness:* For neck pain, clients usually describe muscles that are sore, tight, and achy. There is often interscapular pain, from local strains and as a referral from the neck.
  - *Decreased ROM in the neck:* The degree of lost motion often predicts the degree of injury. Severe loss of motion due to muscle splinting is a poor prognosis. Certain movements may elicit acute, sharp pain, which implicates joint involvement of the capsular ligaments, the cartilage, or both.
  - *Headache:* May result from a variety of causes. Loss of short-term memory may occur if there is minimal traumatic brain injury (MTBI).
  - *Referral of pain,* numbing, or tingling into the shoulders, arms, and hands may occur.
  - *Vertigo,* dizziness, tinnitus, and visual disturbances from irritation of the cervical sympathetic nerves may occur.
  - *Emotional distress* such as irritability, depression, etc. may be experienced.
- *Signs:* Hypertonic and tender musculature, which is often due to an acute reflex contraction caused by damaged fibers, may occur. Superficial and deep anterior and posterior muscles of the neck will be painful. Swelling in the soft tissues; painful restriction of motion; and neurologic signs, such as loss of reflexes and muscle weakness, may occur.
  - *Treatment:* RI MET and CR MET are begun in the acute phase, always within comfort. Gentle manual release of the hypertonic muscles, minimizing the rocking, and gentle figure-eight mobilization are begun in the acute phase, even if only as micromovements. Isometric exercises are given for a home program. Active motion is encouraged, even if uncomfortable, as long as the client can relax into the discomfort. One of the unfortunate outcomes I have been treating for years is the degeneration and subsequent loss of motion in the cervical spine after improper treatment of a neck injury. In the author's opinion, this sequela is associated with the adhesions that have deposited owing to the lack of movement in the initial phases after a whiplash injury.

Fixation or Subluxation of the Vertebral Facets (Facet Syndrome)

- *Cause:* Trauma, sustained muscle contraction, and postural faults.
- *Symptoms:* Facet syndrome may be completely asymptomatic. In acute episodes, however, the client typically reports a sudden onset of sharp pain in his or her neck, with a significant loss of motion in certain directions, especially rotation, lateral bending, and extension. Pain is usually well-localized, but pain, numbing, and tingling may radiate to the arm and hand.
- *Signs:* The neck usually has some loss of motion. Active and passive motion is restricted and painful at a specific spot. Joint-play assessment identifies loss of normal passive glide of the involved facet. Taut and tender muscles have a thin-membraned rigidity due to acute spasticity.
- *Treatment:* The entire protocol of MET, manual release, and mobilization is described in this chapter. It is important to remember that fixations or subluxations can be completely asymptomatic. Fixations in the vertebrae are common, and in the author's opinion, a chiropractor or an osteopath should assess patients who have any dysfunction in the cervical region.

Arthrosis (Arthritis)—Degeneration of Vertebral Facets

- *Causes:* Previous trauma, FHP, and sustained muscle contraction. The degeneration begins as restriction of the joint capsule.[6] The articular cartilage needs movement to maintain lubrication on the surface. It also needs cycles of decompression that are inherent in moving the joint to allow the cartilage to imbibe its nutrition.

- *Symptoms:* Arthrosis may be asymptomatic. Gradual onset of dull, achy neck, shoulder or interscapular pain might occur. The neck is typically stiff and achy in the morning, feels better after it warms up with movement, and then worsens again at the end of the day due to fatigue. Extension and lateral bending aggravate the stiffness and pain.
- *Signs:* Signs of arthritis are a loss of motion in lateral bending and extension or a more complete loss of all motions except flexion with more serious degeneration in multiple joints. Loss of passive motion (joint play) in the involved facets with a capsular or bony end feel may occur.
- *Treatment:* These clients need to move. There will be some discomfort with increasing movement, but this discomfort is necessary to recover function in the joint. The general rule is that the client should be able to relax completely into the discomfort of moving the involved area. Begin massage therapy with CR MET and manual release and progress to PIR MET, especially directed to increase rotation, as this provides the greatest change in the client's function in daily activities. Further work focuses on the deep posterior muscles and the joint capsules.

Spondylosis—Disc Degeneration

- *Causes:* Whether the degeneration is a natural aging process or the result of previous trauma, sustained muscle contraction, or faulty posture is controversial.
- *Symptoms:* Disc degeneration may be painless, or there may be a dull and achy neck pain, worsened by sudden movements. Diffuse neck stiffness and decreased ROM are also possible, as are headache and arm pain. Typically, the pain is worse in the morning.
- *Signs:* Usually deep musculature of the neck is thick and has a fibrous feel. Ligaments and joint capsules are also thickened and gristly. Active and passive ROM is limited in most directions, especially lateral bending and extension.
- *Treatment:* Improve posture, and perform CR MET—the entire massage protocol of strokes in this chapter—and mobilization.

Cervical Disc Herniation

- *Cause:* Traumatic injury, cumulative stresses caused by postural strain, sustained muscle contraction, joint dysfunction caused by fixation of the facets, adhesions of the ligaments or stresses through the region caused by muscle imbalance.
- *Symptoms:* Disc herniation has two categories: one, internal herniation or derangement, which would cause constant deep gripping pain in the neck or interscapular region; and two, external herniation, also called a disc bulge or protrusion. This protrusion typically compresses or stretches the nerve roots, causing pain that is sharp or gripping as well as numbing and tingling into the arms and hands, in a dermatomal and myotomal distribution. The pain, numbing, and tingling worsen with movements of the neck, especially extension and lateral flexion. Typically, the neck is painful even with rest and disturbs sleep.
- *Signs:* Cervical disc herniation painfully limits most movements, especially lateral flexion and extension. If the motor root of the nerve is affected, it leads to loss of muscle strength in the affected myotome. A positive foraminal compression test elicits pain, numbing, and tingling into the arms.
- *Treatment:* CR MET is used to reduce sustained muscular contraction, and gentle manual release is performed within the client's comfortable limits. **Deep work is contraindicated, as some of the muscle tension is stabilizing the disc.**

Scalenus Anticus Syndrome (Anterior Scalene Syndrome)

- *Causes:* Previous strain to the scalenes, such as whiplash or other cervical trauma; FHP, which shortens the anterior scalene; or dysfunctional respiratory pattern of chest breathing in which the scalenes are overused, which is associated with periods of emotional and psychological stress.
- *Symptoms:* Pain, numbness, and tingling may occur, usually on the ulnar side of hand but may affect the entire hand.
- *Signs:* Anterior scalene syndrome elicits pain that is often brought on with arm elevation, the elevated-arm stress test (EAST). Digital pressure on scalenes may produce pain, numbing, or tingling that radiates to the ulnar border of hand.
- *Treatment:* CR MET and manual release of the scalenes. Improve posture, instruct the client in abdominal breathing, and strengthen lower trapezius and abdominals.

Temporomandibular Joint Dysfunction

- *Causes:* FHP; emotional stress creating sustained contraction of the muscles that close the jaw; malocclusion of the teeth; trauma, such as a whiplash.

- *Symptoms:* Decreased motion of the jaw and insidious onset of dull, aching pain in the area of the TMJ, often radiating to the face, head, neck and shoulders are indicators of TMJ dysfunction (TMJD). TMJD may lead to OA in the elderly.
- *Signs:* Muscle tenderness, especially the masseter; decreased ROM in the ability to open the jaw; deviation in the mandible while opening; and clicking in the joint while opening and closing, which typically indicates derangement of the disc, may occur.[12]
- *Treatment:* Improve posture and perform CR MET and manual release of the muscles of the jaw.

Assessment

HISTORY QUESTIONS SPECIFIC FOR NECK PAIN CLIENTS

- **Do you have neck pain that is worse at night?**
  - Localized, constant, gripping neck pain that is worse at night are symptoms that need immediate referral to a doctor. These symptoms may indicate a tumor, as the cervical spine is a common site for metastatic tumors from the breast, lung, and prostate.[2] Pain can be worse at night with significant inflammation as a result of the pooling of inflammatory waste products, but it typically is not localized, constant, or gripping.
- **Is the pain, stiffness, or ache better or worse in the morning?**
  - Pain that is worse in the morning or at night implies inflammation. These clients typically take longer to respond to treatment, as there is a chemical, not just a mechanical, basis to their pain, and that requires a longer healing time.
  - Chronic morning stiffness implies a degenerative condition. These clients need postural and exercise instruction, including stretching of the muscles of the spine.
  - Pain that is better in the morning and worsens during the day implies fatigue as a contributing factor. This fatigue could result from postural stresses, tension from emotional stress, or a functional problem with a soft-tissue basis.
- **Do you have pain, numbing, or tingling in the arm(s) or hand(s)?**
  - If the client has arm or hand pain that is sharp and localized in a dermatome, it may be a result of a nerve-root irritation in the neck. Perform the foraminal compression test (see "Foraminal Compression Test," below) and the active ROM tests to the area of referral and isometric muscles tests to the area of pain. If the pain is being referred, the ROM of the extremity is full and pain-free. It is not uncommon for a client to present with arm or hand pain that is worse than the neck pain, indicating a nerve-root irritation. If the client can lie comfortably on the table, proceed with your massage, but strokes should be light, and rocking should be gentle. Pain-free CR for the hypertonic muscles may also be performed.
- **Do you have headaches, blurred vision, or dizziness?**
  - Headaches may be caused by muscle tension or an upper cervical facet syndrome, and is usually responsive to OM. If the client has throbbing headaches, unrelated to activity, associated with blurred vision and nausea, they need a referral to a doctor. As mentioned, after a neck injury, symptoms of nausea, blurred vision, tinnitus, and dizziness often are associated with an irritation of the sympathetic nervous system.

OBSERVATION: CLIENT STANDING

- Notice any signs of inflammation such as redness or swelling or signs of previous trauma or surgery such as bruising or scars, in all views described below.

Front View

- Is head held in a tilted or rotated position? A neck or head held in a sustained, painless rotation, flexion, or lateral flexion may be caused by muscle imbalances, fixation of a vertebral facet, or degenerative joint disease (DJD). If the neck is painful, it may be a herniated disc, entrapped fibromeniscus in the joint, or an acute spasm caused by soft-tissue injury.

Side View

- Does the client stand in a forward-head, rounded-shoulder posture? As mentioned in the beginning of this chapter, this posture is a major source of neck pain because of the excessive demand on the soft tissues.
  - Correct the client's posture in the standing position as described in Chapter 3, p. 100, by first correcting the lumbar curve and then bringing the head back so that the opening of the ear is in line with the upright acromion.

OBSERVATION: CLIENT SITTING

Side View

- Observe the client's posture when seated (Fig. 5-12). With correct posture, the opening of the ear should be over the upright shoulder. If the client is slumping, instruct him or her in correct posture by first introducing the normal lumbar curve, and then bring the head so that the opening of the ear is in line with the upright acromion.

MOTION ASSESSMENT

To assess **active movements,** stand, facing the seated client. Note the ROM, and ask the client whether the movement is painful, where it is painful, and the quality of pain. Perform the most painful movements last, as movement into pain may irritate the other structures.

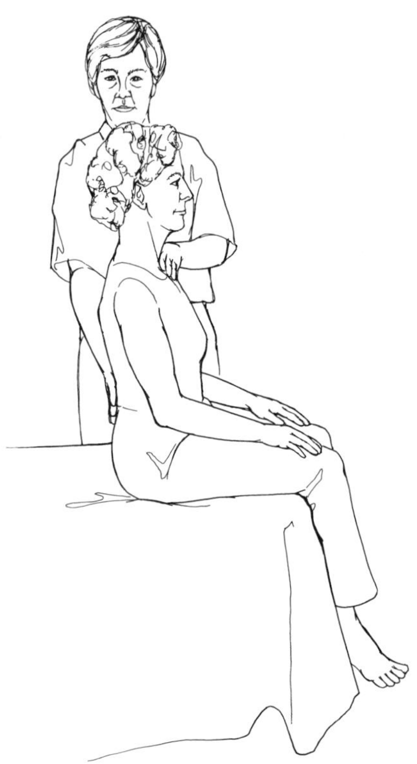

Figure 5-12. If the client has slumped posture, instruct her in the correct posture by first introducing a slight curve in the lumbar spine. Next, have her lift her sternum and then bring the head upright, so that the opening of the ear is over the acromion.

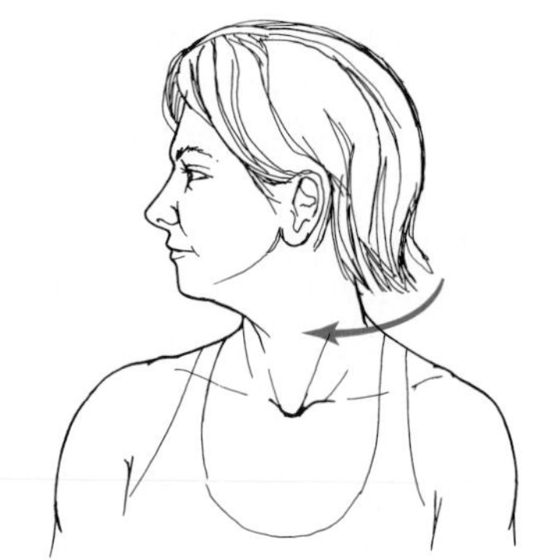

Figure 5-13. Active cervical rotation to the right.

Rotation

- ***Action:*** Ask the client to turn his or her head as far as comfortable to one direction, and then to the other.
- ***Observation:*** The range of rotation is approximately 70°, that is, not quite to the plane of the shoulder (Figs. 5-13 and Fig. 5-14). A line or area of tension indicates muscle hypertonicity. A diffuse area of pain indicates soft-tissue irritation or inflammation. A sharp, local pain indicates a facet syndrome, including irritation of the joint capsule.

Extension

- ***Action:*** Ask the client to look up as far as comfortable.
- ***Observation:*** In active cervical extension, the client should be able to look at the ceiling comfortably (Fig. 5-15). Extension closes the facet joints and the IVF and elicits a sharp, local pain in the neck if there

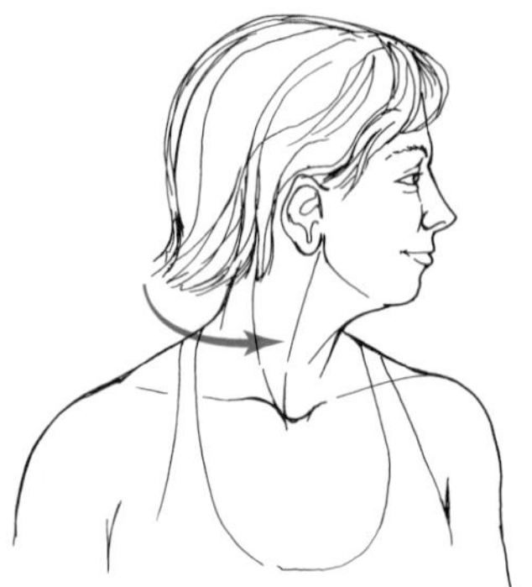

Figure 5-14. Active cervical rotation to the left.

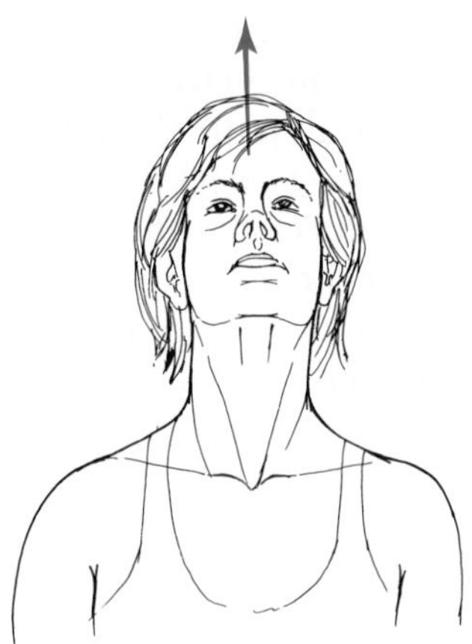

Figure 5-15. Active cervical extension.

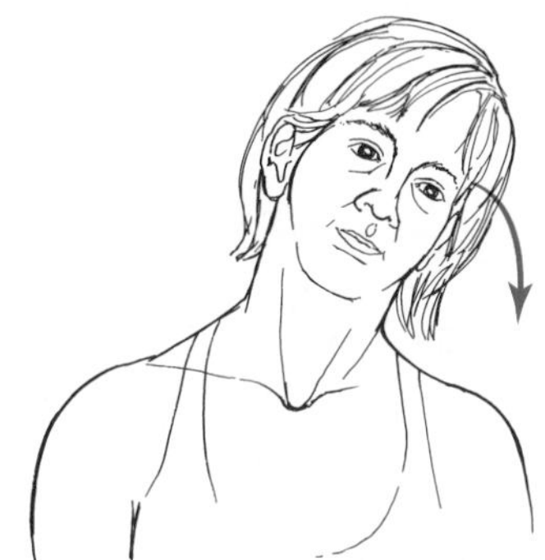

Figure 5-17. Active side bending to the left.

is a fixation of the facet or irritation of the joint capsule. This motion often elicits a soreness or pain in the suboccipital region due to compression of tight suboccipital muscles or a pain in the front of the neck if there has been injury to the anterior neck muscles. Sometimes this movement elicits suboccipital pain and pain in the front of the neck. A referral of pain to the top of the shoulder or scapular area indicates irritation of the joint, and referral of a sharp dermatomal pain into the arm or hand indicates a nerve root problem.

Flexion

- *Action:* Ask the client to bend his or her head as far as is comfortable to the chest.
- *Observation:* In active cervical flexion, two-fingertips distance between the chin and the chest is within normal limits (WNL) (Fig. 5-16). Flexion opens the vertebral facets and provides relief for joint problems. However, this motion stretches the muscles of the back of the neck and shoulders, including the cervical extensors and trapezius and often elicits a pulling sensation or pain in the scapular region caused by muscle injury or hypertonicity.

Lateral Flexion

- *Action:* Ask the client to bring his or her ear toward the shoulder to the comfortable limit (Figs. 5-17 and 5-18).
- *Observation:* The normal range is approximately 45°, that is, approximately halfway to the shoulder. A spot of pain on the side of bending usually indicates a joint problem. A line of pain or tension on the opposite side usually indicates muscle injury or hypertonicity. Lateral bending closes the facets and the IVF on that side. It may elicit a diffuse referral of pain to the top of the shoulder or to the scapular region with joint irritation; or it might elicit sharp dermatomal pain, numbing, or tingling into the arm or hand with nerve root irritation. Chronic limited side bending is indicative of capsular fibrosis or DJD.

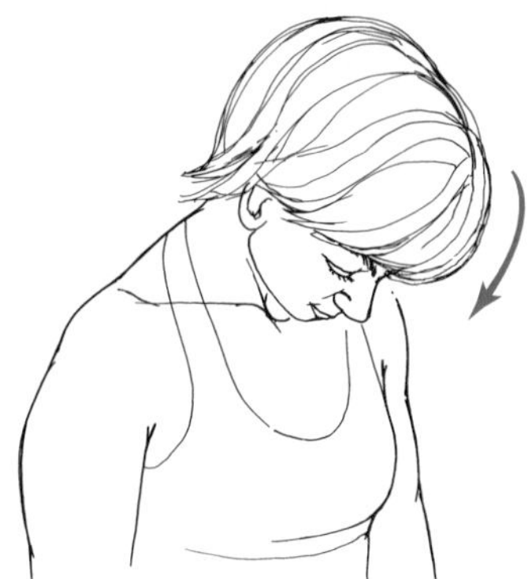

Figure 5-16. Active cervical flexion.

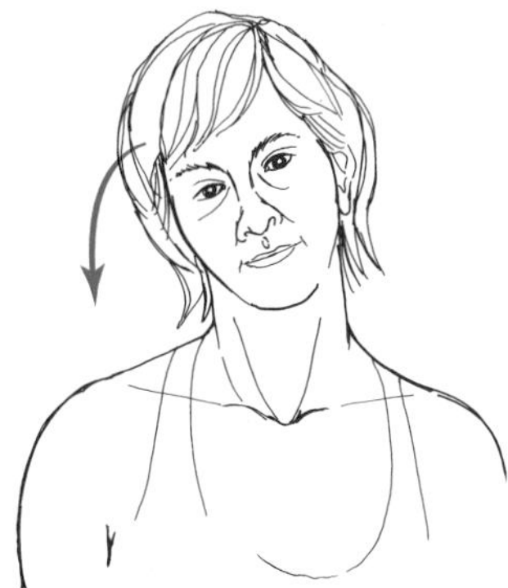

Figure 5-18. Active side-bending to the right.

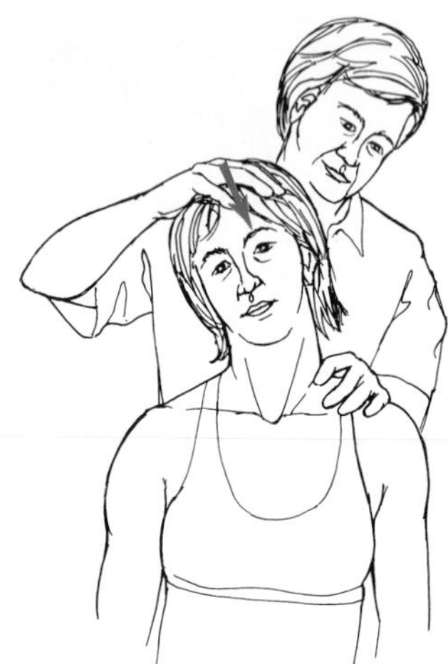

Figure 5-19. Foraminal compression test. Client laterally flexes neck to the painful side. Press down gently into the crown of the head. Localized pain in the neck usually indicates a joint problem. Referral of pain, numbing, or tingling into the arm indicates irritation of the nerve root.

SPECIAL TESTS: CLIENT SITTING

Foraminal Compression Test

- *Intention:* The foraminal compression test is performed if there is referral of pain, numbing, or tingling into the shoulder or arm. To differentiate whether if the injury is a joint problem or nerve root irritation (Fig. 5-19).
- *Action:* Client laterally flexes head to one side and the therapist carefully pushes straight down into head. Do not proceed with this test if positioning the neck in lateral flexion elicits sharp, local pain or referral of symptoms into the shoulder or arm.
- *Observation:* This test closes the IVF, compresses the facets, and reproduces the client's symptoms if the joint is injured or the nerve root is irritated. If pain, numbing, or tingling radiates into the arm or hand or there is increased radiation in a dermatomal pattern, it indicates a nerve-root irritation. A diffuse referral of pain into the top of the shoulder or scapular region indicates a facet joint irritation. A sharp pain local to the neck may indicate a subluxation or fixation of the facet.

Elevated Arm Stress Test

- *Intention:* The EAST test is performed if there is numbing or tingling in the hand(s). The intention is to determine if the client has compression of the neurovascular bundle in the area of the thoracic outlet.
- *Action:* Have client sit. Flex the client's elbows to 90° and abduct and externally rotate the client's shoulders to 90°. Have the client open and close his or her hands for 3 minutes (Fig. 5-20).
- *Observation:* This test stretches the neurovascular bundle that travels under the clavicle. If the brachial plexus, artery, or vein is compressed, the client will feel numbing, tingling, coldness, or weakness in the hands. This compression may be due to injury; postural stresses; or muscle hypertonicity of the scalenes, subclavius, or pectoralis minor. Weakness

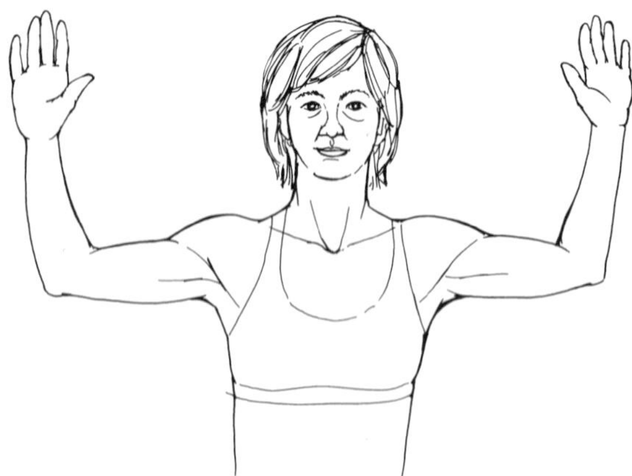

Figure 5-20. Elevated-arm stress test (EAST). This helps determine if the client has compression of the neurovascular bundle in the area of the thoracic outlet.

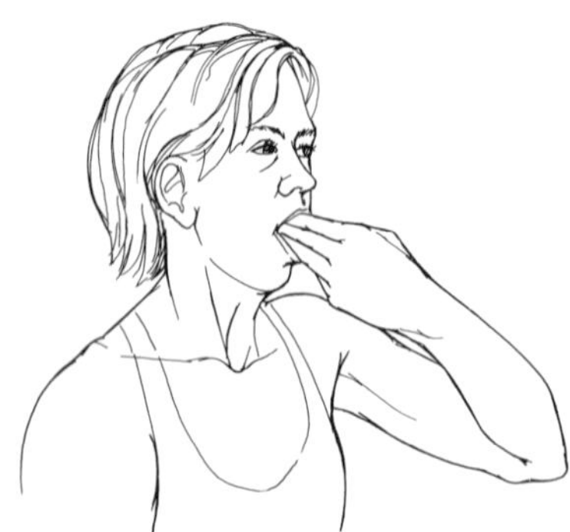

Figure 5-21. To determine if the client has a normal opening of the jaw, ask her to place three fingers into the opening of the mouth. Limited motion or pain is an indication of temporomandibular dysfunction.

in the arms manifests as unconscious lowering of the arm as he or she performs the test.

Assessment of the Temporomandibular Joint Range of Motion

- *Action:* Have the client open his or her mouth to the comfortable limit. Ask the client to place three fingers between the front teeth (Fig. 5-21).
- *Observation:* Limited motion or pain is an indication of TMJ dysfunction. A person should be able to place the width of three fingers in the opening of the mouth. Loss of motion may be caused by pain, muscle hypertonicity, disc derangement, or OA. Notice if there are deviations of the mandible to the side when the client opens the jaw. Deviations may be caused by muscle hypertonicity, subluxation of the TMJ, or disc derangement.

SPECIAL TESTS: CLIENT SUPINE

Assessment of Cervical Extensors Length (Chronic Only)

- *Action:* Gently lift client's head and passively flex toward the client's chest to the resistance barrier (Fig. 5-22).
- *Observation:* Performing an assessment of the cervical extensor muscle length is **contraindicated** for the client in acute pain. Client's chin should be able to touch the area above the sternum. Perform PIR for cervical extensors if there is a limitation of motion (see Fig 5-32).

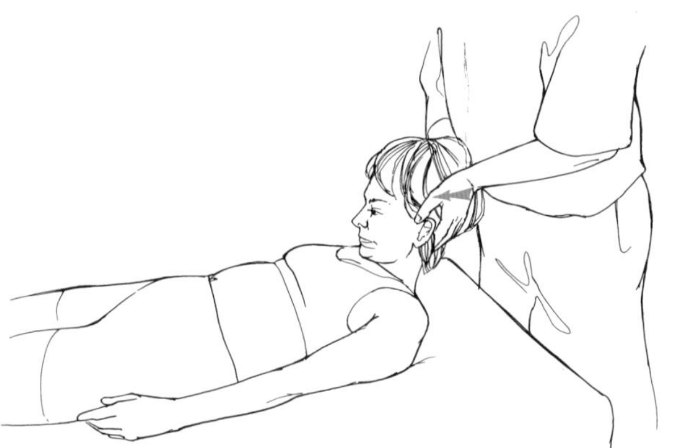

Figure 5-22. Assessment of the cervical extensor muscles length. Slowly lift the head toward the sternum. It is **contraindicated** to perform this on a client in acute pain.

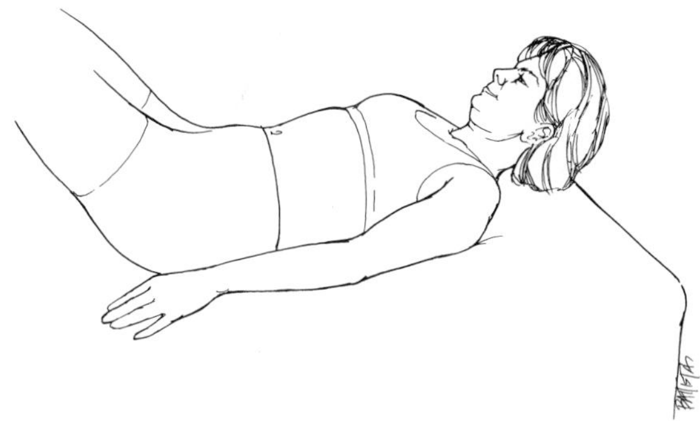

Figure 5-23. Cervical flexion test. In clients who have weak deep cervical flexor muscles, the chin juts away from the throat.

Cervical Flexion Test to Assess the Deep Cervical Flexor Strength (Chronic Only)

- *Action:* Ask your client to bend his knees, and bring his feet flat on the table. Ask him to raise his head off the table to look toward his feet (Fig. 5-23).
- *Observation:* Watch to see if the head is extending on the neck; that is, if the chin is jutting away from the throat or if the head is being flexed with the neck and the chin moves closer to the throat. If the deep neck flexors are of normal strength, the chin moves toward the throat and not up to the ceiling. If the deep cervical flexors are weak, the SCM and scalenes substitute, extending the head, jutting the chin toward the ceiling.

PALPATION

Soft-Tissue Palpation

- Perform a brief scan of the soft tissue as part of the assessment, and perform a much more precise palpation in the context of the strokes. Palpate the soft tissue on either side of the vertebrae, in the suboccipital region, and on the superior border of the scapulae. Note any heat, swelling, or muscle hypertonicity. Ask the client if it hurts and if there is referral of pain. If it is painful, ask if it is mild, moderate, or severe. If pain is severe, refer the client to a doctor.

Vertebrae Palpation

- Put the fingertips of one hand on each SP from C7 to C2 and push posterior to anterior (P–A) to assess tenderness of the vertebrae. If tenderness is severe, refer the client to a doctor.

ASSESSMENT OF VERTEBRAL FACET JOINT MOBILITY

- Passive glide in a joint is called *joint play,* and to function properly, each joint in the spine needs to have this play (Fig. 5-24).
- ***Intention:*** The intention is to induce a passive glide gently into the vertebral facets from C7-C2, one joint at a time, to assess whether the joints have normal motion.
- ***Action:*** Find the vertebral facets 1 inch lateral to the SP, over the muscle bundle. Place your fingertips on the facets, and press in a medial direction, one side at a time. Move up to the next vertebrae, and perform this motion in rhythmic oscillations.
- ***Observation:*** A normal, painless gliding motion is present in a healthy joint. Localized restriction indicates a fixation of the facet joint or localized degeneration. Diffuse hypomobility indicates more generalized degeneration. Localized pain or local pain that refers to the scapular region indicates irritation or inflammation of the vertebral facet.

ISOMETRIC TESTS

- Isometric tests are performed to determine if muscles are strong and pain free, weak, or painful. Isometric tests of the cervical spine and CR MET are performed simultaneously. The muscles should be strong and pain-free to isometric challenge. Ask the client if the resisted motion is painful. If it is painful, ask the client the location and the quality of the pain.

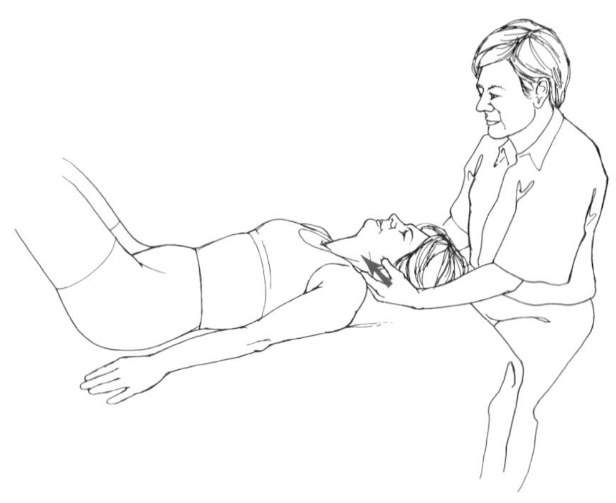

Figure 5-24. Joint play to assess the passive mobility of the vertebral facets. This is an assessment and a treatment.

Techniques

MUSCLE ENERGY TECHNIQUE

Muscle Energy Technique for Acute Neck Pain

1. Contract-Relax Muscle Energy Technique for the Cervical Extensors

- ***Intention:*** The intention is to release cervical extensors. Cervical extensors are typically hypertonic in acute neck pain.
- ***Position:*** Client is supine. If the client is in acute distress, a pillow may be placed under the head to give it extra support. Place both your hands under the skull (Fig. 5-25).
- ***Action:*** Instruct the client to resist as you gently attempt to lift the head straight off the table for approximately 5 seconds.

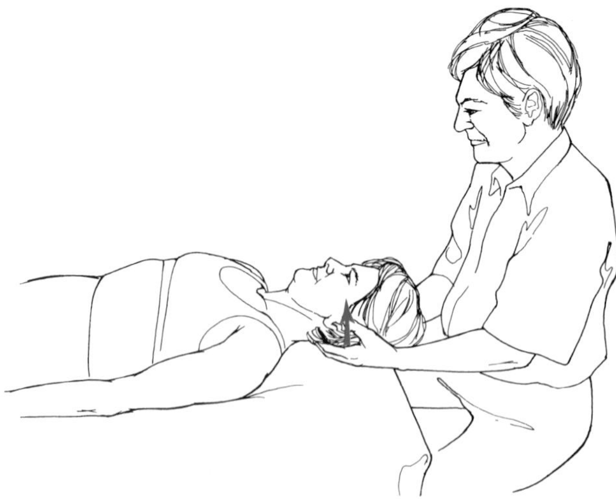

Figure 5-25. CR MET for the cervical extensors.

2. Contract-Relax Muscle Energy Technique for the Suboccipital Muscles

- ***Intention:*** The intention is to perform CR MET to release the suboccipital muscles. The suboccipital muscles are typically short and tight owing to FHP. If these muscles are injured, the client might feel suboccipital pain and posterior cranium pain. In addition, injuries to these muscles can contribute to disturbances in balance and position sense (proprioception).

- ☐ ***Position:*** Hold the base of the client's head (occipital bone) and ask the client to rotate the head backwards approximately 1 inch, as if looking overhead (Fig 5-26).
- ☐ ***Action:*** Instruct the client to resist as you attempt to roll the head back into flexion.

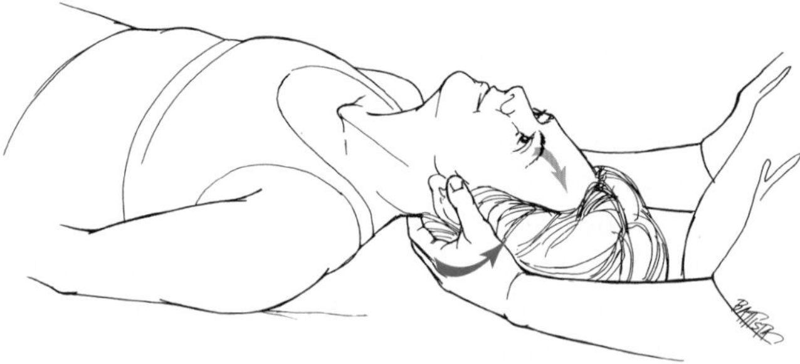

Figure 5-26. CR MET for the suboccipital muscles.

3. Contract-Relax Muscle Energy Technique for the Cervical Flexors

CAUTION: **This motion may be painful after a cervical strain. Do not perform this movement if it is painful.**

- ☐ ***Intention:*** The intention is to perform light CR of the flexors to help normalize cervical flexor function and also to create greater relaxation by reciprocally inhibiting hypertonic extensors. Cervical flexors are often injured in cervical trauma. They are typically weak as a result of chronic dysfunction and pain and owing to injury.
- ☐ ***Position:*** Tuck one hand under the skull and place the other hand on the forehead to stabilize the head (Fig. 5-27).
- ☐ ***Action:*** Lift the client's head off table an inch or two, and rotate the cranium slightly to move the chin toward the throat. If this position is not painful, have the client resist as you attempt to press the head back to the table.

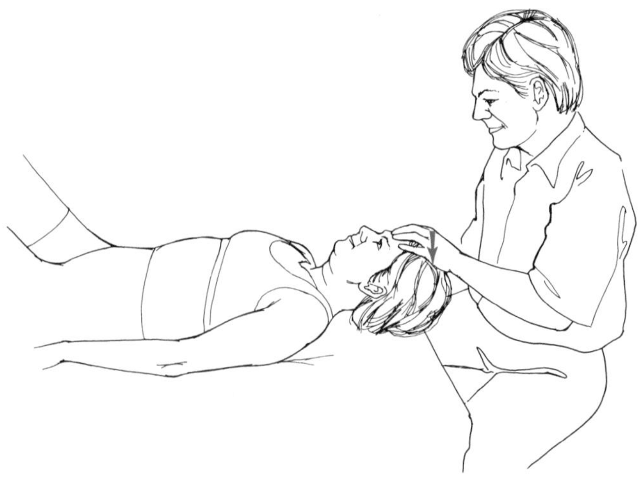

Figure 5-27. CR MET for the cervical flexors.

4. Contract-Relax Muscle Energy Technique for the Lateral Flexors

- ☐ ***Intention:*** The intention is to perform CR MET to release the lateral flexors. Lateral flexors are typically short and tight.
- ☐ ***Position:*** Client is supine, with the head in neutral. Place the palm of your hand on the mastoid processes, with your index and ring fingers behind the ears (Fig. 5-28).
- ☐ ***Action:*** Instruct the client to resist as you press gently into the side of the head. Hold for 5 seconds, and repeat on the opposite side. This cycle of CR on one side and then the other is repeated for 3 to 5 times.

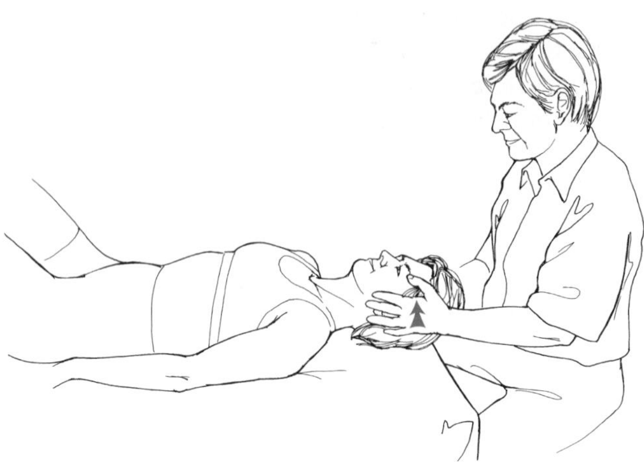

Figure 5-28. CR MET for the lateral flexors.

Muscle Energy Technique for Subacute and Chronic Neck Pain

5. Contract-Relax Muscle Energy Technique for the Anterolateral Flexors, Especially the Sternocleidomastoid

- ☐ ***Intention:*** The intention is to perform CR MET for the anterolateral flexors and especially for the SCM. The SCM is one of the most commonly injured muscles. It is typically short and tight and contributes to FHP.

- *Position:* Hold the client's head at the mastoid processes (Fig. 5-29).
- *Action:* Lift the client's head and rotate it to one side. Have the client resist as you attempt to press the head back toward the table. Hold for approximately 5 seconds, and rotate the head to the opposite direction, and repeat. RI is to have client press into your lower hand.

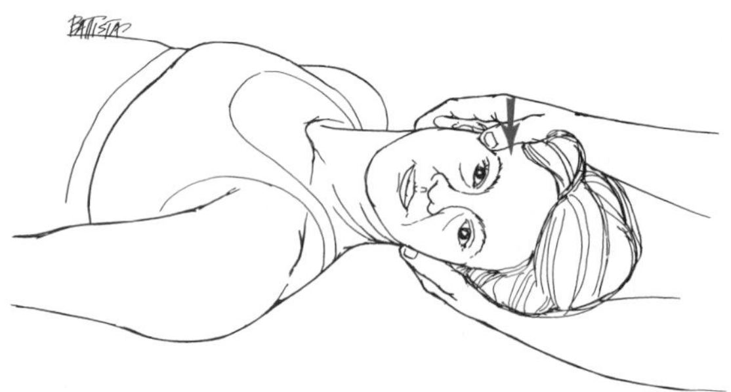

Figure 5-29. CR MET for the anterolateral flexors, especially the SCM.

6. Postisometric Relaxation Muscle Energy Technique for the Upper Trapezius and the Levator Scapula

- *Intention:* The intention in performing PIR MET is to relax and lengthen the more lateral fibers of the levator scapula and upper trapezius. The upper trapezius and levator are typically short and tight.
- *Position:* Tuck one hand under the skull, and place the fingers of one hand on the mastoid bone behind the ear. Place the other hand on top of the shoulder (Fig. 5-30).
- *Action:* Instruct the client to resist as you attempt to pull the head and shoulder apart. Hold for 5 seconds, relax, and then move the head toward the opposite shoulder until a resistance barrier is felt. Have the client resist as you attempt to pull the head and shoulder away from each other again. Repeat this CR–lengthen cycle several times, and then perform it on the other side.

7. Variations in Postisometric Muscle Energy Technique for the Upper Trapezius, Levator Scapula, and Scalenes

- *Intention:* The scalenes, levator scapula, and upper trapezius are typically short and tight and need to be lengthened. The intention is to use PIR MET to isolate these muscles more specifically.
- *Position:* For the left levator, lift the client's head into cervical flexion with your left hand, and stabilize the shoulder with your right hand. Have client rotate the head to the right (Fig. 5-31). For left trapezius and middle scalenes, keep the client's face toward the ceiling. For the left anterior scalenes, have client rotate the head toward the left shoulder.
- *Action:* Instruct the client to resist as you pull the client's head into greater flexion and to the right; that is, away from the shoulder. Hold for 5 seconds, relax for a couple of seconds, and move the head away from the held shoulder until a new resistance barrier is felt. Repeat several times, and perform on the other side.

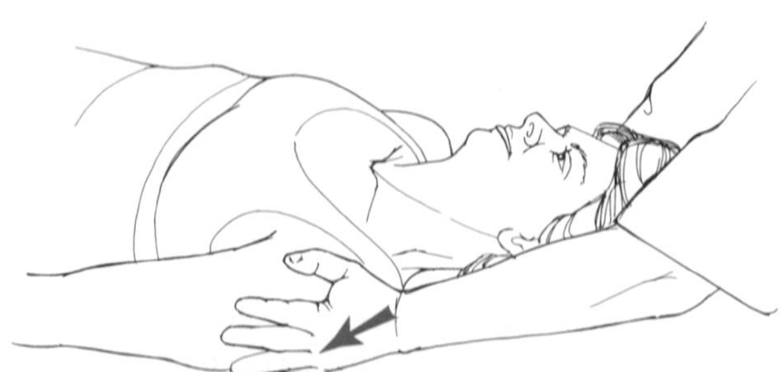

Figure 5-30. PIR for the upper trapezius and the levator scapula. This MET is used to relax and lengthen the more lateral fibers of the upper trapezius and the levator scapula.

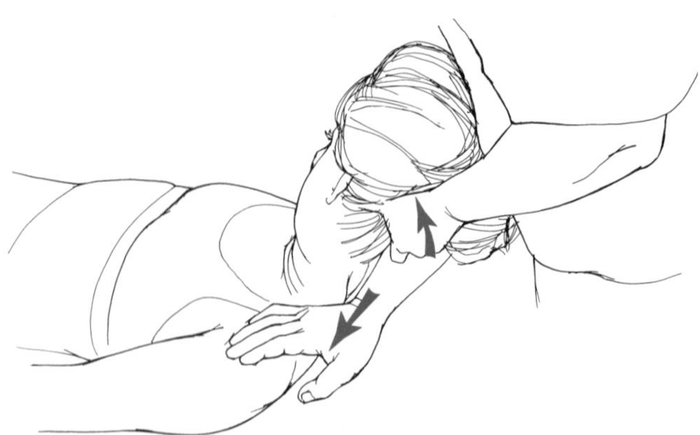

Figure 5-31. Variations in PIR MET for the upper trapezius, the levator scapula, and the scalenes. This MET is used to isolate the muscles more specifically. This figure shows the head turned away from the stabilizing hand for the levator scapula.

Muscle Energy Technique for Chronic Neck Pain or Loss of Range of Motion

8. Postisometric Relaxation Muscle Energy Technique to Increase the Length of the Cervical Extensors

- *Intention:* The intention is to use PIR MET to lengthen the cervical extensors. The cervical extensor muscles are typically short and tight, due to chronic forward head posture, and as a consequence of prior injury (Fig. 5-32).
- *Position:* Place both hands under the client's skull.
- *Action:* Lift the client's head toward his or her chest (into flexion) until pain or a resistance barrier is felt. Instruct the client to resist as you attempt to lift the head into further flexion. Hold for 5 seconds, have the client relax for a few seconds, and then flex the neck further, until a new resistance barrier is felt. Repeat several times, and after the last relaxation, have the client resist as you attempt to push the head back toward the table. This "sets" the extensors at their new length.

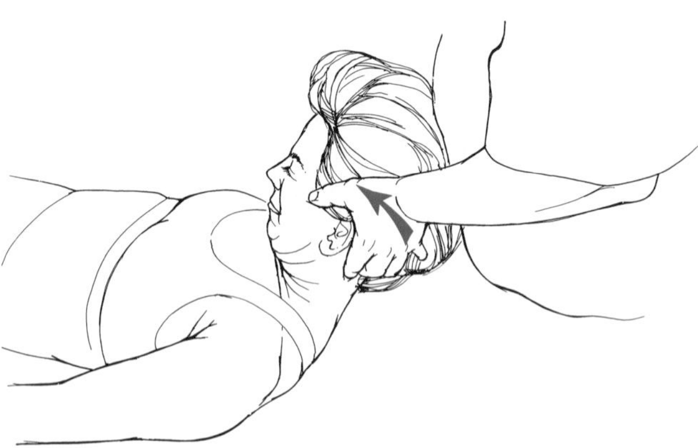

Figure 5-32. PIR MET to lengthen the cervical extensors. It is common for the extensors to shorten in chronic neck problems. This MET effectively lengthens the connective tissue of the extensors.

9. Contract-Relax-Antagonist-Contract to Increase the Cervical Spine Rotation

- *Intention:* The intention is to use contract-relax-antagonist-contract (CRAC) MET to increase cervical spine rotation. Cervical rotation is typically limited by chronic muscular or ligamentous problems or from degeneration of the joints (Fig. 5-33).
- *Position:* Place one hand on the client's mastoid processes, and the other hand over the ear.
- *Action:* Have the client rotate his or her head to the right to the comfortable limit. Have the client resist as you attempt to lift the head further off the table. As the client is resisting, have him or her rotate the head further to the right. Have the client relax, and after a few seconds, have the client resist as you attempt to rotate further to the right. Repeat this CRAC cycle several times. Repeat in the other direction.

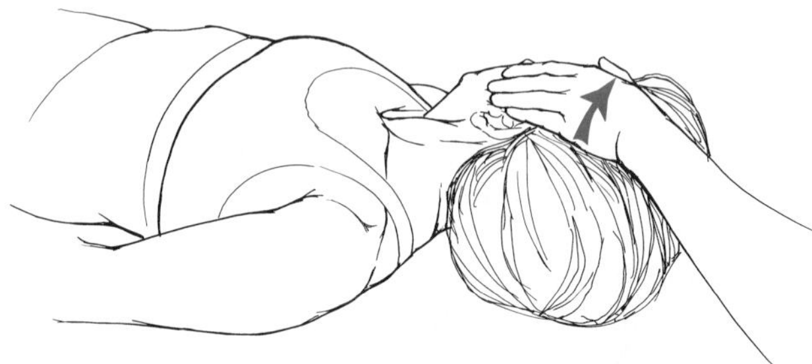

Figure 5-33. CRAC MET to increase the rotation of the cervical spine. Rotation is often limited due to shortening of the connective tissue in the muscles and joint capsules.

Muscle Energy Technique for the Temporomandibular Joint Muscles

10. Contract-Relax Muscle Energy Technique to Release the Muscles Primarily Responsible for Opening of the Jaw (Digastrics and Lateral Pterygoids)

- *Intention:* The digastrics and the lateral pterygoids—the muscles chiefly responsible for opening the jaw—can be released by CR MET (Fig. 5-34).
- *Position:* Place the fingertips under the client's mandible. Have the client open the jaw to its resting position, approximately one-finger width.
- *Action:* Instruct the client to resist as you gently attempt to close the jaw. Hold for approximately 5

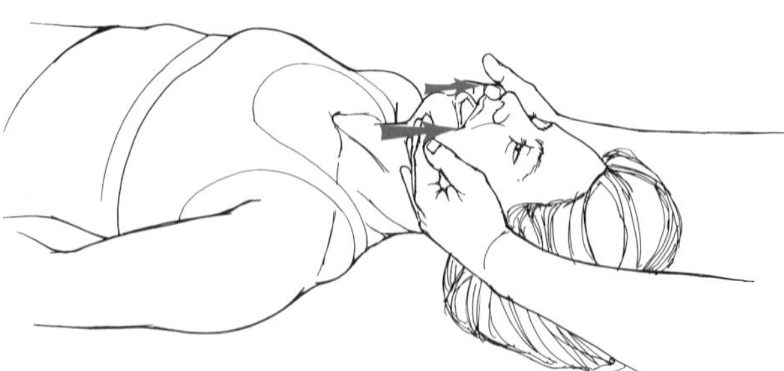

Figure 5-34. CR MET to release the muscles primarily responsible for opening the jaw, the digastrics, and the lateral pterygoids.

seconds. Relax, and perform the next two METs in the jaw sequence. Repeat this cycle several times, and instruct the client in how to do this at home.

11. Contract-Relax Muscle Energy Technique to Release the Muscles Primarily Responsible for Closing the Jaw (Masseter, Temporalis, Medial Pterygoid)

- □ *Intention:* The masseter, temporalis, and medial pterygoid—the muscles chiefly responsible for closing the jaw—can be released with CR MET (Fig. 5-35).
- □ *Position:* Place the shaft of both thumbs on the anterior aspect of the client's mandible, with the tips of your thumbs nearly touching under the client's lower lip.
- □ *Action:* Instruct the client to keep the jaw open approximately one-finger width into the resting position of the TMJ and to resist as you attempt to open it further.

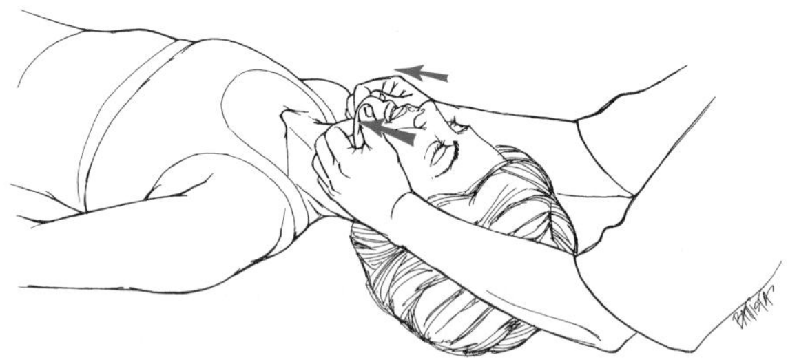

Figure 5-35. CR MET to release the muscles primarily responsible for closing the jaw, the masseter, the temporalis, and the medial pterygoid.

12. Contract-Relax Muscle Energy Technique to Release the Muscles Primarily Responsible for Lateral Movement of the Jaw (Medial and Lateral Pterygoids)

- □ *Intention:* The medial and the lateral pterygoids—the muscles chiefly responsible for lateral jaw movement—can be released with CR MET (Fig. 5-36).

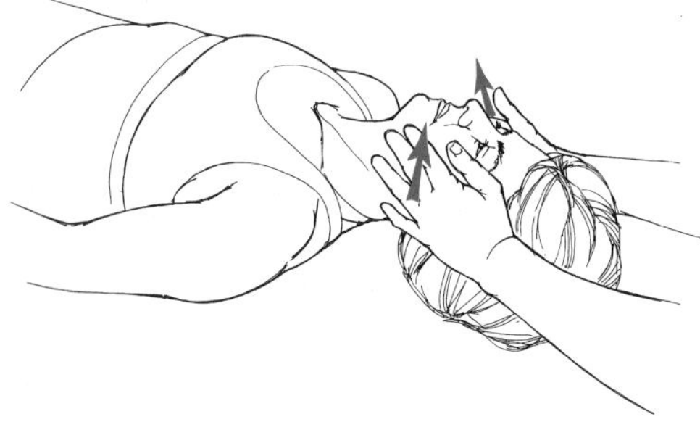

Figure 5-36. CR MET to release the muscles primarily responsible for lateral movement of the jaw, the medial and lateral pterygoids.

- □ *Position:* Place the palm and fingertips on the lateral side of the client's mandible.
- □ *Action:* Instruct the client to open the jaw slightly into the resting position and to resist as you press into one side of the jaw. Make sure the client keeps the jaw in neutral and does not jut it to one side. Repeat on the opposite side.

ORTHOPEDIC MASSAGE

Level I – Cervical Spine

1. Release of the Soft Tissue Between the Spinous and the Transverse Processes

- *Anatomy*: Splenius capitis and cervicis, erector spinae, semispinalis cervicis and capitis, rotatores, multifidi (Figs. 5-37A and B).
- *Dysfunction*: Extensor muscles of the cervical spine, except the suboccipitals, tend to contract eccentrically with FHP, becoming taut (i.e., tight and long). With FHP, the suboccipital muscles become tight and short, and the extensor muscles develop an abnormal medial torsion and need to be stroked away from the SPs.

Position

- TP—standing, facing headward for longitudinal strokes, facing the table for transverse strokes
- CP—side-lying, with the chin tucked and the shoulder near the therapist at the edge of the table

Strokes

Your supporting hand is on the scapula. Move the scapula in the direction of your stroke as this brings the superficial tissue into slack.

1. With your body facing 45° headward, use a single-thumb technique to perform short, scooping inferior to superior (I–S) strokes from C7 to C2 (Fig. 5-38). Your fingertips are placed underneath the neck, and they gently squeeze the neck with each stroke. This is nurturing, adds stability, and disperses the pressure throughout the entire hand. Perform this stroke in three lines: one, at the SP; two, at the lamina groove 1 inch laterally; three, on the posterior surface of the transverse process, approximately 1 inch lateral to the second line. Be cautious at C1, approximately one-finger's breadth under the skull, as direct pressure on this vertebra may sublux it (shift its position) and cause headaches.
2. With your body facing perpendicular to the table, use your thumb to perform short scooping strokes,

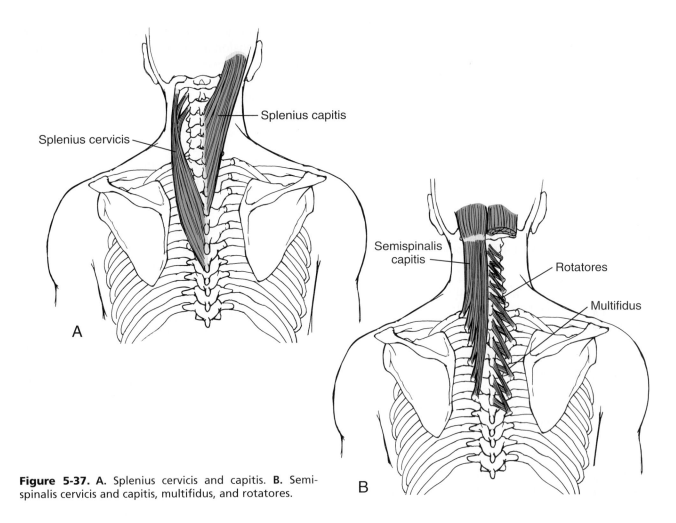

Figure 5-37. **A.** Splenius cervicis and capitis. **B.** Semispinalis cervicis and capitis, multifidus, and rotatores.

in the P–A and medial to lateral (M–L) direction (Fig. 5-39). Begin at the SPs and proceed in 1-inch segments from C7 to C2. The same stroke is repeated in a second line in the area of the lamina groove beginning approximately 1 inch lateral to the SPs.

3. Turn your body to face 45° headward again. The transverse processes are found in a line between the ear and the shoulder. Using a single-thumb technique, feel for the bony protuberance of the transverse process, then slide your thumb to its posterior surface (Fig. 5-40). Perform a series of 1-inch, scooping strokes in an anterior to posterior (A–P) direction over the transverse process. This is an unwinding stroke, rolling the soft tissue posteriorly

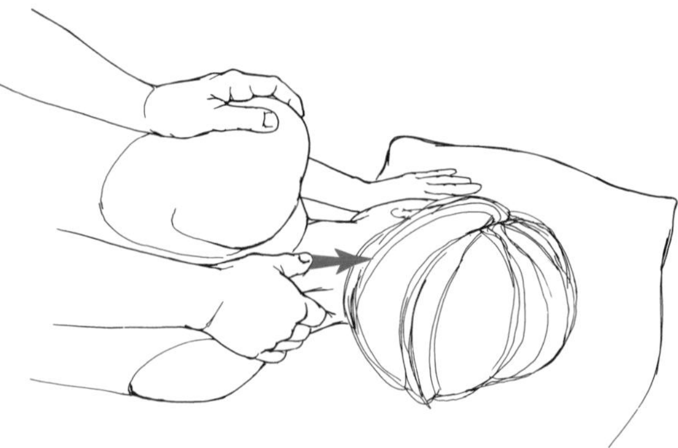

Figure 5-38. Thumb release of the cervical soft tissue in an inferior to superior direction. Keep your wrist in neutral, and gently squeeze the neck with each stroke.

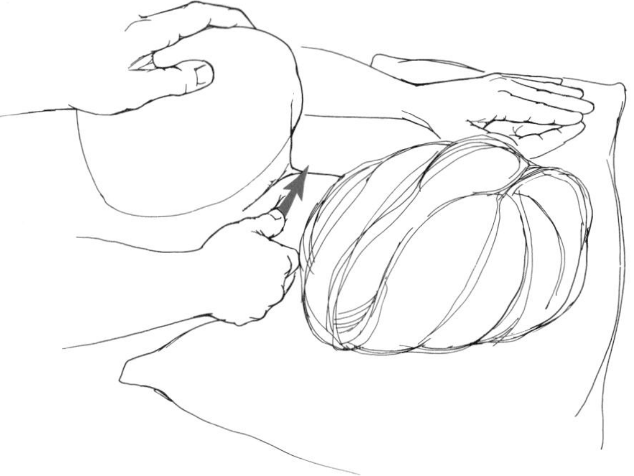

Figure 5-39. Thumb release in the medial to lateral direction.

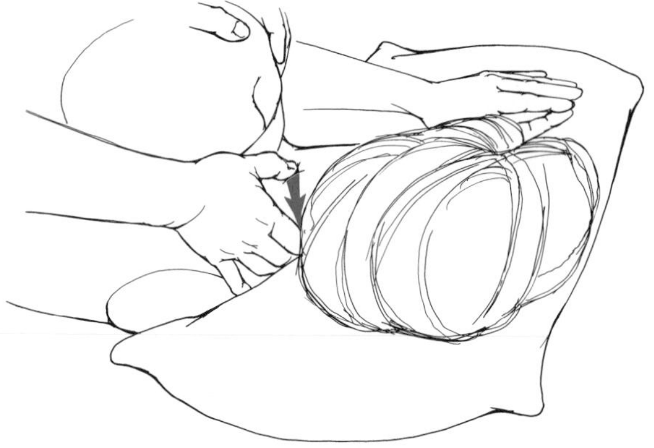

Figure 5-40. Thumb release of the soft tissue from the area of the posterior surface of the transverse process.

and toward the table. Begin at C7 and proceed inch-by-inch to C2. Keep an even smooth rhythm. Do not slide over the skin.

2. Release of the Muscle Attachments on the Base of the Skull

- ***Anatomy***: Trapezius, longissimus capitis, semispinalis and splenius capitis, rectus capitis posterior minor and major, SCM, obliquus capitis superior, greater occipital nerve (Fig. 5-41)
- ***Dysfunction***: Muscle attachments on the skull tend to thicken and become fibrotic with sustained tension in the cervical extensors and suboccipital muscles. This is commonly caused by FHP, previous injury, or emotional tension. This sustained muscle tension can lead to tension headaches. The rectus capitis posterior minor interweaves with the fibrous covering of the brain (the dura), and special attention to this muscle is indicated. The greater occipital nerve can become entrapped in the semispinalis capitis fascia.

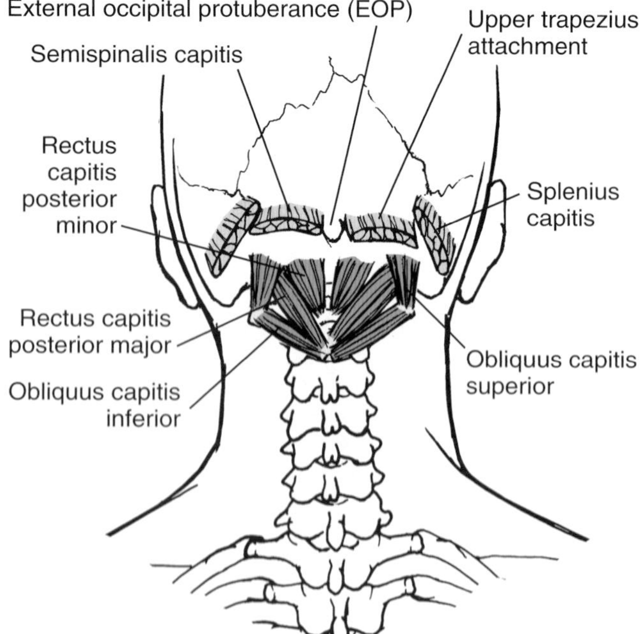

Figure 5-41. Muscle attachments to the base of the skull.

Position

- TP—standing, facing headward
- CP—side lying, neck flexed

Strokes

Use short, scooping strokes with the thumb or braced thumb from the mastoid to the midline. Move the scapula with the inferior hand in a superior motion to feed the area. It is important not to dig into the skull. Rather, take the tissue into tension, and using the bone as a guide, scoop it medially. Gently pull the skin back 1 inch, scoop in, and move approximately 1 inch. When you encounter an area of thickening in the soft tissue, you may use strokes that are shorter and more brisk. Three lines of strokes are described below. Remember that for attachment points, it is not necessary to be concerned with positional correction, but rather with dissolving fibrosis, and therefore, use transverse strokes in both directions.

1. Locate the EOP in the center of the posterior skull at the level of the top of the ear. The area from the EOP to the top of the ear is called the superior nuchal line. Release the attachments of the SCM on the mastoid and the trapezius in the midline of the occiput on this superior nuchal line. These muscles have thin, flat tendons at their attachments (Fig. 5-42).

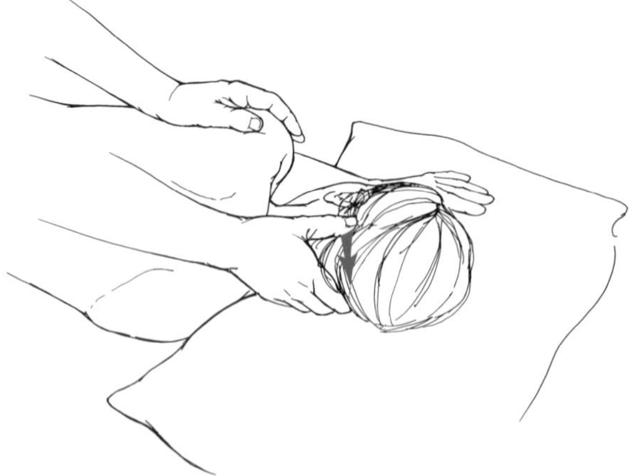

Figure 5-42. Release of the muscle attachments in the area of the superior nuchal line.

2. Working on the mastoid 1 inch inferior to your previous series in the area of the middle nuchal line, release the splenius capitis and longissimus capitis. Continue a series more medially on the occiput for the obliquus capitis superior and the semispinalis capitis muscles.
3. As you follow the contour of the bone of the skull, turn your thumb to face superiorly and perform a third line of strokes. Begin approximately 1 inch inferior to the previous series on the medial third of the inferior nuchal line to release the rectus capitis posterior minor and major.

3. Release of Soft Tissue Between the Clavicle and the Supraspinous Fossa of the Scapula

- *Anatomy*: Scalenus anterior, medius, and posterior; levator scapula, upper trapezius, and supraspinatus (Fig. 5-43)
- *Dysfunction*: These muscles tend to develop torsion as they roll forward and shorten with an FHP or as a result of spinal trauma. In the client with rounded shoulders, this soft tissue shortens and thickens. The upper trapezius is commonly short and tight owing to emotional tension or FHP.

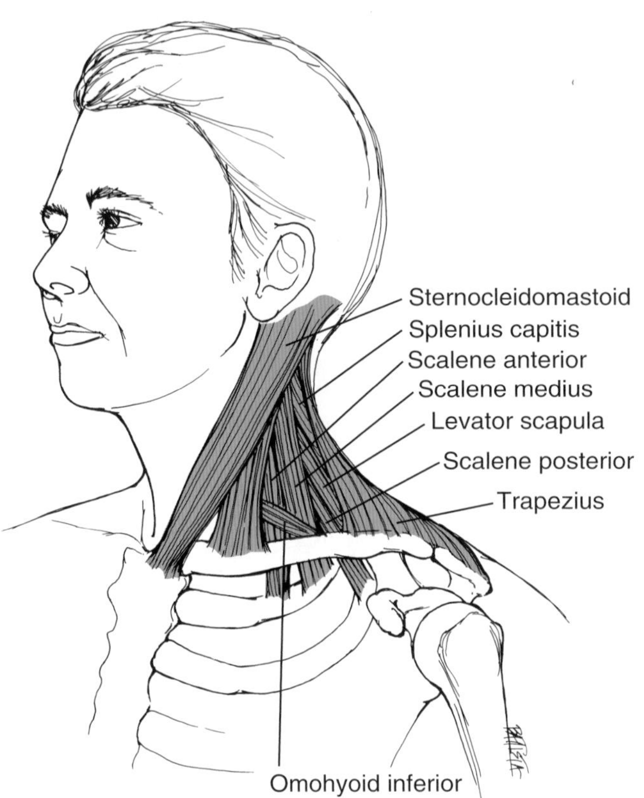

Figure 5-43. Muscles between the clavicle and the scapula.

Position

- TP—standing, facing table
- CP—supine

Strokes

1. In this stroke we have two intentions: one, to unwind the abnormal torsion of the scalenes, levator scapula, trapezius, and supraspinatus; two, to dissolve any fibrosis within these muscles.
   - Begin by placing the client's flexed elbow on his or her chest so that the arm rests across the chest (Fig. 5-44).
   - With your inferior hand, grasp just above the client's elbow and gently impulse the arm headward and posteriorly toward the superior hand.
   - At the same time, with the thumb of your superior hand, perform 1-inch scooping strokes in the A–P direction in the area between the clavicle and the scapula.
   - To repeat the stroke and return to the starting position, release the thumb of your superior hand, and lift the scapula and the arm anteriorly and inferiorly. Reposition the thumb of your superior hand to a new position, and scoop as the arm is pulsed.

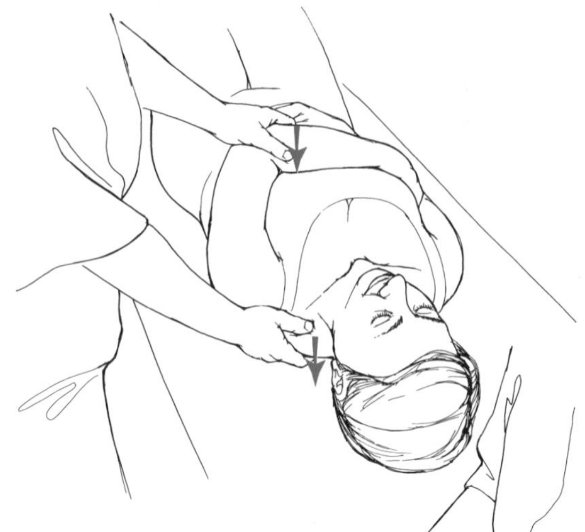

Figure 5-44. Thumb release of the soft tissue between the clavicle and the supraspinous fossa of the scapula. Move the arm in an oscillating rhythm coordinated with the strokes. Each stroke works in a slightly different area.

2. Release the soft tissue between the upper third of the scapula and the upper thoracic and C7 SPs. Your inferior hand remains in the same position. The fingertips of your working hand scoop the soft tissue at the superior angle of the scapula, moving it headward, coordinating it with the upward movement of the client's arm in short, oscillatory strokes.

4. Release of the Sternocleidomastoid Muscle

- *Anatomy*: SCM (Fig. 5-45)
- *Dysfunction*: The SCM is one of the most commonly injured muscles in the cervical region, especially with whiplash injuries. The SCM is typically short and tight, and pulls the head into an FHP. It can be a source of headaches and chronic neck tension.

Position

- TP—seated at the head of the table
- CP—supine

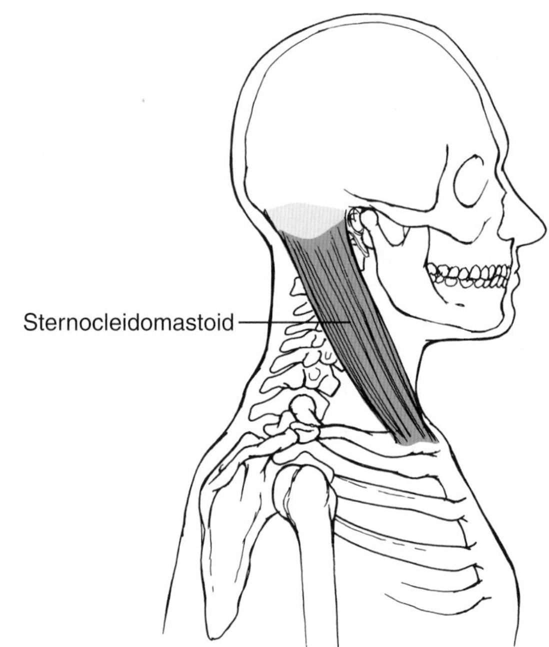

Figure 5-45. SCM muscle.

Strokes: To identify the SCM, have the client rotate his or her head to one side and begin the motion of lifting the ear toward the ceiling. The SCM will protrude from the side of the neck. Have the client bring his or her head back to neutral, and then rotate it slightly toward the side on which you will be working.

1. Place your thumb on top of the SCM and your flexed fingers underneath (Fig. 5-46). Gently squeeze the SCM, and perform a 1-inch stroke from A–P and from superior to inferior (S–I), inducing a subtle spiral from M–L as you perform the stroke. Rock your whole body forward and laterally with the stroke. Place the nonworking hand under the opposite mastoid, cupping the head, and roll the head slightly with the stroke.

Note: If this stroke refers pain to the head, it may indicate a trigger point in the SCM. As mentioned, MET relieves trigger points, so perform CR MET, and then return to the strokes.

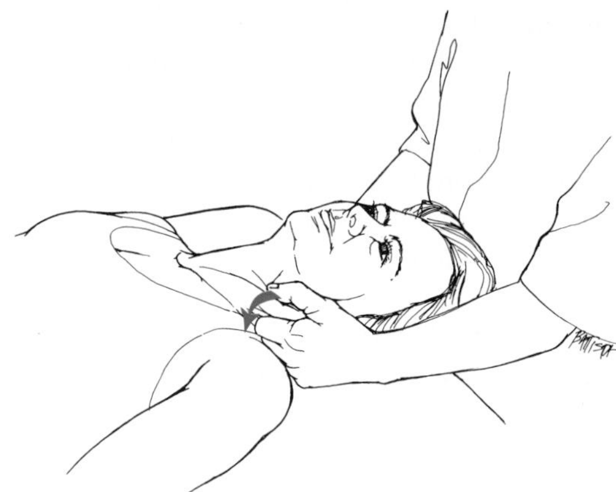

Figure 5-46. Release of the SCM. Gently squeeze the muscle between your thumb and flexed index finger and unwind the muscle laterally.

5. Release of the Scalenes

- *Anatomy*: Anterior, medial and posterior scalenes (Fig. 5-47)
- *Dysfunction*: These muscles often contract after a whiplash or other spinal trauma or with chronic tension and tend to develop an anterior and medial tor-

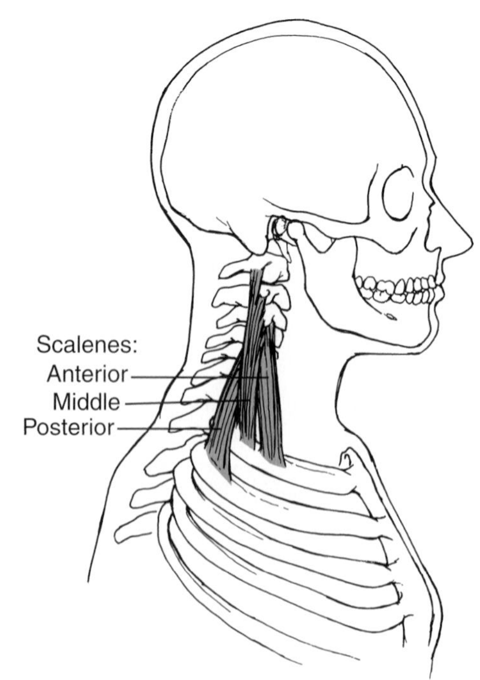

Figure 5-47. Anterior, middle, and posterior scalenes.

sion. They need to be moved from A–P and from M–L. This sustained contracture can entrap the brachial plexus and axillary artery, causing pain, numbing, and tingling into the arm, especially the ulnar side of the hand. This is called *scalenus anticus syndrome.*

Position

- TP—seated at client's head
- CP—supine

Strokes

There are three lines of strokes, one each for the anterior, medial, and posterior scalenes.

1. Place the flat surface of the shaft of your thumb on the scalenes by tucking it under the SCM and finding the lateral aspect of the posterior surfaces of the transverse processes (Fig. 5-48). Perform gentle, 1-inch-long, scooping strokes in an M–L, A–P direction, transverse to the line of fiber. This is also an unwinding stroke, like moving around a cylinder. Gently supinate your forearm with the stroke. Start near the attachments on the transverse processes of C2 and work down to the area above the clavicle. Roll the client's head toward the side you are working with each stroke. Roll it back to center on release. Rock your entire body laterally as you stroke. The fingertips rest underneath the neck. Gently squeeze the neck as you are stroking. This stroke should feel nurturing.
2. To release the anterior scalenes, perform the same strokes described above, but on the anterior surface of the cervical transverse processes. To contact the anterior scalenes and bring them into slack, rotate and laterally bend the client's head slightly toward your working hand. Gently tuck the pad of your thumb under the SCM and place it on the anterior surface of the cervical transverse processes. Perform slow, gentle scooping strokes in the A–P and M–L planes, unwinding the tissue, transverse to the line of the fiber of the anterior scalene. Proceed inch-by-inch down the neck, covering the area from the muscle's origin at C3 to the first rib area under the clavicle.

   Note: Mention to the client that it is normal for some people to feel a slight tingling in the arm while they undergo this treatment. It indicates that the nerves are under tension and that the area needs release. This sensation is relieved a few minutes after the strokes. Do not work more than 1 minute in this area if there is a referral of pain, numbing, or tingling into the extremity.

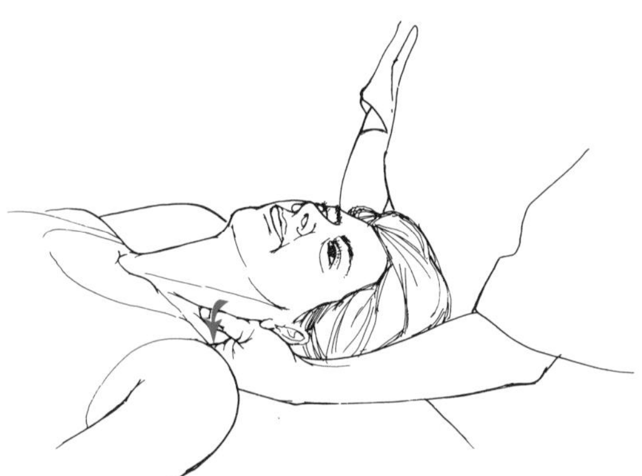

Figure 5-48. Release of the scalenes. Place your flat thumb posterior to the SCM, and gently scoop the muscles posteriorly. This should be a nurturing stroke.

6. Transverse Release of the Cervical Soft Tissue

- ***Anatomy***: Posterior cervical muscles (Fig. 5-49) and the suboccipital muscles at C1 to C2 and at occiput (See Fig. 5-41)
- ***Dysfunction***: The posterior cervical muscles, including the suboccipital muscles are typically short and tight. They thicken and become fibrotic because of chronic irritation caused by poor posture, emotional tension, or inflammation from injury.

Position

- TP—seated, at client's head
- CP—supine

Strokes

1. With the fingertips of one hand on the lateral side of the SP, scoop 1 inch laterally to clear any residual tension not released in prior work (Fig. 5-50). Because of the position of function of your hand, the fingertips scoop approximately 45° headward. Treat one side of the neck at a time. Rotate the client's head slightly to the side you are working on and bend it slightly laterally, as this will put the superficial soft tissue into slack. Typically, you rock the client's head into the direction of the stroke, but you may also allow the client's head to roll in the opposite direction as you stroke. Move your fingertips up the cervical spine one vertebra at a time, covering the entire area between the SPs and the transverse processes.
2. Perform the same series of strokes in 1-inch segments under the skull at the OCC-C1 junction. Your strokes move medially to laterally, covering the en-

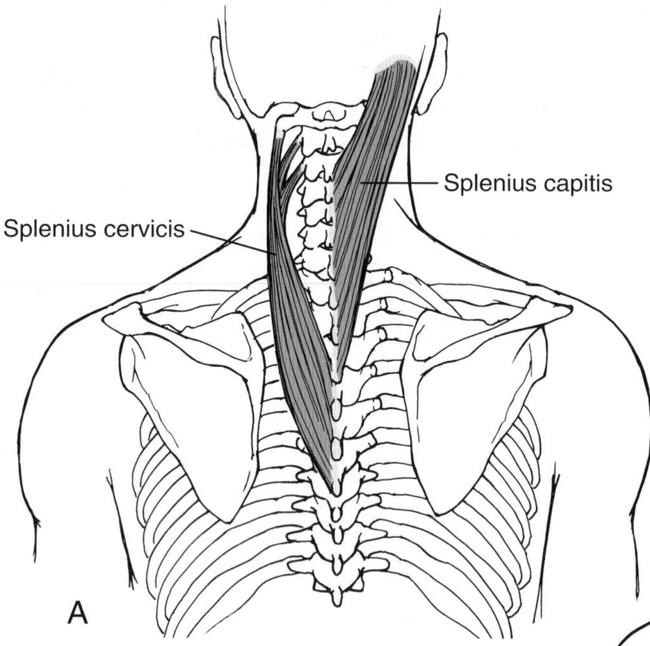

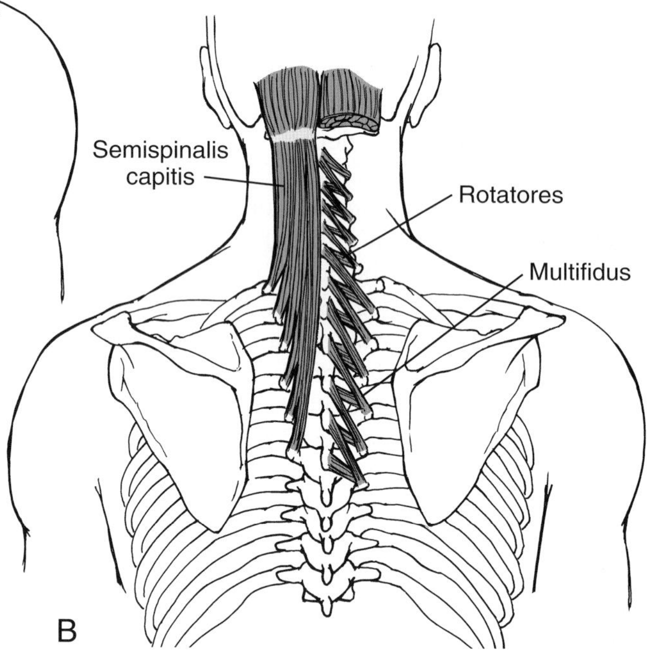

Figure 5-49. A. Splenius cervicis and capitis. **B.** Semispinalis cervicis and capitis, multifidus, and rotatores.

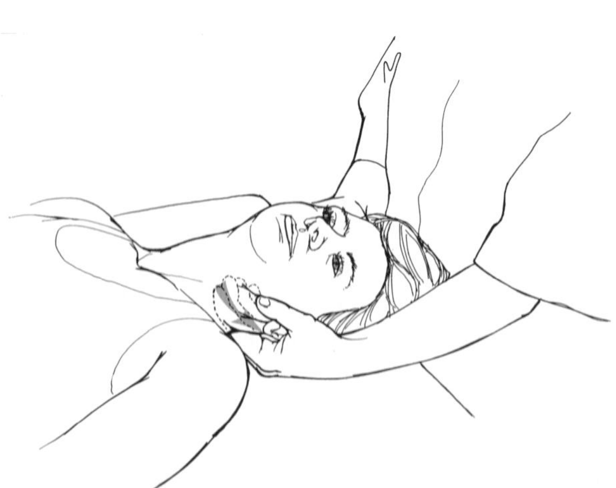

Figure 5-50. Fingertip release of the soft tissue in the posterior neck. This position places the superficial tissue into slack and allows for work on the deeper layers. This is also the best position for work on the area of the atlas-occipital region.

tire area. Do not press into the bone of the atlas (C1). Rather, take the tissue into tension and scoop it laterally, using the bone as your guide.

3. Perform the same series of strokes on the three nuchal lines described in the second stroke of Level I. Lift the skull with one hand and rotate it to the side of the working hand. Using fingertips, scoop the soft tissue in an M–L direction as you rock the head in the direction of the stroke.

Level II – Cervical Spine

1. Release of the Transversospinalis Group

- *Anatomy*: Semispinalis cervicis, semispinalis capitis, multifidus and rotatores (Fig. 5-51)
- *Dysfunction*: These muscles tend to shorten and develop fibrosis. The multifidus is attached to the joint capsule and is typically held in a sustained contraction when there is dysfunction or injury to the facet joint. Sustained tension in the multifidi can cause a

loss of motion in the vertebral facets. All chronic neck pain must be assessed for fibrosis in this group of muscles. Injuries to the neck can cause eventual fibrosis and thickening of the capsular ligaments, which interweave with the multifidi.

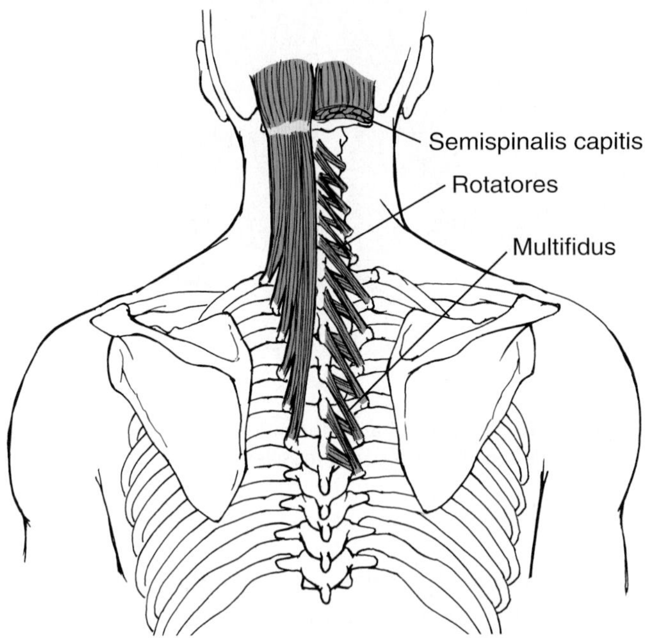

Figure 5-51. Semispinalis capitis, multifidus, and rotatores.

Position

- TP—standing
- CP—side-lying, neck propped on a pillow to allow some slack in the tissue

Strokes

1. Use a single-thumb technique to perform 1-inch, scooping strokes in an M–L, 45° headward direction (Fig. 5-52). Tuck the thumb under the erectors to contact the underlying transversospinalis group. Begin your strokes next to the SP of the C7 vertebrae and work to C2. Use your inferior hand to cup the scapula, and gently move it headward while you are stroking to help bring the tissue into slack.

2. Release of Muscle Attachments on the Posterior Cervical Spine

- *Anatomy*: *Spinous process attachments* from superficial to deep—trapezius, spinalis cervicis, rhomboids, semispinalis cervicis insertion, splenius cervicis and capitis and multifidus insertion; *transverse processes attachments* from superficial to deep—levator scapula, semispinalis capitis origin, iliocostalis cervicis insertion, origin of the multifidus, longissimus cervicis and capitis origins, and joint capsule (capsular ligaments) (Fig. 5-53)

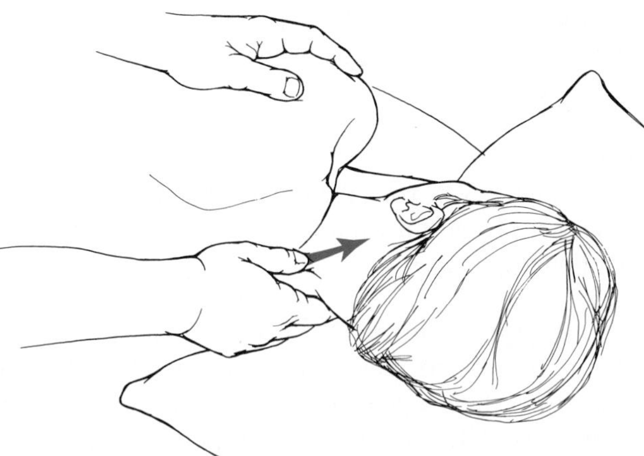

Figure 5-52. Release of the transversospinalis group. Tuck your thumb under the more superficial erector spinae group. Direct your stroke 45° headward, perpendicular to the line of the fiber of these muscles.

- *Dysfunction*: These attachment sites tend to thicken as the result of previous inflammation or because of chronic dysfunction, such as FHP. As mentioned in the previous stroke, the fascia of the deepest layers of the cervical muscles interweave with the capsular ligaments. These areas of the tenoperiosteal insertions are thick and fibrotic in nearly all patients who have chronic neck pain or loss of motion.

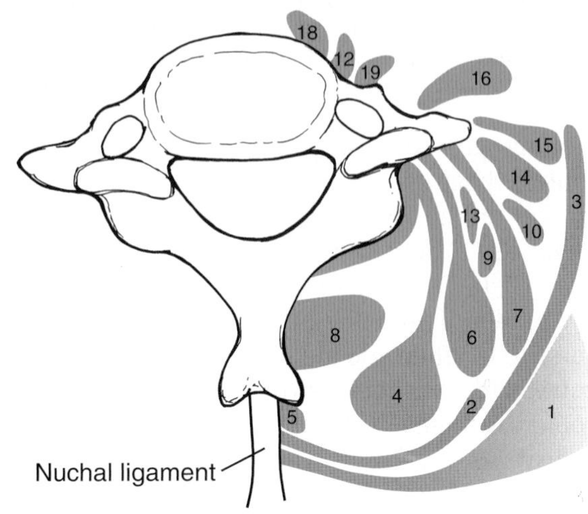

Figure 5-53. Muscle attachments to the posterior cervical spine. 1: Trapezius m, 2: Splenius capitis m, 3: Sternocleidomastoid m, 4: Semispinalis capitis m, 5: Interspinalis cervicis m, 6: Longissimus capitis m, 7: Levator scapulae m, 8: Semispinalis cervicis m, 9: Longissimus cervicis m, 10: Splenius cervicis m, 11: Multifidus m, 12: Rotatores muscles, 13: Iliocostalis cervicis m, 14: Scalene posterior m, 15: Scalene medius m, 16: Scalene anterior m, 17: Longus capitis m, 18: Longus colli m

Position

- TP—standing, facing headward
- CP—side-lying

Strokes

Hold the neck with your fingertips and gently squeeze the neck to support it while your thumb is performing the following strokes.

1. SP—Beginning at the C7 SP, use the fleshy pad of your thumb to perform gentle back-and-forth strokes in the I–S plane on the lateral side of the SPs (Fig. 5-54). If the tissue is fibrous, perform a series of gentle, transverse friction strokes. Work on each SP from C7 to C2. The supporting hand moves the shoulder headward with your strokes.

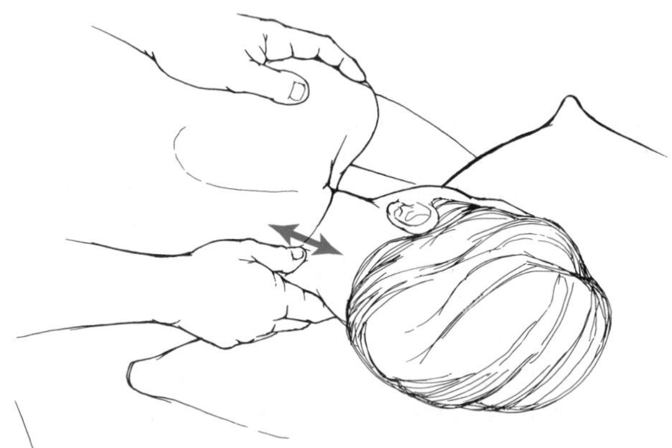

Figure 5-54. Release of the soft-tissue attachments in three areas: the SP, the lamina groove, and the transverse process. These are gentle, deep, back-and-forth strokes to release any fibrosis at the attachments to the periosteum covering the bone.

2. Lamina groove—Using the fleshy pad of your thumb, begin a series of gentle, back-and-forth strokes on the area of the lamina–pedicle junction. Begin at C7, and work on one vertebra at a time from C7 to C2. Work in the P–A and the I–S planes. Try to identify the line of the fiber and work transverse to it. When you are perpendicular to the fiber, you will feel the fibers "strum" under your fingers as you cross them.
3. Transverse processes—Using either fingertips or thumb, perform a series of gentle back-and-forth strokes in the I–S plane on the posterior surface of the transverse processes. Begin at C7 and proceed to C2.

3. Release of the Superficial Muscles of the Anterior Neck

- *Anatomy*: *Suprahyoids*—digastric, mylohyoid, stylohyoid, geniohyoid; *Infrahyoids*—thyrohyoid, sternothyroid, sternohyoid, omohyoid (Fig. 5-55)

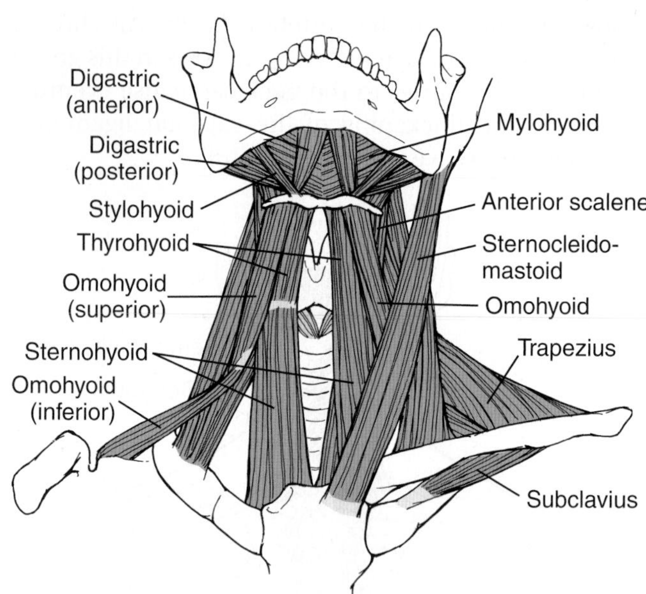

Figure 5-55. Superficial anterior muscles of the neck are the suprahyoid and the infrahyoid muscles.

- *Dysfunction*: Typically, in a whiplash injury, the head is hyperextended, overstretching and traumatizing the anterior cervical soft tissue. You may begin this work immediately after an injury if severe injury has been ruled out. Typically, the hyoid muscles are short and tight.

Position

- TP—standing, facing headward
- CP—supine

Strokes

Find the hyoid bone by first placing your thumb and index finger on the thyroid cartilage in the center of the anterior neck. As you gently walk your fingers up the cartilage, you will come to a space and then to another solid structure. This is the hyoid bone.

CAUTION: Never squeeze the hyoid bone, as it is thin and delicate.

1. Suprahyoid muscles: If you are standing on the client's right side, hold fingertips of your left hand gently against the right side of the hyoid bone to stabilize it (Fig. 5-56). With the index finger of your right hand, gently perform back-and-forth strokes on the superior surface of the left side of the hyoid bone to release the stylohyoid and the mylohyoid on the anterior-medial surface. Perform a series of strokes until you reach the midline.

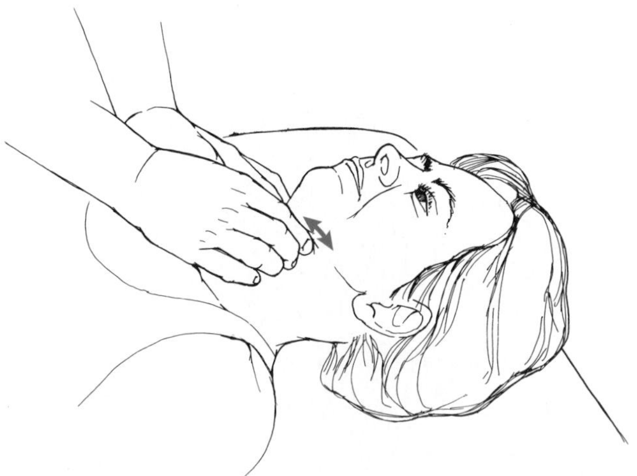

Figure 5-56. Fingertip release of the superficial muscles of the anterior neck.

2. Infrahyoid muscles: Place the index finger of your right hand on the inferior lateral surface of the client's left hyoid bone. Perform gentle, back-and-forth strokes to release the sternohyoid and the omohyoid superficially and the thyrohyoid more deeply.
3. Muscles over the thyroid cartilage: Place the fingertips of your left hand on the lateral surface of her right thyroid cartilage. Release the sternohyoid superficially and the sternothyroid and thyrohyoid more deeply on the anterior surface of the left thyroid cartilage with gentle back-and-forth strokes. Gently stroke across the thyroid cartilage; however, be careful not to press down into the throat. You may elicit the coughing reflex if you press too hard or if the area is particularly tense. If the client remains comfortable, you may proceed, but be gentler.

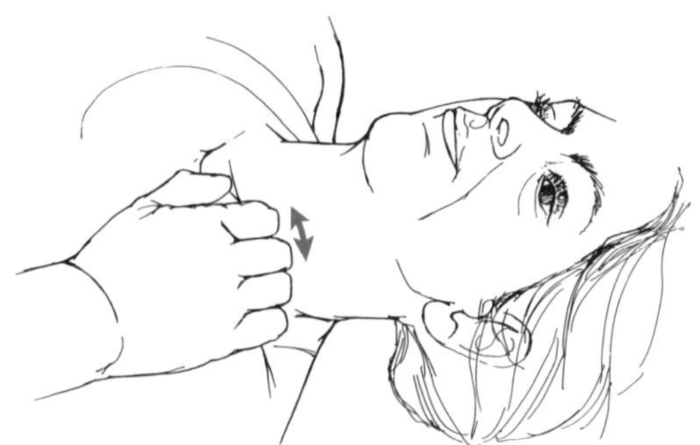

Figure 5-57. Fingertip release of the attachments to the clavicle and sternum.

4. Muscles attaching to the clavicle and sternum: Move your body to the opposite side of the table, facing 45° headward (Fig. 5-57). Cupping your fingertips around the top surface of the sternum, release the lower attachment points of the sternohyoid and the sternothyroid by performing back-and-forth strokes in the M–L plane. Perform the same stroke on the posterior surface of the clavicle.

4. Release of Deep Anterior Cervical Musculature

- ***Anatomy***: Longus capitis, longus colli, and cervical sympathetic nerves (Fig. 5-58)
- ***Dysfunction***: These muscles tend to shorten after spinal trauma, causing a loss of cervical curve, called "military neck." This may lead to entrapment of the sympathetic nerves that travel through these muscles, producing various symptoms, including tinnitus, dizziness, blurry vision, and nausea.

Position

- TP—standing, facing headward
- CP—supine

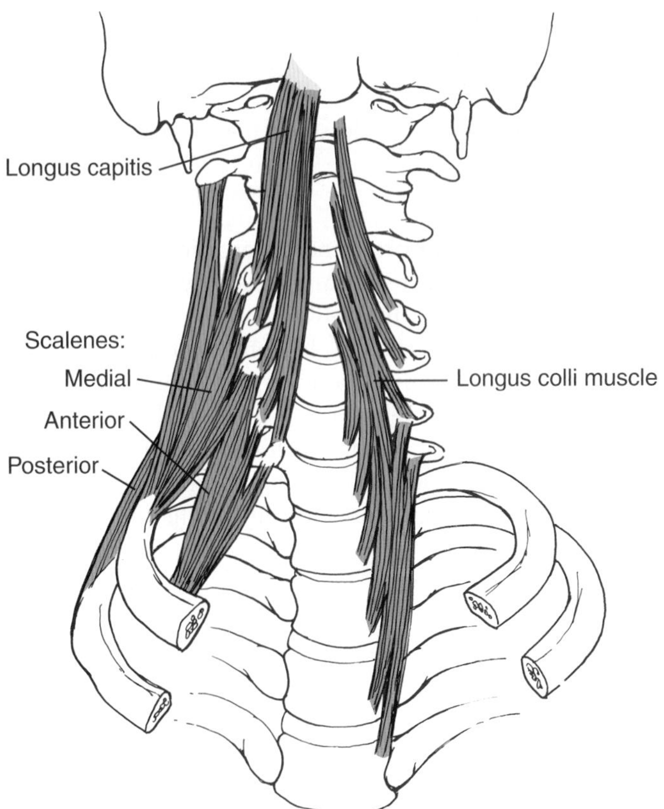

Figure 5-58. Muscles on the deepest aspect of the anterior neck are called the prevertebral muscles.

Strokes

1. Stand on the right side of the table. Gently grasp the trachea with your right thumb and index finger and move it toward you to give some slack to the soft tissue (Fig. 5-59). Place the index finger of your left hand next to your right thumb. Move the trachea to the client's left so that your index finger is nearly at the midline. Slowly and gently press posteriorly, superiorly, and medially with your left index finger until you make contact with the muscles on the anterior surface of the cervical vertebrae. The carotid artery will be lateral to your fingertips; remember, never put pressure on a pulse. Gently move your finger and thumb as a unit, back-and-forth, transverse to the midline. Release the pressure on the fingers and move inferiorly 1 inch and repeat the same strokes. Continue in 1-inch segments until approximately 2 inches above the clavicle. Repeat on the other side.

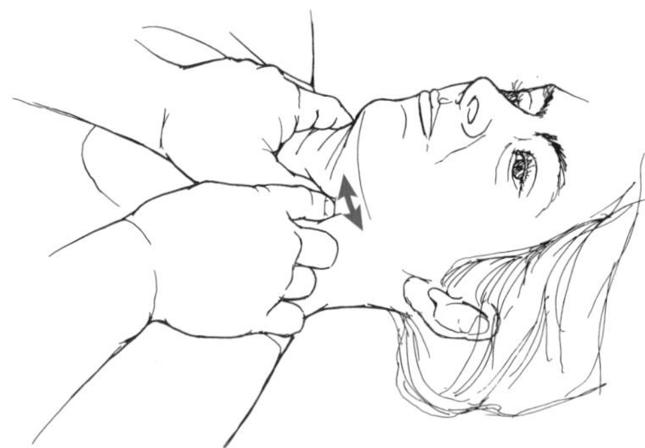

Figure 5-59. Fingertip release of the deep anterior neck muscles.

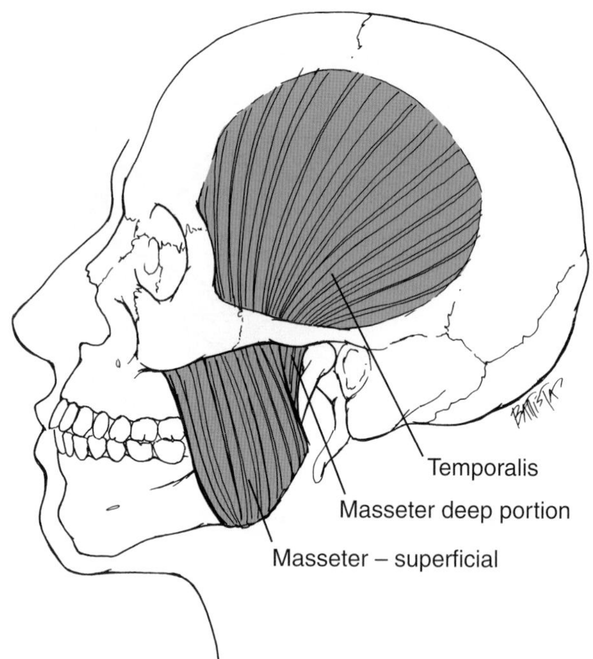

Figure 5-60. Temporalis and masseter muscles.

5. Release of Temporomandibular Joint

- *Anatomy*: Masseter, temporalis, medial pterygoid, lateral pterygoid (Fig. 5-60)
- *Dysfunction*: These muscles tend to shorten and become fibrotic with chronic tension (e.g., grinding or clenching of the teeth) or with cervical trauma. The jaw moves forward in a whiplash, rolling the masseter and temporalis into an anterior and medial torsion. The masseter and temporalis are typically short and tight.

Position

- TP—seated
- CP—supine

Strokes

1. To release the masseter, use your fingertips to perform a series of 1-inch, scooping strokes, in the A–P direction in three lines (Fig. 5-61). The first line begins under the zygomatic arch, near the ear. The second line is in the mid-belly, 1 inch inferior to the first line, and the third line is on the mandible.
2. To release the temporalis, use single-thumb technique or fingertips to perform short, scooping strokes in an A–P direction, covering the entire temporal fossa. Concentrate your attention on the tendon immediately superior to the zygomatic arch.
3. Release the medial pterygoid, mylohyoid, and the proximal attachments of the suprahyoids by cupping your fingertips under the mandible at the angle of the jaw to contact its posterior surface (Fig. 5-62). Perform a series of short, scooping strokes in a posterior direction to release these muscles. Begin each new stroke approximately 1 inch more anteriorly and scoop posteriorly.

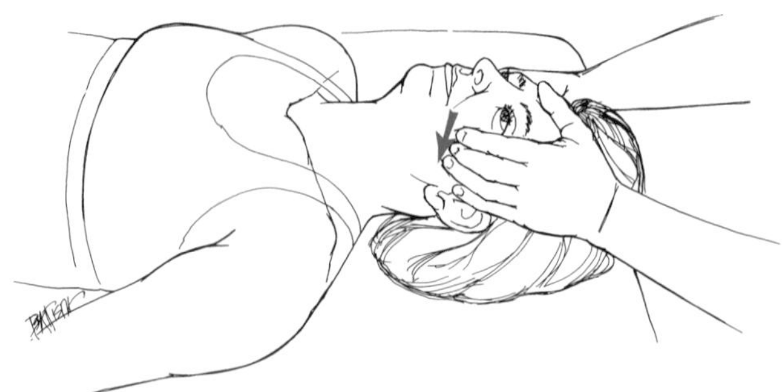

Figure. 5-61. Fingertip release of the masseter. Perform gentle scooping strokes in an anterior to posterior direction.

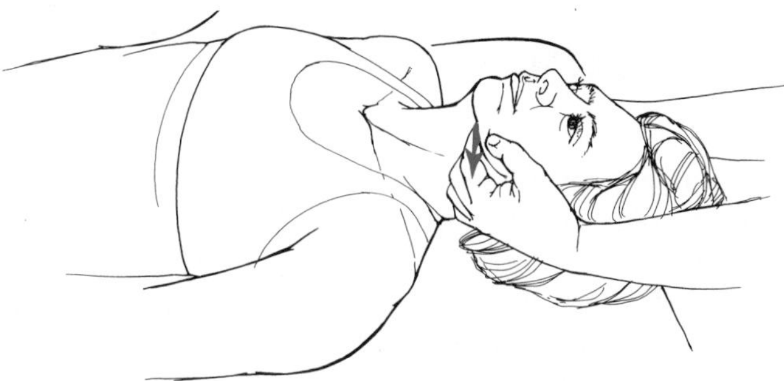

Figure 5-62. Fingertip release of the medial pterygoid, mylohyoid, and proximal attachments of the suprahyoid muscles.

6. Mobilization of the Cervical Spine

- *Anatomy*: The cervical facets are oriented in a plane facing anteromedially (Fig. 5-63).
- *Dysfunction*: The facets of the cervical spine are often inhibited from their normal gliding characteristics by sustained muscle contraction. This not only can be a source of local pain but also can cause an arthrokinetic reflex that contracts the musculature further, leading to increased inhibition of the normal motion of the joint.

Position

- TP—seated
- CP—supine

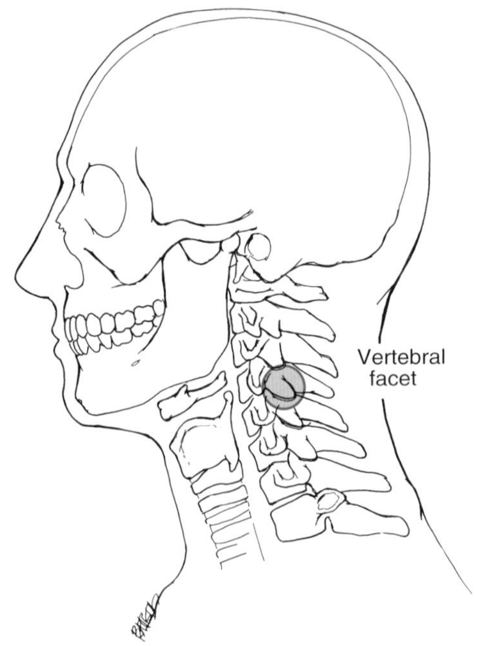

Figure 5-63. Vertebral facets of the cervical spine are located lateral and deep to the soft-tissue bundle next to the SPs.

Strokes

1. Lateral to medial (L–M) mobilization of the cervical vertebrae: Find the vertebral facets by first locating the SPs in the midline. Move slightly laterally to touch the medial extensor muscles. Move your fingertips over that muscle bundle, and you will feel a bony indentation, which is the facet. To assess motion in one vertebra relative to the next, gently push in an L–M direction on one side of the vertebra, and then in the same L–M direction on the other side of the same joint (Fig. 5-64). A healthy joint has a resilient end feel. A hypomobile joint has a thickened, dry, stiff or bony-block end feel, depending on the cause of resistance. An analogy that is useful to patients is that the joints can become like a rusty hinge and that by moving it we "oil" or lubricate it. Move up to the next joint, and repeat from C7 to T1 to the C1 to C2 area.
2. Figure-eight mobilization of the cervical vertebrae: With your fingertips placed at the vertebral facets starting at the C7 to T1 area, gently induce a slight movement with the hands in a figure-eight pattern. For example, the client's head is rotated to the right, then side flexed to the left, while the fingertips of your left hand push on the left facets. Then rotate the client's head left, laterally flex it right, etc. This is a slow, extremely gentle procedure, and there should be no pain. For a client with acute injuries, you can perform this mobilization as micromovements, using extremely gentle and small amplitude movements. Chronic conditions need bigger-amplitude movements.

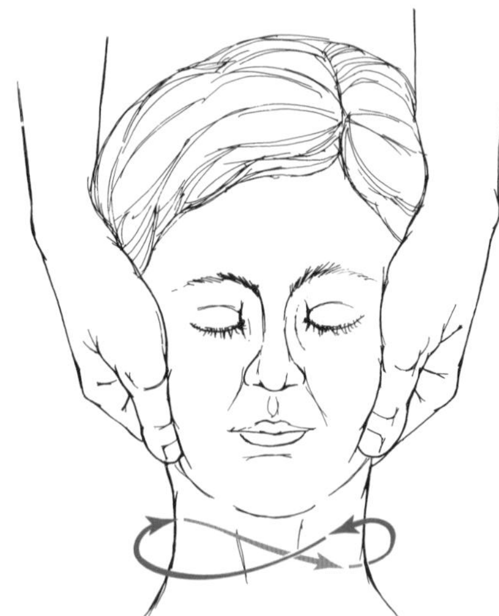

Figure 5-64. Figure-eight mobilization of the cervical facets. For acute conditions, move slowly and gently. For chronic conditions, the ROM of the mobilization may be increased.

CASE STUDY

PH is a 40-year-old, 5'1", 100-lb, female management executive who presented to my office in October 1993 for complaints of neck pain and limited ROM in her neck, with occasional sharp pain and muscle spasms. Her complaints began in October of 1992 after a serious injury in which she fell off her horse and landed on her head. A computerized axial tomography (CAT) scan showed that she had fractured her right occipital condyle. It also revealed many congenital anomalies in her neck, including a hemivertebra, in which only one-half of the vertebral body is present, and multiple fusions from C3 to C7. She was placed in a rigid collar and given muscle relaxants and pain medication.

Examination on the first visit revealed an elevated right ilium in standing, a left thoracic scoliosis, and a positive Adam's test. Lumbar ROM was normal. Cervical range of motion was 75% of normal in flexion and right rotation, 25% of normal in extension and left rotation, and 50% of normal in right and left lateral flexion. Reflexes and isometric testing of the neck and upper extremity muscles were normal. To palpation, PH had spastic and tender cervical and upper thoracic musculature and a significant loss of normal joint play at multiple levels in the cervical spine.

A diagnosis was made of cervical somatic dysfunction, which describes the altered joint mechanics and soft-tissue hypertonicity. As PH had been through such a serious injury, the session began with CR MET with a neutral spine, that is, without any side bending or rotation. MET was used to increase the ROM in four primary directions: flexion, extension, lateral flexion, and posterior rotation of the head. After the MET, OM was performed on the cervical paraspinals.

After two sessions, she said she was feeling slightly better and was taking fewer muscle relaxants. Our next sessions began with PH supine, and the CR MET was repeated in neutral spine. After the tissue was warmed up, CR MET for rotation was introduced. She was asked to rotate her head to her comfortable limit in one direction and to resist as I attempted to lift her head off the table. As she was pressing into extension, she was instructed to rotate further. Her ability to rotate was greater if she was simultaneously extending. This was repeated to the other side. She was then asked to lie on her side, and deeper massage strokes were performed on her upper thoracic and cervical musculature, including the transversospinalis group and the joint capsules.

PH reported that she was without pain, that her ROM was dramatically better, and that she wanted to continue treatments on a weekly basis. Reevaluation showed that her cervical ROM was normal in flexion, right rotation, and right lateral flexion; was 75% of normal in extension and left rotation; and was 50% of normal in left lateral flexion.

STUDY GUIDE

Cervical Spine, Level I

1. List the four suboccipital muscles.
2. Describe the difference in symptoms between cervical disc degeneration and herniation.
3. Locate the facet joints on a skeleton and on a fellow student.
4. Describe how to perform CR MET for acute neck pain.
5. Describe the possible symptoms of a whiplash injury.
6. Describe the symptoms of anterior scalene syndrome.
7. What is the direction of our stroke for the scalene muscles?
8. List which muscles are tight and which muscles are weak in the upper crossed syndrome.
9. What is the stroke direction for the medial group of erector spinae muscles in the neck?
10. List four factors that predispose a person to developing neck pain.

Cervical Spine, Level II

1. List the suprahyoid, infrahyoid, prevertebral, and TMJ muscles.
2. Describe the basic origins and insertions of the following muscles: scalenes, SCM, suboccipital muscles, longus capitis, longus colli, temporalis, and masseter.
3. What are the ranges of normal motion of the cervical spine?
4. Describe what a positive EAST test indicates.
5. Demonstrate PIR MET for the cervical region and CR MET for the TMJ.
6. List the muscle attachments on the cervical SPs and transverse processes from superficial to deep.
7. Describe FHP and its effects on the facet joints.

8. Describe a common site of entrapment of the cervical sympathetic nerves, and describe the massage and MET techniques to release them.
9. Describe the foraminal compression test and its significance.
10. Describe the postural signs of an upper crossed syndrome.

REFERENCES

1. Bovim G, Schrader H, Sand T. Neck pain in the general population. Spine 1994; 19:1307–1309.
2. Porterfield JA, DeRosa C. Mechanical Neck Pain. Philadelphia: WB Saunders, 1995.
3. Cailliet R. Neck and Arm Pain, Philadelphia: FA Davis, 1991.
4. Kendall F, McCreary E, Provance P. Muscles: Testing and Function. 4th Ed. Baltimore: Williams & Wilkins, 1993.
5. Grieve G. Common Vertebral Joint Problems. Edinburgh: Churchill Livingstone, 1981.
6. Richmond FJ, Abrahams VC. What Are the Proprioceptors of the Neck? Prog Brain Res 1979;50:245–254.
7. Blakney M, Hertling D. The cervical spine. In: Hertling D, Kessler RM, Kessler E, eds. Management of Common Musculoskeletal Disorders. 3rd Ed. Baltimore: Lippincott, Williams & Wilkins, 1996:528–558.
8. Cole A, Farrell J, Stratton S. Functional rehabilitation of cervical spine athletic injuries. In: Kibler WB, Herring S, Press J, eds. Functional Rehabilitation of Sports and Musculoskeletal Injuries. Gaithersburg, Maryland: Aspen Publication, 1998:127–148.
9. Barnsley L, Lord S, Bogduk N. Critical review: whiplash injury. Pain 1994;58:283–307.
10. Kraus SL. Influences of the cervical spine on the stomatognathic system. In: Donatelli R, Wooden MJ, eds. Orthopedic Physical Therapy. 2nd Ed. New York: Churchill Livingstone, 1994:61–76.
11. Perry JF. The temporomandibular joint. In: Norkin CC, Levangie PK, eds. Joint Structure and Function. 2nd Ed. Philadelphia: FA Davis, 1992:193–206.
12. Hertling D. The temporomandibular joint. In: Hertling D, Kessler RM, Kessler E, eds. Management of Common Musculoskeletal Disorders. 3rd Ed. Baltimore: Lippincott, Williams & Wilkins, 1996:444–488.

SUGGESTED READINGS

Cailliet R. Neck and Arm Pain. Philadelphia: FA Davis, 1991.

Calais-Germain B. Anatomy of Movement. Seattle: Eastland Press, 1991.

Chaitow L. Muscle Energy Techniques. New York: Churchill Livingstone, 1996.

Clemente C. Anatomy: A Regional Atlas of the Human Body. 4th Ed. Baltimore: Williams & Wilkins, 1997.

Corrigan B, Maitland GD. Practical Orthopaedic Medicine. London: Butterworths, 1983.

Kendall F, McCreary E, Provance P. Muscles: Testing and Function. 4th Ed. Baltimore: Williams & Wilkins, 1993.

Kessler R, Hertling D. Management of Common Musculoskeletal Disorders. 3rd Ed. Baltimore: Lippincott, Williams & Wilkins, 1993.

Magee D. Orthopedic Physical Assessment. 3rd Ed. Philadelphia: WB Saunders, 1997.

Norkin C, Levangie P. Joint Structure and Function. 2nd Ed. Philadelphia: FA Davis, 1992.

Platzer W. Locomotor System, vol 1. 4th Ed. New York: Thieme Medical, 1992.

Porterfield JA, DeRosa C. Mechanical Neck Pain. Philadelphia: WB Saunders, 1995.

Reid DC. Sports Injury and Assessment. New York: Churchill Livingstone, 1992.

oulder

houlder girdle is common in
th a prevalence of 15 to 25%
ige group.[1] Disorders of the
for 30 to 40% of industrial
reased sixfold in the past
to the shoulder girdle ac-
sports injuries, they repre-
entage of physician visits,
perceived as being serious
[2] The shoulder region may
al from the cervical and the
visceral diseases, such as
blems.[3]

ion, and Dysfunction of the Shoulder Complex

GENERAL OVERVIEW

- The bones of the **shoulder complex** includes the bones of the shoulder girdle; the clavicle and scapula; and the humerus, sternum, and rib cage (Fig. 6-1). These bones form four typical joints: the glenohumeral joint (shoulder joint), the sternoclavicular, the acromioclavicular, and the scapulothoracic joints. There is a fifth functional joint, the coracoacromial arch, which describes the region where the head of the humerus is covered by the acromion and the coracoacromial ligament. All these joints must be considered together in discussing the shoulder, as any motion of the glenohumeral joint also occurs at each of the other joints. The shoulder is the most mobile joint in the body with the least stability; therefore, it is one of the most frequently injured joints in the body.
- The function of the shoulder is influenced by many joints. The function and position of the cervical and the thoracic spine influence mobility of the arm. The upper thoracic vertebrae must be able to extend, rotate, and side bend to accomplish full elevation of the arm.[1] There must also be mobility in the upper ribs, as well as mobility in the acromioclavicular and sternoclavicular joints for full range of motion (ROM) in the arm, stability of the scapula is necessary to allow proper positioning of the head of the humerus in the glenoid fossa of the scapula.

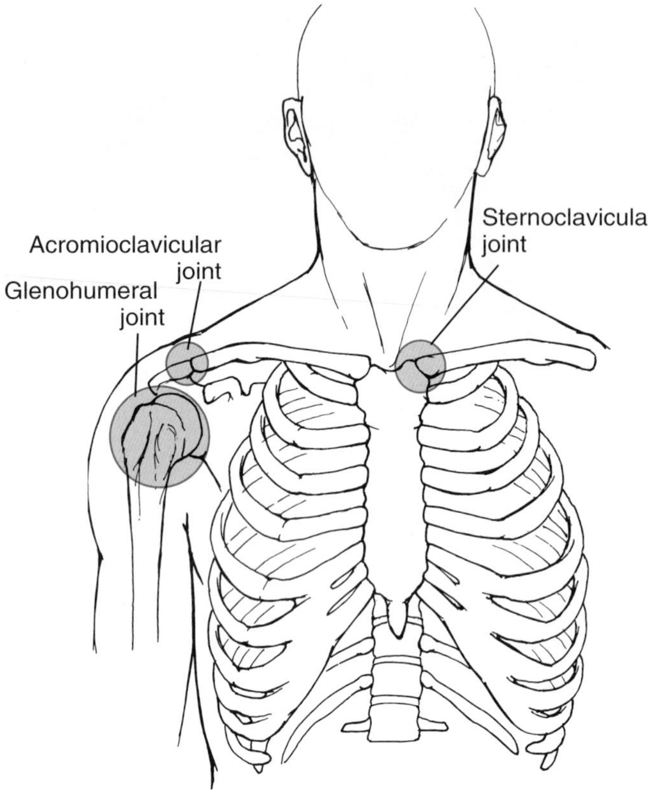

Figure 6-1. Anterior view of the bones and joints of the shoulder complex.

SHOULDER GIRDLE BONES AND JOINTS

Scapula

- The scapula or shoulder blade is a flat, triangular bone (Fig. 6-2). The resting position of the scapula covers the second to seventh ribs, and the vertebral border is approximately 2 inches from the midline. The posterior aspect has a bony ridge called the spine of the scapula that extends laterally as a bulbous enlargement called the acromion. The acromion articulates with the clavicle, forming the acromioclavicular (AC) joint. Above the spine is a deep cavity or fossa that contains the supraspinatus muscle belly. Below the spine are the infraspinatus and the teres minor and major. On the anterior surface is a fossa where the subscapularis muscle attaches. There are 15 muscles that attach to the scapula.
- On the anterior-superior surface of the scapula is a bony process called the coracoid process, which is a point of attachment for three muscles and three ligaments. The muscles are the pectoralis minor, the short head of the biceps brachii, and the coracobrachialis. The three ligaments are the coracoclavicular, the coracohumeral, and the coracoacromial.
- The glenoid fossa is a shallow cavity on the lateral aspect of the scapula that serves as the articulation for the head of the humerus. In the normal resting position, the glenoid fossa faces laterally, anteriorly, and superiorly.

Clavicle

- The clavicle or collarbone is an S-shaped bone, convex anteriorly in the medial two-thirds and concave anteriorly in the lateral one-third. It articulates with the sternum medially, connecting the upper extremity to the axial skeleton, forming the sternoclavicular joint. It articulates with the acromion of the scapula, forming the acromioclavicular joint. It is the attachment site of six muscles and a number of ligaments.
- ***Dysfunction and injury:*** The brachial plexus, the group of nerves from the neck that innervates the arm, travels under the clavicle in what is called the **thoracic outlet.** A broken collarbone or other injuries leading to fibrosis in the fascia attaching to the clavicle or a rounded-shoulders, forward-head

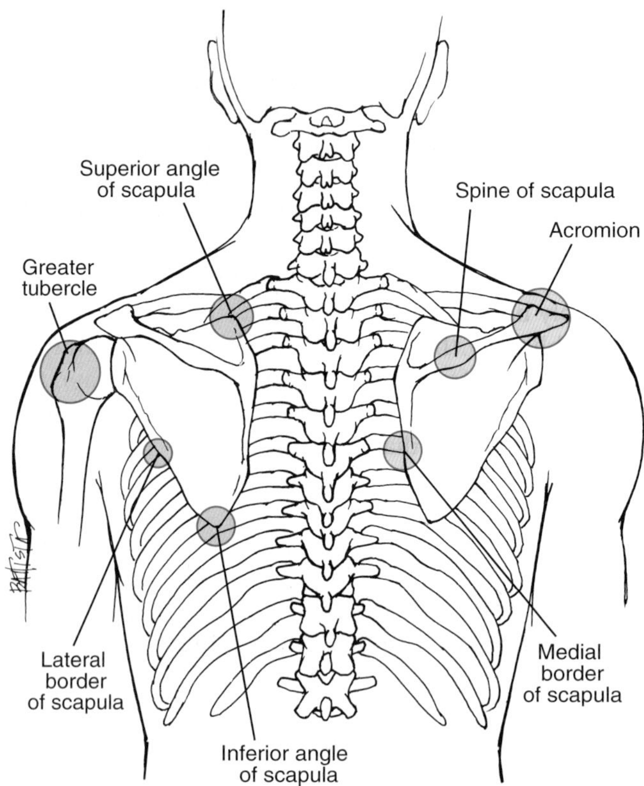

Figure 6-2. Posterior view of the bones and bony landmarks of the shoulder complex.

posture (FHP) closes down this space and contributes to **thoracic outlet syndrome** (TOS).

Sternum

- The sternum or breastbone is a flat bone located in the center of the chest. It is divided into three parts: the manubrium, body, and xiphoid. The manubrium articulates with the clavicle and first rib at its superior-lateral aspect and with the second rib at the inferior-lateral aspect. The body provides an attachment site for the other ribs, forming the sternocostal joint. The xiphoid is the inferior tip. The sternum functions to protect the heart and lungs.

Sternoclavicular Joint

- The sternoclavicular joint is a synovial joint in which the sternal end of the clavicle articulates with the upper lateral edge of the sternum, as well as the first rib (See Fig. 6-1).
- ***Structure:*** The sternoclavicular joint has a strong joint capsule, an articular disc, and three major ligaments.
  - The three ligaments of the sternoclavicular joint are the costoclavicular ligament, the interclavicular ligament, and the anterior and the posterior sternoclavicular ligaments.
  - The articular disc, or meniscus, is a fibrocartilage that helps distribute the forces between the two bones. It is attached to the clavicle, first rib, and the sternum.
- ***Function:*** The sternoclavicular joint has five possible motions: elevation, depression, protraction, retraction, and rotation.
- ***Dysfunction and injury:*** The sternoclavicular joint is so strong that the clavicle will break or the AC joint will dislocate before the sternoclavicular joint dislocates.[1]

Acromioclavicular Joint

- The AC joint is a synovial joint in which the lateral aspect of the clavicle articulates with the acromion of the scapula (see Fig. 6-5).
- ***Structure:*** It has a weak joint capsule, a fibrocartilage disc, and two strong ligaments.
- The ligaments are the superior and the inferior acromioclavicular ligaments and the coracoclavicular ligament, which is divided into the lateral trapezoid and medial conoid portions. These ligaments function to suspend the scapula from the clavicle and to prevent posterior and medial motion of the scapula, as in falling on an outstretched hand (FOOSH) injury.
- ***Function***: Approximately 30° of rotation of the clavicle can occur at the AC and the sternoclavicular joints as the arm is elevated. The clavicle rolls superiorly and posteriorly after approximately 90° of abduction.
  - The rotation of the scapula and hence the upward and downward movement of the glenoid fossa, occurs at the AC joint.
- ***Dysfunction and injury:*** A fall on the shoulder can tear the acromioclavicular ligament and cause the clavicle to ride on top of the acromion, which is called a **shoulder separation.** This is visible when observing the client from the anterior view and is called a **step deformity.**

Scapulothoracic Joint

- The scapulothoracic joint describes the relationship of the scapula to the rib cage (see Fig. 6-2). It is not a true joint with a synovial capsule, but a functional joint, as the scapula moves on top of the thoracic cage.
- ***Function:*** The critical functions of the scapulothoracic joint are to allow for proper positioning of the glenoid fossa for arm motion and to stabilize the scapula for efficient arm motion. The scapula makes approximately a 30° to 45° angle anteriorly as it rests on the thoracic cage. This angle is called the **scapular plane.**
  - There are six motions of the scapulothoracic joint: elevation, depression, adduction, abduction, and upward and downward rotation, which describes the movement of the inferior angle of the scapula moving away from or toward the vertebral column.
  - The scapula has **static** and **dynamic stabilizers.** The static stabilizers are the joint capsule and ligaments, and the principle dynamic stabilizers are the rhomboids, the trapezius, levator scapula, and the serratus anterior. The static and dynamic stabilizers work in concert to provide a stable position of the scapula to allow optimum arm motion.
- ***Dysfunction and injury:*** It is common for the dynamic stabilizers of the shoulder to be weak. During our assessment, this is manifested as winging of the scapula and excessive scapular motion when the client does a pushup (see "Shoulder Assessment," p. 221). Decreased scapular stability contributes to protracted scapula (i.e., the scapula moves away from the spine). As the scapula slides laterally, the

optimal length–tension relationship of the muscles of the glenohumeral joint is lost, which results in weakness of the muscles of the arm. This is often caused by rounded-shoulders, and a FHP. As the scapula rides forward on the rib cage, the superior portion rotates downward, and the glenoid fossa no longer faces upward. This inhibits the normal abduction of the arm, contributing to impingement of the rotator cuff, subacromial bursa, and biceps tendon between the greater tuberosity of the humerus and the acromion or coracoacromial ligament. For many other clients who have FHP, the scapula is held in a retracted position owing to short and tight rhomboids. These clients typically do not develop impingement syndrome.

GLENOHUMERAL JOINT BONES AND SOFT-TISSUE STRUCTURES OF THE

Glenohumeral Joint

- *Structure:* The glenohumeral joint is a ball and socket synovial joint consisting of the shallow glenoid fossa of the scapula and the large, rounded head of the humerus (Fig. 6-3). It contains a joint capsule, a fibrocartilage rim called a labrum, and numerous ligaments.
- *Function:* The glenohumeral joint has the greatest ROM of any joint in the body, but it sacrifices stability for mobility. It is described as an incongruous joint, meaning that the humerus and glenoid fossa barely make contact with each other at rest. It is held in the normal resting position by the superior joint capsule and the coracohumeral ligament. This is different from the hip joint, in which two-thirds of the head of the femur is within the acetabulum, and the two articulating surfaces fit closely together.
- Because the glenohumeral joint is incongruous, the muscles play a dual role of support and motion. The muscles must maintain the proper alignment of the head of the humerus to the glenoid fossa as the arm is moving.[3]
- The glenohumeral joint has six basic motions: flexion, extension, abduction, adduction, and medial and lateral rotation. Abduction is easier in the plane of the scapula, which is 30° to 45° of forward flexion, because the joint capsule is more lax, and the greater tuberosity of the humerus is not abutting against the acromion at this angle.[4] It is the most natural and functional position of abduction. Patients who have shoulder pain typically abduct their arm in this plane.
- Abduction of the humerus is a combination of rolling and inferior sliding of the humeral head in the glenoid fossa. As the deltoid muscle abducts the arm, the supraspinatus pulls the head of the humerus into the glenoid fossa, and the infraspinatus, teres minor, and subscapularis contract and pull the humeral head inferiorly. This action creates enough room for the humeral head to slide under the acromion. If the cuff muscles are dysfunctioning and weak, the humeral head migrates superiorly and impinges against the acromion and coracoacromial ligament.
- ***Scapulohumeral rhythm:*** The first 15° to 30° of arm motion happens solely at the glenohumeral joint. Beginning at 15° to 30° of abduction, the scapula moves to contribute to arm elevation. The relationship of scapular movement to arm motion is called scapulohumeral rhythm. For every 10° movement of the humerus, there is 5° of scapular movement. These combined movements allow for 160° of abduction. To achieve 180° of abduction, the upper thoracic and lower cervical spine bends. Thus, thoracic hypomobility prevents full abduction.[5]
- ***Dysfunction and injury to the glenohumeral joint:*** Because of the poor congruency of the humeral head in the glenoid fossa, this joint is susceptible to dislocation and subluxation (partial dislocation). The massage therapist treats the consequences of previous dislocations, which usually result in shoulder instability. Acute traumatic dislocation is predominantly an injury of young adults, caused by forced external rotation and extension of the arm, dislocat-

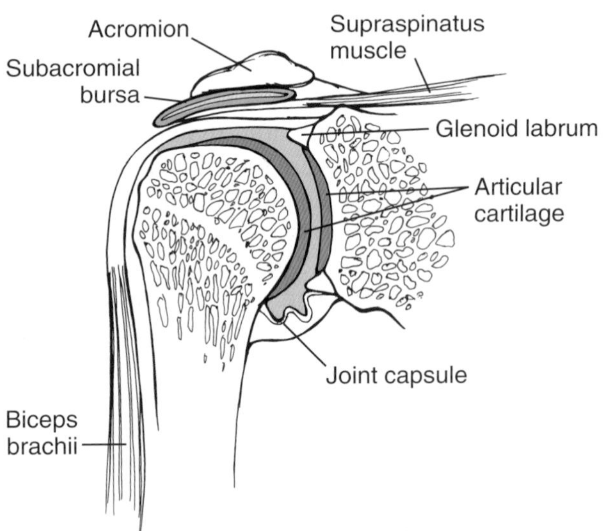

Figure 6-3. Glenohumeral joint showing the articular cartilage, joint capsule, subacromial bursa, supraspinatus, and long head of the biceps.

ing the humerus in the forward, medial, and inferior direction.[1] Instability of the glenohumeral joint is a common problem, and anterior instability is the most common direction. The instability may be attributable to traumatic dislocation, rotator cuff injury or weakness, or acquired or congenital joint laxity. Acquired instability is caused by prior or recurrent dislocations or by treatment failure of the initial injury.[2]

- *Treatment implications:* It is important for the massage therapist to appreciate that certain conditions require stabilization and strengthening rather than to assume that all clients need release of muscle tension. If your assessment findings or doctor's diagnosis indicate glenohumeral instability, use contract-relax (CR) muscle energy technique (MET) in the rotator cuff and muscles stabilizing the scapula to help facilitate their normal function. These clients typically require treatment with a physical therapist or a personal trainer to guide them in proper exercise.

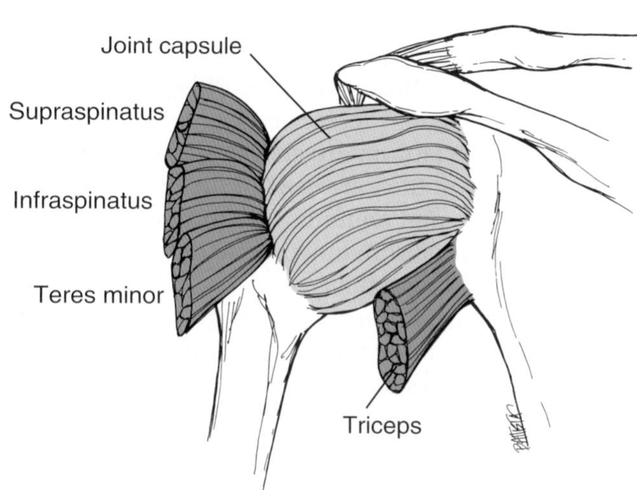

Figure 6-4. Joint capsule, interweaving rotator cuff muscles and long head of the triceps.

Humerus

- The humerus or arm bone consists of a body and upper (proximal) and lower (distal) ends. The humeral head forms the upper end. On the anterolateral surface is the greater tubercle, and on the anteromedial surface is the lesser tubercle. Between these two bony prominences is the intertubercular groove, which contains the tendon of the long head of the biceps. The greater tubercle is an attachment site for the supraspinatus, infraspinatus, and teres minor. The lesser tubercle is the attachment site for the subscapularis. The distal end of the humerus articulates with the radius and ulna to form the elbow.

Joint Capsule

- *Structure:* The joint capsule originates from the glenoid labrum and attaches to the periosteum of the shaft of the humerus (Fig. 6-4). There is a synovial lining throughout the capsule[3] that is reinforced posteriorly and superiorly by the rotator cuff muscles and anteriorly by the subscapularis tendon, pectoralis major, teres major, and the coracohumeral and glenohumeral ligaments. The fibers of the joint capsule have a medial and forward twist with the arm hanging at the side in its resting position.
- *Function:* The twist in the joint capsule is increased with abduction and decreased with flexion. The tension in the capsule in abduction pulls the humerus into external rotation, which allows the greater tubercle of the humerus to clear the coracoacromial arch.[1] The posterior capsule tightens when the arm rotates medially (internally), and the anterior capsule tightens when the arm rotates laterally (externally). The joint capsule is also involved in the **instability syndrome** and in **rotator cuff tendinitis,** which are addressed later in the chapter (see the sections "Instability Syndrome of the Glenohumeral Joint" and "Rotator Cuff Tendinitis").
- *Dysfunction and injury:* A common problem to the joint capsule is called **frozen shoulder,** or **adhesive capsulitis.** The joint capsule becomes fibrotic; the anterior portion of the capsule develops adhesions to the humeral head, and the folds in the capsule can adhere to themselves. This fibrosis and thickening shortens the capsule and prevents external rotation of the shoulder, which, in turn, restricts abduction. External rotation is necessary in abduction to allow the greater tuberosity to clear the coracoacromial arch. Thoracic kyphosis may be a causative factor.[3]
- *Treatment implications:* The treatment of frozen shoulder is a tremendous challenge. Passive traction and MET provide the most comfortable and effective therapy. The first motion to introduce for frozen shoulder is inferior glide, which reduces sustained muscle tension and stretches the joint capsule. Next, perform CR MET to increase external rotation, as this allows the greater tuberosity to roll under the coracoacromial arch for abduction. Finally, perform postisometric relaxation (PIR) or eccentric MET to increase flexion and abduction, first in the sagittal plane, then the scapular plane, and finally in the coronal plane.

Labrum

- *Structure:* The labrum is a fibrocartilage lip that surrounds the glenoid fossa (see Fig. 6-3). The outer surface of the labrum attaches to the joint capsule. The tendons of the long head of the biceps and triceps attach to and reinforce the labrum.
- *Function:* The labrum functions to deepen the glenoid cavity, adding stability.
- *Dysfunction and injury:* Injuries to the labrum can result from shearing forces if the humerus is forced through extremes of motion or through repeated or excessive traction of the long head of the biceps tendon from its attachment to the superior labrum.[8]

Ligaments

- The **ligaments** of the glenohumeral joint are the glenohumeral, the coracohumeral, the coracoacromial, and the transverse humeral (Fig. 6-5). The joint capsule thickens in bands that are sometimes referred to as capsular ligaments. As in all joints, there is a reflex from the mechanoreceptors within the joint capsule and ligaments to the muscles surrounding the joint.[6]
  - The **glenohumeral ligament** lies underneath the coracohumeral ligament, reinforcing the joint anteriorly and tightening on external rotation of the humerus.
  - The **coracohumeral ligament** is further divided into the superior, middle, and inferior portions. It is a broad band reinforcing and interweaving with the upper part of the joint capsule. It attaches to the lateral border of the coracoid process, passing laterally to blend with the tendon of the supraspinatus, capsule, and transverse humeral ligament.
  - The **coracoacromial ligament** is a strong triangular band attached to the edge of the acromion just in front of the articular surface for the clavicle and to the entire length of the lateral border of the coracoid process.
  - The **transverse humeral ligament** crosses the intertubercular groove to stabilize the tendon of the long head of the biceps.

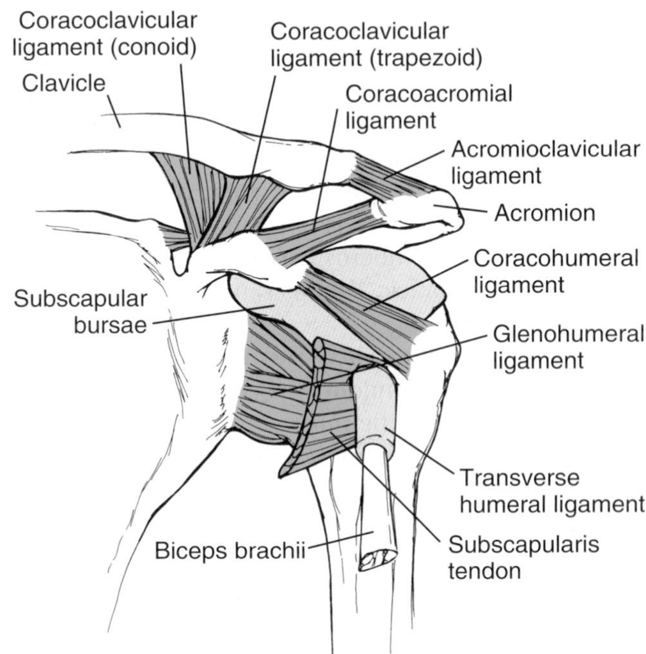

Figure 6-5. Ligaments of the glenohumeral and the acromioclavicular joints and of the subscapular bursa.

Coracoacromial Arch

- *Structure:* The coracoacromial arch consists of the coracoid process anteriorly, the acromion posteriorly, and the coracoacromial ligament in between them (see Fig. 6-5). In the arch space lie: the head of the humerus below; the coracoacromial ligament and acromion above; and the joint capsule, supraspinatus and infraspinatus tendons, the bicipital tendon, and the subdeltoid bursa in between.
- *Function:* The coracoacromial ligament prevents dislocation of the humeral head superiorly, and along with the acromion and coracoid process, it forms an important protective arch. It also acts as a soft-tissue buffer between the rotator cuff and the bony surface of the acromion. The coracoacromial arch may be described as an accessory joint that is lined with the synovial membrane of the synovial bursa.[7]
- *Dysfunction and injury:* The greater tubercle of the head of the humerus may impinge or compress the supraspinatus and infraspinatus tendons, the joint capsule, the bicipital tendon, or the subdeltoid bursa against the coracoacromial ligament and anterior acromion. This is called **impingement syndrome.** The causes of this syndrome are diverse but include postural causes such as thoracic kyphosis, or a habitual rounded-shoulders and a FHP. It may also be caused by muscle weakness from the scapular stabilizers or the rotator cuff muscles and the long head of the biceps, which provide a downward force on the humerus.
- *Treatment implications:* The first intention is to correct the client's posture, if indicated. Next, use CR MET to facilitate and strengthen the external rota-

tors. Then, perform transverse massage on the coracoacromial arch, to reduce any adhesions and scar tissue in the coracoacromial ligament and to correct any positional dysfunction in the deltoid and rotator cuff muscles.

Bursae

- *Structure:* A bursa is a synovial-lined sac filled with synovial fluid.
- *Function:* The function of a bursa is to secrete a lubricant to neighboring structures, which decreases friction.
- Of the eight or nine bursae that are about the shoulder, only the subacromial bursa is commonly involved clinically, and two others are occasionally involved.
  - The **subacromial** or **subdeltoid bursa** lies over the greater tubercle of the humerus and supraspinatus tendon and under the coracoacromial ligament, acromion, and deltoid muscle (Fig. 6-6).
  - The **subscapular bursa** lies over the anterior joint capsule and under the subscapularis muscle attachment to the lesser tubercle of the humerus.
  - The **subcoracoid bursa** lies between the coracoid process and the clavicle.
- *Dysfunction and injury:* The subacromial bursa can become inflamed due to overuse, postural stresses, or trauma and can become impinged under the acromial arch. Because of its closeness to the supraspinatus tendon, any scarring or calcium deposits in the body of the tendon can irritate this bursa. It is also susceptible to irritation from a type III acromion, also called a *hooked acromion.* This type of acromion has a bony protuberance on the undersurface, which can irritate the supraspinatus tendon that travels underneath it.
  - The subscapular bursa can become irritated because of increased tension in the pectoralis minor and subscapularis muscles.
  - The subcoracoid bursa can become irritated because of the forward tipping of the scapula caused by pectoralis minor hypertonicity.
- *Treatment implications:* Lauren Berry, RPT, taught that the bursae can be manually drained if they are swollen. They can also be manually pumped to increase their synovial fluids, if they are dried out because of adhesions. These techniques are clinically effective for both conditions.

CAUTION: **When treating an acute bursitis be extremely gentle, or you may aggravate the condition.**

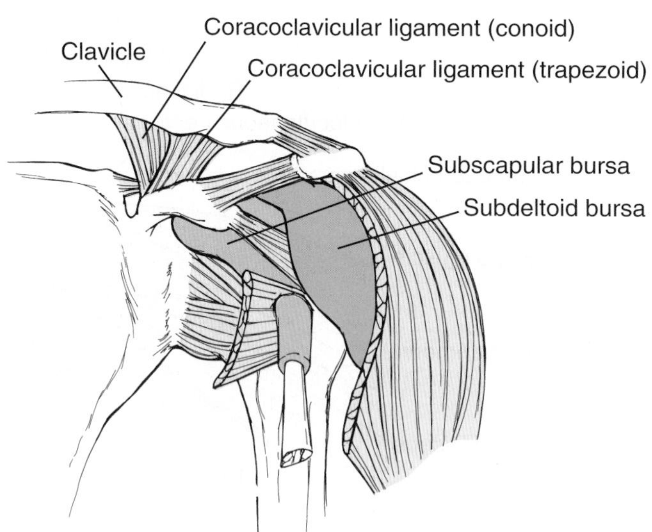

Figure 6-6. Subdeltoid and subscapular bursa.

Shoulder Region Nerves

- Most of the nerve supply of the shoulder and arm arise from the **brachial plexus,** which begins as five nerve roots from C5 to C8 and T1 (Fig. 6-7). As mentioned in Chapter 5, "Cervical Spine," these nerve roots travel through the anterior and the middle scalenes. The roots of the brachial plexus unite just above the clavicle to form the superior, middle, and inferior trunks. The middle part of the clavicle is convex anteriorly, and the axillary artery and vein and brachial plexus pass posterior to this.
- The brachial plexus then travels over the first rib and under the clavicle and subclavius muscle. This costoclavicular space can become compromised because of previous trauma, such as a fractured clavicle, or because of postural imbalances, such as rounded shoulders.
- The nerves then travel between the pectoralis minor and the rib cage, medial to the coracoid process. At the level of the pectoralis minor, the brachial plexus forms the medial, lateral, and posterior cords. Distal to the pectoralis minor, the three cords divide into many branches, including the radial, median, and ulnar nerves that travel into the arm and down to the hand.
- The medial and ulnar nerves travel along the medial arm in the medial bicipital groove, bounded by the biceps and triceps. The radial nerve leaves this groove at the margin of the proximal and middle third of the arm and travels to the posterior surface of the humerus in the radial groove.
- In addition to the brachial plexus, there are two branches in the shoulder region that we address in

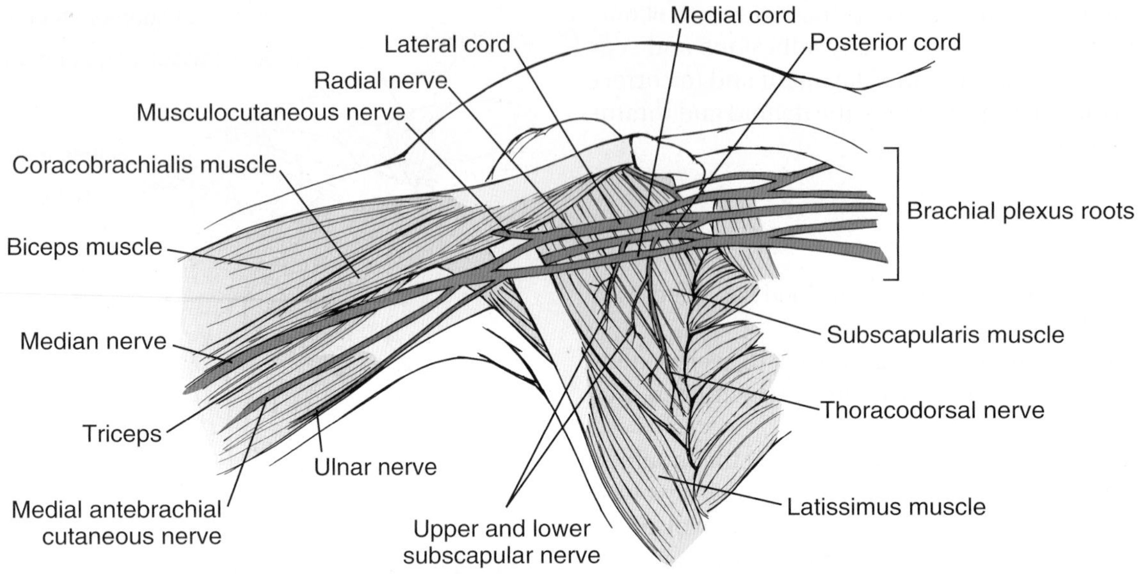

Figure 6-7. Brachial plexus leaves the neck between the anterior and the middle scalenes. It then travels under the clavicle, subclavius, and pectoralis minor and enters the medial arm.

the treatment section of this chapter. The long thoracic nerve travels on the thoracic wall over the serratus anterior; the subscapular and thoracodorsal nerves lie on the subscapularis muscle. Both these nerves can become entrapped due to shortened fascia or to sustained contraction in the muscles.

- ***Dysfunction and injury:*** As mentioned in Chapter 5, **TOS** is a result of compression or entrapment of the brachial plexus. As Kendall et al.[8] point out, the diagnosis of TOS is often ambiguous because it includes many similar entities, including costoclavicular, anterior scalene, hyperabduction, and pectoralis minor syndromes.
- Nerves become compressed for several reasons—poor posture and faulty alignment of the neck, upper back, and shoulders. A forward head, rounded-shoulder posture, creates a forward depression of the coracoid process, shortening the pectoralis minor and weakening the lower trapezius. This posture also predisposes to an adduction and internal rotation of the shoulder. This leads to compression. Brachial plexus compression may also result from prolonged overhead activities, such as painting, in which the clavicle rotates posteriorly, compressing the nerves between the clavicle and the first rib.
- Clinically, the brachial plexus can become compressed at several different sites:
  - Between the anterior and the middle scalenes.
  - Between the clavicle and the first rib, called a *costoclavicular syndrome.* This syndrome is caused by rounded-shoulders posture; thoracic kyphosis; or previous trauma to the clavicle, AC joint, or glenohumeral joint.
  - At the pectoralis minor, as the plexus travels between the muscle and the rib cage.
- Brachial plexus compression symptoms include a generalized numbing, tingling, and pain. The medial cord, the most inferior part of the brachial plexus, is most vulnerable to compression, and therefore ulnar nerve symptoms along the ulnar border of the forearm and hand are most commonly reported.[3]
- ***Treatment implications:*** Four distinct areas must be released when the therapist considers peripheral entrapment of the brachial plexus—the region of the scalenes, the supraclavicular space, the infraclavicular space, and the pectoralis minor. Scalenes were discussed in Chapter 5.
  - Begin with instruction in postural awareness. Next, perform CR MET to reduce the hypertonicity in the tight muscles. Then use PIR MET to lengthen the short anterior muscles and fascia and use CR MET and home exercises to strengthen the weak lower trapezius. Treat the pectoralis minor, pectoralis major, and subscapularis first. After facilitating the lower trapezius, perform manual release on the supraclavicular and infraclavicular spaces.

Shoulder Region Muscles

- ***Structure:*** The muscles of the shoulder region may be divided into two major groups: muscles that stabilize the scapula and muscles of the rotator cuff.

- Four main muscles stabilize the scapula: the rhomboids, trapezius, levator scapula, and serratus anterior (Figs. 6-8 and 6-9). To perform elevation of the arm, these muscles must contract first to stabilize the scapula against the rib cage. Then the rotator cuff muscles and the deltoids contract to elevate the arm.[3]
- The four muscles of the rotator cuff are the supraspinatus, infraspinatus, teres minor, (Fig. 6-10) and subscapularis (see Fig. 6-9). They attach to the posterior, superior, and anterior head of the humerus as a continuous cuff and not as discrete tendons. The fibers of the cuff blend with the articular joint capsule.

- ***Function:*** The chief function of the rotator cuff muscles is dynamic stabilization of the glenohumeral joint. In most joints, the close fit of the articulating bones and the ligaments and joint capsule offer primary stability. As mentioned, there is little congruency between the humeral head and the glenoid fossa. When the arm hangs at the side, little contraction of the deltoid or cuff muscles is required, as the

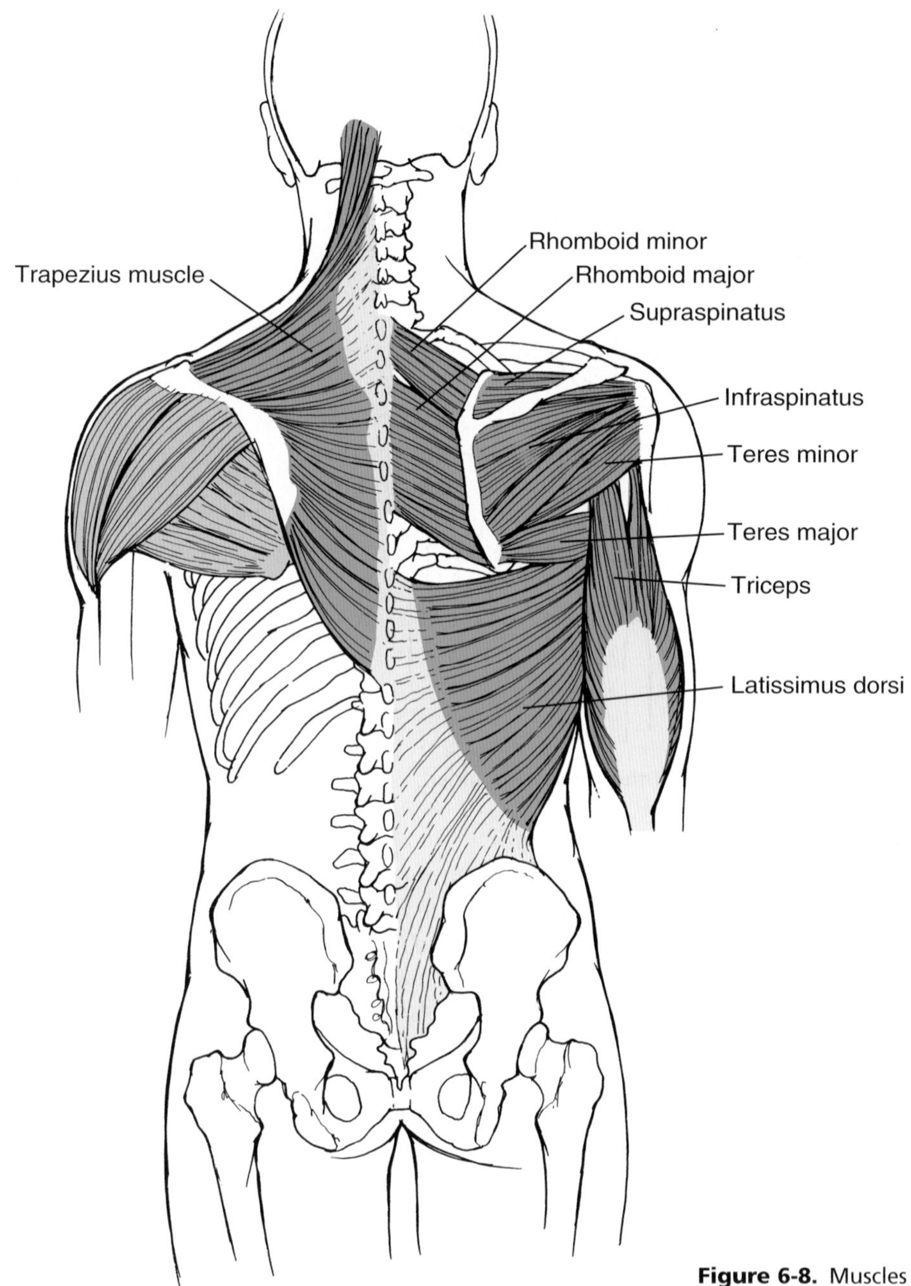

Figure 6-8. Muscles of the posterior shoulder region.

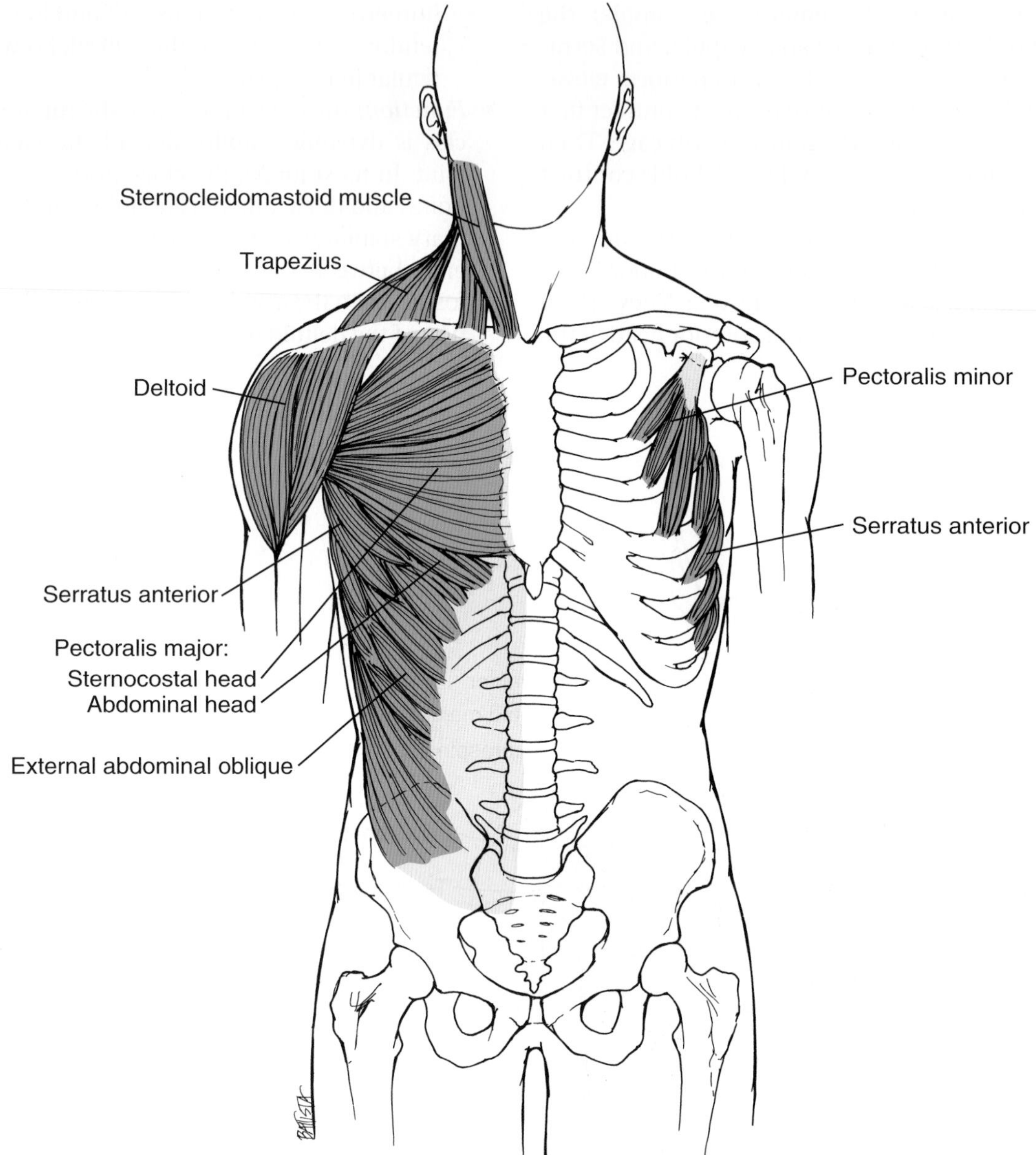

Figure 6-9. Muscles of the anterior shoulder.

superior joint capsule and the coracohumeral ligament provide a reactive tensile force that pulls the humeral head against the glenoid cavity.[5] When the arm is elevated, the superior joint capsule is lax and no longer stabilizes the joint, so the muscles of the rotator cuff must hold the humerus in proper orientation to the glenoid, playing an essential role in stabilizing the joint. They create joint compression and downward depression, creating a fixed fulcrum, so that the deltoid can rotate the arm upward. If the cuff muscles are weak or dysfunctioning, the contraction of the deltoid causes an abnormal upward movement of the humeral head, causing an impingement of the soft tissue into the coracoacromial arch.

- ***Dysfunction and injury:*** The rotator cuff is a common site of injury, usually of a degenerative nature caused by cumulative stresses. The most commonly affected muscle is the supraspinatus. The supraspinatus should receive its primary blood supply from the thoracoacromial artery. This artery is frequently absent, leaving the tendon hypovascular.[5] The infraspinatus may also be hypovascular, but to a much lesser extent. This decreased blood supply makes the area susceptible to fatigue and degeneration.

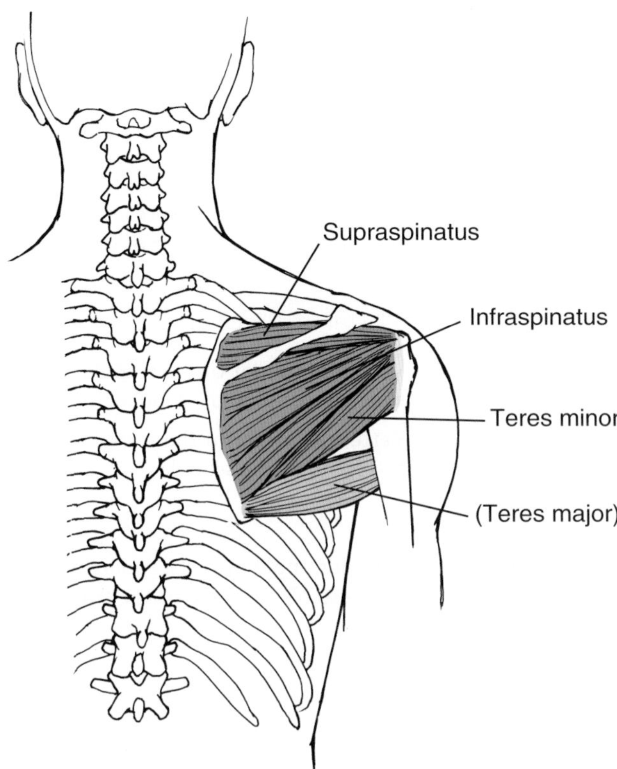

Figure 6-10. Supraspinatus, infraspinatus, and teres minor are three of the four rotator cuff muscles.

- Two common conditions decrease the stability of the joint:
  - Thoracic kyphosis, which causes the tension in the superior joint capsule to be lost, and the rotator cuff muscles must maintain constant contraction to stabilize the arm, making it susceptible to fatigue and degeneration.[5]
  - Weakness in the scapular stabilizing muscles, especially the serratus anterior and the lower and middle trapezius. This allows the acromion to migrate forward, into a position of greater impingement.
  - As mentioned previously, according to Janda,[9] there are predictable patterns of muscle dysfunction. In the upper body, he describes this as the **upper crossed syndrome.**[9] Below are listed the muscles of the shoulder girdle complex that are typically imbalanced and participate in the upper crossed syndrome.

Shoulder Region Muscle Imbalances

- **Muscles that tend to be tight and short:** Pectoralis major and minor, upper trapezius, subscapularis, and levator scapula. Overdevelopment of the pectoralis and the subscapularis result in a protracted scapula and a stretch weakness of the rhomboids and middle trapezius.[10]
- **Muscles that tend to be inhibited and weak:** Lower and middle parts of the trapezius, rhomboids, and serratus anterior, supraspinatus,[11] infraspinatus, and teres minor. Weakness in the scapular stabilizing muscles allows lateral sliding of the scapula and results in anterior motion of the humeral head during abduction and external rotation, stressing the anterior joint and contributing to impingement.

Positional Dysfunction of Shoulder Region Muscles

- The shoulder internally rotates and adducts. In dysfunction, the humeral head migrates superiorly, leading to impingement. Also, this internally rotated position can cause the bicipital tendon to track abnormally against the medial side of the intertubercular groove, irritating it.[10]
- The anterior and posterior deltoid, and infraspinatus and teres minor tend to drop into an inferior torsion

- ***Treatment implications:*** To treat muscular dysfunction, it is important to treat the short and tight muscles first, as they have an inhibiting effect on their antagonists. Regarding the positional dysfunction, Lauren Berry, RPT, theorized that the humeral head migrates upward after an injury or cumulative stress to the rotator cuff muscles and that the anterior and posterior deltoid and the rotator cuff muscles tend to roll into an inferior torsion, parting the midline. The treatment implication is that the humerus must be mobilized inferiorly and that the anterior and posterior muscles about the head of the humerus must be lifted superiorly. As mentioned, it is also important to assign home exercises to strengthen the external rotators and thus help depress the humerus. It is also important to strengthen the scapular stabilizers, especially the lower trapezius, and the serratus anterior.

Shoulder Muscle Anatomy

See Muscle Table 6-1.

Muscular Actions of the Shoulder

See Table 6-2.

Muscular Actions of the Shoulder Girdle

See Table 6-3.

TABLE 6-1 ANATOMY OF THE MUSCLES OF THE SHOULDER

Scapular Stabilizing Muscles *(See Fig. 6-8)*

Muscle	*Origin*	*Insertion*
Trapezius	External occipital protuberance, spinous processes of C7 and all thoracic vertebrae.	Spine and acromion processes of scapula and lateral third of clavicle.
Rhomboid Minor	Spine of C7 and T1.	Vertebral border of the scapula, superior to spine of scapula.
Rhomboid Major	Spines of T2, 3, 4, 5.	Vertebral border of the scapula below the spine of the scapula.
Levator Scapula	Posterior tubercles of the transverse processes of C1, 2, 3, 4. This attachment site is significant as there are four major muscles that blend into each other at this point: the splenius cervicis, posterior scalene, longissimus capitis, and the levator.	Superior angle of the scapula and to the base of the spine of the scapula.
Serratus Anterior (see Fig. 6-9)	Surface of the upper nine ribs at the side of the chest.	Costal aspect of the whole length of the medial border of the scapula.

Rotator Cuff Muscles

Muscle	*Origin*	*Insertion*
Supraspinatus (See Fig. 6-10)	Supraspinous fossa of the scapula.	Superior facet of the greater tubercle of the humerus.
Infraspinatus	Lower margin of the spine of the scapula, infraspinatus fossa.	Middle facet of the greater tubercle of the humerus.
Teres Minor	Caudal section of the infraspinatus fossa and lateral margin of the scapula.	Lower facet of the greater tubercle of the humerus.

Action	Dysfunction
The upper fibers elevate the scapula, the lower fibers depress it, and the middle fibers retract the scapula.	The upper fibers tend to be tight and short, while the lower fibers tend to be weak and long, allowing the scapula to migrate headward, decreasing stability of the scapula for movement of the arm.
(Both major and minor) draws the scapula upward and medially; holds the scapula to the trunk along with the serratus anterior muscle; retracts the scapula along with the fibers of the middle trapezius.	Rhomboids tend to be weak, which contributes to a rounded shoulders posture.
Pulls the scapula upward and medially (along with the trapezius); if the scapula is fixed, pulls the neck laterally; acts similar to the deep fibers of the erector spinae in helping to prevent forward shear due to cervical lordosis.	Tends to be short and tight, but is in an eccentric contraction in the forward-head posture.
It is a major stabilizer of the scapula, holding the scapula against the rib cage. It performs abduction (protraction), i.e., draws the medial border of the scapula away from the vertebrae. Also provides upward rotation. The longer, lower fibers tend to draw the inferior angle of the scapula farther from the vertebrae, thus rotating the scapula upward slightly. It is the antagonist of the rhomboids.	The serratus tends to be weak, demonstated by winging of the scapula during the push-up test. Weakness of the serratus leads to instability of the scapula, contributing to impingement.

Action	Dysfunction
Initiates abduction by compressing the head of the humerus into the glenoid fossa, stabilizing the humerus, so that the deltoid can rotate the arm upward.	The most commonly injured muscle of the shoulder. It is predisposed to degeneration due to hypovascularity. This contributes to a poor repair after an injury, and also predisposes it to fatigue that develops from sustained contraction. This sustained contraction develops from an altered position in the glenohumeral joint from rounded-shoulder posture, or thoracic kyphosis. Tends to be weak, which prevents humeral head from being seated properly in the glenoid fossa during arm movements, leading to instability of the glenohumeral joint.
Lateral rotation; dynamic stabilizer of the glenohumeral joint by compressing and pulling the humeral head down during elevation of the arm. The infraspinatus is more active than the supraspinatus with the arm abducted 120-150°, which explains why it is commonly irritated with excessive overhead activities.	As with the supraspinatus, the infraspinatus has a diminished blood supply relative to the other muscles of the shoulder, and therefore is commonly involved clinically. The infraspinatus tends to be weak either due to irritation or injury, or due to inhibition from the short and tight subscapularis, which allows the humeral head to migrate superiorly, contributing to impingement syndrome.
Lateral rotation and adduction; dynamic stabilizer of the glenohumeral joint by compressing and pulling the humeral head down during elevation of the arm.	Tends to be weak, which allows the humeral head to migrate superiorly, contributing to impingement syndrome.

(Continued)

TABLE 6-1 ANATOMY OF THE MUSCLES OF THE SHOULDER—cont'd

Rotator Cuff Muscles—cont'd

Muscle	*Origin*	*Insertion*
Subscapularis (See Fig. 6-9)	Entire anterior surface of the subscapular fossa.	The lesser tubercle of the humerus, and the joint capsule.

Additional Muscles

Muscle	*Origin*	*Insertion*
Deltoid (See Fig. 6-9)	Outer third of the clavicle, border of the acromion, and lower edge of the spine of the scapula.	Deltoid tubercle on the lateral surface of the humerus.
Biceps Brachii	Short head from the coracoid process; long head from the supraglenoid tubercle above the glenoid cavity, and the superior labrum.	Radial tuberosity of the radius and bicipital aponeurosis, which is a broad sheet of fascia that blends with the deep fascia of the medial forearm.
Triceps Brachii (See Fig. 6-8)	Three heads: long head from the tubercle below the glenoid; lateral head from the lateral posterosuperior shaft of the humerus; and medial head from the posterior shaft of the humerus.	Olecranon process of the ulna at the elbow.
Teres Major	Lower third of the lateral border of the scapula.	Inner lip of the intertubercular groove of the humerus, and blends with the anterior joint capsule.
Coracobrachialis	Coracoid process of the scapula.	Medial surface of the humerus, in mid-shaft.
Pectoralis Major	Medial half of the anterior surface of the clavicle, anterior surface of the costal cartilages of the first six ribs, and adjoining portion of the sternum insertion: flat tendon 2″ or 3″ wide to outer lip of the intertubercular groove of the humerus, and blends with the anterior joint capsule.	
Pectoralis Minor	3rd to the 5th ribs.	Coracoid process of the scapula.
Subclavius	From the junction of bone and cartilage of the first rib.	Into the sulcus for the subclavius muscle on the lower surface of the clavicle.

Action	Dysfunction
Medial rotation and adduction; dynamic stabilizer of the glenohumeral joint by compressing and pulling the humeral head down during elevation of the arm.	Tends to be short and tight, leading to a sustained adduction and medial rotation of the arm, and contributing to inhibition of the external rotators.

Action	Dysfunction
The deltoid joins with the rotator cuff muscles to act as a force couple during elevation of the arm. The deltoid elevates the humerus, as the infraspinatus, teres minor, and subscapularis pull inward and down. As the origin of the deltoid is on the scapula, which raises during elevation of the arm, this provides an optimal length/tension relationship for the strongest muscle contraction throughout the range of motion. The anterior fibers provide flexion and medial rotation. The posterior fibers provide extension and lateral rotation.	According to Lauren Berry, R.P.T, the fascicles of the deltoid roll into an abnormal anterior and inferior torsion with a rounded-shoulders posture. This posture tends to promote adduction and internal rotation of the humerus, contributing to this torsion.
Primarily a flexor and supinator of the forearm. Long head is involved in abduction, the short head in adduction. The tendon of the long head is fixed, and the humerus moves relative to it. Also acts like a cuff muscle as a dynamic stabilizer of the humeral head during abduction, aiding in humeral depression. In fact, Cailliet states that the greatest downward glide of the humerus has been attributed to the mechanical force of the contracting bicipital tendon.	
Primarily an elbow extensor; also extends the arm and adducts it.	
Extension—draws the arm from the front horizontal position down to the side. Inward rotation—as it depresses, it rotates the humerus inward. Adduction—draws the arm from the side horizontal position down to the side and rotates inward as it adducts.	
Flexes and adducts arm.	
Contraction of both the sternal and clavicular heads produces adduction and medial rotation.	
Depression of shoulder girdle, so that the glenoid cavity faces more inferiorly; abduction of the scapula—draws the scapula forward and tends to tilt the lower border away from the ribs.	Tends to be tight and short, leading to rounded-shoulder posture, creating an excessive load on the thoracic extensors, leading to thoracic pain. A short, tight pectoralis minor can also compress the brachial plexus against the rib cage, leading to pain, numbing and tingling down the arm, a type of thoracic outlet syndrome.
Pulls the clavicle toward the sternum and so stabilizes the sternoclavicular joint.	

TABLE 6-2 MUSCULAR ACTIONS OF THE SHOULDER

- Flexion (1/2 as strong as extension[10]).
  - Deltoid (anterior)—also causes abduction and medial rotation
  - Pectoralis major (clavicular part)—also causes horizontal flexion, adduction, and medial rotation; and the sternal portion of the pectoralis causes shoulder adduction, horizontal flexion, and medial rotation
  - Biceps brachii—short head also assists in horizontal flexion and medial rotation; long head also assists in abduction; and biceps also flexes and supinates the elbow
  - Coracobrachialis—also assists in adduction
- Extension (2× stronger than flexion)
  - Teres major—also adducts and medially rotates
  - Latissimus dorsi—also adducts and medially rotates
  - Triceps (long head)—also adducts and extends the elbow
  - Deltoid (posterior part)—also abducts and laterally rotates
- Horizontal flexion (horizontal adduction)
  - Deltoid (anterior)
  - Pectoralis major
  - Coracobrachialis
  - Biceps (short head)
- Horizontal extension (horizontal abduction)
  - Deltoid (posterior)
  - Triceps (long head)
  - Latissimus dorsi
  - Teres major
- Adduction (3× stronger than abduction)
  - Pectoralis major
  - Latissimus dorsi
  - Teres major
  - Triceps brachii (long head)
- Abduction (1/3 as strong as adduction)

The primary muscles of abduction are the middle and anterior deltoid and the supraspinatus. There is debate in the literature as to the function of the supraspinatus. It is easiest to test the supraspinatus at 15° abduction and the deltoid at 90° abduction.

  - Deltoid—middle and anterior
  - Supraspinatus—may assist in lateral rotation
  - Biceps brachii (long head)
- Medial (internal) rotation (2× stronger than lateral rotation)
  - Subscapularis—also adducts
  - Pectoralis major
  - Teres major
  - Latissimus dorsi
- Lateral (external) rotation (1/2 as strong as medial rotation)
  - Infraspinatus—performs greater lateral rotation than the teres minor, deltoid (posterior), and supraspinatus combined
  - Teres minor
  - Deltoid (posterior)
  - Supraspinatus

TABLE 6-3 MUSCULAR ACTIONS OF THE SHOULDER GIRDLE

- Elevation
  - Levator scapula—also laterally flexes the neck
  - Trapezius (upper)
  - Rhomboid major—also retracts the shoulder girdle and rotates the scapula downward
  - Rhomboid minor—same as the rhomboid major
- Depression
  - Pectoralis minor—rotates the scapula downward and abducts it
  - Serratus anterior (lower)
  - Trapezius (lower)
- Protraction (abduction)—scapula moves away from spine
  - Serratus anterior—also rotates the scapula upward
  - Pectoralis major and minor
- Retraction (adduction)—scapula moves toward the spine
  - Rhomboid major
  - Rhomboid minor
  - Trapezius (middle)
- Upward rotation—the lower part of the scapula moves away from the spine, as in lifting the arm overhead
  - Serratus anterior
  - Trapezius (upper and lower)
- Downward rotation—in the anatomic position the scapula is almost to maximum downward rotation
  - Levator scapula
  - Rhomboid major
  - Rhomboid minor

Shoulder Dysfunction and Injury

FACTORS PREDISPOSING TO SHOULDER PAIN

- Instability of the glenohumeral joint
- Weakness in the scapular stabilizing muscles
- Previous injury, including previous dislocation of the glenohumeral joint or separation of the acromioclavicular joint
- Hypomobility of the cervical or thoracic spine, which limits full ROM of the glenohumeral joint
- Postural dysfunction, such as rounded-shoulders, FHP, thoracic kyphosis
- Muscle imbalances

DIFFERENTIATION OF SHOULDER PAIN

- Once you have ruled out pathology and pain from visceral diseases such as gallbladder irritation and cardiac problems (see the section "Contraindications to Massage Therapy: Red Flags" in Chapter 2, "Assessment & Technique), shoulder pain that hurts at night or pain that increases at night, indicates that there is an active inflammation. It may be caused by a rotator cuff tendinitis, bursitis, capsulitis, or nerve root irritation, called a cervical radiculitis (meaning, root inflammation).
- Dysfunctions and injuries of the cervical facets and disc degeneration commonly refer to the interscapular region. Scapular motion rarely increases the pain, but active motion examination of the cervical spine reveals limited motion that may refer pain to the scapular region at the end ranges. As mentioned in Chapter 5. "The Cervical Spine," irritation of a sensory nerve root elicits sharp pain, numbing, and tingling in a specific area of skin called a dermatome. The cervical dermatomes include the shoulder region. A myotome includes those muscles innervated by a specific motor nerve. Cervical nerves innervate the shoulder muscles. Irritation of the motor nerve elicits a deep aching in the corresponding muscle and a weakness in that muscle. The shoulder is also a referral site from the fascia, ligaments, and joint capsules in the cervical spine that are innervated by the same segmental nerve. This is called sclerotomal pain and is described as deep and aching and poorly localized.
- To help differentiate shoulder pain from pain that is being referred from the neck, there are certain guidelines:
  - pain originating from the neck is often elicited or increased from neck motion;
  - pain originating from the shoulder is typically elicited or increased from active shoulder motion and is relieved by rest;
  - isometric challenge of the muscles of the shoulder will be painful with a localized lesion in the shoulder;
  - often, a painless weakness occurs in the arm and shoulder muscles that has a motor nerve root problem from the cervical spine.
- Pain that originates in the glenohumeral joint is rarely felt at the joint, but over the lateral brachial region. This is explained by the concept of sclerotomal pain, because the tissue that is irritated is mainly the joint capsule and interweaving tendons of the rotator cuff.

COMMON DYSFUNCTIONS AND INJURIES OF THE SHOULDER

Supraspinatus Tendinitis

Tendinitis of the rotator cuff most commonly involves the supraspinatus tendon and then the infraspinatus.

- *Cause:* The supraspinatus tendon has a poor blood supply, and the demands of the muscle may overwhelm the nutritional supply.[5,12] This ischemia, or low oxygen in the tissue, combined with mechanical stress, leads to a breakdown of fibrils, which leads to an inflammatory response with the consequent scar tissue and potential calcium deposits. This lesion is common in swimmers, tennis players, and baseball pitchers, as well as clients who have poor posture. In the rounded-shoulders posture, the supraspinatus is under constant tension, leading to fatigue and degeneration.
- *Symptoms:* Clients experience a generalized, dull, toothache-like pain that refers to the lateral aspect of the humerus and that often is worse at night. Calcific tendinitis can cause a hot, burning pain.
- *Signs:* Tendinitis signs are a painful arc, which can be sharp, during active abduction between 60° and 120°, painful resisted abduction at 15°, positive supraspinatus test ("empty-can test").
- *Lesion Sites:* Tendinitis lesions occur at the tenoperiosteal junction and the musculotendinous junction. The tenoperiosteal junction will have the above signs, whereas the musculotendinous lesion will have a painful resisted abduction, but will not have a painful arc or impingement tests.
- *Treatment:* Perform transverse friction massage (TFM) at the tenoperiosteal junction, CR MET to reduce any sustained hypertonicity in the muscle belly, and manual release of the muscle belly and musculotendinous junction. Exercises should be assigned to strengthen the rotator cuff muscles.

Infraspinatus Tendinitis

- *Cause:* Infraspinatus tendinitis commonly occurs in musicians, carpenters, swimmers, tennis players, and others who perform activities that involve sustained abduction and external rotation and overhead activities. The infraspinatus is more active than the supraspinatus with the arm abducted 120° to 150°, which explains why it is commonly irritated with repetitive overhead activities.[6]

- *Symptoms:* Clients typically experience pain at the insertion over the posterior aspect of the greater tuberosity at the myotendinous junction, or anywhere in the belly of the muscle.
- *Signs:* Pain on resisted lateral rotation is a sign of infraspinatus tendinitis.
- *Treatment:* Perform CR MET to strengthen the infraspinatus, which is typically weak, and PIR MET to lengthen the subscapularis; perform manual release to lift the fibers superiorly, as the fibers are typically in a sustained inferior torsion.

Subscapularis Tendinitis

- *Cause:* Causes of subscapularis tendinitis are activities involving repetitive or excessive internal rotation and adduction, as in carpentry, or cleaning; or in throwing or racquet sports.
- *Symptoms:* Clients typically experience pain at the lesser tuberosity.
- *Signs:* Pain on resisted medial rotation is a sign of subscapularis tendinitis as are: painful arc—lesion at upper site of insertion point; and painful passive horizontal adduction—as it is pinched against the coracoid process.
- *Treatment:* Perform PIR MET to lengthen the subscapularis, which is typically short; perform manual release to broaden, hydrate, and reset the fibers.

Adhesive Capsulitis (Frozen Shoulder)

- *Cause:* Adhesive capsulitis is an inflammatory lesion of the anterior and inferior portion of the glenohumeral joint capsule that leads to its thickening and shortening. There is no known cause. It affects women more than men, and the middle-aged and elderly more than younger clients. Hertling and Kessler[5] theorize that thoracic kyphosis and the consequent alteration in the scapulohumeral alignment is the predisposing factor.[5]
- *Symptoms:* Adhesive capsulitis symptoms develop in three stages.[7] The ***first stage*** is a gradual onset of stiffness in the shoulder that elicits pain in the lateral brachial region with movement. The ***second stage*** may be a constant, dull ache, present at night or painful only with movement. The pain may disturb the client's sleep, especially when the client rolls onto that shoulder, and the pain may radiate to the elbow. The ***third*** stage is a much more pronounced stiffness and minimal pain at rest. Also, muscles may atrophy.
- *Signs:* In the ***first stage,*** active and passive lateral rotation may be limited, but this movement is usually painless. Active and passive abduction is the next most limited motion. A thick, capsular end feel with passive lateral rotation and abduction is present. Resisted movements are not painful. In the ***second stage,*** active and passive movements may be limited and painful, but resisted movements are painless. In the ***third stage,*** active and passive motion may be restricted in all planes and painful only at the end ranges of movement.
- *Treatment:* Inferior glide of the humerus is helpful in relieving muscle spasms. PIR MET is performed next to increase lateral rotation. Finally, PIR or eccentric MET is used to increase elevation, first in the sagittal plane, then in the scapular plane, and finally in the coronal plane. If indicated, provide instruction in postural awareness, including retracting and depressing the scapula and engaging the lower and middle trapezius. Encourage the client to use the arm as much as possible within comfortable limits to minimize disuse atrophy.

Impingement Syndrome

- *Cause:* Impingement syndrome is defined as a compromise of the space between the coracoacromial arch and the proximal humerus. The rotator cuff, subacromial bursa, and biceps tendon are compressed between the humeral head and the acromion or coracoacromial ligament. Impingement syndrome has structural and functional causes. Structural causes include thickening of the rotator cuff tendons, inflamed bursa, and hooked acromion. Functional causes include rotator cuff weakness, scapular instability, thoracic kyphosis, and muscle imbalance. Typically, the client presents with the upper crossed syndrome, which includes tight upper trapezius and levator scapula, weakness in the lower trapezius, tight internal rotators and weak external rotators. Neer[13] describes three stages: an initial overuse syndrome; the development of thickening and fibrosis; and the development of bony changes, including spurs.
- *Symptoms:* Clients usually experience a gradual onset of pain at the anterior acromion or greater tuberosity, but this pain may refer down the C5 to C6 sclerotomes.[5] It also may present as sharp twinges, especially with abduction.
- *Signs:* Painful arc of abduction between 90° and 120° and a positive Neer's impingement test are signs of impingement syndrome.
- *Treatment:* The principle treatment is strengthening of the rotator cuff muscles. CR MET may be

applied to these muscles to help strengthen (facilitate) them and increase sensory awareness. Perform manual release of any fibrosis palpated in the cuff tendons and the coracoacromial ligament. It is important that the client has a home exercise program in cuff strengthening.

Instability Syndrome of the Glenohumeral Joint

- *Cause:* Instability may result from rotator cuff weakness; lack of scapular stabilization; damage to the anterior capsule, glenohumeral ligament, and glenoid labrum. Instabilities are classified as traumatic, nontraumatic, and acquired. Traumatic usually involves a history of shoulder dislocation or rotator cuff injury, such as a fall on an outstretched hand. Nontraumatic causes involve rotator cuff weakness. Acquired instability describes either congenital laxity in the ligaments or poor treatment outcome after a dislocation.[2]
- *Symptoms:* Clients experience diffuse pain in the shoulder region with the feeling of the shoulder "going out."
- *Signs:* A positive relocation test indicates glenohumeral joint instability syndrome.
- *Treatment:* Instability often involves sustained contraction in the pectoralis minor and subscapularis, pulling the humerus forward, and weakness in the external rotators. Although the client needs active care to strengthen the rotator cuff, it is often helpful to perform CR MET on the pectoralis minor and subscapularis to reduce any hypertonicity and on the external rotators to facilitate them and increase the sensory awareness in these muscles. As the shoulder is too loose, it is important to work selectively on the tighter muscles rather than creating a generalized release in the shoulder region.

Bicipital Tendinitis

- *Cause:* Bicipital tendinitis is usually the result of repetitive microtrauma as a result of overhead activities that involve flexion and internal rotation, such as swimming, tennis, or throwing. As the long head attaches to the supraglenoid labrum, an acute or cumulative trauma to the biceps can tear the labrum.
- *Symptoms:* Clients experience pain over the anterior aspect of the humerus at the bicipital groove (tenosynovitis) and at the superior labrum with insertional tendinitis of the long head.
- *Signs:* Pain on resisted forward flexion of the shoulder with the elbow extended and the forearm supinated (Speed's test) and pain on resisted supination.
- *Treatment:* Perform CR MET to reduce any sustained hypertonicity and perform manual release of the bicipital groove and attachment points, if indicated by palpation.

Subacromial (Subdeltoid) Bursitis

- *Cause:* Excessive overhead activities can irritate the bursa, leading to an acute bursitis in which the bursa swells. This is a rare condition. Typically, the supraspinatus tendon is involved. Over time, calcific deposits from this tendon, which lies under the bursa, may irritate or even rupture the bursa.[5]
- *Symptoms:* Clients experience the following symptoms with acute or chronic subacromial bursitis:
  - Acute: Pain can be excruciating, and the patient loses the ability to move the arm.
  - Chronic: Pain can be diffuse and achy over the proximal humerus and is often painful at night.
- *Signs:* Acute and chronic subacromial bursitis signs are as follows:
  - Acute: All active ROM is painful. Heat and swelling may be palpable. Resisted abduction is painful. To passive motion testing there is an empty end-feel; that is, the client reports pain, but you do not feel the tension barrier in the tissue.
  - Chronic: A painful arc in the middle of active and passive abduction. Resisted movements are usually painful.
- *Treatment:* Perform manual draining of the bursa, but use extreme caution. If the bursitis is chronic, assess the rotator cuff muscles. Often an underlying tendinitis in the supraspinatus is found, and any fibrosis at the tenoperiosteal junction must be released.

Acromioclavicular Joint Sprain

- *Cause:* AC joint sprain is usually a traumatic event, such as a fall on an outstretched hand or a direct fall onto the shoulder.
- *Symptoms:* Clients experience well-localized pain over the AC joint.
- *Signs:* Pain at the AC joint from 90° to the end range of active abduction and pain at the AC joint on passive horizontal adduction are signs of AC joint sprain.
- *Treatment:* Perform TFM to the AC ligaments.

Suprascapular Nerve Entrapment

- *Symptoms:* Clients experience pain at the posterolateral edge of the spine of the scapula or in the lateral aspect of the suprascapular notch. The pain may radiate down the arm.
- *Signs:* Weakness without pain to resisted tests of supraspinatus and infraspinatus, possible pain at the posterolateral aspect of the scapula with overpressure in passive adduction of the arm, and pain after application of digital pressure on the nerve in the suprascapular or the spinoglenoid notch are signs of suprascapular nerve entrapment.

Costoclavicular Syndrome (Part of Thoracic Outlet Syndrome)

- *Cause:* Costoclavicular syndrome is defined as a compromise of the space between the clavicle and the first rib. It may be caused by a rounded-shoulders posture or previous trauma to the clavicle, AC joint, or glenohumeral joint, which lead to fibrous adhesions in the costoclavicular space.
- *Symptoms:* Clients experience a generalized pain, numbing, or tingling down the arm, especially to the ulnar border.
- *Signs:* A positive elevated-arm stress test (EAST) (see Cervical Assessment section, Chapter 5).
- *Treatment:* Perform manual release of the supra- and infraclavicular spaces and postural correction, including strengthening the lower trapezius.

Pectoralis Minor Syndrome (Part of Thoracic Outlet Syndrome)

- *Cause:* Pectoralis minor syndrome is caused by sustained contraction of the pectoralis minor, which causes forward depression of the coracoid process, narrowing the space between the pectoralis minor and the rib cage, compressing the brachial plexus.
- *Symptoms:* Clients experience generalized pain, numbing, or tingling down the arm, especially to the ulnar border.
- *Signs:* Symptoms are elicited with the application of digital pressure over the pectoralis minor and with the EAST test (see Cervical Assessment, Chapter 5).
- *Treatment:* Perform CR or PIR MET to reduce the hypertonicity of the muscle and to lengthen it. Also perform manual release to the muscle in a superior direction, as the pectoralis minor rolls into a sustained inferior torsion in dysfunction.

Shoulder Assessment

HISTORY QUESTIONS SPECIFIC TO SHOULDER PAIN

- Where is the pain? What is the quality of the pain?
  - Strains of the rotator cuff are usually a dull ache that worsens at night, referred to the anterior and lateral shoulder, often down to the deltoid tuberosity. Shoulder pain from emotional stress manifests as a dull pain in the upper trapezius and levator muscles. Persistent gripping pain in the arm and elbow—even at rest and especially if there is also numbing and tingling in the hands—may be a nerve root irritation from the cervical spine. An acute onset of throbbing pain that worsens at night indicates an acute bursitis. Chronic, severe, gripping pain that worsens at night needs a referral to a doctor.
- Is there a loss of motion in the arm?
  - Rotator cuff injuries are most inhibited in abduction. Impingement syndrome is reproduced with active flexion with the arm in medial rotation. Adhesive capsulitis can present as a drastic loss of external rotation and abduction, with or without pain. Acute bursitis presents as a drastic loss of motion with pain, especially at night.

OBSERVATION: CLIENT STANDING

Anterior View

- Are the clavicles level? Shoulder height even? The shoulder often is elevated in rotator cuff and frozen shoulder conditions. The shoulder or clavicle is normally lower on the dominant side. Look for redness, swelling, and atrophy.
- Notice if there is a smooth contour to the area of the lateral shoulder or the clavicle lies superior to the acromion at the AC joint. This is called a step deformity and indicates a previous AC separation.
- Is there a sulcus sign (i.e., an indentation below the acromion) resulting from a flattening of the normally round deltoid? This indicates an instability of the glenohumeral joint, a weak deltoid muscle, or an inferior subluxation.

Posterior View

- Is there scapular winging? If the inferior angle (or angles) of the scapula juts away from the thoracic wall, there may be a loss of scapular stabilization. Winging of the scapula in the resting position on the arm may be caused by scoliosis. It may also result from muscular injury; inhibition (weakness) of the scapular stabilizers, which are tested below (see "Scapular Stabilization Test"); or a nerve injury.

MOTION ASSESSMENT

Active Movements: Observe the ROM and ask the client if the motion is painful. There may be an arc of pain; that is, there is pain during one part of the movement and then the pain disappears while the client continues the motion. If the motion is painful, ask the client to describe the location and quality of the pain. If the client knows what the painful motions are, ask him or her to perform these motions last.

Scapular Stabilization Test

- *Position:* Have the client stand at arm's distance from the wall and place his or her hands on the wall at shoulder level. Stand behind the client (Fig. 6-11).
- *Action:* Ask the client to lean into the wall to perform a push-up against the wall.
- *Observation:* When performing the push-up, the inferior angle of the scapula should not wing off of the thoracic cage, and the medial borders of the scapula should not move more than approximately an inch. Winging indicates a weak serratus anterior or an injury to the long thoracic nerve. Excessive movement of the scapula indicates weakness of scapular stabilizers, including the serratus anterior, middle trapezius, or rhomboids.

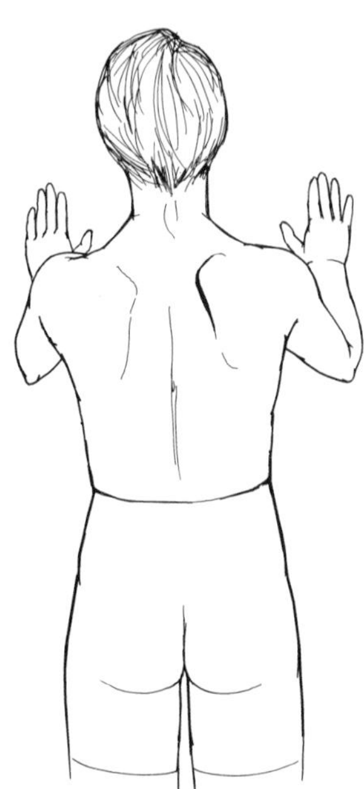

Figure 6-11. Scapular stabilization test. Notice the slight winging of the right scapula, indicating a slight weakness of the serratus anterior.

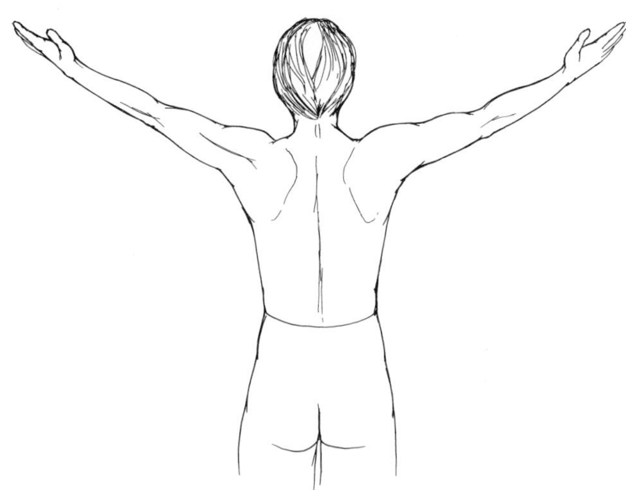

Figure 6-12. Shoulder abduction test. Notice if the top of the shoulder hikes toward the ear as the arm is abducted. This would indicate a tight upper trapezius and a weak lower trapezius.

Abduction

- *Position:* Client stands with his or her back to you (Fig. 6-12).
- *Action:* Instruct the client to rotate his arms externally by turning the palms out. Then have the client raise his or her arms, trying to touch the palms together overhead.
- *Observation:* Notice if the top of the shoulder hikes upward at the beginning of the motion. This hiking typically indicates that there is a tight and short upper trapezius and levator scapula and a weak lower trapezius, serratus anterior, and supraspinatus. This muscular imbalance predisposes to impingement syndrome. Also notice if the client needs to move in the scapular plane; that is, approximately 30° of forward flexion. This position is assumed with acute and chronic problems. An arc of pain indicates supraspinatus tendinitis, subacromial bursitis, calcific deposits, or an AC joint irritation. Abduction is the best motion to indicate a rotator cuff tear. It may be impossible to perform the motion beyond 90° if there is a significant tear.

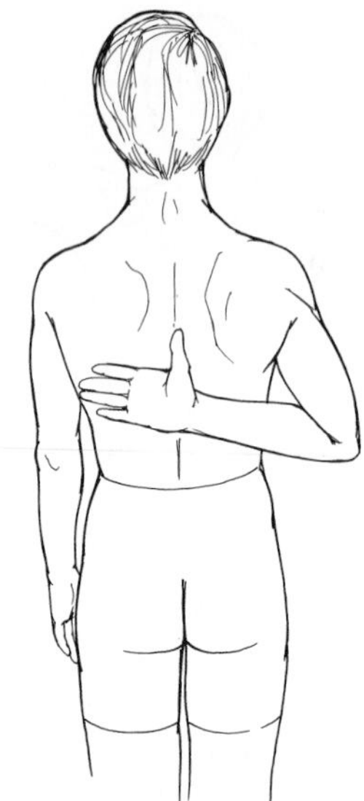

Figure 6-13. Active medial rotation. Notice how far up the spine the client can reach. Compare sides.

Medial Rotation

- ☐ ***Position:*** Client stands with his or her back to you (Fig. 6-13).
- ☐ ***Action:*** Beginning with the non-involved side, ask the client to reach his or her hand up the back and try to touch the scapula. Measure the vertebral level that the fingertips or thumb touches. If measuring with the thumb, have the client place the thumb in the "hitch hiking" position. Compare with the other side.
- ☐ ***Observation:*** It is normal to be able to reach to approximately T5 to T10. Client may only be able to reach the greater trochanter or sacrum on one side. This motion elicits pain in the anterior shoulder with an impingement syndrome, as you are forcing the greater tuberosity against the coracoacromial ligament. If the movement is not painful, have the client attempt the "lift-off" test, lifting the hand off the back. This tests the strength of the subscapularis.

Flexion with Internal Rotation (Neer's Impingement Test)

- ☐ ***Position:*** Client faces you and medially rotates the arm so that the thumb faces posteriorly.
- ☐ ***Action:*** Ask the client to raise both arms up to the sides of the head. The thumb now faces anteriorly.
- ☐ ***Observation:*** The range is normally approximately 170° to 180°. With the arm medially rotated, the supraspinatus, which attaches to the greater tuberosity, needs to slide under the coracoacromial ligament. If there is irritation, swelling, or scarring of the tendon, it impinges against this ligament.

Lateral Rotation

- ☐ ***Position:*** Client faces you (Fig. 6-14).
- ☐ ***Action:*** There are two actions. Ask the client to clasp his or her hands behind the head, with elbows pulled as far back as possible. If this is difficult, have the client place his or her arms at her sides, with the elbows at 90°, and laterally rotate the arms.
- ☐ ***Observation:*** The first motion allows for easy comparison of both sides. It combines elevation and external rotation, a position of function for daily activities, such as getting dressed. In the second motion, the normal range is approximately 75° to 90°. Compare both sides. Lateral rotation is the first motion to be lost in adhesive capsulitis.

Horizontal Flexion (Adduction)

- ☐ ***Position:*** Client faces you.
- ☐ ***Action:*** Client is instructed to elevate his or her arm to 90° and move the arm across the front of the body, attempting to place the hand on the opposite shoulder.

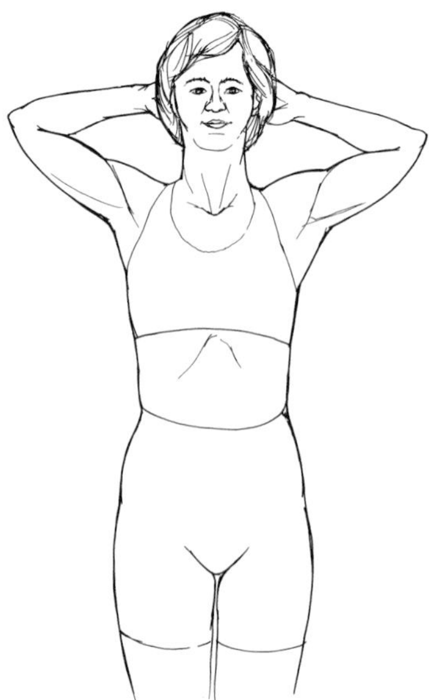

Figure 6-14. Lateral rotation with abduction performed bilaterally is an easy way to compare the ROM of both sides at the same time.

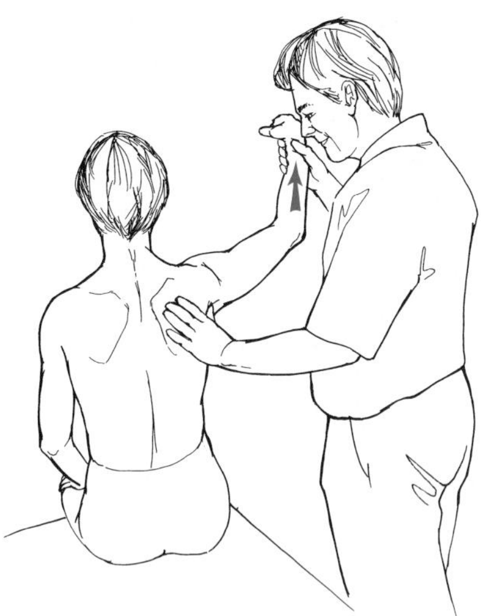

Figure 6-15. Passive abduction. Therapist places one hand on the scapula to detect when it moves. If the scapula moves before approximately 90° of abduction, then adhesion in the joint capsule is indicated.

- ***Observation:*** If there is pain at the top of the shoulder, it implicates the AC joint; pain at the posterior shoulder implicates the posterior-inferior capsule; anterior joint pain may be the anterior labrum, subcoracoid bursa, or the subscapularis tendon. If there is anterior joint pain, differentiate bursitis from tendinitis by first performing the same movement passively, which would typically be painful with bursitis, but not tendinitis. Isometrically challenge the subscapularis, which may be painful with tendinitis, but not bursitis.

Passive Movements

Passive movements are performed for those movements that do not have full and pain-free active ROM. Note the range, pain, arc of pain, pain with overpressure, and end-feel. The following passive shoulder movements are performed with the client sitting.

Abduction

- ***Position:*** Stand to one side of the client. Hold the lower scapula with your thumb and index finger with one hand and the distal forearm with your other hand (Fig. 6-15).
- ***Action:*** Slowly abduct the client's arm until the resistance barrier is met or until the arm is against the client's head, and feel for when the scapula begins to move.
- ***Observation:*** Normally, the range is approximately 170° to 180°. The scapula should not move until 90° of abduction. If there are adhesions of the joint capsule, anchoring the scapula to the humerus, the scapula begins moving before 90°. If there is no pain in passive abduction and active abduction was painful, it indicates a tendinitis of the rotator cuff, typically the supraspinatus. If there is pain in passive abduction before there is tissue tension, this is the "empty" end-feel of bursitis, in this case, of the subacromial bursa.

Lateral Rotation

- ***Position:*** Stand to one side of the client and place one hand on the client's elbow to stabilize it against his or her body and the other hand on the client's distal forearm, holding it.
- ***Action:*** Slowly pull the forearm laterally, which laterally rotates the arm.
- ***Observation:*** Lateral ROM is limited in adhesive capsulitis, as the anterior capsule has developed fibrotic adhesions. The end feel is thick and leathery. It may or may not be painful.

Circumduction

- ***Position:*** Stand behind and to one side of the client. Place one hand on the top of the glenohumeral joint and hold the distal forearm with the other hand (Fig. 6-16).

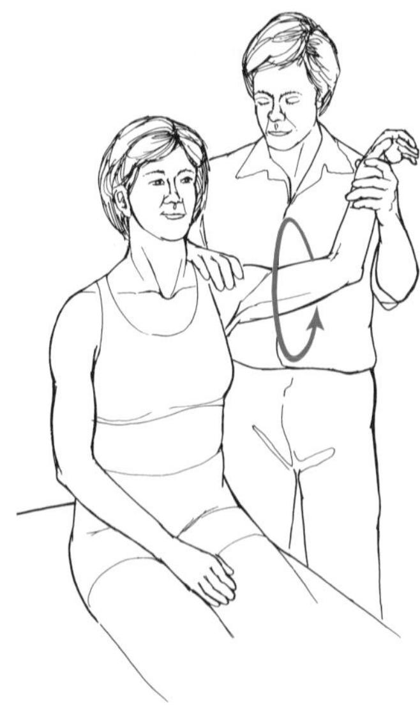

Figure 6-16. Passive circumduction. This test is Lauren Berry's, RPT, preferred method to determine if the shoulder complaint is muscular, capsular, or articular.

- *Action:* Slowly draw the arm backwards to begin a circumduction motion. Move the arm in a swimming motion.
- *Observation:* Circumduction motion helps differentiate joint, muscle, and ligament lesions. There will be a loose feel or clunking with joint instability. You will feel crepitus (grinding sounds) with calcific deposits or arthrosis. There is a thickened feel and limited range with capsular lesions. With muscle hypertonicity, fascicular torsion, and soft tissue misalignment, there is a "cogwheel" pattern (i.e., there are resistances and dips in an otherwise smooth motion). Over time you can learn to feel the subtleties of resistance under your hand.

Isometric Tests

The client should be able to provide strong resistance to the following tests. Note if the client has difficulty in providing resistance, ask if the resisted action is painful. If it is painful, ask about the location and quality of pain. Remember that the shoulder and arm are common referral sites for neck problems. Painless weakness may be indicative of a nerve-root problem. If the client remains weak after treatment, he or she needs a referral to a chiropractor or an osteopath. All of the following muscles are innervated by C5 and C6.

Middle Deltoid

- *Position:* The client's arm is placed at 90° of abduction, with the elbow flexed 90° (Fig. 6-17).
- *Action:* Instruct the client to resist as you press down on his or her elbow.

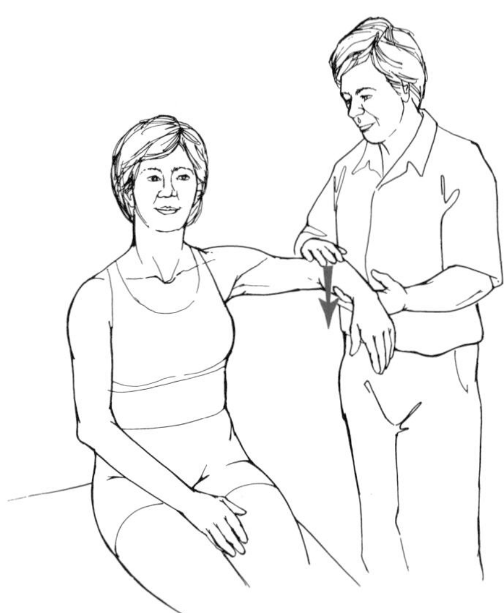

Figure 6-17. Isometric test for the middle deltoid.

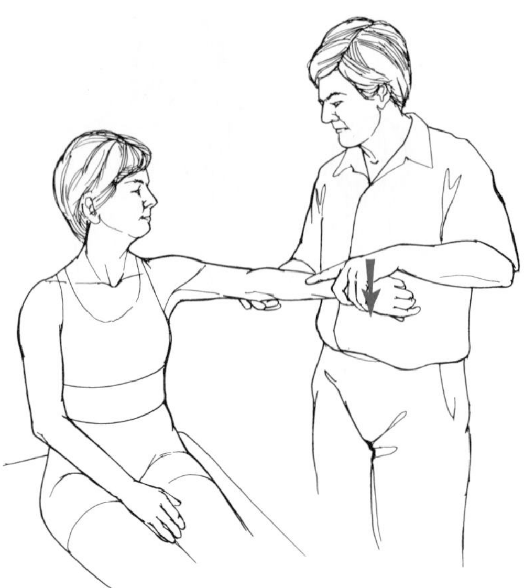

Figure 6-18. "Empty-can" test to isolate the supraspinatus.

- *Observation:* Pain indicates irritation or injury in the middle deltoid.

Supraspinatus (Empty-Can Test)

- *Position:* The client's arm is abducted 90°, 30° forward flexion, and maximally internally rotated, that is, with the thumb turned down (Fig. 6-18).
- *Action:* Press down on the distal forearm.
- *Observation:* The empty-can test isolates the action to the supraspinatus, and pain at the lateral and anterior shoulder indicates irritation, injury, or scarring of the supraspinatus tendon.

Long Head of Biceps (Speed's Test)

- *Position:* The client's arm is flexed 30° in the scapular plane, with the elbow extended and the forearm supinated (Fig. 6-19).
- *Action:* Press down on the client's forearm.
- *Observation:* Pain in the anterior humerus implicates the long head of the biceps.

Resisted Lateral Rotation

- *Position:* The client's arm is at his or her side, with the elbow flexed to 90°. Place one hand on the client's elbow to stabilize it and the other at the distal forearm.
- *Action:* Instruct the client to resist as you press medially on the client's distal forearm.
- *Observation:* Pain at the posterior humerus indicates involvement of the infraspinatus and the teres minor.

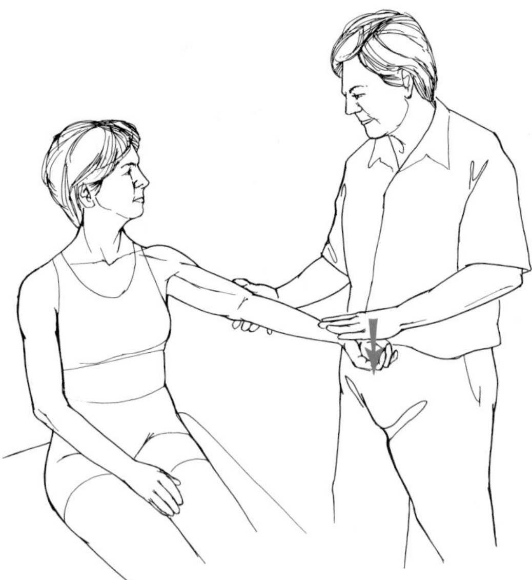

Figure 6-19. Speed's test for the long head of the biceps.

ADDITIONAL TEST

Relocation Test

- *Intention:* The relocation test is performed to help ensure the normal position of the humeral head in the glenoid and to assess instability (Fig. 6-20).
- *Position:* The client is supine with his or her arm at approximately 90° of abduction and elbow flexed to 90°. Hold the distal forearm with one hand and place the palm of the other hand over the head of the humerus.

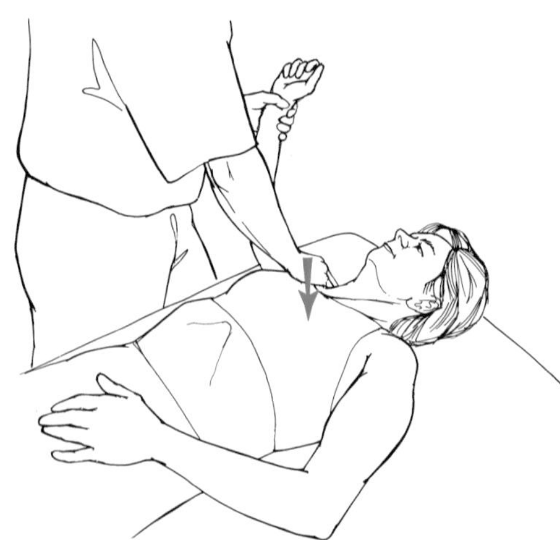

Figure 6-20. Relocation test. The humerus is often sitting slightly anterior in the glenoid fossa owing to rounded-shoulders posture or previous injury. This test ensures that the humerus is seated properly.

- *Action:* Gently push the humeral head posteriorly, while stabilizing the arm with your other hand.
- *Observation:* The typical positional dysfunction of the head of the humerus is a forward position. Mobilizing the head of the humerus posteriorly in this position helps reestablish its normal position. Excessive movement of the humeral head indicates joint instability.

Techniques

MUSCLE ENERGY TECHNIQUE

The internal rotators are typically short and tight, and the external rotators are weak and long. We will first assess their length. Next we will assess and treat the muscles that tend to be tight that were described in the upper crossed syndrome of Janda. In the muscles of the shoulder in the upper crossed syndrome, we usually find the pectoralis major and minor and subscapularis short and tight. Next, we will assess and facilitate the muscles of the rotator cuff that tend to be weak, the supraspinatus, infraspinatus, and teres minor.

Assessment of Muscle Length and of Glenohumeral Joint Passive Range of Motion

1. Assessment of the Range of Motion of Glenohumeral Joint Lateral Rotation and of the Medial Rotator Length

- *Intention:* For full external rotation, there must be normal length in the medial rotators, the pectoralis major, the latissimus, the teres major, and the subscapularis (Fig. 6-21).
- *Position:* Client is supine, with the knees flexed and the feet on the table and with the low back flat on the table. Client then rests his or her arm at shoulder level (90° abduction) and lowers the

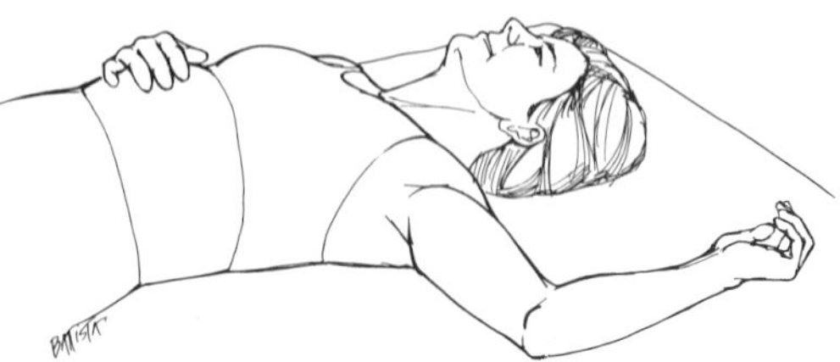

Figure 6-21. Assessment of the ROM of glenohumeral joint in lateral rotation and of the medial rotator length.

forearm toward the head of the table without lifting the low back off the table.

- *Observation:* The normal ROM allows the forearm to lie flat on the table (90° of external rotation). This motion is drastically reduced in frozen shoulder and slightly reduced with shortness on the medial rotators.

2. Assessment of the Range of Motion of the Glenohumeral Joint in Medial Rotation and of the Lateral Rotator Length

- *Intention:* For full internal rotation, there must be normal length in the lateral rotators, teres minor, infraspinatus, and posterior deltoid.
- *Position:* Client is supine, with the knees flexed and the feet on the table and with the low back flat on the table. Client then rests his or her arm at shoulder level (90° abduction) and lowers the forearm toward the foot of the table without lifting the low back off the table.
- *Stabilization:* Hold the shoulder down to prevent the shoulder from moving forward.
- *Observation:* The normal range of medial rotation is 70° (i.e., for the forearm to be 20° from the table). This motion may be reduced in impingement syndrome, bicipital tendinitis, and supraspinatus tendinitis.

Contract-Relax and Postisometric Relaxation Techniques

3. Contract-Relax and Postisometric Relaxation Muscle Energy Technique for the Medial Rotators of the Shoulder

- *Intention:* The goal is to relax the medial rotators, to increase the strength of the medial rotators if they test weak, and to increase their length if they were found short by the previous assessment (Fig. 6-22).
- *Position:* Client is supine, with the knees flexed and the feet on the table and with the low back flat on the table. Client then rests his or her arm at shoulder level (90° abduction) and lowers the forearm into lateral rotation as far to the table as comfortable, without lifting the low back off the table.
- *Stabilization:* Hold the shoulder down at the glenohumeral joint, to prevent the shoulder from moving forward. As the arm is being moved into lateral rotation, clients with a history of dislocation may feel apprehensive. It is critical that you prevent the humeral head from moving anteriorly while you place the arm in lateral rotation.

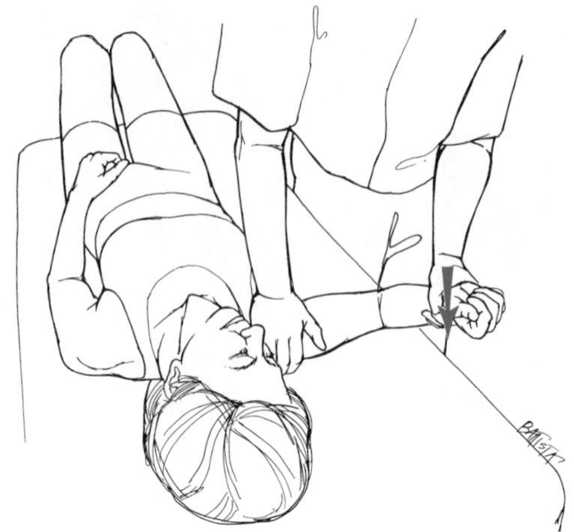

Figure 6-22. CR and PIR MET of the shoulder medial rotators.

- *Action:* To release the medial rotators, have the client resist as you attempt to press into further lateral rotation for approximately 5 seconds on the distal forearm. Relax and repeat to reduce hypertonicity. To lengthen the muscle, move the arm into further lateral rotation, and have client resist again for 5 seconds. Repeat three to five times.

4. Contract-Relax and Postisometric Relaxation Muscle Energy Technique of the Lateral Rotators of the Shoulder

- *Intention:* The goal is to relax tight lateral rotators, to increase the strength of the lateral rotators if they test weak, and to increase the length of these muscles if they were found short by the previous assessment (Fig. 6-23).
- *Position:* Client is supine, with the knees flexed and the feet on the table and with the low back flat on the table. Client then rests his or her arm at shoulder level (90° abduction) and lowers the forearm into medial rotation as far to the table as comfortable, without lifting the low back off the table.
- *Stabilization:* Hold the shoulder down at the glenohumeral joint, to prevent the shoulder from moving forward.
- *Action:* Have the client resist as you attempt to press into further medial rotation on the distal forearm for approximately 5 seconds. Relax and repeat to reduce hypertonicity. To lengthen the muscle, move the arm into further medial rotation and have the client resist again for 5 seconds. Repeat three to five times.

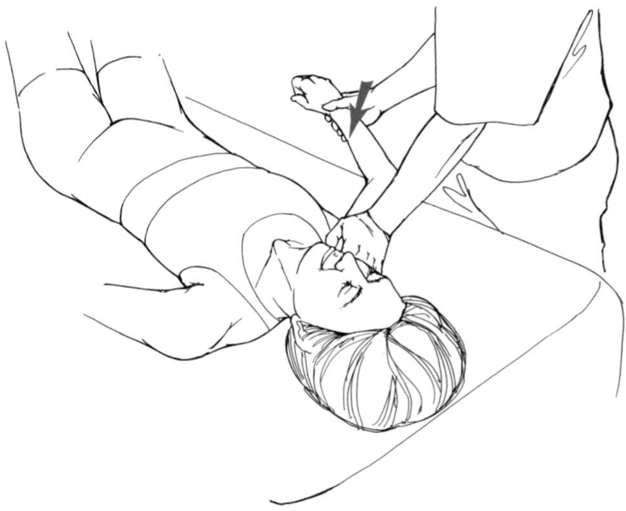

Figure 6-23. CR and PIR MET of the shoulder lateral rotators.

5. Contract-Relax and Reciprocal Inhibition Muscle Energy Technique in the Side-Lying Position for the Posterior Scapular Muscles

- *Intention:* The goal is to reduce the hypertonicity of the infraspinatus, teres minor, and teres major with the client in a position that allows for massage of the region after the MET (Fig. 6-24).
- *Position:* Client is in the side-lying position. Place the client's arm on the side of his or her body with the elbow flexed to 90°. Place one hand on the client's elbow to stabilize the arm and the other hand on the distal forearm.
- *Action:* Have the client resist as you press down on the distal forearm for 5 seconds. To engage the teres major, which is an internal rotator of the arm, have the client resist as you pull up on the distal forearm for 5 seconds. Repeat these two METs several times and throughout your session as needed.

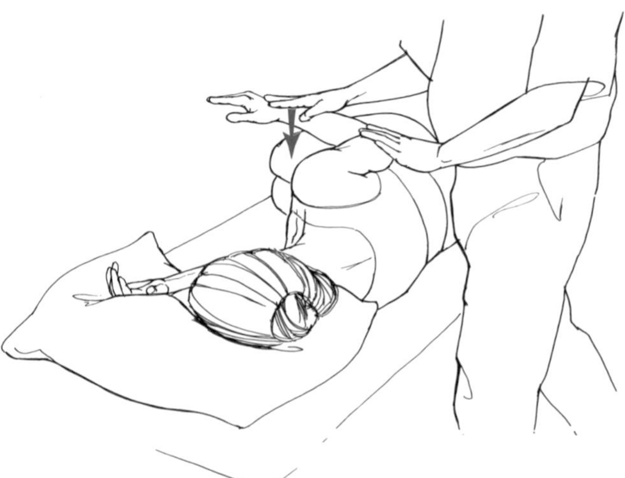

Figure 6-24. Side-lying position CR and RI MET for the posterior scapular muscles.

6. Contract-Relax Muscle Energy Technique for the Pectoralis Major

- *Intention:* The goal is to reduce hypertonicity with CR-MET if the pectoralis major palpates as tight (Fig. 6-25).
- *Position:* Client is supine with knees bent, feet on the table. Place the client's arm in 90° of flexion.
- *Action:* Hold the client's distal forearm and have the client resist as you attempt to pull the arm away from the body (abduction) for approximately 5 seconds. Have the client relax, and then repeat the procedure. To reciprocally inhibit the pectoralis major, have the client resist as you press the arm toward the body.

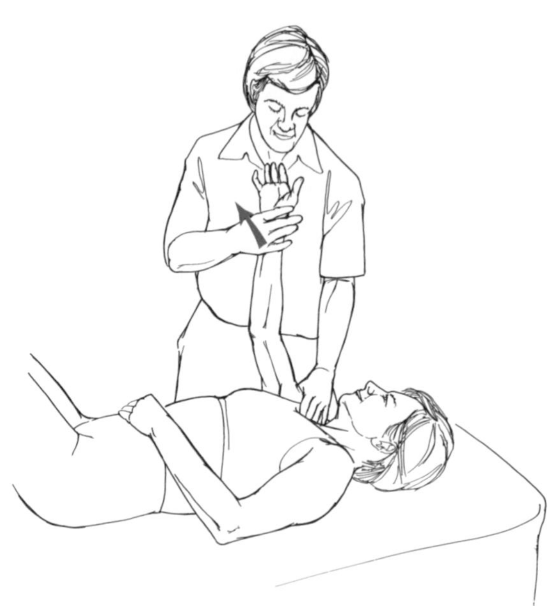

Figure 6-25. CR MET for the pectoralis major.

7. Postisometric Relaxation Muscle Energy Technique for the Pectoralis Major

- *Intention:* The intention is to lengthen the pectoralis major using PIR MET (Fig. 6-26).
- *Position:* Client is supine with the knees bent, feet on the table. To lengthen the upper fibers, place the client's arm at 90° of abduction, and to lengthen the lower fibers, place the arm at 135° of abduction.
- *Stabilization:* Place one hand on the opposite clavicle when working with the upper fibers; place

one hand on the glenohumeral joint on the same side when working with the lower fibers.

- *Action:* To lengthen the upper fibers, hold the client's distal forearm and slowly move the arm to its tension barrier. Have the client resist as you press the arm toward the floor. Repeat this series until the arm can hang over the side of the table at 90° abduction.

  For the lower fibers, move the arm overhead at approximately 135° abduction to its tension barrier and have the client resist as you press the arm toward the floor. Relax, move the arm to a new length, and repeat.

CAUTION: If the stretch of this muscle causes numbing and tingling, you are stretching the brachial plexus and need to perform CR technique without the stretch.

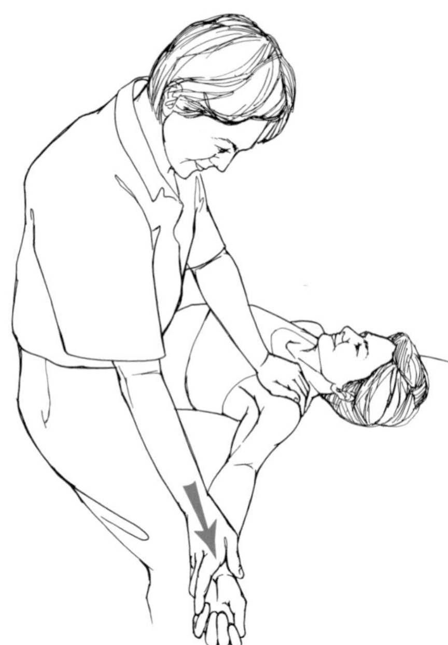

Figure 6-26. PIR MET of the pectoralis major.

8. Contract-Relax Muscle Energy Technique of the Pectoralis Minor

- *Intention:* The intention is to relax the pectoralis minor (Fig. 6-27).
- *Position:* Client is supine with the knees bent, feet on the table. Place the palm of one hand over the coracoid process and place the other hand under the posterior humerus. Lift the shoulder forward and medially, bringing the origin and insertion of the pectoralis minor toward each other.
- *Action:* Have the client resist as you press on the coracoid process, attempting to press it back to the table. Hold for approximately 5 seconds, relax, and repeat. RI is to place the shoulder back on the table and have the client resist as you attempt to lift the scapula off the table.

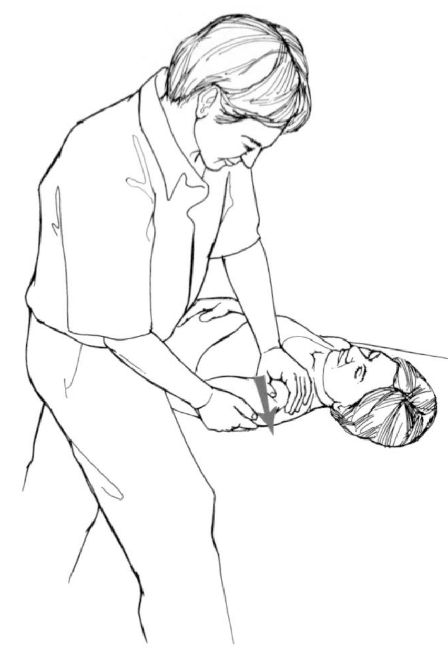

Figure 6-27. CR MET of the pectoralis minor.

9. Contract-Relax Muscle Energy Technique of the Supraspinatus

- *Intention:* The intention is to relax the supraspinatus.
- *Position:* Client is supine, with his or her arms at the sides. Bring one arm away from the client's body approximately 6 inches, to approximately 15° abduction. Place one hand on the client's distal forearm and the other hand on the belly of the supraspinatus in the supraspinous fossa of the scapula.
- *Action:* Have the client resist as you press toward the client's body. Hold for 5 seconds, relax, and repeat. Tap on the belly of the muscle and say "feel this muscle working" to bring sensory awareness to the muscle. RI is to have the client resist as you attempt to pull the arm away from the body.

10. Postisometric Relaxation Muscle Energy Technique for the Supraspinatus

- *Intention:* The intention is to lengthen the connective tissue of the supraspinatus. This procedure is for chronic conditions only (Fig. 6-28).
- *Position:* Client is sitting and places one hand on his or her low back. Hold one hand on the client's

distal forearm and stabilize the client's trunk with the other hand.

- *Action:* Have the client resist as you attempt to pull his or her arm toward you, across the back. Hold for 5 seconds. Relax for a few seconds, and while the client is completely relaxed, pull her arm slowly into a further stretch across the back. Repeat three to five times.

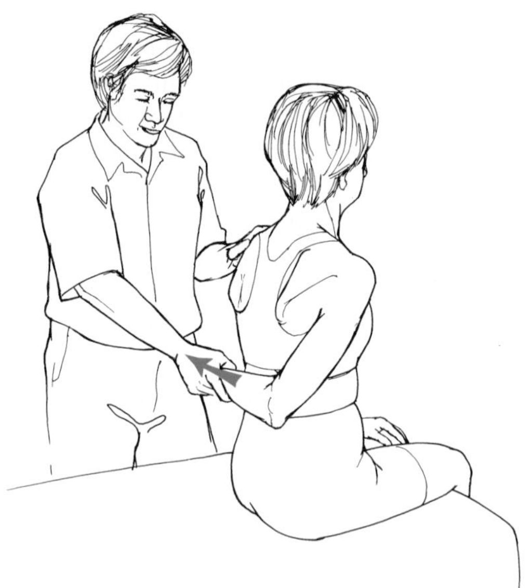

Figure 6-28. PIR MET for the supraspinatus.

11. Postisometric Relaxation Muscle Energy Technique to Increase Medial Rotation

- *Intention:* The intention is to increase medial (internal) rotation of the glenohumeral joint and to stretch the posterior capsule and subscapularis (Fig. 6-29).
- *Position:* Client is sitting, and places one hand on his or her low back. If this is difficult, the hand is placed on the sacroiliac joint (SIJ) or the greater trochanter area. Hold one hand on the client's elbow and one hand on the distal forearm.
- *Action:* Have the client resist as you attempt to pull the distal forearm away from his or her lower back (i.e., into greater medial rotation). Hold for 5 seconds. Relax for a few seconds, and while the client is completely relaxed, pull the distal forearm slowly away from the lower back into a new resistance barrier or until it begins to be painful for the client. This is usually only approximately 1 inch. If it is painful, release the pull until it is comfortable again. Repeat three to five times.

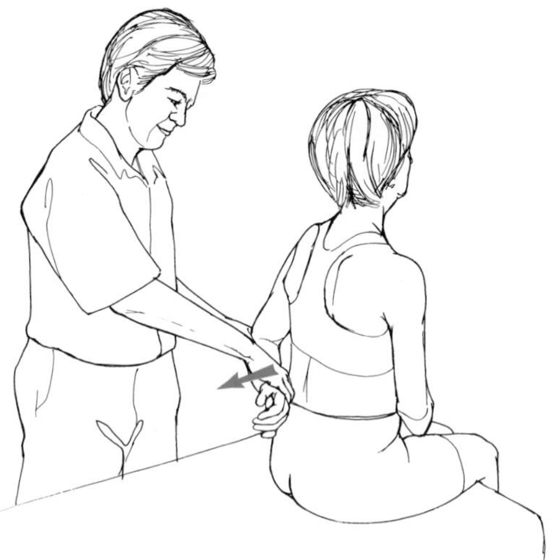

Figure 6-29. PIR MET to increase internal rotation.

12. Muscle Energy Technique to Increase Inferior Glide of the Glenohumeral Joint

- *Intention:* The intention is to reduce the hypertonicity of the muscles of the shoulder, to relieve pain, and to stretch the joint capsule (Fig. 6-30).
- *Position:* Client is supine, with the involved arm at his or her side. Stand in the 45° headward position, tuck the client's forearm against your body, and hold it there with your arm. Place one hand in the client's axilla to stabilize the shoulder, and your other hand holds the distal humerus.
- *Action:* While the client is completely relaxed, press headward slightly with the stabilizing hand

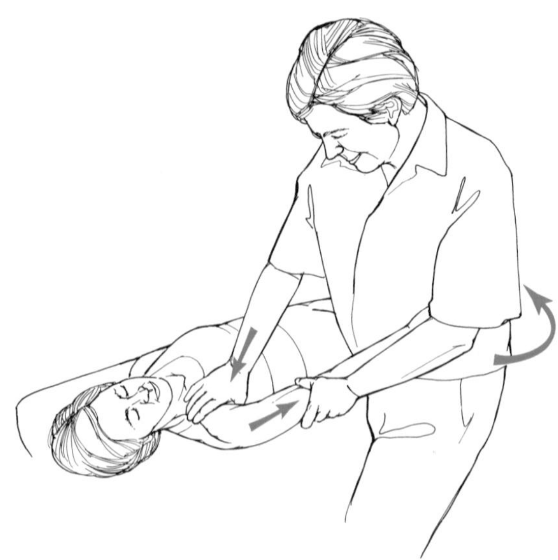

Figure 6-30. MET to increase inferior glide of the glenohumeral joint.

while you rotate your trunk away from the table, gently pulling the humerus inferiorly (toward the feet). Hold for 30 to 90 seconds.

- *Alternate Method:* This MET movement is performed with the therapist sitting. Take your shoe off and place your foot in the axilla of the client and hold the distal forearm. Lean back to traction the client's arm. Hold for 30 to 90 seconds.

Treatment for Loss of Shoulder Motion

13. Postisometric Relaxation Muscle Energy Technique to Increase External Rotation in Abduction

- *Intention:* The goal is to increase the ROM and the length of the internal rotators. In chronic shoulder problems, clients lose the ability to abduct and externally rotate the shoulder fully. This technique is a comfortable way to correct these problems (Fig. 6-31).
- *Position:* Client is supine, with the feet on the table and with the low back against the table. Place a pillow under the head if the arms cannot rest comfortably at the end of their tension barrier. Have the client interlace his or her fingertips and place the hands under her head. Face 45° headward and place your palms on the client's elbows.
- *Action:* Have the client resist as you attempt to press the elbows toward the pillow or table.
- *Home exercise:* To increase the ROM of the shoulder, have the client perform the following exercise at home: The client should attempt to pull the elbows into the pillow for 5 seconds, relax, and repeat five times.

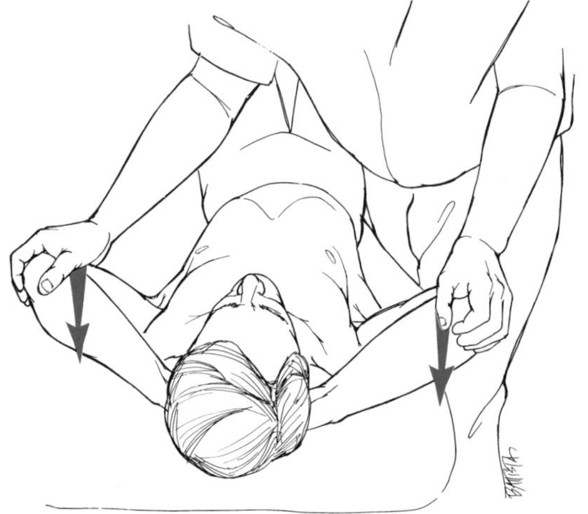

Figure 6-31. PIR MET to increase external rotation in abduction.

14. Eccentric Muscle Energy Technique to Increase Shoulder Elevation

CAUTION: This technique is not to be performed on geriatric clients.

- *Intention:* The goal is to help dissolve adhesions in the anterior joint capsule, as elevation of the shoulder is one of the primary motions lost in frozen shoulder (Fig. 6-32).
- *Position:* Client is supine, and elevates his or her arm to the comfortable limit. Hold the distal humerus and place one hand on the forearm.
- *Action:* Have the client resist as you attempt to move the arm overhead with moderate pressure. Tell the client, "Let me win, and allow me to move your arm very slowly, as long as it is not painful." Move the arm slowly to the pain-free limit for approximately 10 seconds. Relax, but hold the arm in its new range if it is not painful. Bring it back slightly if it is painful. Repeat three to five times, and rest the arm. Repeat another three to five times.
- *Variations:* Eccentric MET movement can be performed at increasing degrees of abduction, up to approximately 80°.

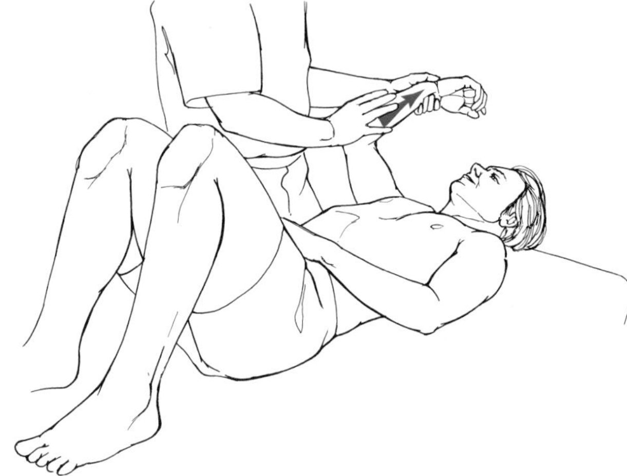

Figure 6-32. Eccentric MET to increase shoulder elevation.

ORTHOPEDIC MASSAGE

Level I—Shoulder

1. Release of Serratus Anterior and Subscapularis

- *Anatomy*: Subscapularis (Fig. 6-33), serratus anterior, long thoracic nerve, and median and ulnar nerves (See Fig. 6-7).

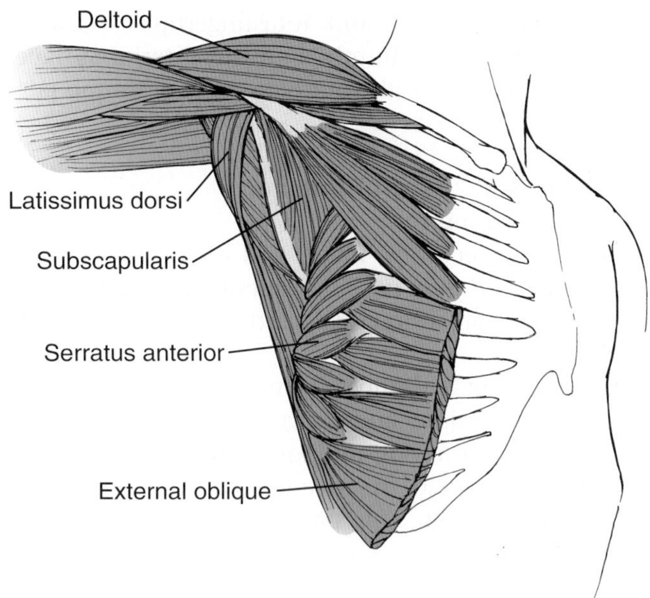

Figure 6-33. Serratus anterior and subscapularis.

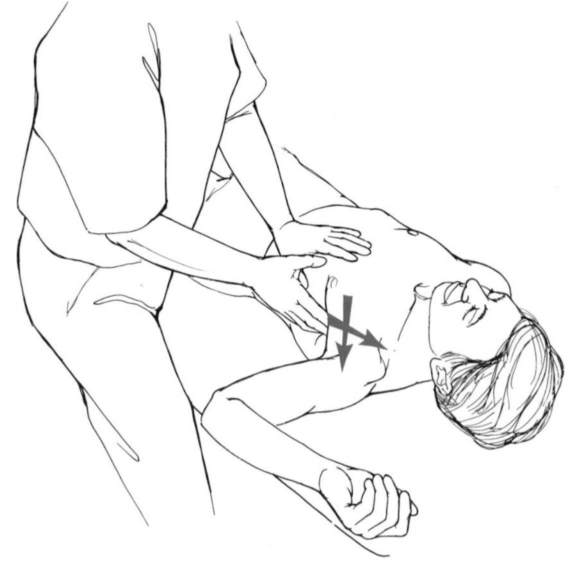

Figure 6-34. Fingertip release of the serratus anterior.

- *Dysfunction*: The typical position of dysfunction of the shoulder is a forward and internally rotated position. The subscapularis is typically short and tight. It holds the humerus in an adducted, internally rotated position. The serratus is typically weak in a head-forward, kyphotic posture. The long thoracic nerve lies over the serratus anterior, and the subscapular nerve lies over the subscapularis. These nerves may be entrapped in the overlying fascia.

Position

- TP—standing, facing 45° headward or facing the table
- CP—supine, with arm abducted and externally rotated. If this position is difficult or painful, place a supporting pillow under the client's arm.

Strokes

1. If the shoulder cannot reach 90° of external rotation, perform PIR MET to increase external rotation (see "Muscle Energy Technique" section above).
2. With the client's arm abducted and externally rotated, use fingertips to perform a series of short, scooping strokes on the lateral rib cage to release the serratus anterior and long thoracic nerve (Fig. 6-34). Perform the strokes both posteriorly and toward the axilla. Cover the entire lateral rib cage.
3. Using your superior hand to hold the client's distal forearm, place the fingertips of your inferior hand on the anterior scapula and perform short, scooping strokes in a headward direction on the subscapularis as you rock her arm in a backstroke-type motion (Fig. 6-35).
4. With the client's arm in the abducted and externally-rotated position, place the thumb of your superior hand on the anterior surface of the scapula, and perform short, scooping, headward strokes to release the subscapularis (Fig. 6-36). Grasp the entire

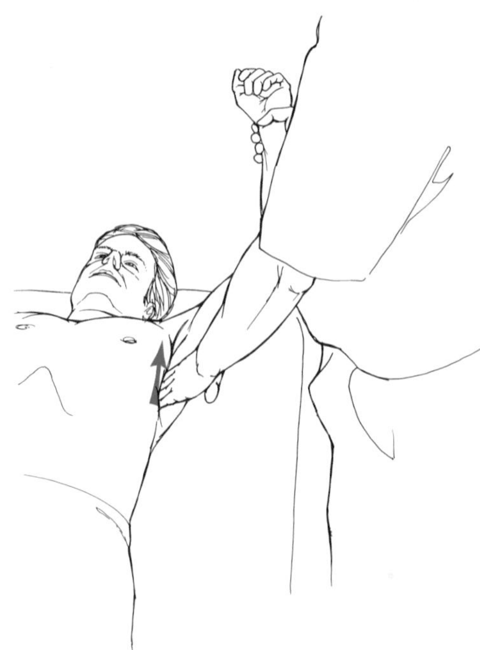

Figure 6-35. Fingertip release of the subscapularis. The fingertips scoop headward as the arm is rocked into a backstroke motion.

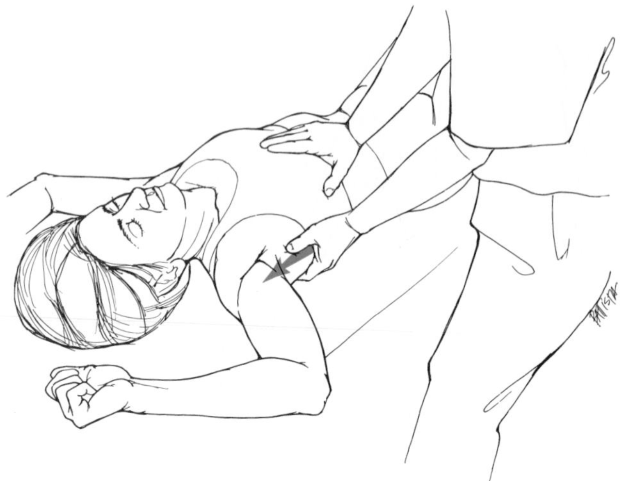

Figure 6-36. Thumb release of the subscapularis.

scapula with your hand. Your fingertips are underneath, and your thumb is on the anterior surface. Gently squeeze with your hand as your thumb performs the stroke.

2. Rolling Soft Tissue of Anterior Shoulder Superiorly

- ***Anatomy***: Pectoralis major and minor, rotator cuff muscles and joint capsule, anterior and middle deltoid, and coracobrachialis and biceps (short head) (Fig. 6-37).
- ***Dysfunction***: With most dysfunctions, the pectoralis major and minor and the anterior deltoid tend to roll into an anterior, inferior, medial torsion as the humerus is held in an adducted and internally-rotated position. This pattern is present in head-

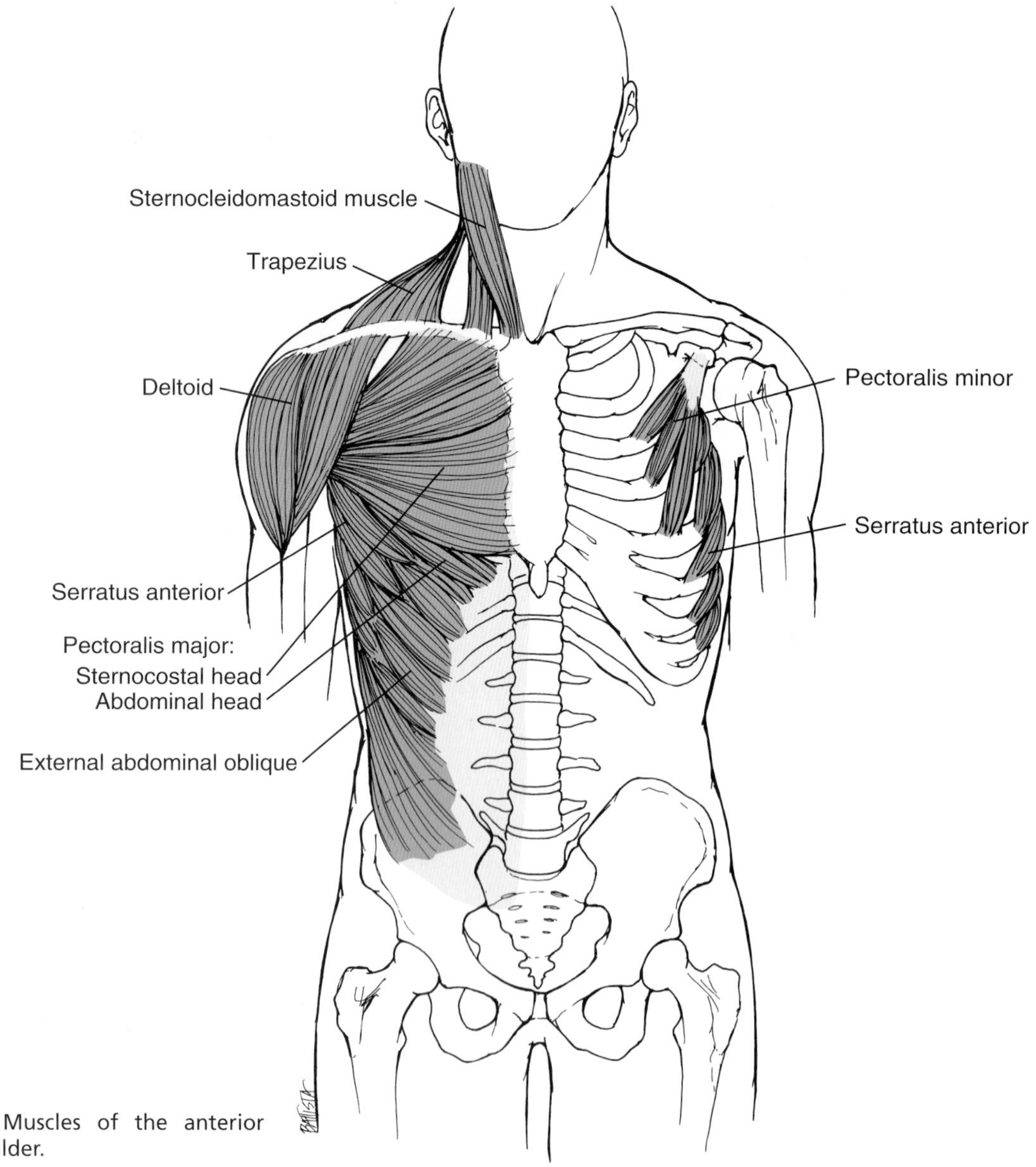

Figure 6-37. Muscles of the anterior chest and shoulder.

forward, slumped posture; in kyphotic thoracic spine; and in anterior subluxations. The pectoralis minor is typically tight and can entrap the neurovascular bundle that travels under it.

Position

- TP—standing
- CP—supine

Strokes

1. Hold the client's distal forearm with your superior hand and move his or her arm into small arcs of external rotation as you perform 1-inch, scooping strokes with the fingertips of your other hand on the upper part of the pectoralis major, the pectoralis minor, and the anterior deltoid (Fig. 6-38). Sink into the tissue until you take it into tension, and then scoop the fibers headward in a rhythmic, oscillating fashion, coordinated with the movement of the arm. Change the angle of your strokes so that you are working perpendicular to the line of the fiber.
2. To reset the entire segment into an externally-rotated position from the dysfunctional internally-rotated position, perform a backstroke-type circular motion with the arm as you perform several additional strokes in this area. The arm is adducted slightly as the backstroke begins and abducted and externally-rotated as it finishes.
3. An alternate method is to release the superficial muscles, and as a method to release the deeper rotator cuff and joint capsule, switch hands, and hold the deltoid muscle with your superior hand such that the shaft of your thumb is in line with the shaft of the humerus (Fig. 6-39). Hold the client's arm with your inferior hand at 90° abduction, and then lift it off the table slightly to bring the superficial tissue into slack. Perform a series of short, scooping strokes in a superior direction with your thumb as you rock the client's arm in a small arc of external rotation. Imagine rolling the tissue around the bone, unwinding it. Cover the entire area of the anterior and superior glenohumeral joint.

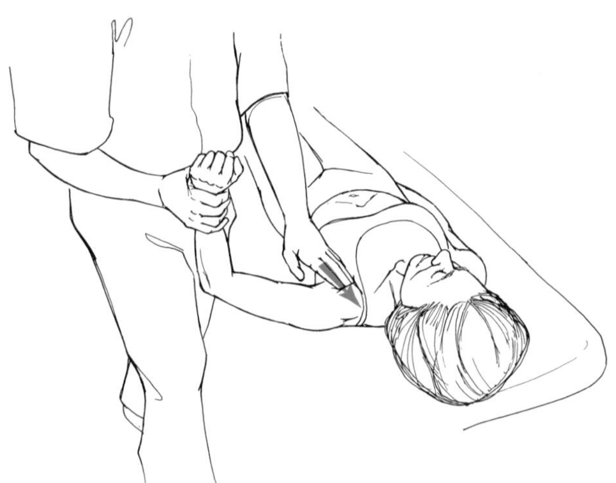

Figure 6-38. Fingertip release of the anterior shoulder muscles. This stroke releases the torsion and unwinds the tissue in a superior and posterior direction.

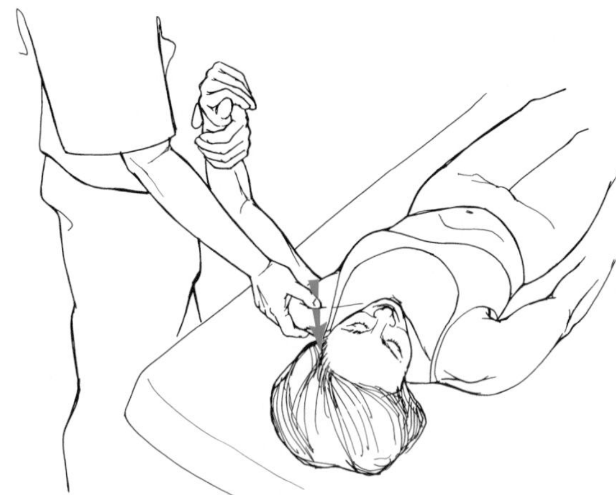

Figure 6-39. Scooping strokes with the thumb for the anterior shoulder muscles.

3. Unwinding the Soft Tissue and Mobilization of the Glenohumeral Joint

- *Anatomy*: Superficially—the pectoralis major, anterior and middle deltoid, coracobrachialis, and biceps brachii (Fig. 6-40); deeply—the joint capsule (see Fig. 6-4).

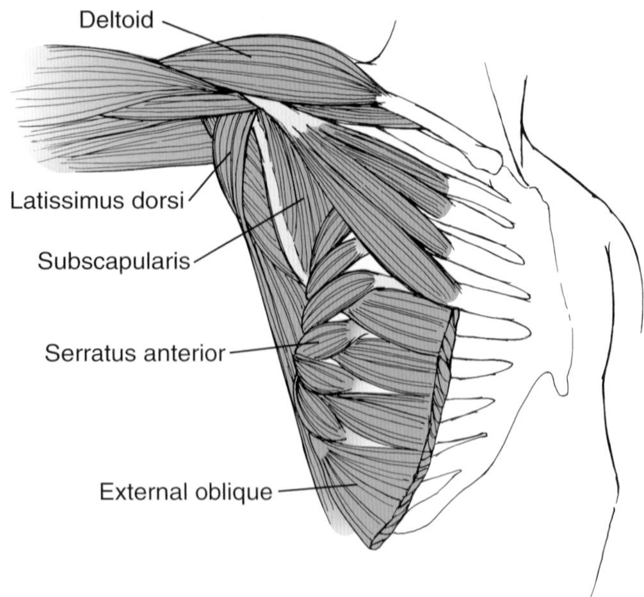

Figure 6-40. Anterior shoulder muscles.

- *Dysfunction*: The position of dysfunction is for the humerus to sustain an internally rotated position. The soft tissue "winds" into an abnormal internal torsion, decreasing the normal lubricant between the fascicles. Eventually the glenohumeral joint may develop adhesions and begin drying out, losing full ROM, which leads to calcific deposits.

Position

- TP—standing. Place the client's arm under your axilla. If the client's shoulder is stiff, it may be more comfortable in your inferior axilla. Otherwise, the arm is better placed on your superior side. If the arm is too heavy, place a pillow under the elbow.
- CP—supine

Strokes

1. Hold the proximal humerus with both hands and compress it slightly into the glenoid cavity to bring the superficial tissues into slack (Fig. 6-41). In this series of strokes the entire surface of both hands is used to unwind the soft tissue of the anterior and the middle humerus. We externally rotate the tissue around the bone. The thumbs of both hands lie next to each other and also perform short scooping strokes. Cover the anterior and middle portions of the proximal humerus down to the deltoid tuberosity.
2. Mobilize the shoulder. Perform circumduction to help normalize the movement characteristics of the glenohumeral joint and to rehydrate the joint by stimulating the synovial microvilli. Hold the arm as described in the first stroke. Move the entire humerus in a superior direction and then posteriorly, inferiorly, anteriorly, and superiorly again. Repeat this motion either in slow, gentle small amplitude circles for acute conditions or in more vigorous, brisk, larger-amplitude circles for chronic conditions. If there is a loss of normal external rotation, you may externally rotate the humerus as you move it superiorly. This stroke is an assessment and a treatment. Perform this movement gently and in small circles if the client is hypermobile or unstable.

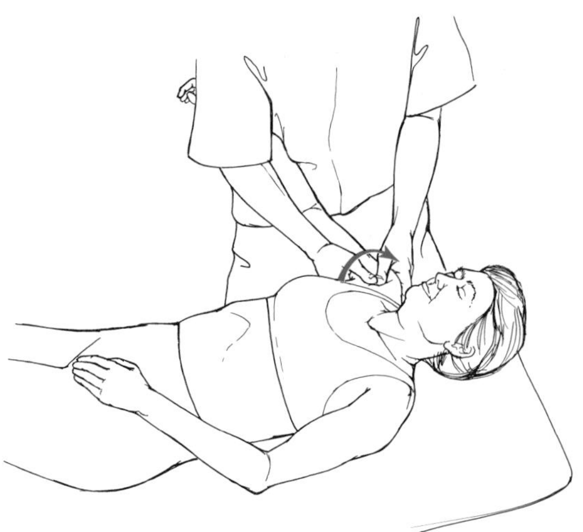

Figure 6-41. Hands used to unwind the torsion that develops in the soft tissue of the glenohumeral joint.

4. Release of the Supraspinatus

- *Anatomy*: Supraspinatus and coracoacromial ligament (Fig. 6-42).
- *Dysfunction*: This is the only muscle of the rotator cuff that travels through a tunnel and is therefore susceptible to loss of oxygen when inflamed, as the swelling compresses the tissue, and can leave a scar on the tendon. The tendon can impinge under the acromion when the arm is abducted or during flexion, especially when combined with internal rotation. The coracohumeral ligament blends with the superior joint capsule and the supraspinatus tendon.

Position

- TP—standing
- CP—supine

Strokes

1. Release the supraspinatus muscle belly and myotendinous junction using single-thumb or fingertips technique. Place the client's flexed elbow on his or her chest so that the arm rests across the chest. With your inferior hand, grasp just above the client's elbow and gently impulse the arm headward and posteriorly in the scapular plane. At the same time,

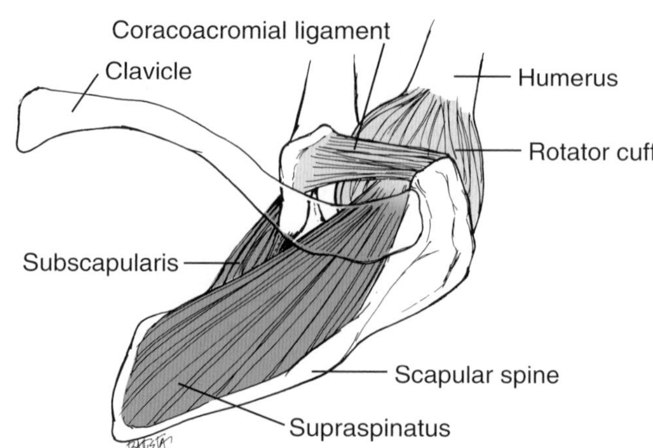

Figure 6-42. Superior view of the supraspinatus and the coracoacromial ligament.

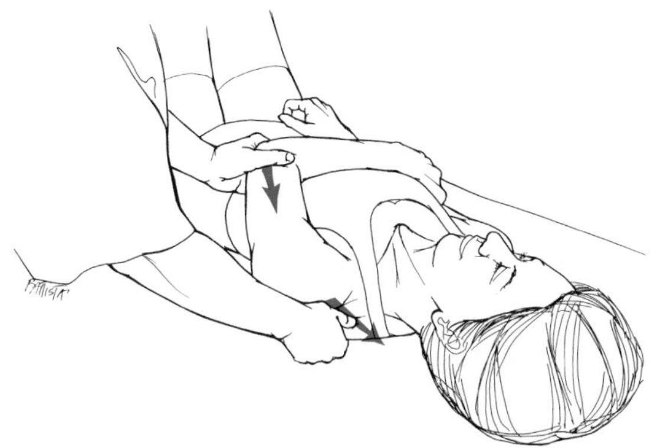

Figure 6-43. Thumb release of the belly and myotendinous junction of the supraspinatus muscle.

the thumb or fingertips of your superior hand perform a 1-inch, scooping stroke in the anterior to posterior direction in the supraspinous fossa (Fig. 6-43). Reposition the thumb slightly, draw the arm back, and repeat a series of strokes covering the entire supraspinous fossa.

2. To locate the supraspinatus attachment on the greater tuberosity, place your thumb on the anterior-superior portion of the greater tuberosity, just under the anterolateral aspect of the acromion.
3. Using the thumb or fingertips of your superior hand, perform TFM strokes on the tenoperiosteal junction of the supraspinatus tendon (Fig. 6-44). The pressure of a TFM stroke is applied in both directions, transverse to the line of the fiber. Rock the client's arm with each stroke. As the fingertips move forward, the arm moves forward; as the fingertips move back, the arm moves back. This may also be performed as a shearing stroke, with the fingers and arm moving in opposite directions. Palpate for a thickened feel to the tendon, as these strokes are used only as needed. The tendon is usually tender. Perform approximately 6 to 10 strokes on the same spot, and then move to another spot. Work for 3 to 4 minutes per session on the tendon. It often takes 6 to 8 sessions to dissolve the fibrosis. To expose more of the tendon, horizontally adduct the humerus across the client's chest.

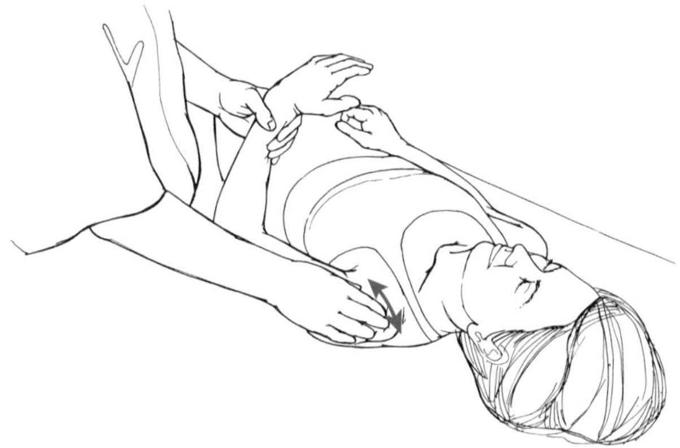

Figure 6-44. Fingertips perform TFM at the tenoperiosteal junction of the supraspinatus. Oscillate the arm with each stroke, which makes the treatment much more comfortable.

5. Release of the Infraspinatus, Teres Minor and Major, and Supraspinatus

- *Anatomy*: Infraspinatus and supraspinatus, teres minor and major, and suprascapular nerve (Fig. 6-45).
- *Dysfunction*: These muscles tend to roll into an inferior torsion as the humeral head migrates superiorly in dysfunction. The external rotators are usually weak, losing their normal function, which is to depress the humerus during arm elevation. This inferior torsion is also created with slumping posture, kyphosis, and weak scapular stabilizers. The suprascapular nerve travels under the infraspinatus on top of the scapula. A site of potential injury to this nerve is under the lateral aspect of the spine of the scapula.

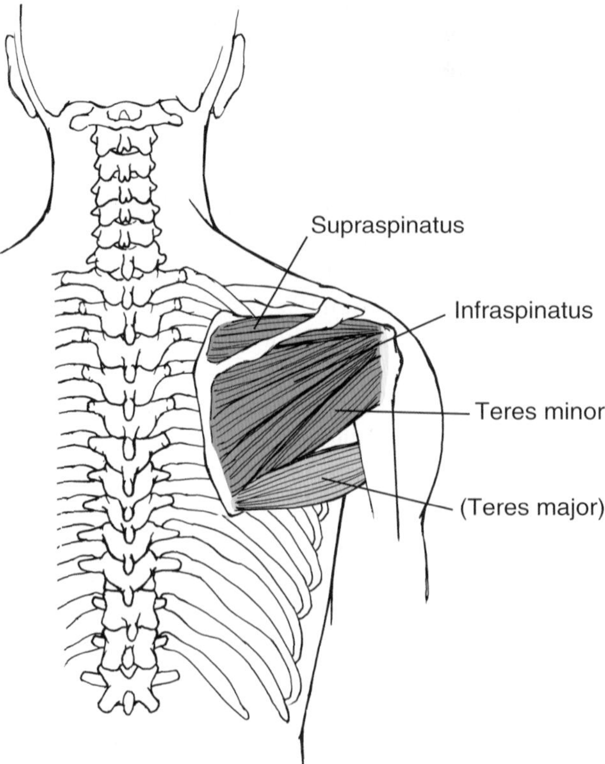

Figure 6-45. Teres minor, infraspinatus, and supraspinatus.

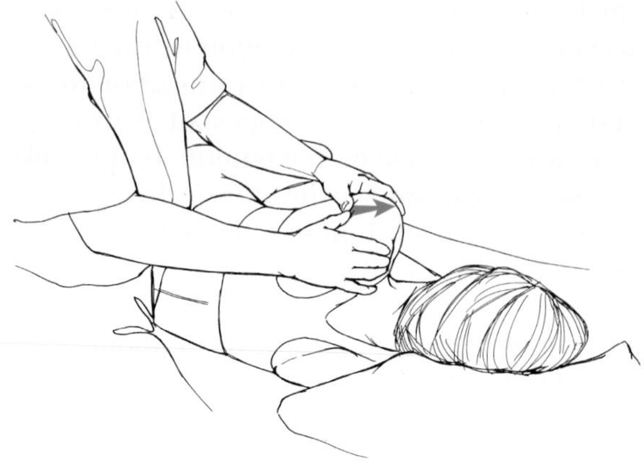

Figure 6-46. Double-thumb technique to release the infraspinatus and the teres minor.

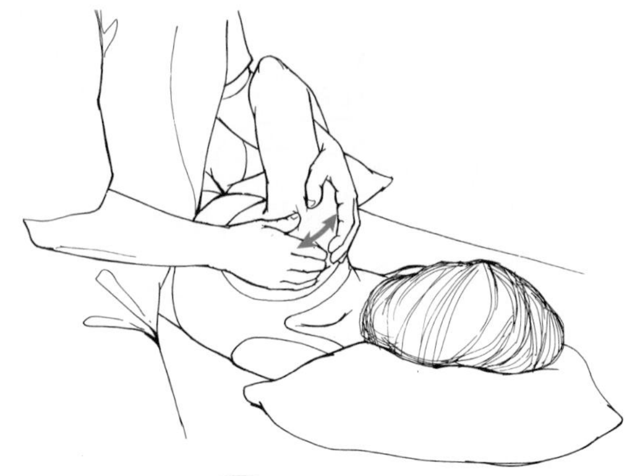

Figure 6-47. Fingertip release of the belly and myotendinous junction of the supraspinatus.

Position

- TP—standing
- CP—side-lying, with elbows flexed, arms and hands resting on each other. Place a pillow between the client's arms to help support and stabilize the arms.

Strokes

There are three lines of strokes: one, on the superior aspect of the scapula inferior to the spine; two, in the middle of the scapula; and three, on the inferior aspect of the scapula. These strokes should be across the bone, not into the bone.

1. To release the hypertonicity or to recruit an inhibited muscle on the posterior scapula, perform CR and RI MET with the client in the side-lying position (see Fig. 6-24, p. 227).
2. Using a double-thumb technique, begin at the superior portion of the scapula inferior to the spine of the scapula, and perform 1-inch, scooping strokes in a superior direction (Fig. 6-46). Begin the series of strokes at the vertebral border and continue to the posterior humerus.

   Note: The suprascapular nerve travels under the infraspinatus and lies on top of the scapula. It is most exposed inferior to the most lateral aspect of the spine of the scapula. A sharp radiating pain is elicited if the nerve is compressed. It can be released with gentle scooping strokes.
3. Begin a second and third line of strokes on the middle and inferior aspects of the scapula, continuing to the posterior humerus.
4. As an alternate method to release the supraspinatus, face 45° headward. Tuck your arm under the client's arm and place both hands on the supraspinous fossa of the scapula (Fig. 6-47). Using your fingertips, perform back and forth strokes in an anterior to posterior direction on the supraspinatus muscle. Move your arms and the client's arm with each stroke. Cover the entire area of the supraspinous fossa.

6. Prone Release of the Posterior Rotator Cuff and Posterior Deltoid

- *Anatomy*: Supraspinatus, infraspinatus, teres minor, and posterior deltoid (Fig. 6-48).
- *Dysfunction*: As mentioned, the muscles of the posterior shoulder tend to roll into an inferior torsion

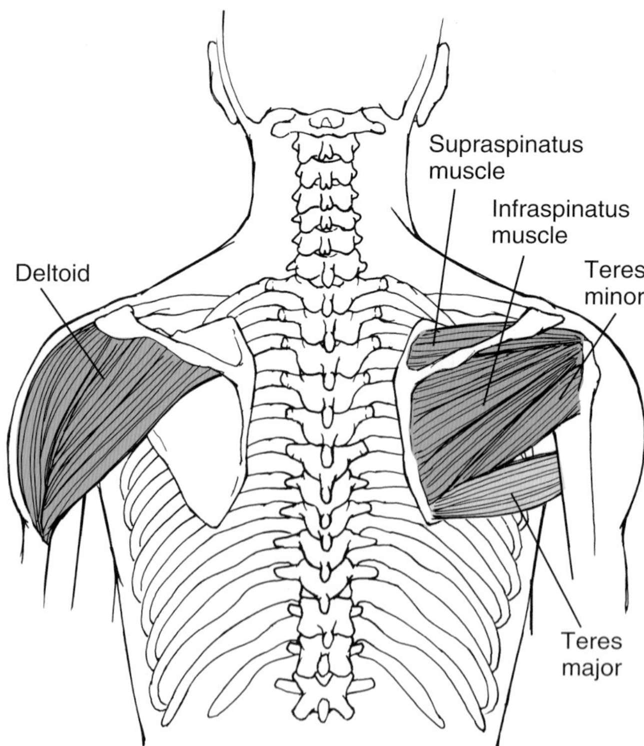

Figure 6-48. Posterior rotator cuff muscles, the posterior deltoid, and teres major.

and need to be moved superiorly. With a loss of the normal thoracic curve and a retracted scapula, the posterior cuff muscles and joint capsule shorten.

Position

- TP—standing
- CP—prone

Strokes

1. Place both thumbs on the posterior aspect of the proximal humerus, and perform a series of gentle, scooping strokes, rolling the soft-tissue fibers superiorly (Fig. 6-49). The intention is to unwind the tissue around the bone. This releases the adhesions that develop from a sustained contraction and inferior torsion. Grasp the entire arm with your hands and move all the soft tissue that wraps around the humerus with each stroke. Release the pressure at the end of each stroke, place your hands in a slightly new location, and perform another stroke. Cover the entire posterior humerus.

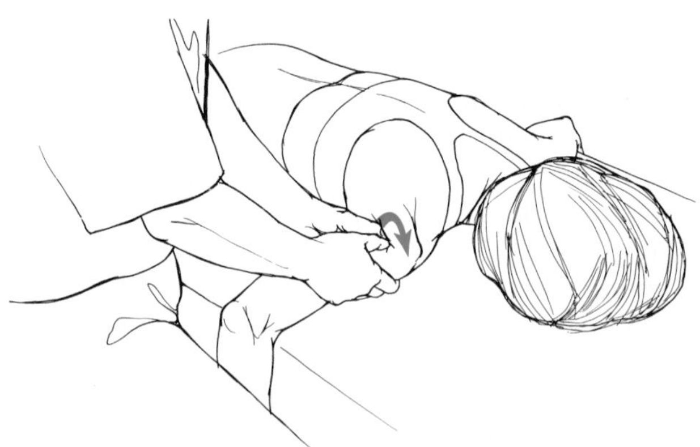

Figure 6-49. Release of the posterior shoulder muscles. Both hands wrap around the soft tissue of the posterior shoulder and roll the tissue in a headward direction.

Level 2—Shoulder

1. Release of the Clavicle and the Coracoid Process Attachments

- *Anatomy*: Pectoralis major and minor, anterior deltoid, subclavius, and coracobrachialis; coracoacromial, coracohumeral, and coracoclavicular ligament (Figs. 6-50**A** and **B**).
- *Dysfunction*: TOS can be caused by a thickening in the fascia and a shortening of the musculature in the areas above and below the clavicle. Causes include forward-head, rounded-shoulders posture or previous injury, such as a fall on an outstretched hand. The ligaments attaching to the coracoid process are often fibrotic because of FHP, rounded shoulders, or impingement syndrome.

Position

- TP—standing, facing the direction of your stroke
- CP—supine

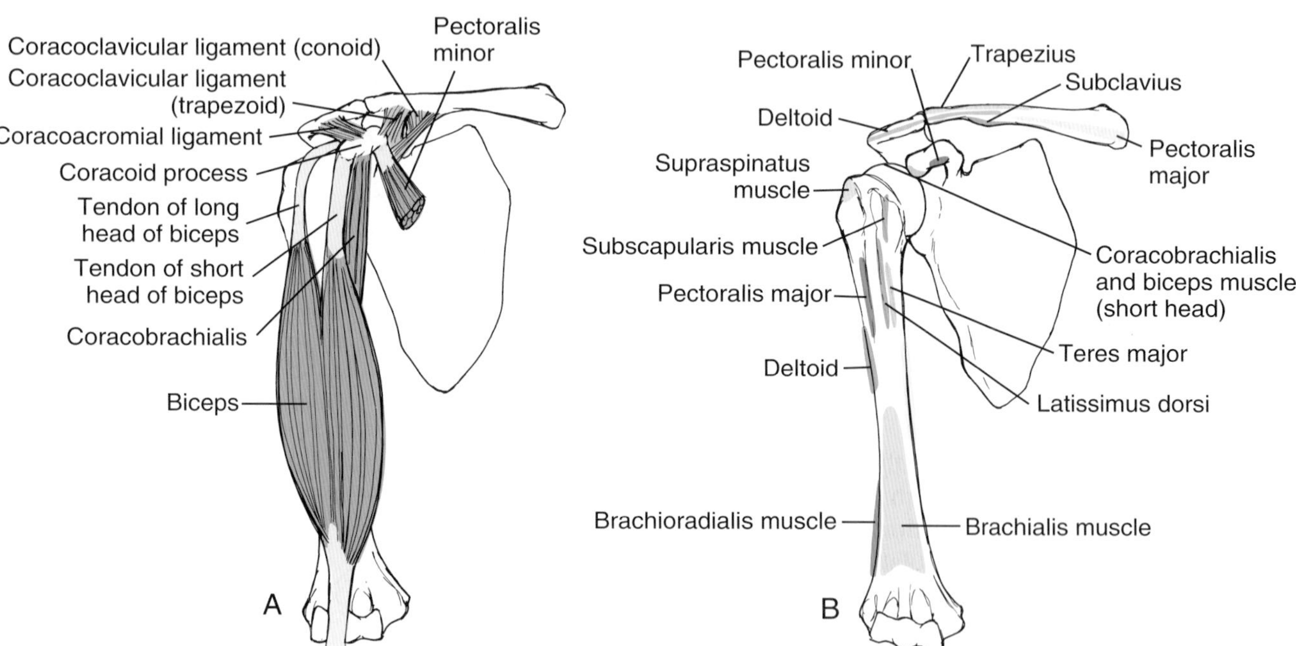

Figure 6-50. **A.** Attachments to the coracoid process. **B.** Attachments to the anterior shoulder complex.

Strokes

1. Press the base of your superior hand under the clavicle as you wrap your fingertips over the sternum or clavicle (Fig. 6-51). Perform a series of short, back-and-forth strokes in the medial to lateral plane. Rock your body with your strokes. This technique cleans the superior and posterior portions of the medial clavicle and sternum for the sternocleidomastoid and superficial and deep cervical and pectoral fascia. Place your other hand on the lower rib cage. Press posteriorly and superiorly on the lower rib cage with your strokes to give some slack to the area being worked. Alternately, you can hold the client's distal forearm and move the arm up and down with your strokes to help mobilize the clavicle.

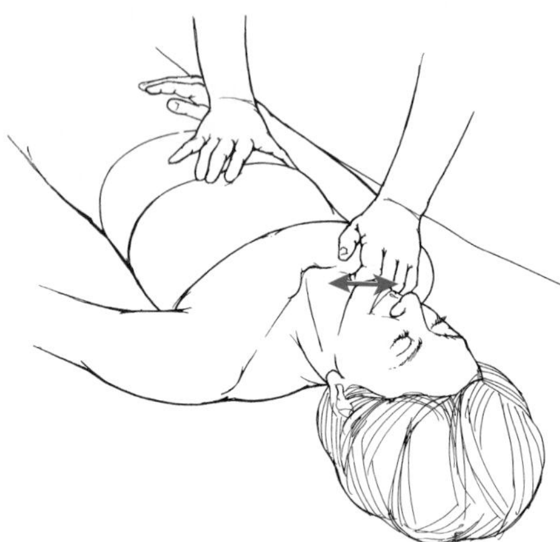

Figure 6-51. Fingertip release of the clavicle attachments.

2. Perform short, back-and-forth strokes in the medial to lateral plane with your thumb on the anterior and inferior clavicle. This technique releases the clavicular portion of the pectoralis major, the anterior deltoid, and the subclavius on the inferior portion of the clavicle.
3. Using the thumb of your superior hand, perform back-and-forth strokes on the inferior border of the coracoid process to release the pectoralis minor, coracobrachialis, and short head of the biceps (Fig. 6-52). Hold the client's distal forearm to abduct the arm, and elevate it slightly to bring the tissue into slack.
4. Holding the client's arm as in the previous stroke, perform transverse strokes with the thumb or fingertips on the superior portion of the coracoid process for the coracoclavicular and coracoacromial ligaments. Rock the client's arm in the direction of your stroke and coordinate the movement of the arm with the stroke.

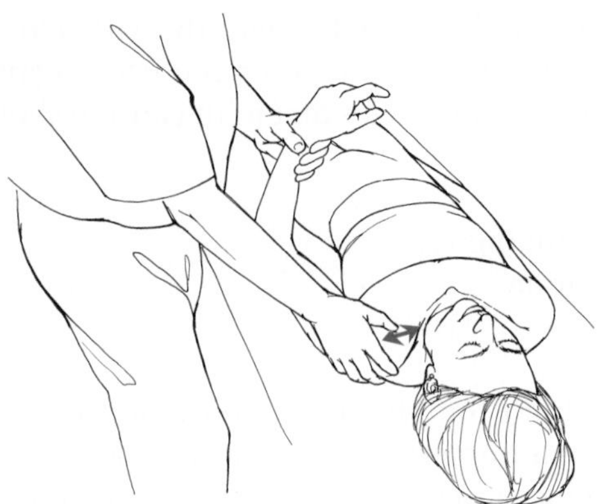

Figure 6-52. Thumb release of the inferior border of the coracoid process.

2. Transverse Release of the Anterior Humerus Muscle Attachments

- *Anatomy*: Subscapularis, long head of the biceps in the bicipital groove, pectoralis major, teres major, latissimus dorsi, and transverse humeral ligament (Fig. 6-53).
- *Dysfunction*: The muscles attaching to the anterior humerus are usually short and tight, pulling the arm into an adducted and internally rotated position. The tenoperiosteal and myotendinous junctions become fibrotic from the cumulative stress of poor posture, previous inflammation caused by overuse, or injury. The long head of the biceps is irritated with an internally rotated humerus, because it forces the tendon to rub against the medial aspect of the groove.

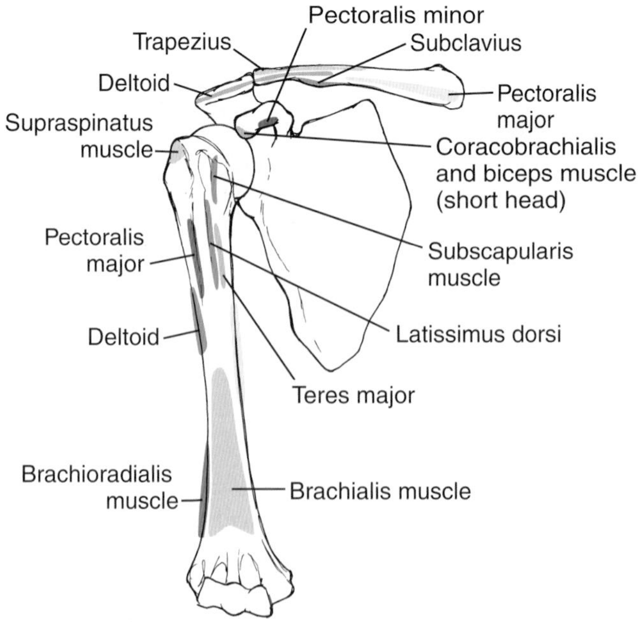

Figure 6-53. Attachments to the anterior shoulder complex.

Position

- TP—standing
- CP—supine

Strokes

1. Facing 45° headward, use a single-thumb technique to release the transverse humeral ligament by moving in the inferior to superior (I–S) plane on both sides of the bicipital groove (Fig. 6-54). Rock the client's arm as you rock your entire body with each stroke. Let your hand and thumb stay relaxed, and let the thumb move with the arm motion. Next, release any adhesions to the bicipital tendon by keeping your thumb on the bicipital tendon and moving the client's arm into medial and lateral rotation, letting the tendon roll under your thumb.
2. With the client's arm at his or her side and the elbow flexed to 90°, place your thumb or fingertips to the most medial part of the lesser tuberosity. You can palpate the subscapularis by having your client resist as you attempt to pull out on the distal forearm. Perform a series of back-and-forth strokes approximately 30° headward on the broad, tendinous attachment of the subscapularis. To expose the tendon more fully, move the arm into more external rotation.
3. From the lesser tuberosity, slide your thumb distally along the humerus to find the attachments of the teres major, latissimus, and coracobrachialis. Perform back-and-forth strokes in the I–S place on the medial side of the humerus to release these muscles. Lift the arm off the table slightly to bring the tissue into slack. In this technique, the strokes are along the bone, and not into the bone. With each stroke, rock the entire arm in the direction of your stroke.

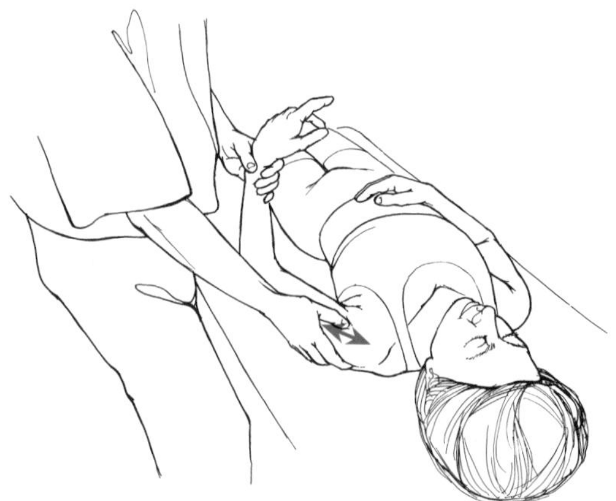

Figure 6-54. Release of the muscle attachments to the anterior humerus.

4. Using single-thumb technique, release the attachment of the pectoralis major on the lateral side of the bicipital tendon with short back-and-forth strokes in the I–S plane.

3. Release of the Attachments of the Rotator Cuff, Posterior Joint Capsule, Long Head of the Triceps, and the Radial Nerve

- *Anatomy*: Attachments of the posterior rotator cuff, posterior joint capsule, triceps, and radial nerve (Figs. 6-55**A** and **B**).
- *Dysfunction*: With an irritation or inflammation of the infraspinatus or teres minor, the tenoperiosteal attachment points thicken and become fibrotic. As these muscles interweave with the posterior joint capsule, the capsule also thickens. Thickening of the posterior joint capsule manifests as limited medial rotation.

Position

- TP—standing
- CP—prone, with forearm over edge of table, in 90° of abduction

Strokes

1. Place both thumbs next to each other and wrap your hands around the proximal portion of the humerus (Fig. 6-56). Use the thumbs to penetrate through the muscle to perform short, back-and-forth strokes transverse to the shaft of the humerus to release the attachments of the infraspinatus, teres minor, and joint capsule on the posterior glenoid fossa and proximal humerus.
2. To palpate the attachment of the long head of the triceps at the infraglenoid tubercle of the scapula, place the fingertips of one hand on the inferior aspect of the glenoid fossa and have the client resist as you attempt to press his or her elbow into flexion. Using a double-thumb technique, perform a series of back-and-forth, transverse strokes on the attachment site.
3. Release the radial nerve, triceps, posterior deltoid, and the posterior brachialis attachments on the posterior humerus. Use the same double-thumb technique described in the first stroke (Fig. 6-56). Beginning at the proximal humerus, perform a series of short, scooping strokes transverse to the shaft of the humerus. To release the posterior deltoid with CR MET, have your client lift his or her arm slightly off the table and resist as you press the arm lightly toward the table.

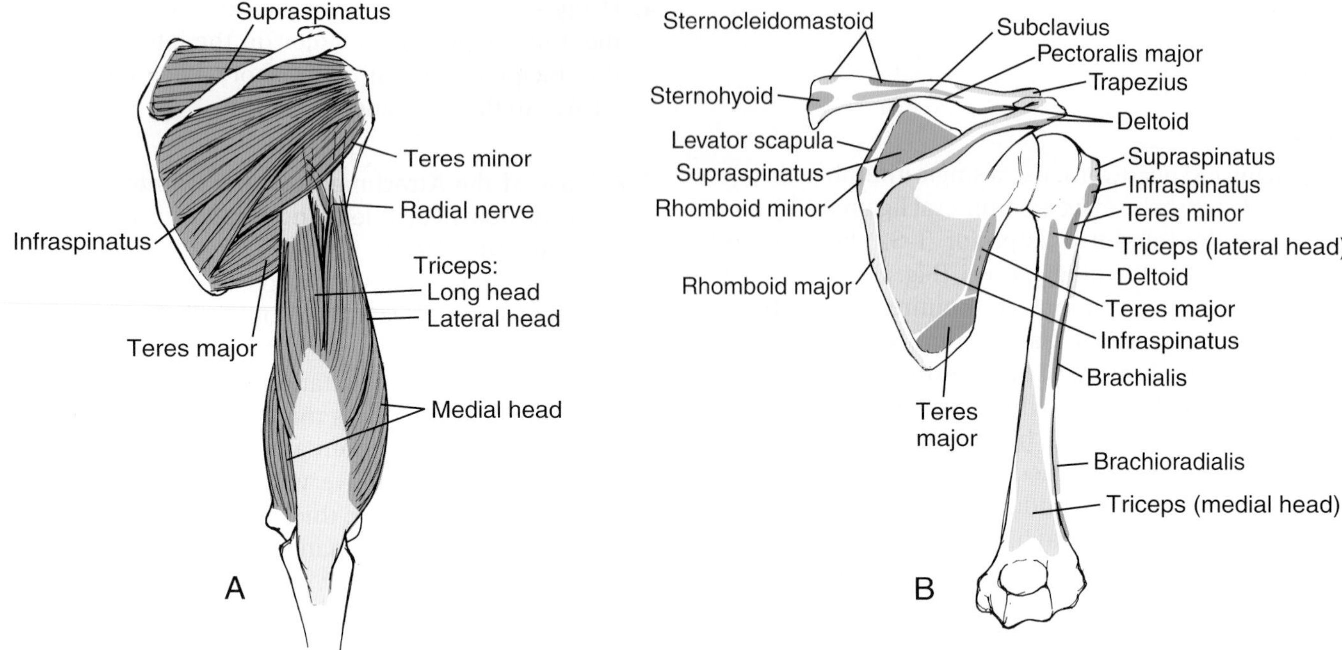

Figure 6-55. **A.** Posterior rotator cuff muscles, the triceps, and radial nerve. **B.** Muscle attachments to the posterior shoulder complex.

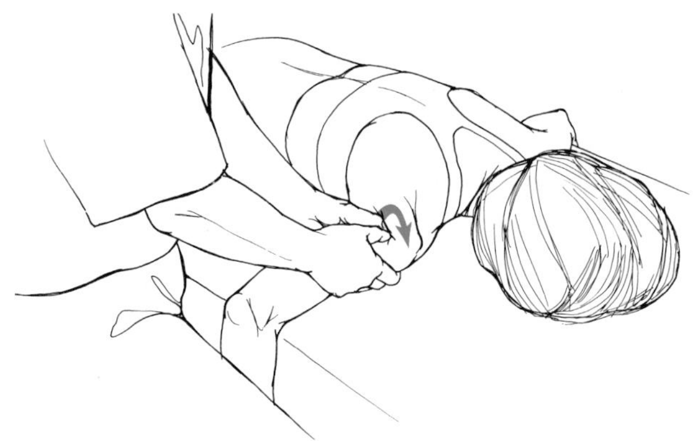

Figure 6-56. Double-thumb release of the rotator cuff muscles, posterior joint capsule, the triceps, and the radial nerve.

4. Repositioning of the Rotator Cuff Muscles and Deltoid in the Seated Position

- *Anatomy*: Deltoid, supraspinatus, infraspinatus, teres minor, and subscapularis (Figs. 6-57**A** and **B**).
- *Dysfunction*: The most common dysfunction of the glenohumeral joint is for the humeral head to sit high in the glenoid fossa. The rotator cuff muscles tend to part at the top of the joint, and roll inferiorly as the humeral head is held in this sustained superior position. The technique is performed in the sitting position with the arm at 90° abduction, as this is a position of function for eating, reaching, etc.

Position

- TP—standing, facing the table at 45° angle. For treatment, place your front foot on the table. If you have a tall client, have the client sit in a chair.
- CP—sitting on the table or a chair, a few inches from the lateral edge

Strokes

These strokes often follow the passive circumduction assessment technique. Your assessment findings help you determine which of the following strokes to use.

1. Place your foot on the edge of the table or chair and rest the client's forearm on your thigh, with the humerus in the scapular plane. To help reestablish normal function and position, perform CR MET with special attention to areas of restriction.
   a. Abduction—Lift the client's arm off your thigh, and have the client resist as you press down on the elbow.
   b. Adduction—Tuck your fingers under the client's elbow, and have the client resist as you attempt to lift the arm off your leg.

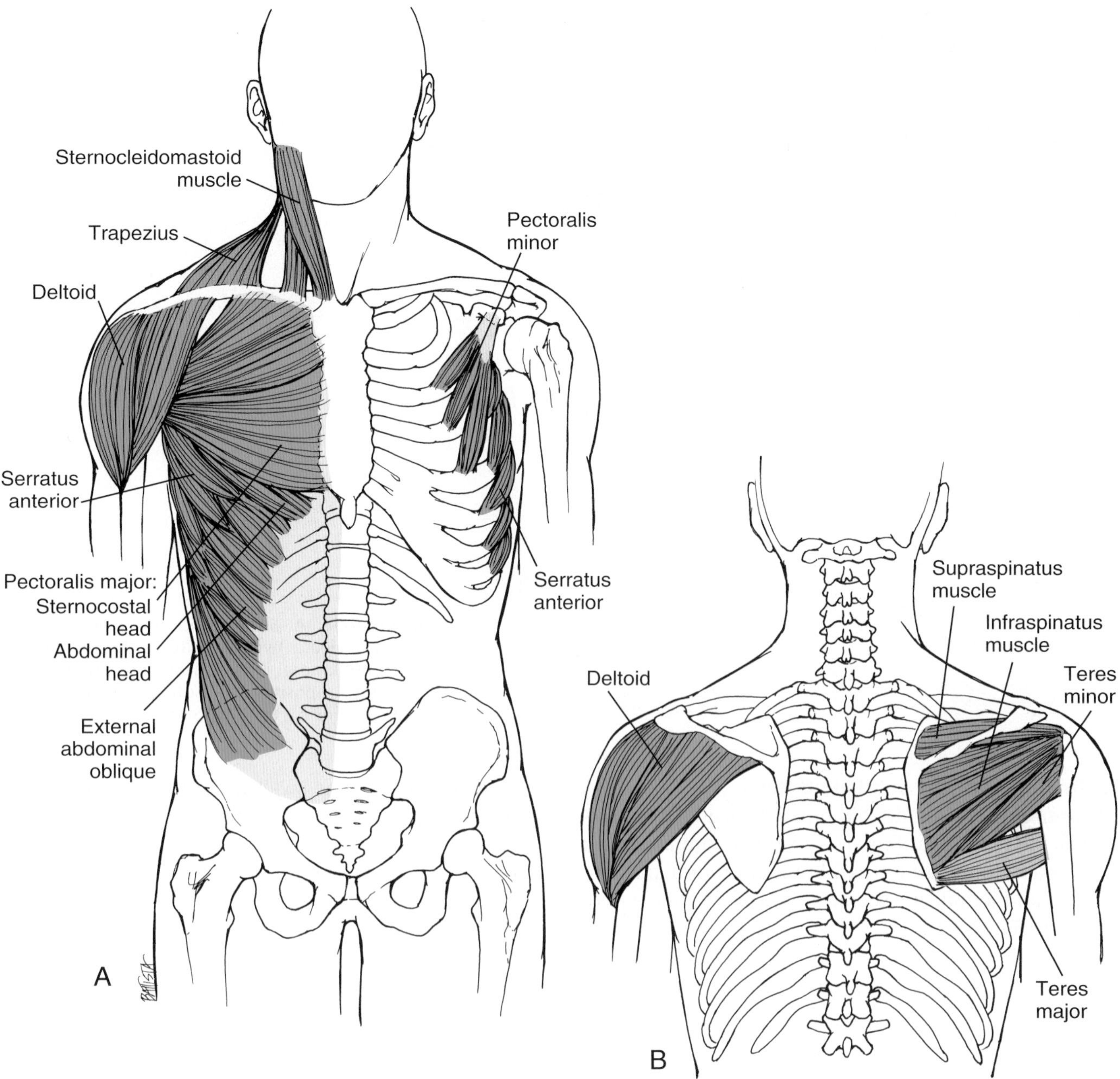

Figure 6-57. **A.** Muscles of the anterior shoulder complex. **B.** Posterior deltoid, supraspinatus, infraspinatus, and teres minor, and teres major.

c. Internal rotation—Tuck your hand under the client's distal forearm. Have the client resist as you attempt to lift the arm.
d. External rotation—First, lift the wrist a few inches off your leg. Have the client resist as you attempt to press down on the distal forearm (Fig. 6-58).
e. Horizontal flexion or extension—Have the client resist as you pull the humerus posteriorly or press anteriorly into the client's elbow.

2. After each MET is performed, use either your fingertips on the anterior muscles or your thumbs on the posterior muscles to scoop the soft tissue superiorly and toward the midline of the superior glenohumeral joint (Fig. 6-58B). The intention is to lift the soft tissue toward the highest point of the shoulder. You may perform more brisk, back-and-forth strokes if you find areas of fibrosis.

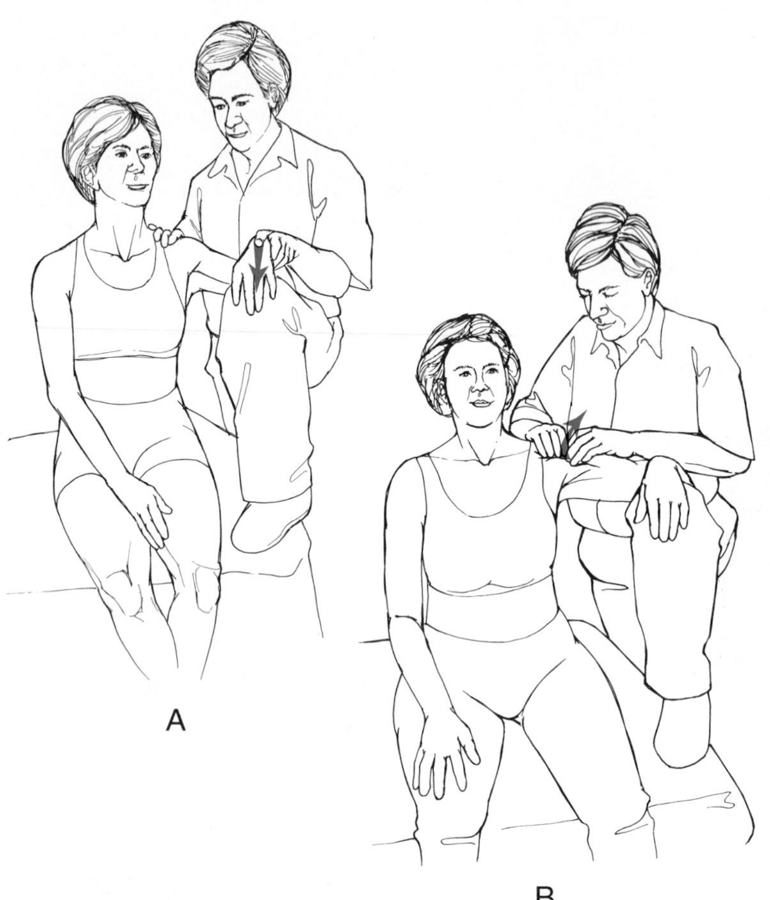

Figure 6-58. A. Sitting MET and OM. Perform METs to release hypertonicity in the muscles of the glenohumeral joint. **B.** Next, use fingertips or thumbs to reposition the soft tissue toward the most superior part of the joint.

5. Treatment of the Subdeltoid Bursa

- *Anatomy*: The subdeltoid bursa is located deep under the deltoid and inferior to the acromial arch. It acts as a lubricant during shoulder motion, particularly abduction, and secretes synovium into the joint space (Fig. 6-59).

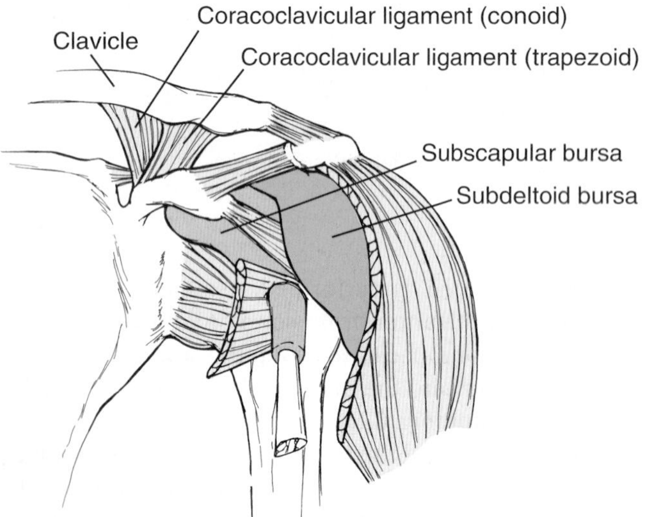

Figure 6-59. Subdeltoid (subacromial) bursa.

- *Dysfunction*: Bursae swell when they are inflamed, whether as a result of acute trauma or of cumulative stress, such as repetitive overhead activities. They dry out and form adhesions and migrate inferiorly during chronic shoulder dysfunction.

Position

- TP—standing
- CP—sitting

Strokes

Apply some oil or lotion to the client's upper arm so that you can easily slide on the skin. Hold the client's distal forearm with one hand and pull the arm into a gentle traction (Fig. 6-60). Place the shaft of your thumb a few inches distal to the acromion on the lateral arm. Using the fleshy portion of the entire shaft of your thumb and webspace, perform a slow, gentle, continuous stroke toward the acromion. When you reach the acromion, traction the arm and lift it slightly into abduction as you use your thumb to press into the arm gently. Coordinate the movements of the arm and the stroke, so that the arm is lifting as the thumb is pumping the excess fluid from the bursa under the

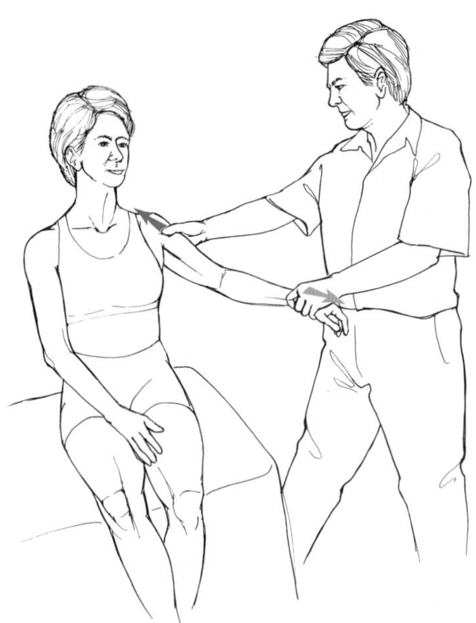

Figure 6-60. Using the web space of the hand, perform slow, gentle strokes on the subdeltoid bursa.

acromion. Repeat this pumping a few times. Then begin the stroke again by placing your hand a few inches below the acromion, and perform another long, continuous stroke. In chronic conditions in which the area has a dry and gristly feel, you may use deeper pressure to rehydrate the bursa. For an acute, swollen bursa, begin your stroke close to the acromion, moving superficially. Your next stroke begins a little more distally, milking the excess fluid headward a little bit at a time. Repeat the stroke.

CAUTION: **In acute bursitis, use gentle pressure, and do not repeat this stroke more than ten times.**

CASE STUDY

RA is a 33-year-old, 5'8", 155-lb, female minister who presented to my office complaining of acute right shoulder pain. She reported that the pain began a few days earlier after lots of sanding and painting. She described that a throbbing pain in the midarm was awakening her at night.

Relevant to the case is that RA has been a patient under my care for several years. Her original complaints were an aching, numbing, and tingling in the left arm, elbow, and hand, and significant weakness in the left arm. She was diagnosed with cervical radiculitis and treated with OM and manipulation. After six treatments the pain was resolved and the strength in the arm was normal. That was 4 years prior to the recent episode. Although she has occasional flare-ups, they resolve with one or two treatments.

Examination revealed a nearly complete inability to elevate the arm. Active abduction was approximately 20°, at which point pain was elicited in the left mid-humerus region. Passive abduction was the same. Modified isometric tests were performed on the rotator cuff muscles and the long head of the biceps. They were all painful with minimal effort. Palpation revealed warm and boggy tissue in the area of the middle deltoid. A diagnosis was made of acute subacromial bursitis, with secondary rotator cuff tendinitis.

Treatment began with her sitting. RI and CR MET were performed with minimal resistance in pain-free directions. These included flexion, extension, and adduction. CR MET was then attempted on the internal and external muscles, again with minimal resistance, and she could perform the resistance without pain this time. Finally, the bursa release strokes were performed—slowly, and with minimal pressure. The strokes were begun just below the acromion to create space into which the fluid could move. Further strokes were begun more distally.

RA returned to my office a few days later stating that she was feeling significantly less pain and had increased ROM. Palpation revealed normal temperature in the area of the subacromial bursa, with minimal swelling. I repeated the CR MET treatment to the rotator cuff muscles with her in the seated position. The arm could assume the 90° abduction position, and the MET was pain free using light resistance. RA returned to my office 1 week later, symptom-free, with full ROM and normal strength. She was instructed to call for her next appointment as she needed it.

STUDY GUIDE

Level I

1. List the four muscles of the rotator cuff. Describe their origins, insertions, and actions.
2. List which muscles are tight and which are weak in the shoulder.
3. Describe the MET for the pectoralis minor and the supraspinatus.
4. Describe the common positional dysfunction of the anterior deltoid. Describe the direction of the massage strokes to correct it.
5. Describe the signs and symptoms of a supraspinatus, infraspinatus, and subscapularis tendinitis.
6. Describe the stroke direction for the teres minor and infraspinatus.
7. Describe the MET for the internal and the external rotators.
8. List the scapular stabilizing muscles.
9. List some common causes of TOS.
10. When treating tightness or weakness imbalances, which muscles must be treated first?

Level II

1. Describe how to differentiate rotator cuff symptoms from a nerve root irritation in the neck.
2. Describe the signs and symptoms of bicipital tendinitis, subacromial bursitis, impingement syndrome, and adhesive capsulitis.
3. Describe the "empty-can" test and the Speed's test, and describe the significance of a positive test.
4. List the muscles and ligaments that attach to the coracoid process.
5. Describe the scapular stabilization test.
6. List the muscle attachments to the anterior humerus and their relation to the bicipital groove.
7. Describe what is indicated when the shoulder hikes upward in active abduction.
8. Describe the MET for frozen shoulder.
9. Describe the anatomical boundaries of the coracoacromial arch and the contents within the arch.
10. Describe the consequences of weak rotator cuff muscles.

REFERENCES

1. Boissonnault W, Janos S. Dysfunction, evaluation, and treatment of the shoulder. In: Donatelli R, Wooden M, eds. Orthopedic Physical Therapy. New York: Churchill Livingstone, 1994:169–201.
2. Garrick J, Webb D. Sports Injuries: Diagnosis and Management. 2nd Ed. Philadelphia: WB Saunders, 1999.
3. Cailliet R. Shoulder Pain. 3rd Ed. Philadelphia: FA Davis, 1991.
4. Norkin C, Levangie P. Joint Structure and Function. 2nd Ed. Philadelphia: FA Davis, 1992.
5. Hertling D, Kessler R. The Shoulder and Shoulder Girdle. Management of Common Musculoskeletal Disorders. Baltimore: Lippincott Williams & Wilkins, 1996:165–216.
6. Hammer W. The shoulder. In: Hammer W, ed. Functional Soft Tissue Examination and Treatment by Manual Methods. Gaithersburg: Aspen, 1999:36–135.
7. Corrigan B, Maitland GD. Practical Orthopaedic Medicine. London: Butterworths, 1983.
8. Kendall F, McCreary E, Provance P. Muscles: Testing and Function. 4th Ed. Baltimore: Williams & Wilkins, 1993.
9. Janda V. Evaluation of muscular imbalance. In: Liebenson C, ed. Rehabilitation of the Spine. Baltimore: Williams & Wilkins, 1996:97–112.
10. Halbach J, Tank R. The shoulder. In: Gould J, ed. Orthopedic and Sports Physical Therapy. St. Louis: CV Mosby Company, 1990:483–521.
11. Greenman PE. Principles of Manual Medicine. 2nd Ed. Baltimore: Williams & Wilkins, 1996.
12. Faber K, Singleton S, Hawkins R. Rotator cuff disease: diagnosing a common cause of shoulder pain. The Journal of Musculoskeletal Medicine June 1998:15–25.
13. Neer OS. Impingement lesions. Clin Orthop 1983; 173:70–77.

SUGGESTED READINGS

Chaitow L. Muscle Energy Techniques. New York: Churchill Livingstone, 1996.

Corrigan B, Maitland GD. Practical Orthopaedic Medicine. London: Butterworths, 1983.

Cyriax J, Cyriax P. Illustrated Manual of Orthopedic Medicine. London: Butterworths, 1983.

Garrick J, Webb D. Sports Injuries. 2nd Ed. Philadelphia: WB Saunders, 1999.

Greenman PE. Principles of Manual Medicine. 2nd Ed. Baltimore: Williams & Wilkins, 1996.

Hertling D, Kessler R. The shoulder and shoulder girdle. Management of Common Musculoskeletal Disorders. Baltimore: Lippincott Williams & Wilkins, 1996:165–216.

Hoppenfeld S. Physical Examination of the Spine and Extremities. New York: Appleton-Century-Crofts, 1976.

Kendall F, McCreary E, Provance P. Muscles: Testing and Function, 4th Ed. Baltimore: Williams & Wilkins, 1993.

Magee D. Orthopedic Physical Assessment. 3rd Ed. Philadelphia: WB Saunders, 1997.

Norkin C, Levangie P. Joint Structure and Function. 2nd Ed. Philadelphia: FA Davis, 1992.

Platzer W. Locomotor System, vol. 1. 4th Ed. New York: Thieme Medical, 1992.

Reid DC. Sports Injury and Assessment. New York: Churchill Livingstone, 1992.

The Hip

Dysfunction of the hip joint is a common complaint in all age groups.[1] It is one of the primary causes of impairment of gait in children and in the elderly. The hip joint is much more susceptible to degenerative than to traumatic conditions. The degeneration is more common in the elderly, but it is not uncommon in young athletes or performers. Degenerative joint disease (DJD) of the hip results in significant disability more than any other joint.[2]

Anatomy, Function, and Dysfunction of the Hip

GENERAL OVERVIEW

The hip bone is also called the os coxae or innominate bone and is the fusion of three bones: the ilium, ischium, and pubis (Fig. 7-1). The pelvis includes the two hip bones, the sacrum and coccyx. The hip joint is formed by the articulation of a socket in the hipbone called the acetabulum and the femur head, or thighbone (see Fig. 7-1). Twenty-two muscles surround the hip joint, as well as a dense joint capsule, numerous ligaments, and bursae.

BONES AND JOINTS OF THE HIP

Hip Bone and Acetabulum

- There are three bones that make up the acetabulum: the ilium, ischium, and pubis. The socket forms a hemisphere, but the outer lip of the acetabulum is discontinuous, as it has a deep notch on the inferior portion called the acetabular notch. As in the shoulder, a ring of fibrocartilage called a labrum deepens the socket. The acetabulum faces laterally, anteriorly, and inferiorly.

Femur Head

- ***Structure***: The femur is the longest and strongest bone in the body (see Fig. 7-1). The femoral head is its proximal expansion that sits in the socket formed by the acetabulum. It forms approximately two-

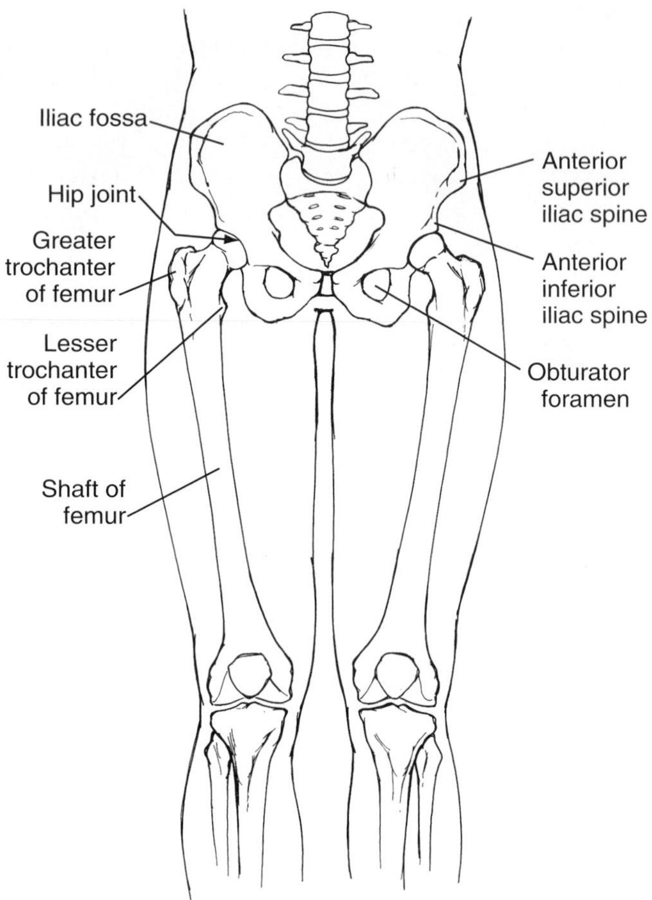

Figure 7-1. Bony landmarks of the hip.

thirds of a sphere and is completely covered by articular cartilage except for a central portion called the fovea. The primary blood supply to the femoral head is intracapsular (i.e., between the capsule and the bone). There are nerve fibers, including pain receptors in the bone under the cartilage (subchondral bone) that potentially communicate with the mechanoreceptors in the joint capsule and ligaments.[3]

- *Function*: The femoral head supports the weight of the trunk and transmits all of the reactive force from the ground up through the leg. While a person stands on one leg and during the support phase of walking, the femoral head sustains as much as six times the body weight. These forces would increase with jumping and carrying weight.
- *Dysfunction and injury:* If intracapsular pressure increases because of acute swelling or chronic tightening, it may lead to loss of blood to the femoral head, called avascular necrosis, and predisposes the joint to the development of degeneration.[2]

Femoral Neck and Shaft

- *Structure*: The femoral neck is a short piece of bone that connects the femoral head to the shaft, between the greater and the lesser trochanters.
- *Function*: In the standing posture, the acetabulum and the femoral neck are directed anteriorly. The femoral neck dictates the angle at which the head fits into the pelvis. There are two important angles that determine the function of the hip:
  - **Angle of inclination:** The axis of the femoral neck to the femoral shaft. In the adult it is normally approximately 125°.
  - **Angle of torsion:** The angle of torsion describes the amount of spiral twist between the femoral neck and the condyles. A line through the femur neck and a line through the condyles form the angle. The angle is normally approximately 15° anterior.
- *Dysfunction and injury:* Developmental changes can create variations in the angles of how the neck and shaft fit together. These variations alter the range of motion (ROM) and function of the hip.
  - An increased angle of inclination is called **coxa valga,** and a decreased angle is called **coxa vara.**
  - An increased angle of torsion is called an **anteverted** hip, and the client tends to walk with a toe-in gait. Lying supine on the treatment table, the foot on the side of the anteverted hip may point straight up or toe in slightly, instead of the normal 15° of external rotation. The client has increased internal hip rotation and decreased external hip rotation.
  - A decreased angle of torsion is called a **retroverted** hip, and the client walks with a toe-out gait. Lying on the treatment table, the foot on the side of the retroverted hip is turned out excessively. The client has increased external rotation and decreased internal rotation.
  - Loss of bone cells in the femoral neck is called **osteopenia** and is common in the elderly. This condition predisposes the region to fracture.[1]
- *Treatment implications:* It is important during the assessment of the hip to determine if a client has lost medial (internal) rotation. This loss of motion is associated with adhesions in the capsule and predisposes the hip joint to degeneration. During the assessment, always compare both sides because the client may have a normal retroversion in the hip and not a loss of medial rotation. With retroverted hips, both sides have a painless, resilient decrease in medial rotation. Painful hips in the elderly are treated with special precautions. Never vigorously mobilize

a geriatric hip because of the potential weakening of the femoral neck owing to osteopenia.

Greater Trochanter of the Femur

- *Structure*: The greater trochanter is a bony projection on the lateral side of the femur where the neck and shaft of the femur meet.
- *Function*: It is the site of attachments of muscles that abduct and externally rotate the hip.

Lesser Trochanter of the Femur

- *Structure*: The lesser trochanter is a bony projection on the posteromedial side of the junction of the neck and the shaft of the femur.
- *Function*: It is the site of the attachment of the iliacus and psoas muscles that are blended into one tendon at their insertion.

Hip Joint

- *Structure*: The hip joint is a synovial, ball-and-socket joint formed by the articulation of the acetabulum of the pelvis and the femoral head. The joint is located approximately 1 inch inferior to the inguinal ligament, approximately midway between the anterior superior iliac spine (ASIS) and the pubic symphysis (Fig. 7-2).

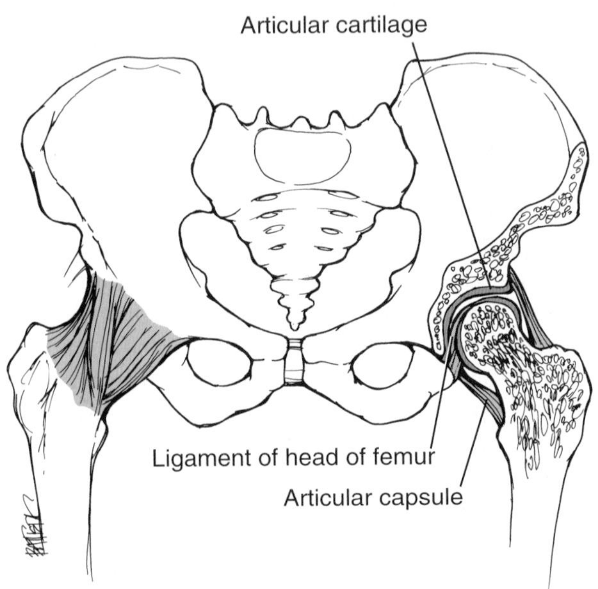

Figure 7-2. Hip joint. Two-thirds of the femur head sits within the acetabulum (socket) of the hip bone.

- *Function*: The primary functions of the hip joint are weight-bearing, walking, and stabilizing the trunk to the lower extremity. It has six possible motions: flexion, extension, abduction, adduction, and medial and lateral rotation. The closed-packed position of the joint is extension and medial rotation, and the open-packed position is flexion, lateral rotation and abduction. The hip joint is stable because two-thirds of the femoral head fits within the acetabulum. This is different from the glenohumeral joint of the shoulder in which the bones have little contact. This stability sacrifices mobility, and the hip has limited range of motion (ROM) compared with the shoulder.
- *Dysfunction and injury:* The hip joint is most susceptible to degenerative rather than traumatic conditions, except the fracture of the femoral neck in senile osteoporosis. Hip joint pain is described as an ache, typically felt in the inguinal region, midpoint between the ASIS and the pubis. The pain can refer to the anterior thigh and knee.
- *Treatment implications:* Assessment reveals loss of passive medial rotation, flexion, and adduction with a hard end-feel in degeneration of the cartilage and a capsular end-feel with fibrosis of the joint capsule. The primary treatment for dysfunction and injuries of the hip joint is to increase the joint ROM. This increase in ROM is accomplished with muscle energy technique (MET). It is also important to balance the length and strength of the muscles crossing the pelvic region, as minor imbalances in joint alignment repeated over a lifetime of use induce wear and tear to the joint.

SOFT-TISSUE STRUCTURES OF THE HIP

Ligament of the Head of the Femur

- *Structure*: The ligament of the head of the femur (ligamentum teres) extends from the nonarticular portion of the acetabular notch to the fovea on the femoral head (see Fig. 7-2).
- *Function*: The ligament forms a sleeve for the ligamentum teres artery that provides nutrition to the femoral head. The ligament is also lined with a synovial membrane, so it spreads a layer of synovium to the joint with hip movement. Lauren Berry, RPT, describes this structure as a "wick" that draws fluid out of the synovial membrane when the ligament brushes against the synovial membrane.
- *Dysfunction and injury:* The ligament of the head of the femur is one mechanism that provides lubrication to the hip joint. Decreased motion in the hip or

any joint eventually causes the joint to dry out. The synovial membrane needs to be stimulated by movement to generate and release the synovial fluid. As most clients do not move their hips in full ROM, the periphery of the cartilage tends to dry out.

- *Treatment implications:* The rhythmic oscillations of orthopedic massage (OM) increase joint lubrication. The mobilization distributes that lubrication into the cartilage surfaces of the femoral head and the acetabulum.

Joint Capsule and Capsular Ligaments

- *Structure*: The joint capsule is a connective-tissue sleeve that attaches proximally around the entire circumference of the labrum and distally around the femoral neck. It is thick and strong and has a spiral orientation as it winds around the femur. It tightens in extension, as in standing upright and in internal rotation, and it becomes slack in flexion and external rotation, as in a cross-legged position. In addition to the capsular sleeve that coils around the hip joint, three capsular ligaments—named according to their bony attachments—spiral around the joint (Figs. 7-3 and 7-4).
    - **Iliofemoral ligament:** It forms an inverted "V," spirals anteriorly and medially, and attaches to the inferior portion of the anterior inferior iliac spine (AIIS) proximally and to the intertrochanteric line inferiorly. It reinforces the capsule anteriorly. It becomes taut in extension, as in standing upright. It is the strongest ligament in the body.[3]

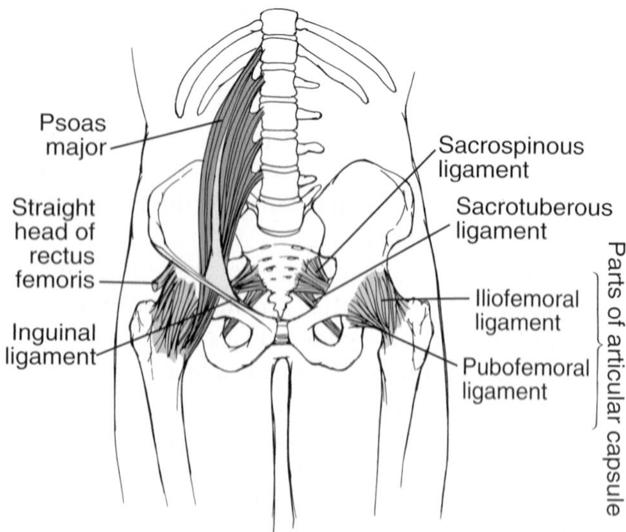

Figure 7-3. Anterior view of the hip joint, showing the joint (articular) capsule that includes the iliofemoral and pubofemoral ligaments and the straight head of the rectus femoris.

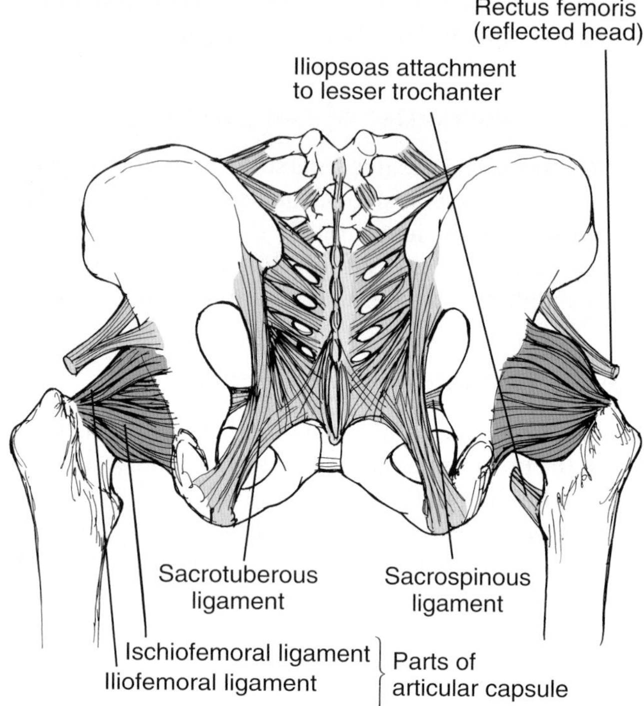

Figure 7-4. Joint capsule and ligaments of the posterior hip. The reflected head of the rectus femoris interweaves with the posterior joint capsule.

    - **Pubofemoral ligament:** It attaches to the pubic ramus and the intertrochanteric line. It reinforces the capsule medially. It becomes taut in hip abduction and extension.
    - **Ischiofemoral ligament:** It forms a spiral weave from the acetabular rim to the inner surface of the greater trochanter. It reinforces the capsule posteriorly. As in the other ligaments, it becomes taut in hip extension and medial rotation and slacker in hip flexion.
- *Function*: The joint capsule and capsular ligaments add passive stability to the joint in standing and moving. The inner layer of the capsule is lined with a synovial membrane that secretes lubricant into the joint with joint movement. The capsule and ligaments provide mechanoreceptor information regarding position, movement, balance, and coordination of the hip. As in all synovial joints, there are reflexive connections between the capsule and the ligaments to the surrounding muscles.
- *Dysfunction and injury:* Unlike the shoulder, the ligaments and joint capsule of the hip are dense and stable. Whereas the shoulder joint is susceptible to instability, the hip joint is susceptible to loss of motion and degeneration. One of the first manifestations of

degeneration is capsular thickening, assessed by painful loss of passive medial (internal) rotation. This is especially true of the iliofemoral ligament. This ligament prevents medial rotation due to the way it spirals around the femur. When it shortens it pulls the joint into external rotation. When the capsule thickens, the joint assumes its more open position (i.e., lateral [external] rotation) and loses its ability to move into medial rotation. Arthrokinetic (regarding movement) and arthrostatic (regarding posture) reflexes are abnormal in degenerating joints.[3] This disturbs normal movement and posture, making the joint more vulnerable to further injury.

- *Treatment implications:* Therapy for capsular swelling is through contract-relax (CR) MET. The muscle contraction causes a tightening or winding of the capsule and ligaments, and the relaxation causes an unwinding of the capsule and ligaments. This winding (tightening) and unwinding (loosening) of the capsule theoretically pumps fluid out of the joint if it is swollen, and stimulates the normal secretion of the synovial fluids if they have dried out. Therapy for capsular and ligamentous thickening is focused on MET to increase medial rotation. This is followed by MET to increase flexion and adduction. Release of the pectineus, rectus femoris, and gluteus minimus is also critical because they interweave with the capsule.

Bursae

- *Structure and function:* A bursa is a synovial-lined sac filled with synovial fluid that functions to decrease friction. Of the many bursae around the hip, only two are commonly involved clinically (Fig. 7-5).
  - **Iliopectineal:** The Iliopectineal bursa is located between the iliopsoas muscle and the joint capsule over the hip joint. The synovial cavity of the hip joint often connects anteriorly with the iliopectineal bursa.
  - **Trochanteric:** The trochanteric bursa lies between the gluteus maximus and the greater trochanter.
- *Dysfunction and injury*: As with all bursae, there are two possibilities of dysfunction and injury. One, the bursa may become inflamed and swell owing to either a traumatic event or cumulative or repetitive stresses. And two, the bursa may develop adhesions and dry out, decreasing its synovial lubricant. Lauren Berry taught that the positional dysfunction of the bursae of the hip is that they migrate inferiorly.
- *Treatment implications:* The bursae need to be stroked superiorly, either with slow, gentle strokes to milk the excess fluid out for an acute bursitis or with deeper strokes in a superior direction to dissolve adhesions and stimulate the secretion of the synovial membrane to rehydrate the bursae.

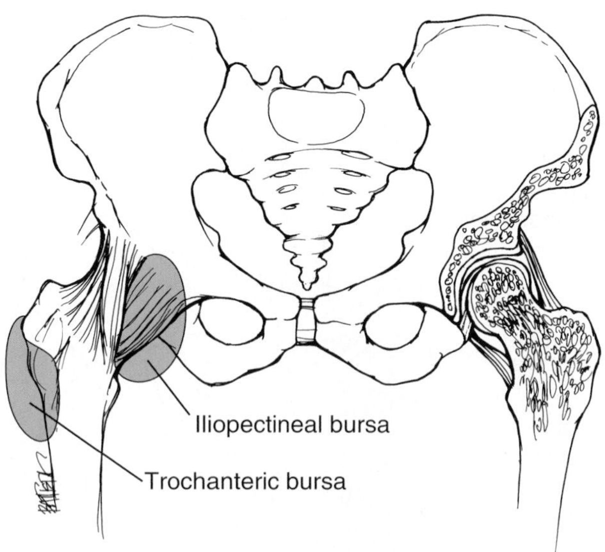

Figure 7-5. Iliopectineal and trochanteric bursae.

Nerves

- The **femoral nerve** is a branch of the lumbar plexus that travels through the psoas muscle and enters the anterior thigh through the **femoral triangle,** medial to the iliopsoas. The femoral triangle is defined as the space between the sartorius, adductor longus, and inguinal ligament. The **femoral nerve** innervates the muscles of the anterior thigh (Fig. 7-6).
- The **lateral femoral cutaneus nerve** enters the thigh under the inguinal ligament, approximately one-half inch medial to the ASIS. It supplies innervation to the skin on the lateral thigh (see Fig. 7-6).
- The **genitofemoral nerve** is a branch of the lumbar plexus that travels through the belly of the psoas major and along the medial border of the psoas. It supplies the scrotum in the male, the labia in the female, and the skin over the femoral triangle (see Fig. 7-6).
- The **obturator nerve** is a branch of the lumbar plexus that travels into the medial thigh under the pectineus and then between the adductor muscles. It supplies innervation to the skin on the medial thigh to the knee (Fig. 7-7).
- The **sciatic nerve** travels just posterior to the hip joint and innervates the muscles of the posterior thigh and the muscles of the leg and foot through the posterior tibial and peroneal nerves (Fig. 7-8).

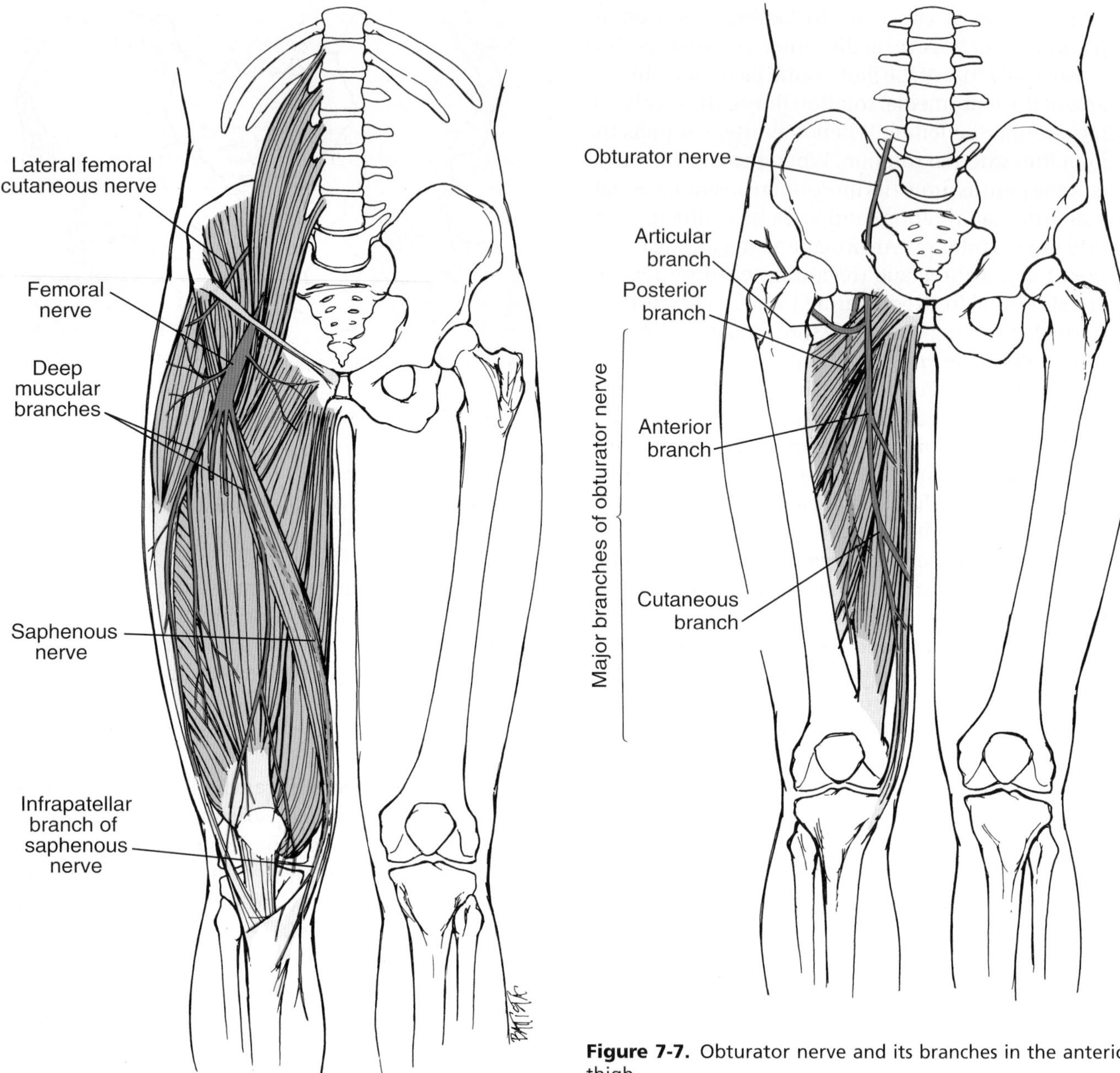

Figure 7-6. Femoral and lateral femoral cutaneous nerves.

Figure 7-7. Obturator nerve and its branches in the anterior thigh.

- ***Dysfunction and injury:*** These nerves can be compressed with sustained muscle contraction, can be entrapped in adhesions resulting from previous inflammation or injury, or can become excessively stretched because of pelvic imbalance. See Chapter 3, "Lumbosacral Spine" for information on nerve root irritation and injury where these nerves originate at the spine.
- ***Treatment implications:*** OM and MET can effectively release peripheral compression and entrapment of the nerves.

Muscles

- ***Function***: As mentioned in Chapter 3, it is important to remember that muscles of the hip region not only

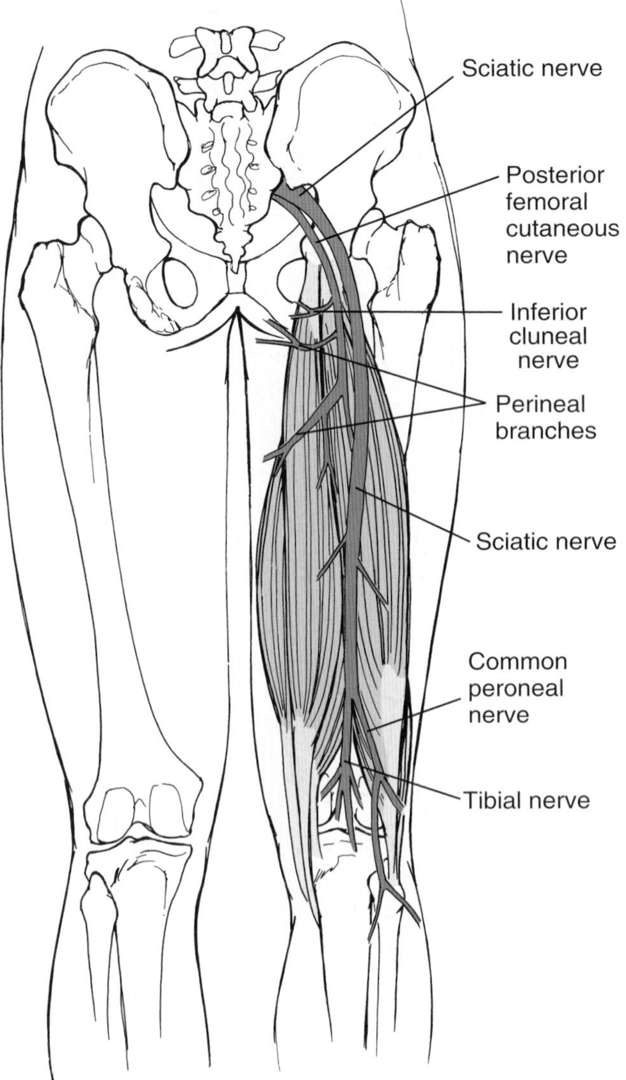

Figure 7-8. Sciatic nerve innervates the posterior thigh, leg, and foot.

affect the hip joint but also have a profound influence on lumbopelvic function.

- Twenty-two muscles surround the hip. These muscles may be divided into five groups:
  - **Flexors:** Iliacus, psoas, rectus femoris, tensor fascia lata (TFL) and sartorius
  - **Extensors:** Gluteus maximus, semimembranosus, semitendinosus, and biceps femoris
  - **Abductors:** TFL and gluteus medius and minimus
  - **Adductors:** Gracilis, pectineus, and adductor magnus, longus, and brevis
  - **Deep lateral rotators:** Piriformis, obturator internus and externus, superior and inferior gemelli, and quadratus femoris
- ***Dysfunction and injury:*** The most commonly injured muscles of the hip region are the two-joint muscles, especially the rectus femoris and the hamstrings. Two-joint muscles incur these injuries because of one of their main functions: eccentric contraction (i.e., to contract while the muscle is lengthening). Muscles are much more prone to injury during eccentric contraction. The rectus femoris must eccentrically contract to decelerate the hip and knee, and the hamstrings eccentrically contract as the knee comes to full extension at heel strike.[4] Muscle dysfunction has two basic categories: muscle imbalance and positional dysfunction. Muscle imbalance describes a condition in which certain muscles usually are weak, and others usually are short and tight. Janda[4a] calls this muscle imbalance in the hip and lumbopelvic region the **lower (pelvic) crossed syndrome.** Muscle imbalances alter movement patterns and therefore add a continuing stress to the joint system.

Muscle Imbalances of the Hip Region (the Lower [Pelvic] Crossed Syndrome)

- **Muscles that tend to be tight and short:** the iliopsoas, piriformis, rectus femoris, TFL, adductors, external rotators, quadratus lumborum (QL), iliotibial band (ITB), and hamstrings
- **Muscles that tend to be weak and inhibited:** the quadriceps (except the rectus femoris), vastus medialis obliquus (VMO), abdominals, and gluteus maximus, medius, and minimus.

Positional Dysfunction of the Hip Region Muscles

- The psoas tends to wind into a medial torsion along with the adductors as the femur becomes internally rotated.
- Pectineus, rectus, sartorius, and TFL all tend to wind into a medial torsion.
- Gluteus maximus and medius, piriformis, and other external rotators tend to roll into an inferior torsion.

Anatomy of the Hip Muscles

See Muscle Table 7-1.

Muscular Actions of the Hip

See Table 7-2.

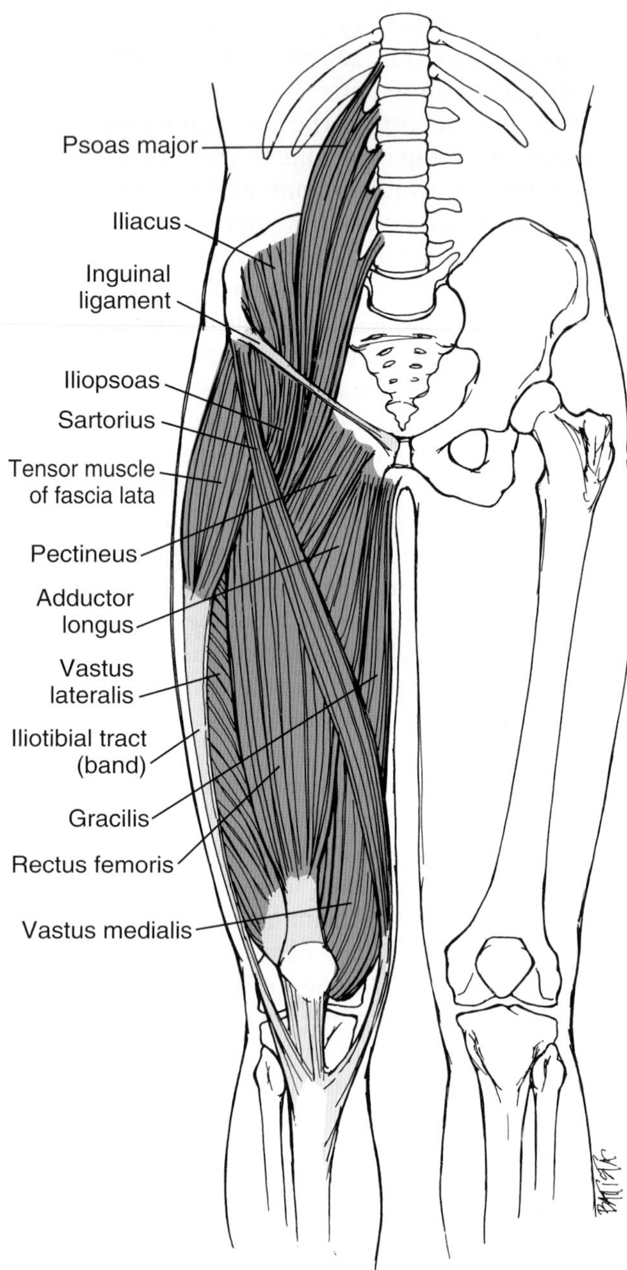

Figure 7-9. Superficial muscles of the anterior thigh.

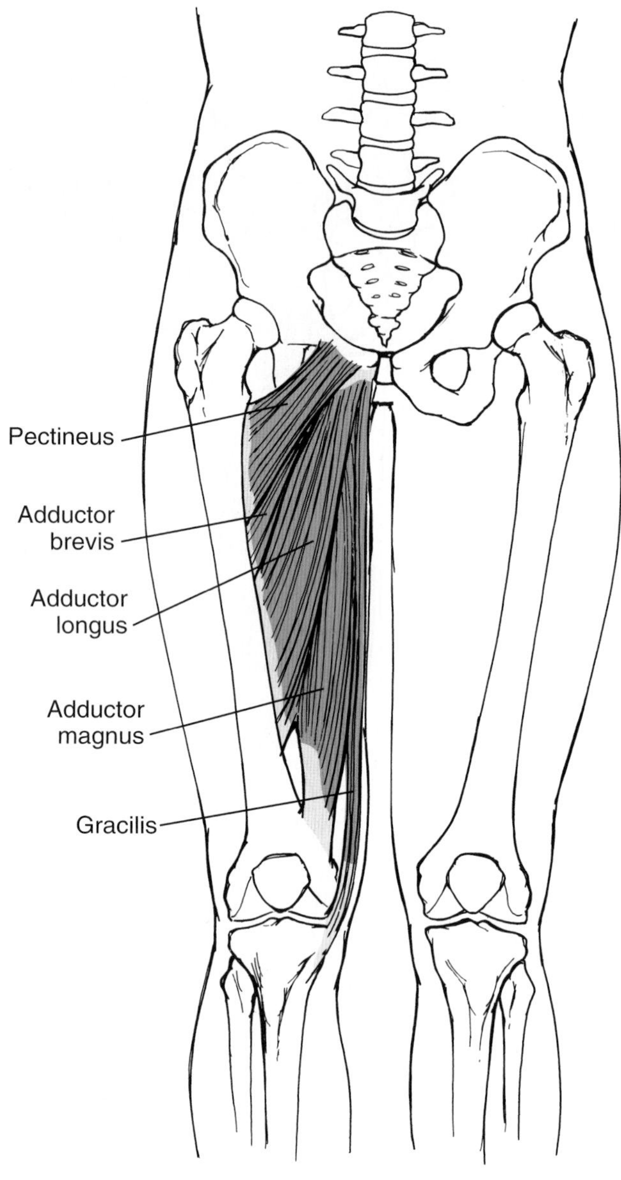

Figure 7-10. Adductor muscles and deep muscles of the anterior thigh.

Hip Dysfunction and Injury

FACTORS PREDISPOSING TO HIP PAIN

- Predisposing factors to hip pain include capsular thickening caused by previous trauma, leg-length inequality, pelvic unlevelling (pelvic obliquity), chronic lower back dysfunction or pain, chronic sacroiliac joint (SIJ) dysfunction or pain, muscle imbalances, anteverted hip, muscle fatigue, obesity, and sedentary lifestyle.
- Leg-length inequality creates pelvic unlevelling and a high ilium relative to the other side. The ilium rolls anteriorly slightly as it elevates, compressing the hip joint on that side. This compression predisposes the joint on the side of the long leg to arthrosis.[7] This unlevelling also creates gait disturbances, which creates uneven stress through the joint, predisposing to degeneration.
- Chronic lower back dysfunction or pain or chronic SIJ dysfunction or pain creates compensations

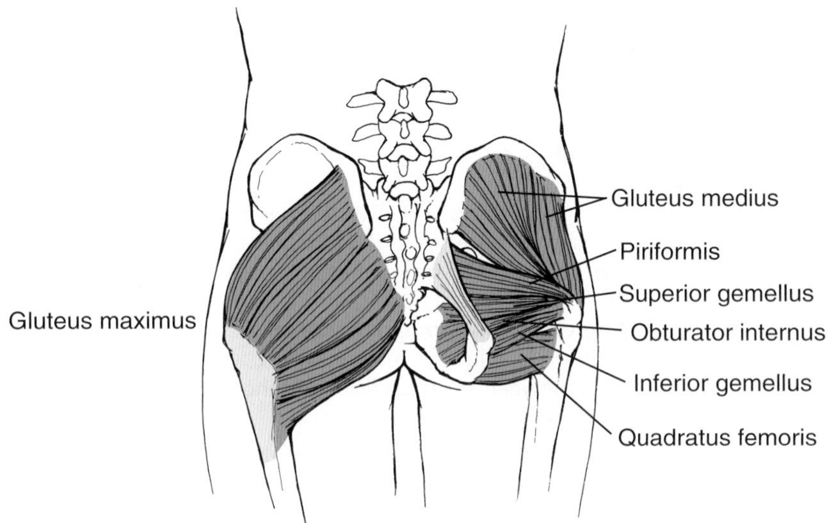

Figure 7-11. Gluteal muscles and deep rotators of the hip.

throughout the hip region, causing uneven distribution of the weight through the cartilage.

- Anteversion in the hip causes the hip to assume its closed-packed position, creating increased compression in the joint and winding the joint capsule into its tightened position.
- Muscle imbalance creates abnormal movement through the joint, which means an imbalanced stress on the cartilage will occur. Tight muscles add a compressive load to the joint, and hypertonic muscles are more easily fatigued and therefore more easily strained.

DIFFERENTIATION OF HIP PAIN

- It is important to realize that on rare occasions hip pain can represent a pathologic condition. See "Contraindications to Massage Therapy: Red Flags" in Chapter 2, "Assessment & Technique" for guidelines on when massage is contraindicated and when to refer. Hip pain can also come from structures other than the hip, most commonly the lumbar spine. Chronic hip pain also requires a thorough examination of the lumbar spine. Assuming that pain in the hip is not pathologic, differentiation may be categorized according to structures involved.
- Myofascial pain of acute onset is described as a sharp, localized pain that is often associated with

Text continued on page 260.

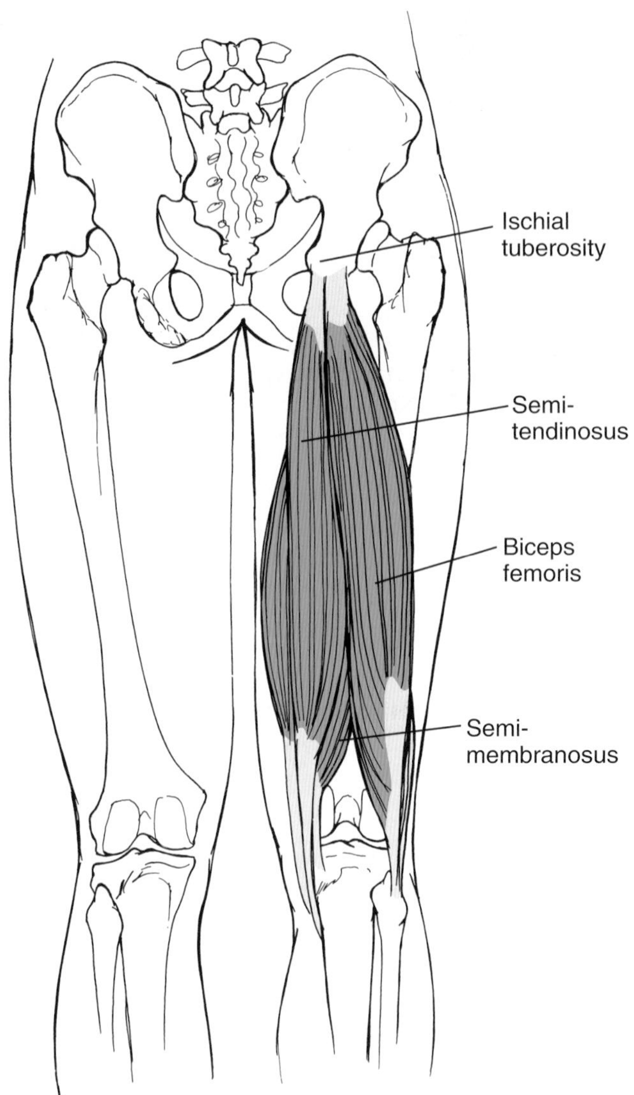

Figure 7-12. Posterior hip and thigh muscles.

TABLE 7-1 **ANATOMY OF THE HIP MUSCLES**

Flexors (Fig. 7-9)

Muscle	*Origin*	*Insertion*
Psoas major	Anterior surfaces and lower border of transverse processes of the lumbar vertebrae and by five digitations, each from the vertebral bodies and intervening discs; psoas interweaves with the diaphragm; lumbar plexus runs between the superficial and the deep part of the psoas major.	Passes behind the inguinal ligament and in front of the joint capsule, ending in a tendon that receives almost all the fibers of the iliacus on its lateral side and attaches to the lesser trochanter of femur.
Psoas minor	Lies in front of psoas major from the sides of T12–L1 bodies and discs.	Ends in long, flat tendon attached to the iliopubic eminence and to the iliopectineal arch, a fascial expansion of the inguinal ligament; psoas minor is absent in approximately 50% of the population.
Iliacus	A triangular sheet of muscle arising from upper two-thirds of iliac fossa; from inner lip of iliac crest, anterior sacroiliac ligaments, and iliolumbar ligaments; and from A–S–lateral surface of sacrum.	Most fibers converge into the lateral side of the tendon of psoas major and insert on lesser trochanter of femur.
Tensor fascia lata (TFL)	Anterior aspect of external lip of iliac crest, lateral surface of ASIS, and border of notch below the ASIS between gluteus minimus and sartorius.	Descends between and is attached to the two layers of the iliotibial tract.
Rectus femoris (for other quadriceps, see Chapter 8, "The Knee."	Arises by two tendinous heads—a straight head from the AIIS and a reflected head from a groove above the acetabulum and from the fibrous capsule of the hip.	Ends in a broad, thick aponeurosis and flattened tendon attached to the upper surface of the patella; superficial, central part of the quadriceps tendon.
Sartorius	A narrow, strap muscle, the longest muscle in the body, arises from tendinous fibers from the medial side of the ASIS.	Ends in a thin, flat tendon that curves forward into a broad aponeurosis attached in front of the gracilis and semitendinosus to the medial surface of tibia.

Adductors of the Hip (Fig. 7-10)

Muscle	*Origin*	*Insertion*
Pectineus	A flat, quadrangular muscle arising from the pectineal line on the superior pubic ramus between the iliopubic eminence and the pubic tubercle.	Fibers pass downward, backward, and laterally to attach on the pectineal line on posterior surface of femur between linea aspera and lesser trochanter; may also interweave with the joint capsule.
Adductor longus	Most anterior of the three adductors; arises by a flat tendon from the front of the pubis in the angle between the crest and the symphysis.	Expands in a broad fleshy belly that is inserted by an aponeurosis into the linea aspera in the middle third of the posterior femur between the vastus medialis and the adductor brevis and magnus.

Action	*Relation*	*Dysfunction*
Flexes the thigh on the pelvis; flexes trunk against thigh, increasing lumbar curve; assists in lateral rotation and abduction of the hip.		If the psoas is contracted or short unilaterally, the trunk is flexed and side bent to the same side.
Flexes thigh on pelvis; flexes trunk against the leg, increasing lumbar curve; performs lateral rotation of hip.	Iliopsoas: lateral to pectineus, medial to sartorius and rectus femoris, anterior to the iliopectineal bursa that lies over joint capsule, and lateral to the femoral artery and vein.	
Assists in abduction and medial rotation and, most important, serves as a stabilizer of the hip.	ITB: deep fascia of lateral thigh that is thicker where the TFL and gluteus maximus are attached to it proximally.	Weakness contributes to bow-legged position; shortness contributes to knock-knees and anterior pelvic tilt.
Assists in flexing the pelvis and extends the leg at the knee; efficiency as a hip flexor increases the more the knee is flexed because flexion lengthens this muscle.		
Flexes thigh on pelvis and leg on the thigh; also helps abduct the thigh and rotate it laterally.		

Action	*Relation*	*Dysfunction*
Flexes the hip and adducts the thigh.	Medial to psoas major, lateral to lateral margin of adductor longus, and medial to the femoral artery.	
Adducts and aids in flexion and lateral rotation of the hip.	Palpation: When the legs are abducted, forms a distinct ridge, extending from the pubic bone just below the crest toward the middle of the thigh.	

Adductors of the Hip—cont'd

Muscle	*Origin*	*Insertion*
Adductor brevis	Posterior to pectineus and adductor longus, arises by a narrow attachment along the external aspect of the body and inferior ramus of the pubis between the gracilis and the obturator externus.	Passes laterally, posteriorly, and inferiorly, attached to femur along a line from lesser trochanter to linea aspera between pectineus and adductor magnus.
Adductor magnus	A massive triangular muscle arising from the lower lateral aspect of the ischial tuberosity, the ischial ramus, and the adjacent pubic ramus.	Pubic fibers, which are short and horizontal, attach to the medial margin of the gluteal tuberosity, medially to gluteus maximus; fibers from the ischial ramus fan out downward and laterally and attach to linea aspera; thigh mass arising from ischial tuberosity descends almost vertically to lower third of thigh in a rounded tendon that attaches to adductor tubercle.
Gracilis	Most superficial of the adductor group; thin and flat, broad above, narrow and tapering below; arises by a thin aponeurosis from the medial margins of the lower pubic body, the inferior pubic ramus, and the adjoining ischial ramus.	Fibers descend vertically into a rounded tendon passing over the medial condyle of the femur behind the sartorius; becomes flattened, curving round the medial tibial condyle and attaching to the medial surface below the condyle, immediately proximal to that of semitendinosus, with its upper edge overlapped by the tendon of sartorius.

Gluteal Region (Fig. 7-11)

Muscle	*Origin*	*Insertion*
Gluteus maximus (see Fig. 7-11 also)	Largest and most powerful muscle, it is the most characteristic feature of the human, associated with bringing the trunk upright; arises from posterior line of ilium, posterior aspect of sacrum, coccyx, and sacrotuberous ligament.	Ends in a thick tendinous lamina, passes lateral to the greater trochanter, and attaches to the iliotibial tract of the fascia lata; deeper fibers of the lower part attach to the gluteal tuberosity of the femur between vastus lateralis and adductor magnus.
Gluteus medius	Broad, thick muscle arises from the outer surface of the ilium, between the anterior and the posterior gluteal lines, and external aspect of ilium.	Fibers converge to a strong, flat tendon that is attached to the superior aspect of the lateral surface of greater trochanter.
Gluteus minimus	Deep to the gluteus medius, smallest of three gluteals; fan-shaped origin arises from outer surface of ilium between ASIS and greater sciatic notch.	Attached to a ridge in the lateral surface of the A–S portion of the greater trochanter and the hip joint capsule.

Deep Lateral Rotators of Hip (See Fig. 7-11)

Muscle	*Origin*	*Insertion*
Piriformis	Anterior surface of sacrum between and lateral to sacral foramina 1–4, the margin of greater sciatic foramen and the pelvic surface of the sacrotuberous ligament.	Passes out of the pelvis through the greater sciatic foramen and attaches by a rounded tendon to the superior-posterior border of greater trochanter; often blended with common tendon of obturator internus and gemelli.

Action	Relation	Dysfunction
Adducts thigh; aids in flexion and lateral rotation of thigh.		
Powerful adductor of thigh; aids in flexion and assists in lateral rotation; lower portion of muscle extends the thigh and rotates it medially; also acts as a dynamic stabilizer of the medial patella, as the VMO inserts into the adductor magnus tendon[5].		With sustained contraction, the hip adductors cause a lateral pelvic tilt, with the pelvis high on the side on contraction[6].
With the knee extended, adducts the thigh and flexes the hip; also flexes and medially rotates the knee.		

Action	Relation	Dysfunction
Extensor and powerful lateral rotator of thigh; inferior fibers assist in adduction and upper fibers are abductors; balances trunk on femur; balances knee joint via ITB.		Weak, inhibited by sustained contraction on the hip flexors, especially the iliopsoas, causing overuse of the hamstrings.
Principal muscle of abduction; anterior fibers medially rotate and may assist in flexion; posterior fibers laterally rotate and may assist in extension of hip.		If weak, leads to lateral pelvic tilt and pelvis is high on the side of weakness; if contracted, pelvis is low on side of contracture.
Acting with gluteus medius, abducts the hip; the anterior fibers of the minimus rotate the hip medially; both may also act as hip flexors.	Nearly vertical course and is completely covered by gluteus medius	Tightness causes abduction and medial rotation of the thigh; in standing, there is a lateral pelvic tilt, low on the side of shortness, accompanied by medial rotation of the femur.

Action	Relation	Dysfunction
Laterally rotates the extended thigh; abducts the hip when hip is flexed.		

Deep Lateral Rotators of Hip—cont'd

Muscle	*Origin*	*Insertion*
Quadratus femoris	Proximal part of lateral border of tuberosity of ischium.	Attaches to posterior femur, extending down intertrochanteric crest.
Obturator internus	Internal or pelvic surface of obturator membrane and margin of obturator foramen, the inferior ramus of pubis and ischium.	Fibers end in 4 or 5 tendinous bands, which make a right-angled bend over the grooved surface of the ischium between the spine and the tuberosity; these unite into a single, flat tendon, passing horizontally across the hip joint capsule, and interweave with the insertions of the gemelli, inserting on medial superior surface of the posterior greater trochanter.
Gemellus superior	External surface of spine of ischium.	Lies on the superior surface of the obturator internus and attaches to the medial surface of greater trochanter.
Gemellus inferior	Upper part of tuberosity of ischium, below groove for obturator internus.	Lies on the inferior surface of the obturator internus and attaches to the medial surface of greater trochanter.
Obturator externus	Flat, triangular muscle covering the external surface of the anterior pelvic wall, arising from bone around the obturator foramen.	Trochanteric fossa of femur.

Hamstrings (See Fig. 7-12)

Muscle	*Origin*	*Insertion*
Biceps femoris (long head)	Ischial tuberosity (blending with the sacrotuberous ligament).	
Biceps femoris (short head)	Middle third of the lateral lip of the linea aspera.	Head of the fibula and lateral condyle of the tibia.
Semitendinosus	From the ischial tuberosity, blended with the long head of the biceps.	Medial margin of the tuberosity of the tibia; together with the sartorius and gracilis, they form the pes anserinus tendons.
Semimembranosus	Ischial tuberosity.	Tendon divides into three parts below medial collateral ligament: first part runs to the posteromedial corner of the tibia, just below the joint line; second, into the fascia of the popliteus; and third, into the posterior wall of the capsule as the oblique popliteal ligament, attaching to the medial meniscus.
Quadriceps (refer to the Chapter 8, "The Knee")		

Action	Relation	Dysfunction
		Lauren Berry, RPT, taught that the obturator rolls into an abnormal inferior torsion in dysfunction and injury to the lumbopelvic region; this torsion puts a tethering or pulling force on the fascia suspending the sciatic nerve; can create irritation of the nerve, and diffuse sciatic pain into the thigh and leg.
		Lateral rotators are nearly three times stronger than medial rotators; if there is lateral rotator weakness, there is a medial rotation of the femur, pronation of the foot, and a tendency for knock-knees; if there is lateral rotator shortness, there is a lateral rotation of the femur and an out-toeing of the foot in standing[6]; piriformis is short and tight as it substitutes for a weak gluteus medius[5].

Action	Relation	Dysfunction
Extension of the hip, flexion of the knee, and lateral rotation of the flexed leg; the only lateral rotator of the knee.		
Extension of the hip, flexion of the knee, and medial rotation of the flexed leg.		
Extension of the hip; flexion and medial rotation of the knee; during knee flexion it pulls the meniscus backwards.		Weakness contributes to an anterior pelvic tilt and to increased lordosis; bilateral contraction causes a posterior pelvic tilt and a decreased lumbar curve; weakness of the medial hamstrings contributes to knock-knees, and a lateral rotation of the femur.

TABLE 7-2 MUSCULAR ACTIONS OF THE HIP

- Flexion
  - Psoas major—also rotates the thigh laterally and assists in trunk flexion
  - Iliacus—flexes the hip and rotates it laterally
  - TFL—flexes, abducts, and medially rotates the hip
  - Rectus femoris—flexes the hip and extends the knee
  - Sartorius—flexes, abducts, and rotates the thigh laterally and flexes and rotates the knee medially
  - Pectineus—also adducts the hip
- Extension
  - Gluteus maximus—also laterally rotates the hip; lower fibers adduct and upper fibers abduct the hip
  - Gluteus medius (posterior fibers)—anterior fibers assist in hip flexion and medial rotation; a strong abductor of the hip
  - Gluteus minimus (posterior fibers)—same as gluteus medius
  - Semimembranosus—also medially rotates the hip and flexes and medially rotates the knee
  - Semitendinosus—also medially rotates the hip and flexes and medially rotates the knee
  - Biceps femoris—also flexes the knee and rotates it laterally
  - Piriformis—acts primarily as an external rotator
- Abduction
  - Gluteus medius
  - Piriformis
  - TFL
  - Obturator internus
  - Gluteus maximus
  - Gluteus minimus
- Adduction
  - Adductor magnus—also flexes hip; lower fibers cause medial rotation
  - Adductor longus—also flexes hip and rotates it laterally
  - Adductor brevis—also flexes hip and rotates it laterally
  - Gluteus maximus—also extends the hip
  - Gracilis—also medially rotates hip and flexes knee
  - Pectineus—also flexes hip
- Lateral rotation (acts like shoulder rotator cuff for fine postural control)
  - Gluteus maximus
  - Quadratus femoris—also adducts hip
  - Obturator internus
  - Gluteus medius and minimus—posterior fibers
  - Iliopsoas
  - Obturator externus
  - All adductors
  - Biceps femoris—also extends the hip
  - Piriformis—also abducts hip
- Medial rotation
  - Gluteus minimus—anterior fibers
  - Gluteus medius—anterior fibers
  - TFL
  - Gracilis—also adducts and flexes the hip and flexes the knee
  - Adductor magnus (which is inserted into adductor tubercle)
  - Semimembranosus and Semitendinosus—also extend the hip

swelling, heat, and redness. The pain is increased with isometric contraction, performed during CR MET, and is better with rest. It is typically localized to the attachment sites or the myotendinous junctions. Gluteus medius tendinitis is well localized to the greater trochanter; adductor strains are localized to the groin; rectus femoris to the AIIS, midbelly, or patellar attachments; hamstrings to the ischial tuberosity or midthigh or at the patellar attachments; iliopsoas elicits a pain in the groin.

- Bursitis is manifested as a diffuse ache or a burning sensation or both. It is worse with movement, or in the case of the trochanteric bursa, worse with lying on it. A swollen bursa elicits an empty end feel on passive motion (i.e., the client feels pain before the tissue is in tension).
- A capsulitis manifests as a deep, diffuse, aching pain and stiffness in the groin. The pain is worse with sitting and climbing stairs and is stiffer in the morning. The first sign of capsulitis of the hip is painful decrease in passive medial rotation. Remember that capsulitis is the precursor of arthrosis (hip degeneration).
- Arthritis is an inflammation of the hip joint, and arthrosis is a degeneration of the joint. Arthritis or arthrosis elicits a deep ache in the groin, greater trochanter, buttock, anterior thigh, and eventually the knee. In the early stages it is painful with excessive movement, but as it progresses, it manifests as a toothache-like pain even at rest. Passive medial rotation and flexion are limited and have a hard end-feel, unlike a chronic capsular shortening which has a thick, leathery end-feel.
- The hip region is a common area for peripheral nerve entrapment. The pain is described as burning or as numbing or tingling or as a combination of the latter two. Peripheral entrapment is typically in a larger area, and the pain is more diffuse.
- The anterior, lateral, and posterior thigh are also common sites of dermatomal pain from nerve root irritation. Nerve root pain is a sharp pain in a well-described patch of skin.

COMMON DYSFUNCTIONS AND INJURIES OF THE HIP

Gluteus Medius Tendinitis

- *Causes:* Pelvic unlevelling stresses the hip abductors on the side of the high ilium; running, dancing, and racket sports all stress the gluteus medius.

- *Symptoms:* Pain is well-localized over the greater trochanter and superior iliac fossa and may radiate down the lateral or posterior thigh. Pain is brought on by hip movements, especially climbing stairs, or prolonged walking or running.
- *Signs:* Pain is reproduced by resisted hip abduction. Pain occurs on tendon stretch with full passive adduction. The gluteus medius usually tests weak, and the TFL becomes hypertonic, substituting for the weak gluteus medius.
- *Sites:* Gluteus medius tendinitis occurs at the tenoperiosteal junction at the lateral aspect of the greater trochanter and the myotendinous junction. The fasciculi in the belly of the muscle tend to roll into an inferior torsion.
- *Treatment:* Perform MET and OM to release any sustained contraction in the adductors first. Perform MET and OM to facilitate the gluteus medius and release its torsion.

Adductor Tendinitis or Groin Strain

- *Causes:* A typical pattern of dysfunction is for the adductors to be tight and short, and for the abductors to be weak. This pattern is associated with anteverted hips, genu valgus, and unlevelling of the pelvis. Sustained contraction fatigues the muscle and makes it more susceptible to injury; the adductor longus is most commonly involved.
- *Symptoms:* Pain is usually well localized to the groin and inner thigh.
- *Signs:* Adductor tendinitis or groin strain signs are pain with resisted hip adduction and possible pain with full passive abduction.
- *Sites:* Groin strain or adductor tendinitis occurs at the tenoperiosteal junction at the anterior pubis and at the musculotendinous junction a few centimeters distally. Adductor fasciculi develop a medial and posterior torsion.
- *Treatment:* Test the length of the adductors, and perform postisometric relaxation (PIR) MET to release the hypertonicity and to lengthen the connective tissue. Release the fibrosis and realign the fibers with OM.

Quadriceps Tendinitis

- *Causes:* The rectus femoris is most commonly involved. Soccer, running, and jumping all stress the rectus femoris. It is more susceptible to injury as it is a two-joint muscle and acts eccentrically to decelerate the hip and knee.[8] It is typically tight and short.
- *Symptoms:* Pain is usually well localized to the AIIS, approximately 3 inches inferior to the ASIS or midbelly or at the patellar attachments either above or below the patella.
- *Signs:* Quadriceps tendinitis signs are pain with resisted knee extension with hip extended (i.e., with the client supine and attempting to lift the straight leg) and pain with passive flexion of the knee >120° (i.e., with the client prone).
- *Sites:* Quadriceps tendinitis occurs at the tenoperiosteal junction at the AIIS, at the insertion of reflected head into the superior aspect of the acetabulum, midbelly, or at the patella.
- *Treatment:* As the rectus is typically tight and short, first perform PIR to lengthen the muscle, and then release the potential fibrosis and realign the fibers with OM.

Hamstring Tendinitis

- *Causes:* The hamstrings are typically short and tight in most people mainly for two reasons. First, we live in a sedentary culture, and sitting shortens the hamstrings and the iliopsoas. The shortened iliopsoas inhibits the gluteus maximus and thus overloads the hamstrings. This overload predisposes the muscle to fatigue. Second, the hamstrings eccentrically contract as the knee comes to full extension at heel strike, making it vulnerable; thus overexertion, such as running, jumping, and racket sports leads to injury. The biceps femoris is most commonly involved.[5]
- *Symptoms:* Pain may be present at three common sites: at the ischial tuberosity, midbelly, and less commonly behind the knee.
- *Signs:* Hamstring tendinitis signs are pain reproduced with resisted knee flexion, possible pain with resisted hip extension, and pain in the muscle with a straight–leg-raising (SLR) test.
- *Sites:* Hamstring tendinitis occurs at the tenoperiosteal insertions at the ischial tuberosity, at the myotendinous junction at various sites on the posterior thigh, and at tenoperiosteal insertions behind the knee.
- *Treatment:* As the hamstrings are typically tight and short, perform PIR or CRAC MET within comfortable limits to help restore normal length. Then release the fibrosis and realign the fibers with OM.

Iliopsoas Tendinitis

- *Causes:* As with the hamstrings, the iliopsoas tends to be short and tight. Repetitive hip flexion, such as stair climbing, can fatigue and strain this muscle. Excessive sitting shortens the muscle.

- *Symptoms:* Pain in the groin, especially with flexing hip, is an iliopsoas tendinitis symptom.
- *Signs:* Iliopsoas tendinitis signs are pain on resisted hip flexion and pain under the inguinal ligament with passive hip flexion and adduction of the hip perpendicular to the inguinal ligament.
- *Sites:* Iliopsoas tendinitis occurs at the tenoperiosteal junction of the lesser trochanter and within the belly of the muscle, especially in the area of the inguinal ligament.
- *Treatment:* Release the hypertonicity with CR or PIR MET to lengthen the connective tissue. Next, release any fibrosis and realign the fibers with OM.

Trochanteric Bursitis

- *Causes:* Trochanteric bursitis occurs as a result of a fall on the side of the hip; a repetitive circular motion of the hip, as in riding a bicycle; or a sustained contraction of the TFL, ITB, and gluteus maximus caused by hip joint pathology or lumbosacral injury or dysfunction.
- *Symptoms:* Clients usually experience an acute onset of diffuse, deep ache and burning sensation over the greater trochanter; this pain may ache and throb down the lateral thigh and may worsen when the client climbs stairs or lays on it at night.
- *Signs:* Resisted abduction and extension may cause pain that is achy and diffuse; passive adduction with hip flexion causes pain. An inflamed bursa is tender to palpation.
- *Sites:* Trochanteric bursitis occurs at the posterolateral aspect of the greater trochanter and down the lateral thigh.
- *Treatment:* Use MET to release any sustained contraction in the TFL, ITB, and gluteus maximus. Normalize the bursa with OM.

Iliopectineal Bursitis

- *Causes:* Repetitive hip flexion, as in stair climbing, dancing, martial arts, etc., or a sustained hip flexion, as in sedentary lifestyle all compress the iliopsoas over the bursa.
- *Symptoms:* Clients experience a diffuse, deep ache in the groin and anterior thigh.
- *Signs:* Passive adduction in flexion compresses the bursa and elicits an empty end-feel or an ache in the groin before the tension barrier; full passive extension reproduces the pain.
- *Sites:* The iliopectineal bursa is located between the psoas muscle and the hip joint capsule.
- *Treatment:* Release any sustained contraction in the iliopsoas with CR or PIR MET. Help reduce the swelling in the bursa with OM.

Hip Capsulitis

- *Causes:* A sedentary lifestyle shortens the anterior capsule of the hip. Repetitive hip flexion, such as stair climbing or hiking, or an overuse of the hip flexors through dance, racket sports, etc. can inflame the area and lead to fibrosis.
- *Symptoms:* Clients experience a sometimes rapid onset of pain and stiffness, made worse with activity, usually localized in the groin, but sometimes in the anterior thigh and knee.
- *Signs:* Medial rotation of the hip is most limited, accompanied by limited flexion and adduction. With acute capsulitis there is an empty end-feel; chronic capsulitis elicits a leathery end-feel with a decreased ROM.
- *Sites:* Hip capsulitis occurs at the capsule between the trochanter and the acetabulum.
- *Treatment:* It is critical to maintain or restore the normal length to the capsule, as a shortened capsule can diminish the blood supply to the femoral head and predisposes the joint to degeneration. Perform MET to increase the length of the capsule by increasing medial rotation and extension.

Hip Arthritis or Arthrosis

- *Causes:* Clients are usually middle-aged or older, often with a history of prior trauma, usually a fall. Arthritis or arthrosis is typically associated with cumulative stress, such as pelvic unlevelling. The side of the high ilium rolls forward slightly, compressing the hip joint on that side. Chronic low back pain (LBP) often leads to gait disturbances and secondary altered weight distribution problems in the hips. Anteverted hip and sedentary lifestyle are also predisposing factors.
- *Symptoms:* Arthrosis or arthritis symptoms usually have an insidious onset of an ache that begins in the groin and extends to the greater trochanter, medial buttock, and anterior thigh and that may refer to the knee. Patients describe being stiff in the morning or after sitting for long periods and having pain after extended walking.
- **Signs:** Medial rotation of the hip is most limited, accompanied by limited flexion. A hard end-feel is evident on flexion and medial rotation.

- *Sites:* Hip arthritis or arthrosis involves a degeneration of the joint cartilage and an eventual dehydration and fibrosis of the capsule; this dehydration and fibrosis diminish blood supply to the femoral head as the artery to the head of the femur is intracapsular.
- *Treatment:* In addition to releasing the hypertonicity and strengthening the inhibited muscles around the hip, it is critical to stretch the joint capsule and to increase medial rotation, flexion, and adduction of the hip with MET.

Snapping Hip Syndrome

- *Causes:* A massage therapist can address three common explanations: (1) the posterior portion of the ITB misaligns over the greater trochanter; (2) the iliopsoas tendon snaps over the iliopectineal eminence; and (3) the iliofemoral ligament snaps over the femoral head.[8]
- *Symptoms:* Clients experience a snapping feeling or pain at the lateral aspect of the hip, or they may experience both.
- *Signs:* When the leg is lowered to the table with the knee extended, the "snap" occurs.
- *Treatment:* Perform OM to roll the soft tissue laterally and posteriorly to reset it.

Entrapment of the Lateral Femoral Cutaneous Nerve

- *Causes:* Pregnancy, obesity, or repetitive hip flexion such as stair climbing, or hiking can entrap the lateral femoral cutaneous nerve of the thigh.
- *Symptoms:* Clients experience burning pain with numbness and tingling over the anterolateral aspect of the thigh to just above the knee.
- *Signs:* Pain brought on by passive hip extension is a sign of entrapment.
- *Sites:* The nerve is usually entrapped under the inguinal ligament approximately one-half inch medial to the ASIS in the fibro-osseous tunnel formed by the iliac fascia and the inguinal ligament.
- *Treatment:* Release the nerve by working transverse to it, medially to laterally, superior and deep to the inguinal ligament.

Entrapment of the Obturator Nerve

- *Causes:* Overuse of the hip adductors, such as riding a horse, or direct pressure on the adductor attachments can irritate the area, leading to fibrosis and peripheral entrapment.
- *Symptoms:* Clients experience burning pain or numbing and tingling in the medial thigh.
- *Signs:* Pain elicited by passive hip adduction may be a sign of obturator nerve entrapment.
- *Sites:* Obturator nerve entrapment occurs medial to the psoas above the inguinal ligament and between the adductor longus and the pectineus immediately distal to the pubis.
- *Treatment:* Release the nerve by working transverse to the nerve at the sites mentioned above.

Entrapment of the Femoral Nerve

- *Symptoms:* Sustained hypertonicity of the psoas is a common source of nerve entrapment. Unlike most nerves, the lumbar plexus, which is the root of the femoral nerve, travels through the body of the psoas, rather than alongside of the muscle.
- *Symptoms:* Clients experience pain, numbing, and tingling in the anterior thigh.
- *Signs:* Pain elicited with passive hip extension is a sign of femoral nerve entrapment.
- *Sites:* Entrapment is usually superior to the inguinal ligament within a psoas contracture.
- *Treatment:* Release the nerve by working transverse to its line, in a medial to lateral (M–L) direction. These are the same strokes as the psoas muscle release, with a different intention.

Entrapment of Sciatic Nerve

- *Causes:* The most common causes are contracture of the piriformis, obturator internus, or biceps femoris. Any inflammation in the gluteal region can create a fibrosis that tethers (pulls) on the loose irregular connective tissue that suspends the sciatic nerve as it travels through the gluteal region.
- *Symptoms:* Clients experience a diffuse ache in the buttock and diffuse pain, numbing, or tingling down the posterior thigh. Symptoms rarely extend to the calf and foot.
- *Signs:* The SLR test may be mildly positive, with diffuse pain, numbing or tingling, in the leg at approximately 70°. If a lumbar disc herniation creates nerve root pressure, it usually creates a sharp, well-localized pain during the SLR test well below 70°.
- *Sites:* Sciatic nerve entrapment can occur at the following sites:
  - Piriformis muscle
  - Greater sciatic notch
  - Lateral-superior aspect of the ischial tuberosity tethered by inferior torsion of obturator internus

- Between the greater trochanter and the ischial tuberosity entrapped under the biceps femoris attachment).
- Adhesions between the adductor magnus and the short head of the biceps femoris.

- *Treatment:* Perform OM strokes to release the above sites.

Note: Sciatic neuritis can be caused by many lesions not listed, including some serious pathologies. The list above represents common entrapment sites that may be addressed safely by the massage therapist.

Hip Assessment

BACKGROUND

One of the primary intentions of the assessment for the massage therapist is to differentiate a shortened joint capsule and degeneration of the joint from muscle dysfunction and injury. This objective is accomplished primarily through passive ROM assessment, addressed in this section. The second goal is to assess the length, strength, and proper firing sequence of the muscles affecting the hip. The third goal is to assess soft tissue accurately after an acute injury. The second and third goals are primarily addressed in the "Muscle Energy Technique" section.

HISTORY QUESTIONS FOR THE CLIENT WHO HAS HIP PAIN

- Where does it hurt? (Ask client to place his or her hand over the area.)
  - Problems in the hip joint itself will be felt in the inguinal region, midway between the ASIS and the pubic symphysis. With worsening conditions, the pain can radiate to the anterior thigh and knee. As the nerves to the knee and hip have the same embryologic origin, dysfunction in one joint can refer pain to the other. Pain over the greater trochanter and lateral thigh is usually pain referred from the lumbar spine or trochanter bursitis. Pain in the buttock may be piriformis or gluteus medius tendinitis or lesions of the SIJ or lumbar spine. Clients often point to the SIJ when asked to locate their hip problem. Pain localized to the SIJ implicates that joint.
- Do you have a history of back problems?
  - Pain in the hip region is often a referral from the lumbosacral spine. Asymmetry in the pelvis can create lower back and hip joint problems due to the abnormal stresses to those joints. These two conditions are differentiated through active and passive ROM studies. Typically, if a client has full and pain-free active and passive ROM in the lumbosacral spine and a full and painless SLR test (see Chapter 3) it eliminates that region as the source of referral.

OBSERVATION

Gait

Observe the client walk around your treatment room. Indications that there may be a hip problem include the following: a limp; guarded weight-bearing, the knee is bent to help absorb the shock of weight-bearing, the stride length is shorter, the hip is stiff during gait, or the trunk is shifted side to side in transferring the weight from one leg to the other.

Posture

- *Position:* The client is standing, facing away from the therapist.
- *Action:* Place your hands on the iliac crests to see if they are level.
- *Observation:* A pelvis that is not level is called a pelvic obliquity. Pelvic obliquity may be caused by leg-length difference, muscle imbalance, SIJ or lumbar spine dysfunction or degeneration, or scoliosis. (See Ch. 3 for further discussion of postural assessment.)

Trendelenburg's Test

- *Intention:* To assess the balance, stability, and strength of the gluteus medius.
- *Position:* Have the client stand with his or her back to you and next to a wall, in case he or she needs to reach out a hand for support.
- *Action:* Ask the client to stand on one leg (the uninvolved leg first).
- *Observation:* Normally, the pelvis on the side of the lifted leg should rise because the gluteus medius pulls the hip down on the standing leg. If the gluteus medius on the standing leg is weak, the pelvis rises on the standing leg side, lowering

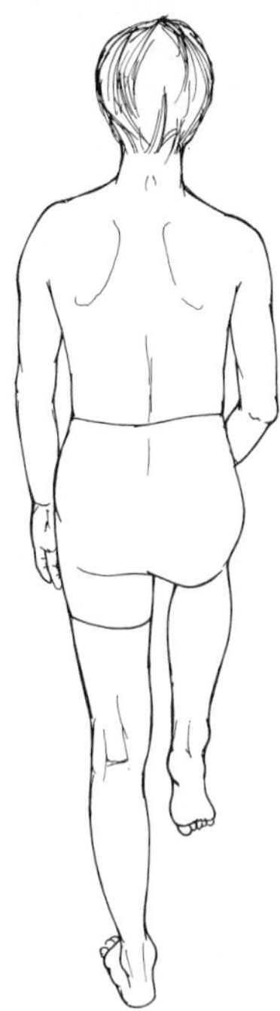

Figure 7-13. Trendelenburg's test. The hip on the standing leg should lower as the opposite leg is lifted. An elevation of the hip on the standing leg side indicates weakness of the gluteus medius on that side.

the pelvis on the lifted side. This is called Trendelenburg's Sign (Fig. 7-13). If the test is negative, have the client repeat the test with eyes closed. This tests balance and the integrity of the proprioceptors. If the client's balance is impaired, standing on one leg for 10 to 30 seconds several times a day is an excellent exercise to help reeducate the proprioceptors.

ACTIVE MOVEMENTS

Observe the ROM. Ask if movement hurts.

Extension

This movement is performed during the lumbar examination. See Chapter 3.

Flexion

- ☐ ***Position:*** Ask the client to stand facing you.
- ☐ ***Action:*** Ask the client to march in place slowly, bringing the thigh as close to the chest as possible. Ask the client not to lean back to perform this action.
- ☐ ***Observation:*** This is a good screening test for hip joint problems and for iliopsoas tendinitis. The normal range is approximately 110° to 120°. With joint involvement, the ROM is limited in flexion. With tendinitis, this movement can elicit pain in the groin.

Abduction

- ☐ ***Position:*** Ask the client to stand facing you.
- ☐ ***Action:*** Have the client bring one leg out to the side to his or her comfortable limit, abducting the hip. Instruct the client to keep the trunk upright and the foot facing forward and not externally rotated as the movement is performed.
- ☐ ***Observation:*** Abduction assessment when the client is standing is a more functional body position than when the client is supine. If there is a dysfunction in the hip, then there is a tendency to bend the trunk to the opposite side as the client attempts to lift the hip, giving a false reading. The normal range is from 30° to 50°. Painless inability to perform this movement may indicate gluteus medius weakness or DJD of the hip. Usually, joint degeneration elicits groin ache with this motion. Pain at the greater trochanter may be a trochanteric bursitis, and pain in the buttock may be a gluteus medius tendinitis.

Lateral Rotation

- ☐ ***Position:*** The client is prone, with one knee bent to 90°.
- ☐ ***Action:*** Place your hand on the sacrum to ensure that it does not move, and ask the client to move the bent leg toward the midline.
- ☐ ***Observation:*** The normal range is from 40° to 60°. Always compare both sides. A person who has retroverted hips has an increased range on both sides of lateral rotation and equal limitation of medial rotation on both sides.

Medial Rotation

- ☐ ***Position:*** The client is prone, with one knee bent to 90°.
- ☐ ***Action:*** Place your hand on the sacrum to ensure that it does not move, and ask the client to move the bent leg away from the midline.
- ☐ ***Observation:*** The ROM is normally approximately 30° to 40°. As with all active and passive tests, compare both sides. A person who has anteverted

hips has an increased range of medial rotation on both sides and equal limitation of lateral rotation on both sides. Loss of medial rotation is one of the key assessment findings in hip degeneration.

PASSIVE MOVEMENTS

Always begin with the "good side," that is, the noninvolved side first. Ask the client to tell you if the movement begins to elicit pain. If there is pain, ask where the pain is felt (location) and what kind of pain or discomfort is felt (quality). Note the ROM and the end feel when you put overpressure on the movement.

Extension

- ☐ ***Position:*** The client is prone, with the knee fully flexed. Place your hand over the client's sacrum to stabilize it and tuck your other hand under the client's distal thigh.
- ☐ ***Action:*** Slowly lift the client's hip into extension until there is pain or until tissue tension. Keep the leg in neutral; do not abduct it as it is extended (Fig. 7-14).
- ☐ ***Observation:*** The normal ROM is approximately 10° to 15°. This movement places a stretch on the iliopsoas and anterior capsule. A tight iliopsoas has a muscle tension end-feel; a tight capsule has a thick, leathery end-feel. This motion is typically limited with DJD of the hip. This is also a *femoral nerve stretch test.* If there is pain, numbing, or tingling in the anterior thigh, there may be a peripheral entrapment within the iliopsoas or a more central lesion at the L2, L3, or L4 nerve roots. If the nerve test is positive, perform MET and manual release of the iliopsoas and femoral nerve for several sessions. If you do not have a significant improvement, refer to a chiropractor or osteopath.

Flexion

- ☐ ***Position:*** The client is supine. Bring client's hip and knee into flexion and place the foot on the table. Place your hand on the client's knee and your other hand on the lateral side of the crest of the ilium.
- ☐ ***Action:*** With your inferior hand, bring the hip into flexion by moving the thigh toward the client's chest until you feel the pelvis move. As soon as you feel the pelvis move, you are at the end range of hip flexion (Fig. 7-15).
- ☐ ***Observation:*** The normal pattern of movement for the thigh is in a straight line toward the chest, independent of movement of the pelvis. The normal range is approximately 140°. A dysfunctional movement pattern for the thigh is to move toward abduction and external rotation as you bring it toward the chest (i.e., toward the open position of the joint) and for the pelvis to move with the thigh. This dysfunctional pattern combined with a limited ROM, typically indicates a shortness of the iliofemoral ligament, fibrosis of the joint capsule, and hip joint degeneration. Pain in the groin at the end of the range indicates psoas tendinitis, and pain in the groin with an empty end feel indicates iliopectineal bursitis. If the range is normal,

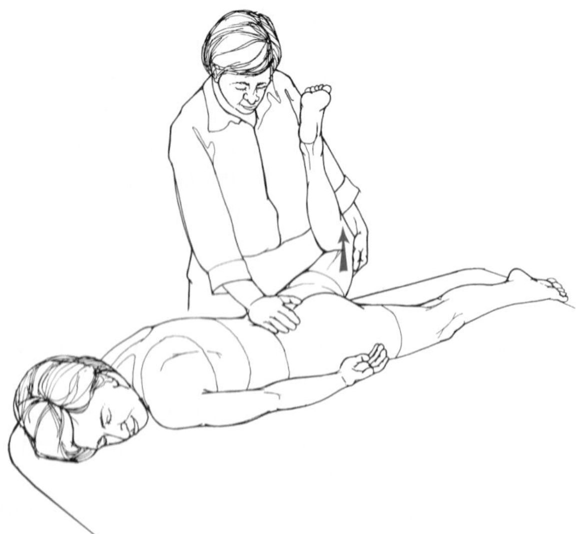

Figure 7-14. Passive extension.

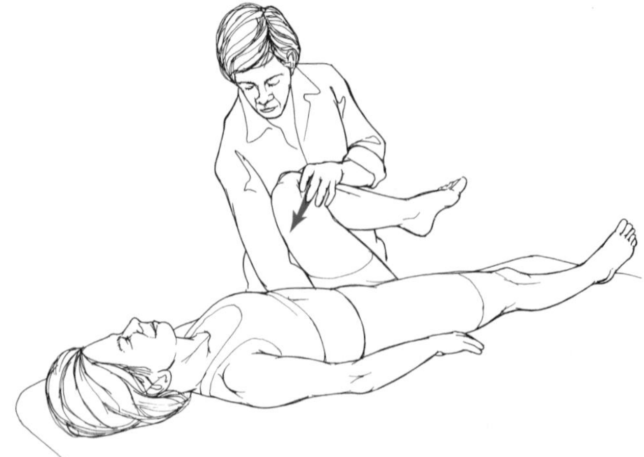

Figure 7-15. Passive flexion.

note whether the opposite leg rises off the table. This indicates a short and tight iliopsoas of the extended leg. Passive hip flexion on one leg to determine psoas tightness on the extended leg is called the **Thomas Test.**

Abduction

- *Position:* For easy comparison, both hips are tested together. The client is supine, with hips in a flexed and abducted position, with the soles of the feet together in the center of the table.
- *Action:* If this position is comfortable, permit the client to rest the legs in this position. If the hips cannot rest in this position comfortably, ask the client to locate the pain and describe its quality. If she or he can rest in this position comfortably, place your hands on the client's knees, and slowly press the knees toward the table, pressing the hips into abduction.
- *Observation:* Compare the height of the knees to determine the ROM of hip abduction. This is a quick screening test that allows you to easily compare the two sides. Discomfort or pain in the groin may indicate a strain of the adductor longus. Pain in the posterior hip may indicate posterior capsule involvement. Loss of motion on one side with a capsular end-feel indicates capsular fibrosis and possible hip joint degeneration. The former condition combined with loss of passive internal rotation would confirm DJD of the hip.

Adduction

- *Position:* The client is supine. Have him or her flex the knee and place the foot on the table. Stabilize the pelvis by placing your hand on the ASIS closest to the client. Place your other hand on the client's knee.
- *Action:* Flex the hip fully, and then move the hip into adduction by pressing the thigh toward the opposite shoulder, 90° to the inguinal ligament (Fig. 7-16).
- *Observation:* This flexion compresses the iliopsoas muscle, the iliofemoral ligament, and the iliopectineal bursa and stretches the piriformis muscle. Groin pain with tissue stretch indicates iliopsoas muscle tension; groin pain with limited motion and capsular end feel indicates iliofemoral ligament fibrosis; and groin pain with an empty end feel indicates iliopectineal bursitis. Buttock pain may indicate piriformis shortness.

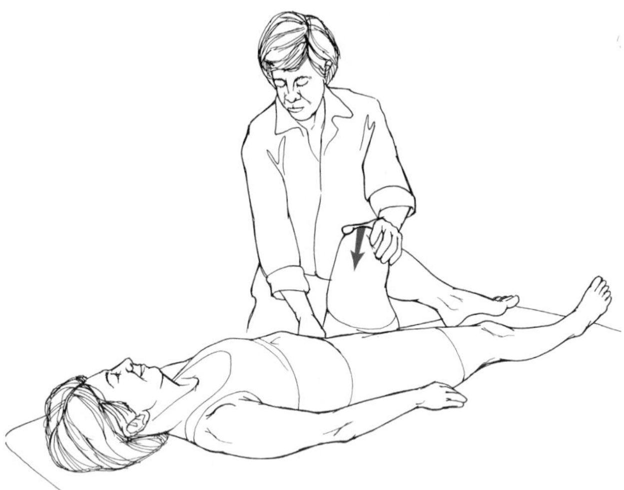

Figure 7-16. Passive hip adduction. The best clinical information is gathered if the hip is pressed into adduction perpendicular to the inguinal ligament.

Medial or Lateral Rotation

- *Position:* The client is supine. Bring the hip and knee to 90° of flexion, with no abduction or adduction of the hip. Hold the ankle in one hand, and place the other hand on the outside of the knee.
- *Action:* Stabilize the knee and slowly pull the ankle laterally, medially rotating the hip joint, and then move the leg medially, laterally rotating the hip joint (Fig. 7-17).
- *Observation:* Lateral rotation should be 10° to 20° greater than medial rotation. Compare both sides. If the client has retroverted hips, there is excessive lateral rotation bilaterally. If the hips are anteverted, there is excessive internal rotation bilaterally. Decreased medial rotation on one side, eliciting groin pain at the end range, is usually indicative of hip joint degeneration or of ligamentous or capsular fibrosis. Joint degeneration has a hard end-feel or a capsular end-feel with decreased ROM. Shortness of the ligaments or capsule has a leathery end-feel. The capsular pattern of the hip is decreased medial rotation and abduction.

PALPATION

- Palpation is performed while you perform the strokes. Be aware that in addition to groin tenderness caused by irritation of the muscle or bursa, the groin is a vulnerable area emotionally. Approach this area with sensitivity.

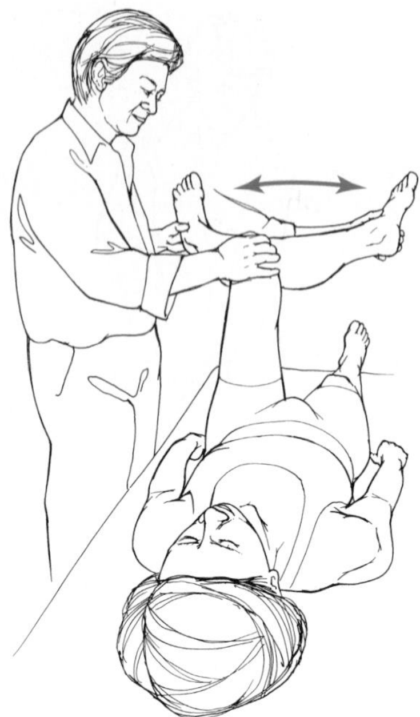

Figure 7-17. Passive medial and lateral rotation. This is one of the most important tests in hip assessment. Medial rotation is the first motion that is decreased in capsulitis, fibrosis of the joint capsule, and degeneration of the articular surfaces. These three conditions are differentiated by the end feel.

Techniques

MUSCLE ENERGY TECHNIQUE

A major goal in performing MET for the hip is to lengthen a shortened joint capsule, as this helps prevent further joint degeneration.

Muscle Energy Technique for Acute Hip Pain

1. Contract-Relax Muscle Energy Technique and Traction for Acute Hip Pain

- *Intention:* The flexors of the hip are most commonly involved in acute hip pain. Use CR MET to help reduce the hypertonicity in the flexors and to help decompress the joint.
- *Position:* The client is supine, with the hip flexed and the foot on the table. Hold the distal thigh with both your hands.
- *Action:* Have the client resist as you pull down on the thigh (toward hip extension) to provide traction on the hip joint for approximately 5 seconds. Relax and repeat 3 to 5 times. After a few cycles, as the client is relaxing, pull the thigh footward for approximately 30 to 90 seconds. Repeat several times (Fig. 7-18).

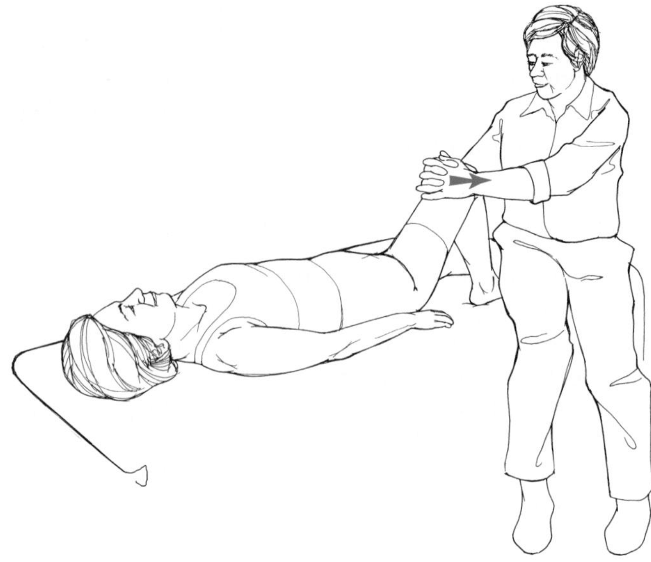

Figure 7-18. CR MET and hip traction for acute hip pain.

Muscle Energy Technique for Hypertonic Muscles

2. Contract-Relax and Postisometric Relaxation Muscle Energy Technique for the Pectineus and Adductors

- *Intention:* The intention is to perform CR and PIR MET to reduce the hypertonicity and lengthen the short adductors and the pectineus—these muscles are often strained, causing a painful limitation of abduction.

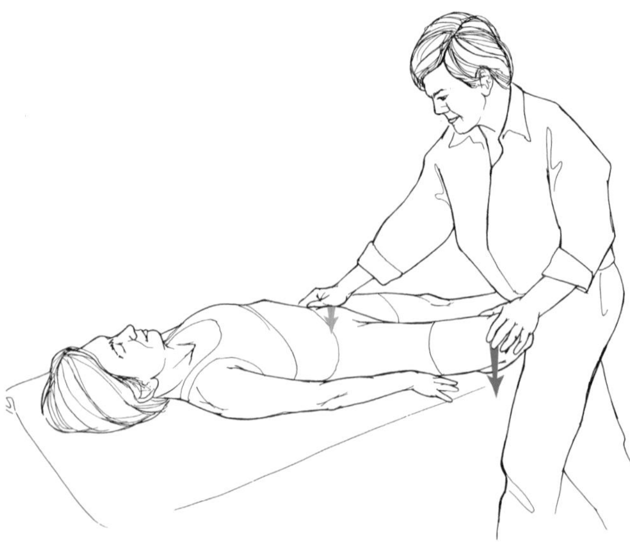

Figure 7-19. CR and PIR MET for the pectineus and adductors.

- *Position:* Client is supine with the involved hip flexed, externally rotated, and abducted to the resistance barrier. Place your flexed knee on the table and have the client rest his or her leg on your thigh, or place a pillow under the abducted thigh.
- *Action:* Place one hand on the distal thigh and the other hand on the opposite ASIS and have the client resist as you press outward at the knee, attempting to move the hip into further abduction for approximately 5 seconds. Have client relax, and then slowly move the hip into further abduction to lengthen the adductors and pectineus. Repeat several times (Fig. 7-19).

3. Contract-Relax Muscle Energy Technique for the Rectus Femoris

- *Intention:* The intention is to release the rectus femoris, which is typically short and tight. As it interweaves with the joint capsule, it is often a cause of dysfunction in the joint.
- *Position:* Place your flexed knee on the table. Client is supine with the hip and knee flexed, resting his or her leg on your thigh.
- *Action:* Place one hand on the client's distal leg and the other hand on the client's knee. Have the client lift his or her foot slightly off the table and resist as you attempt to press the foot back to the table. Relax and rest the foot back on the table. Perform reciprocal inhibition (RI) MET by having the client resist as you attempt to pull the foot off the table. This contracts the hamstrings, reciprocally inhibiting the quadriceps. Repeat several times (Fig. 7-20).

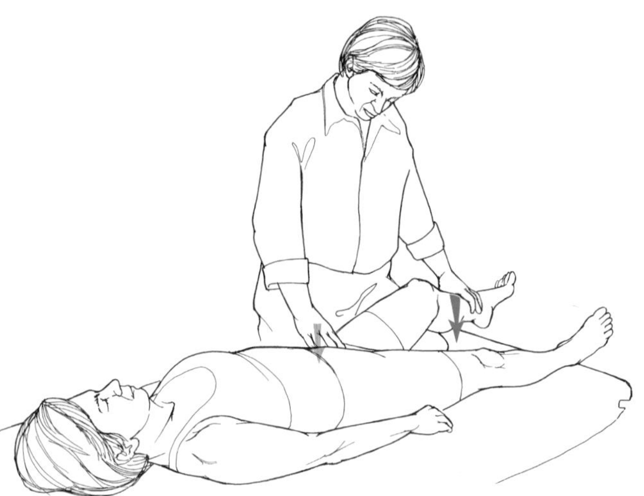

Figure 7-20. CR MET for the rectus femoris.

4. Postisometric Relaxation Muscle Energy Technique for Medial and Lateral Rotators

- *Intention:* If the assessment determined a decrease in medial or lateral rotation of the hip, the intention is to release the medial and lateral rotators. One contributing factor to decrease of hip rotation may be hypertonicity of the muscles.
- *Position:* Client is prone, with one knee flexed. Hold the distal leg with one hand, and place your other hand over the sacrum to stabilize the pelvis to prevent it from rotating.
- *Action: To release the lateral rotators,* move the client's leg laterally, medially rotating the hip, to the resistance barrier. Have the client resist as you pull out at the ankle for approximately 5 seconds. Have the client relax; then move the leg laterally to a new resistance barrier. Relax and repeat. *To release the medial rotators,* move the client's leg toward the opposite leg, externally rotating the hip. Ask the client to resist as you push the leg toward the opposite leg (i.e., into further lateral rotation). Have the client relax; then move the leg medially to a new resistance barrier. Relax and repeat (Fig. 7-21).

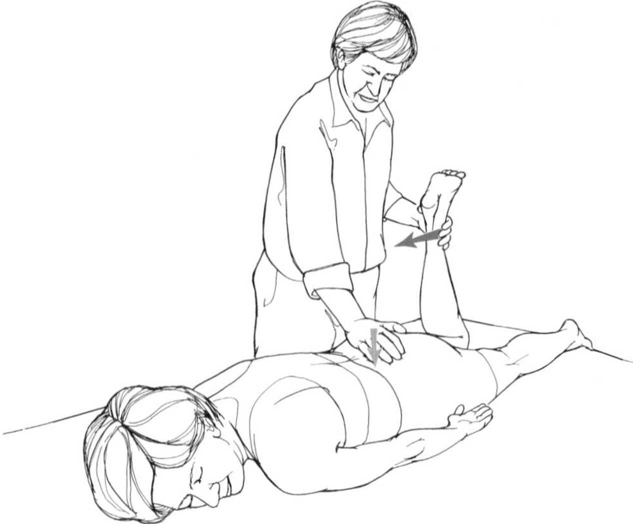

Figure 7-21. PIR MET for the medial and lateral rotators.

5. Contract-Relax Muscle Energy Technique for the Hamstrings

- **Intention:** The hamstrings are typically hypertonic, and the intention is to reduce their hypertonicity. CR MET in conjunction with the massage strokes is a simple way to accomplish this.
- **Position:** Client is prone, with one knee flexed slightly and the foot resting on a pillow. Place one hand on the hamstrings for a sensory cue, and your other hand on the back of the heel.

- ***Action:*** Have the client resist as you attempt to extend the knee by pressing the foot toward the pillow for approximately 5 seconds. Have the client relax; then rest the foot on the pillow. To RI the hamstrings, have the client resist as you attempt to pull the foot off the pillow for approximately 5 seconds. Relax and repeat (Fig. 7-22).

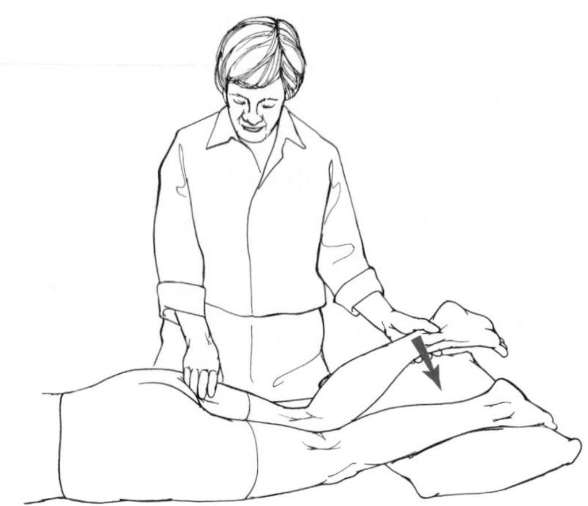

Figure 7-22. CR MET for the hamstrings.

6. Contract-Relax Muscle Energy Technique for the Gluteus Maximus

- ***Intention:*** The gluteus maximus is typically weak, and the intention is to isolate the muscle to test it and to recruit the muscle fibers by use of CR MET.
- ***Position:*** Client is prone with the knee flexed. Place one hand on the gluteus maximus, and your other hand on the posterior thigh.
- ***Action:*** Have the client lift the thigh off the table and resist as you attempt to press the thigh back to the table (Fig. 7-23).

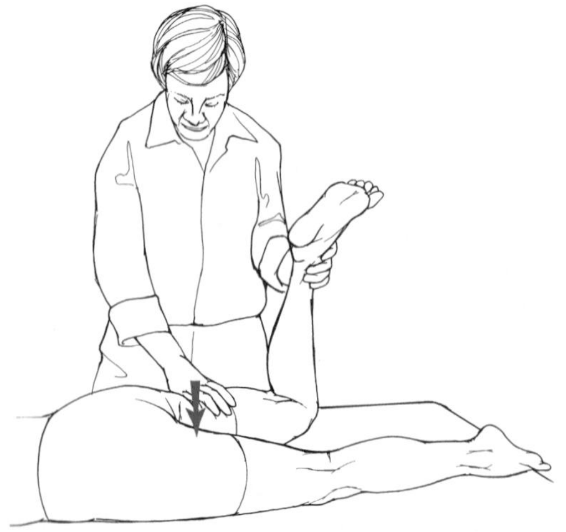

Figure 7-23. CR MET for the gluteus maximus.

- ***Observation:*** If the gluteus maximus is weak, the client will rotate the trunk and elevate the pelvis. Make sure the trunk does not rotate.

7. Contract-Relax Muscle Energy Technique for the Adductors in the Side-Lying Position

- ***Intention:*** The adductors are typically hypertonic, and the intention is to reduce this hypertonicity. This position is an easy way to release the adductors in conjunction with performing the massage strokes.
- ***Position:*** Client is side-lying near the edge of the table, with the top hip and knee flexed resting on a pillow and the bottom leg straight on the table.
- ***Action:*** Have the client raise his or her straight leg off the table for approximately 5 seconds. Make sure the foot is parallel to the table and that the client keeps his or her trunk from rotating. Have the client resist as you gently attempt to press the leg back to the table. Have him or her relax the leg back on the table for a few seconds. To perform RI, have the client resist as you attempt to lift the leg off the table. Relax and repeat several times, and perform on the other side (Fig. 7-24).

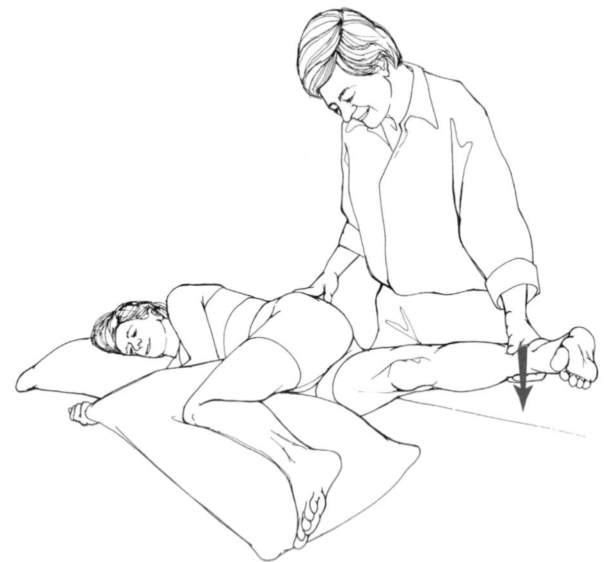

Figure 7-24. CR MET (side-lying position) for the adductors.

Functional Testing and Muscle Energy Technique

8. Assessment of the Muscle-Firing Pattern and Contract-Relax Muscle Energy Technique for the Gluteus Medius

- ***Intention:*** The gluteus medius is often weak, and to compensate for its weakness the TFL will contract first to abduct the hip, causing the hip to flex and internally rotate or the trunk to rotate backwards to allow the TFL to work more efficiently. The intention is to assess the firing pattern of the gluteus medius and to increase gluteus medius strength.

- ☐ ***Position:*** Client is lying on his or her side, without any forward or backward rotation of the trunk. The leg next to the table is flexed to approximately 90°. Stand behind the client.
- ☐ ***Action:*** To assess hip abduction, client is asked to slowly abduct the hip. To perform CR MET on the gluteus medius, the hip is abducted approximately 35° in slight extension and external rotation. Place one hand near the ankle and your other hand on the gluteus medius and TFL. Have the client resist as you press toward the table (toward adduction). To perform CR MET on the gluteus minimus, the hip is in neutral (i.e., the foot is parallel to the table) and not externally rotated. To perform RI MET, have the client straighten the leg and place it on the table and resist as you attempt to lift it off the table (Fig. 7-25).
- ☐ ***Observation:*** It is important to observe two things: (1) an abnormal firing pattern in which the TFL contracts first, causing the hip to flex and internally rotate; (2) whether the trunk rotates posteriorly, allowing for the TFL to flex the hip, substituting for the weak gluteus medius. If you find either one of these patterns, educate the client in using the gluteus medius by having him or her simply slowly initiate abduction to control its motion.

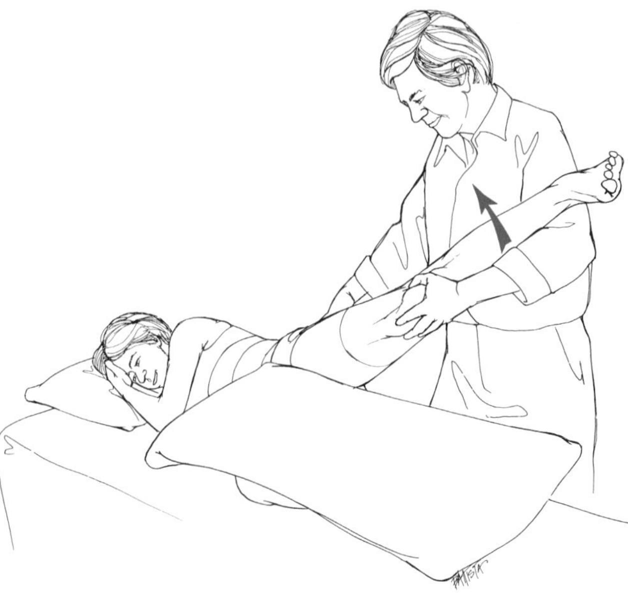

Figure 7-25. CR MET and assessment of the muscle-firing pattern of the gluteus medius.

9. Assessment of the Length and Postisometric Relaxation Muscle Energy Technique for the Medial Hamstrings and Adductors

- ☐ ***Intention:*** The medial hamstrings and adductors are typically short and tight, and the intention of this PIR MET is to assess and to increase their length.
- ☐ ***Position:*** Client is supine with the heel of the supporting leg over the edge of the table to stabilize the body.
- ☐ ***Action:*** Abduct the client's leg and move your body between the table and the tested leg. Keeping the knee extended and the foot in neutral, abduct the client's leg to the tension barrier by moving the leg with your body. Perform PIR MET by having the client resist as you attempt to move the leg into further abduction for approximately 5 seconds. Have the client relax for a few seconds; then slowly abduct the hip to a new tension barrier. Relax and repeat several times, then perform on the other side (Fig. 7-26).
- ☐ ***Observation:*** Normal abduction is approximately 45°. The hip should abduct approximately 25° from the midline in this position, as we are abducting the other hip approximately 20° by placing the heel over the edge of the table.

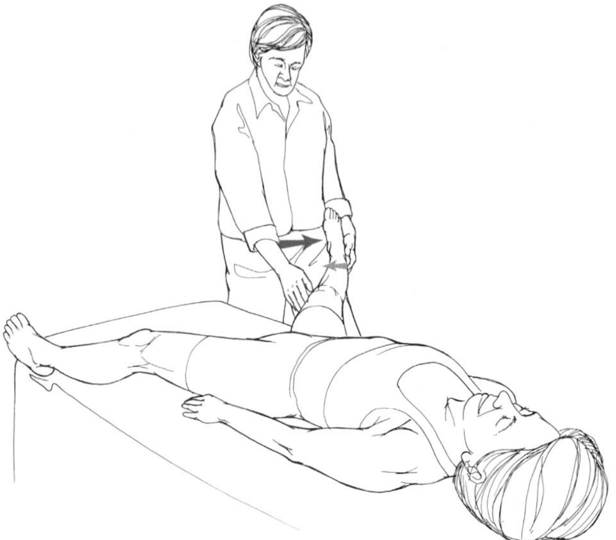

Figure 7-26. PIR MET and assessment of the length of the medial hamstrings and adductors.

10. Assessment of the Length and Contract-Relax-Antagonist-Contract Muscle Energy Technique for the Hamstrings

- ☐ ***Intention:*** The hamstrings are typically short and tight. As they interweave with the sacrotuberous ligament and gluteal fascia, tightness prevents full mobility of the lumbopelvic region. The intention of this CRAC MET is to lengthen the hamstrings. This test is for chronic conditions only.

- *Position:* Client is supine. Place the client's ankle over your shoulder and rest your hands over the client's knee to keep the knee extended.
- *Action:* To assess the length of the hamstrings, perform a modified SLR test by slowly lifting the leg to the resistance barrier. To perform CRAC MET, have the client resist by pressing his or her leg into your shoulder as you attempt to lift the leg toward the head for approximately 5 seconds. Have the client relax, and after a few seconds have him or her actively lift the leg headward while keeping the knee straight. Have the client relax. Repeat the procedure several times, and then perform on the other leg (Fig. 7-27).
- *Observation:* The normal length of the hamstrings should allow for approximately 70° of hip flexion with the opposite leg on the table. With the opposite knee flexed the range is approximately 90°.

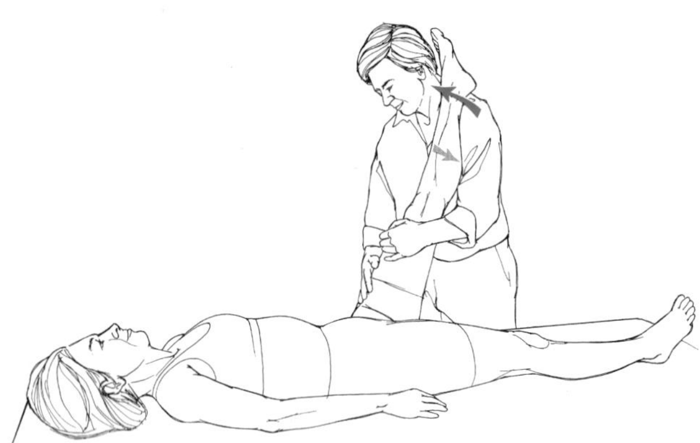

Figure 7-27. CRAC MET and assessment of the length of the hamstrings.

11. Contract-Relax and Eccentric Muscle Energy Technique for Tensor Fascia Lata

- *Intention:* The TFL is typically tight and short. The intention is to reduce the muscle hypertonicity and to lengthen the fascia. CR and eccentric MET is an effective method to accomplish this goal.
- *Position:* Client is supine. Hold the client's leg just above the ankle and assist the client as he or she flexes the hip approximately 45° with slight abduction and medial rotation. Place your other hand on the TFL to give a sensory cue when the muscle is contracting.
- *Action:* To perform CR for more acute conditions, have the client resist as you press toward extension and adduction, that is, toward the other leg. Relax and repeat. To perform eccentric MET for chronic conditions, have the client continue to offer some resistance, but instruct the client to "let me move your leg very slowly." Then slowly move the leg toward the opposite leg. To perform RI MET, have the client hold one foot against the other on the table and resist as you attempt to pull the leg up into flexion and abduction (i.e., to pull the leg back to the beginning position) (Fig. 7-28).

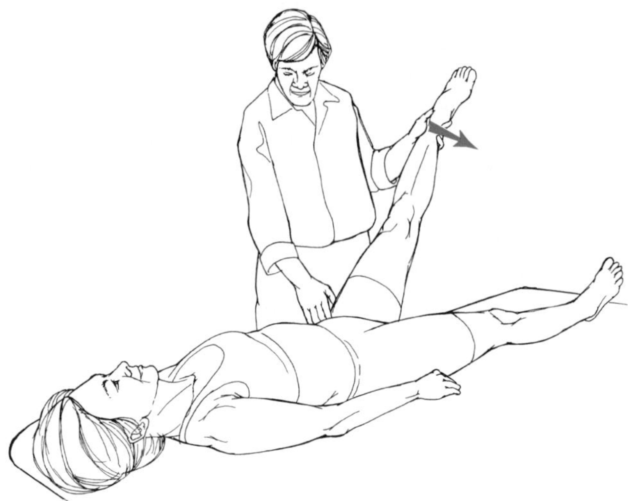

Figure 7-28. CR and eccentric MET for the TFL.

12. Postisometric Relaxation Muscle Energy Technique for the Tensor Fascia Lata, the Iliotibial Band, and the Quadratus Lumborum for Chronic Conditions

CAUTION: **This MET may be challenging for clients with LBP. Do not perform with clients who have had a recent episode of LBP or who have a history of instability or sacroiliac problems. This is for chronic conditions only.**

- *Intention:* The intention is to release the TFL and ITB. These muscles are typically short and tight, contributing to internal rotation of the hip and genu valgus (knock knees).
- *Position:* Client is side-lying near the edge of the table, with the top of the body forward on the table and the pelvis toward the back of the table. The bottom hip and knee are flexed, and the top leg is straight and hanging over the edge of the table. Place one hand on the distal thigh and the other hand on the area of the TFL or the QL.

- *Action:* Have the client resist as you press his or her leg toward the floor for approximately 5 seconds. Have the client relax for a few seconds, and then slowly press the leg toward the floor to a new tension barrier. Relax and repeat several times. Assist the client in lifting the leg back to the table. Perform on the other side (Fig. 7-29).

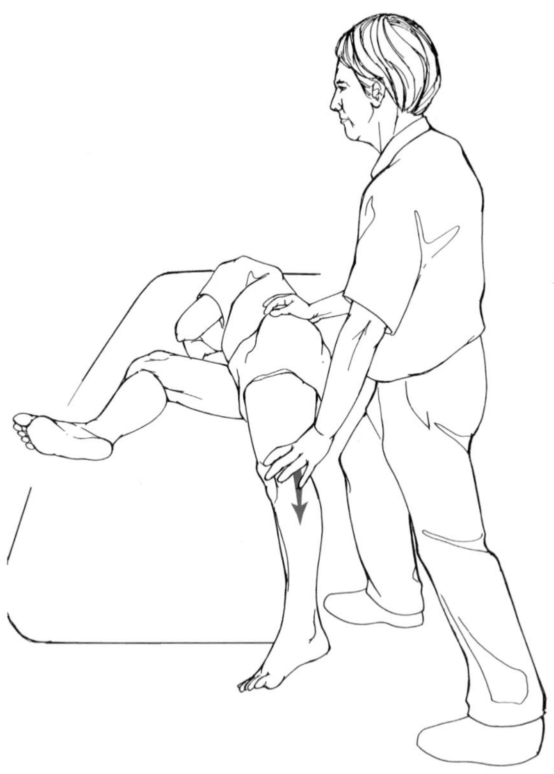

Figure 7-29. PIR MET for the TFL, ITB, and QL.

13. Contract-Relax-Antagonist-Contract Muscle Energy Technique for the Pectineus and Adductors and to Increase Hip Abduction

- *Intention:* The intention is to release the short adductors, which are typically tight in degenerative conditions of the hip, causing limitation of abduction.
- *Position:* Client is supine with both hips flexed, externally rotated, and abducted to their comfortable limit, with the feet on the table in the midline and the soles of the feet touching. Have the client flatten the low back on the table to prevent excessive lordosis. Because with hip dysfunction or degeneration the hip is much more limited in its ability to abduct, begin the MET by placing the "good" hip at the same degree of abduction as the limited hip.
- *Action:* Place both hands on the distal thighs and ask the client to resist as you attempt to press the knees toward the table for approximately 5 seconds. Relax for a few seconds, and then ask the client to squeeze the buttock muscles (gluteals and external rotators) to pull the knees further toward the table. Typically, only about 1 inch of new movement is achieved. Have the client relax. Repeat the CRAC cycle several times (Fig. 7-30).

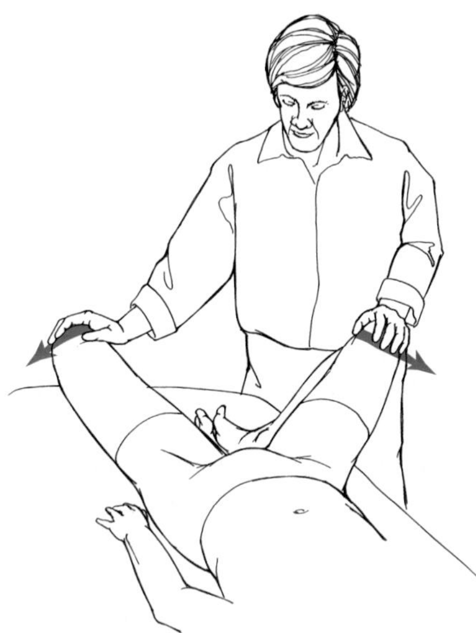

Figure 7-30. CRAC MET for the pectineus and adductors and to increase abduction of the hip.

Muscle Energy Technique for Capsulitis and Hip Degeneration

14. Muscle Energy Technique to Increase Medial Rotation

CAUTION: **This procedure is contraindicated after hip replacement.**

- *Intention:* The intention is to help restore medial rotation, which is the first motion lost in capsulitis and in joint degeneration (arthritis).
- *Position:* Client is supine. Bring the involved hip into 90° of hip flexion and 90° of knee flexion. Do not allow the hip to adduct or abduct. Place one hand on the lateral aspect of the knee and hold the leg just proximal to the ankle.
- *Action:* Pull the leg laterally into the comfortable limit of medial rotation of the hip. Have the client resist as you pull laterally at the ankle, attempting to move the hip into further medial rotation, and press at the knee to stabilize it. Have the client relax. Repeat several times (Fig. 7-31).

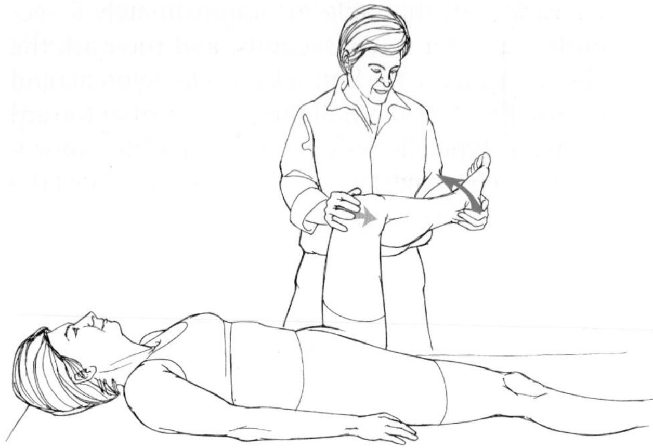

Figure 7-31. MET to increase medial rotation.

15. Muscle Energy Technique to Stretch the Anterior Capsule and to Increase Hip Extension

- ***Intention:*** The intention is to lengthen the anterior capsule, which shortens in chronic capsular conditions and hip joint degeneration.
- ***Position:*** This is the same position as used in the assessment of passive extension. Client is prone. Assume either of two positions. One, tuck one hand under the client's distal thigh, or two, place your flexed thigh on the table and rest the client's thigh on your thigh.
- ***Action:*** Pull the thigh into the limit of passive extension (see Fig. 7-14). Have the client resist as you attempt to pull the thigh further off the table, into further extension. Have the client relax. Then lift their thigh into further extension. If your flexed thigh is on the table, move it headward under the client's thigh, bringing the clients hip into further extension. Repeat several times.

ORTHOPEDIC MASSAGE

Level I—Hip

1. Release of the Gluteals

- *Anatomy*: Gluteus medius and minimus (Fig. 7-32).
- *Dysfunction*: The gluteus maximus tends to be weak and is usually best treated with MET. The gluteus medius and minimus tend to develop tightness weakness. If they test significantly weak, perform MET for the adductors first, as they are usually short and tight and may be inhibiting the gluteus medius. Attachment points usually become fibrotic after injury or sustained overuse. The positional dysfunction is for the gluteals to roll into an inferior torsion.

Position

- TP—standing, facing the direction of the stroke
- CP—side-lying, fetal position

Strokes

Release this area with short, scooping strokes, perpendicular to the line of the fiber. The closer you are to the

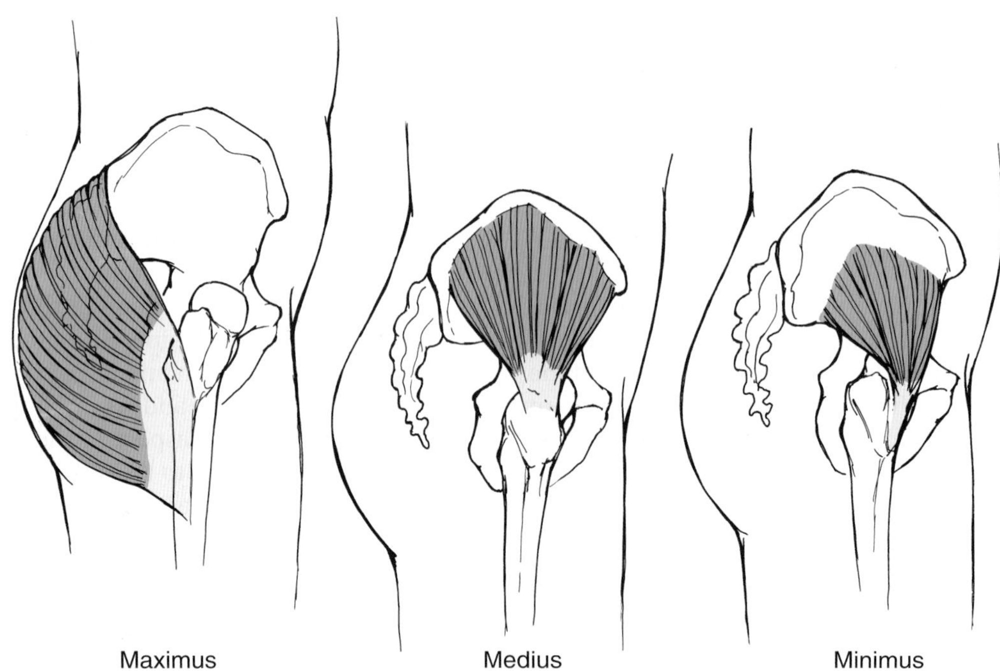

Figure 7-32. Gluteus medius and minimus.

attachment points, the shorter and more brisk your strokes. We use double-thumb, braced-thumb, or the fifth metacarpophalangeal (MCP) joint (knuckle) of a soft fist.

1. As a way to assist palpation, place your fingertips on the superior lateral aspect of the iliac fossa, and perform CR MET on the gluteus medius (see Fig.7-25, p. 271)
2. Have the client bring his or her leg back on the pillow in the fetal position. Perform a series of short, scooping strokes in 1-inch segments, moving transverse to the line of the fiber, medially to laterally on the gluteus medius (Fig. 7-33). Begin your strokes at the most superior portion of the muscle at its attachment under the iliac crest. Continue the strokes to its insertion on the top of the lateral portion of the trochanter. Begin the next line of strokes on the gluteus medius just posterior to the previous line, from the iliac crest to the trochanter. Cover the entire muscle. If the muscle remains hypertonic, perform another series of CR MET on the gluteus medius and the adductors, then come back to the strokes.
3. Palpate the gluteus minimus at its insertion on the anterior aspect of the top of the trochanter as you have your client abduct his or her leg in neutral (i.e., with the foot parallel to the floor).
4. Perform a series of M–L scooping strokes, beginning at the outer surface of the ilium just posterior to the ASIS, and continue to the anterior-superior surface of the trochanter. As the minimus is under the medius except at its insertion, you need to penetrate through the medius to address the minimus.

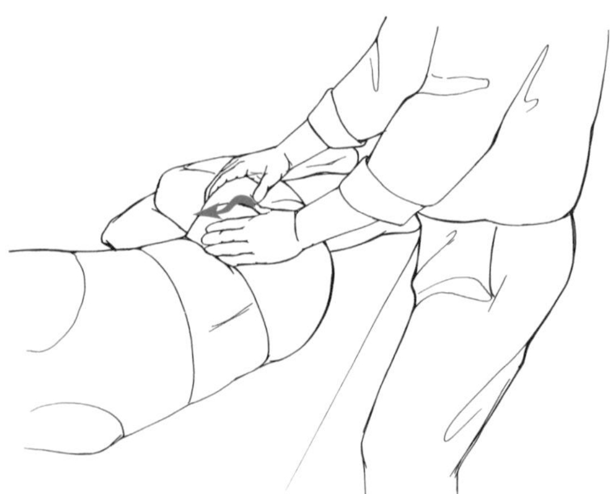

Figure 7-33. Double-thumb release of the gluteus medius and minimus.

2. Release of the Adductors

- ***Anatomy***: Adductor magnus, brevis, and longus (Fig. 7-34).
- ***Dysfunction***: The adductors usually become tight and short, typically held in a sustained medial torsion. This contributes to anteverted hips and genu valgus knees. The positional dysfunction is a medial torsion.

Position

- TP—standing, facing table, or facing headward or standing on opposite side of extended leg to move posterior portion of medial thigh more posteriorly

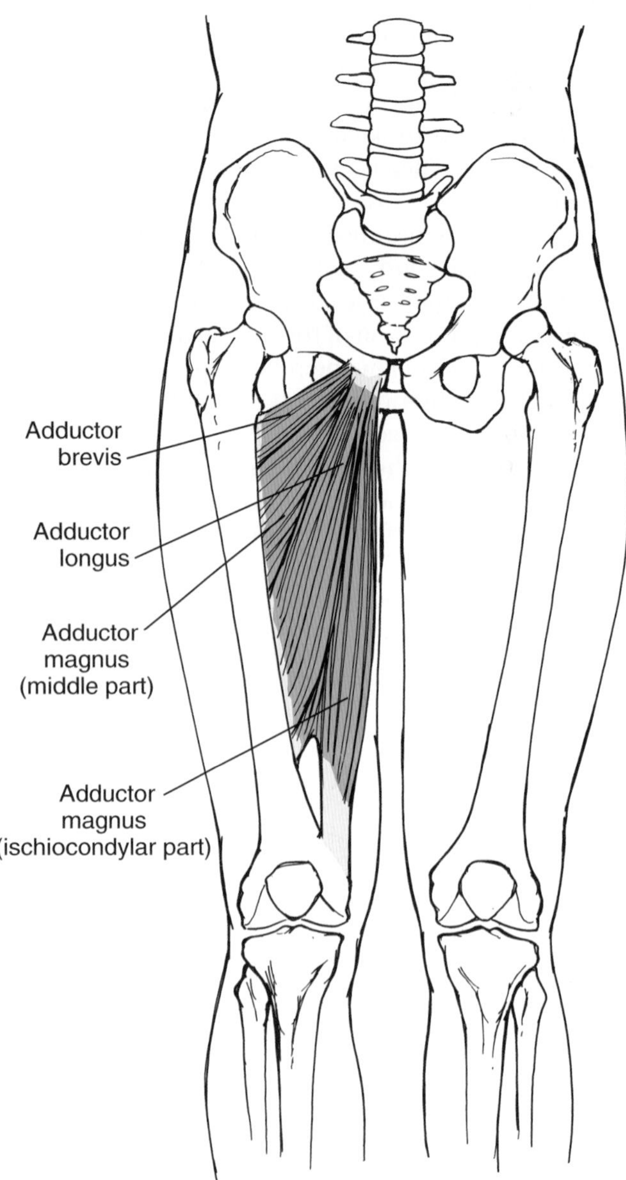

Figure 7-34. Adductor muscles.

- CP—side-lying, with the leg on the table extended and top leg flexed resting on a pillow; have the client's trunk remain in neutral, not allowing it to rotate forward

Strokes

The intention in using these strokes is to "part the midline" of the medial thigh. That is, we move the soft tissue on the posterior half of the medial thigh posteriorly and the tissue on the anterior half of the medial thigh anteriorly. We use fingertips, braced fingertips, and braced thumb.

1. Perform CR MET on the adductors with the client in the side-lying position. (See Fig.7-24, p. 270)
2. Facing 45° headward, wrap your hands around the thigh several inches below the pubic bone, placing your thumbs on the midline of the medial thigh (Fig. 7-35). Perform a short, scooping posterior to anterior (P–A) stroke on the anterior portion of the medial thigh. Begin another stroke just inferior to your last stroke, and continue to the adductor tubercle, a bony prominence on the superior surface of the medial condyle of the femur.
3. Perform another series of short, scooping stokes on the posterior portion of the medial thigh. Beginning several inches below the pubic bone, move the soft tissue from anterior to posterior (A–P). Continue to just above the knee.
4. An alternate method for the first series of strokes is for you to face the table and use a braced-thumb technique to perform a series of short, scooping strokes from P–A on the soft tissue of the anterior portion of the medial thigh (Fig. 7-36). Work from the proximal thigh to just above the knee.

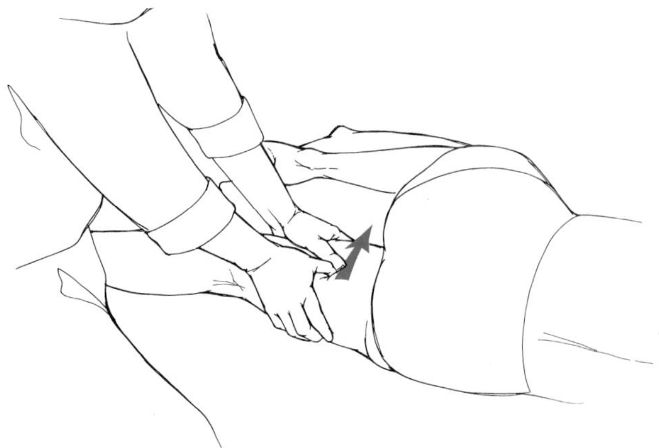

Figure 7-35. Release the adductors. Wrap both hands around the medial thigh and part the midline. Take the posterior tissue more posteriorly and the anterior tissue more anteriorly.

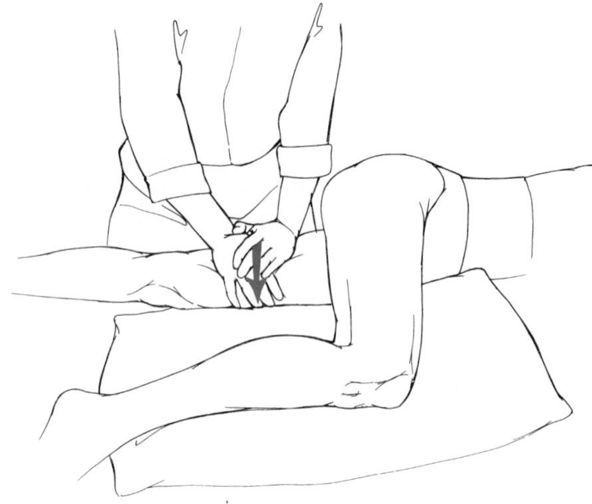

Figure 7-36. Alternate method to release the anterior half of the medial thigh is for the therapist to face the table and use a braced-thumb technique to move the soft tissue anteriorly.

5. An alternate method to release the posterior portion of the medial thigh is to move to the opposite side of the table. Bring the client as close to you as is comfortable to minimize your reach. Face the table, and use a braced-thumb technique as described above to stroke A–P on the soft tissue of the posterior portion of the medial thigh.

3. Release of the Hamstrings

- *Anatomy*: Semimembranosus, semitendinosus, and long head of the biceps (Fig. 7-37).
- *Dysfunction*: Attachment points at the ischial tuberosity and knee tend to thicken and become fibrotic from chronic irritation or injury. The hamstrings are typically tight and short and pull toward the midline in chronic tension. The hamstrings stay in a sustained contraction to counterbalance a forward-tilting pelvis.

Position

- TP—standing, facing headward, or facing the table for alternative technique
- CP—prone, with a pillow under the ankles

Strokes

Our intention is to "part the midline" to release the torsion developed through chronic tension. Use double-thumb or braced-thumb technique.

1. Perform CR MET on the hamstrings with the client in the prone position (Fig.7-22).
2. Facing 45° headward, place your thumbs on the midline of the thigh several inches distal to the is-

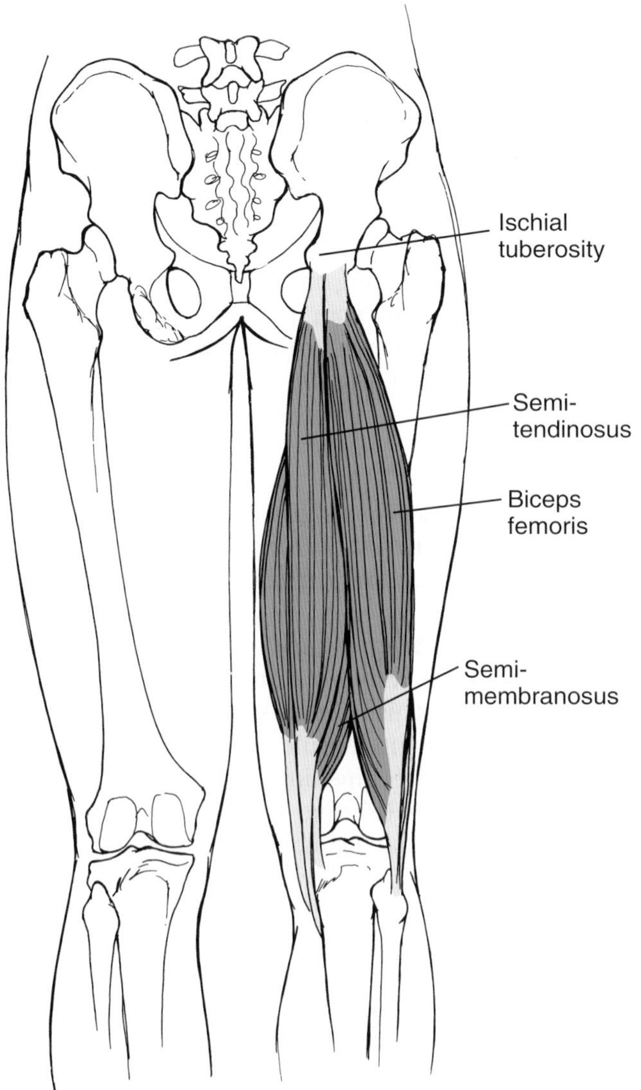

Figure 7-37. Hamstrings, which include the semimembranosus, semitendinosus, and biceps femoris.

chial tuberosity, using the same hand position shown in Fig. 7-35. Perform broad, scooping strokes, unwinding the soft tissue in an M–L direction. Proceed down the entire posterior thigh, following the biceps femoris to its attachment on the fibula.

3. Perform the same scooping strokes from the midline in a lateral to medial direction to release the semimembranosus and semitendinosus. Begin several inches below the ischial tuberosity and continue to the knee.
4. An alternate position to release the medial hamstrings and medial thigh is for you to face the table as shown in the adductor series (See Fig. 7-36). Place your thumb on the midline of the thigh closest to you just below the ischial tuberosity. Using a braced-thumb technique, perform a series of scooping strokes in a medial direction, beginning just below the ischial tuberosity and continuing to the knee.

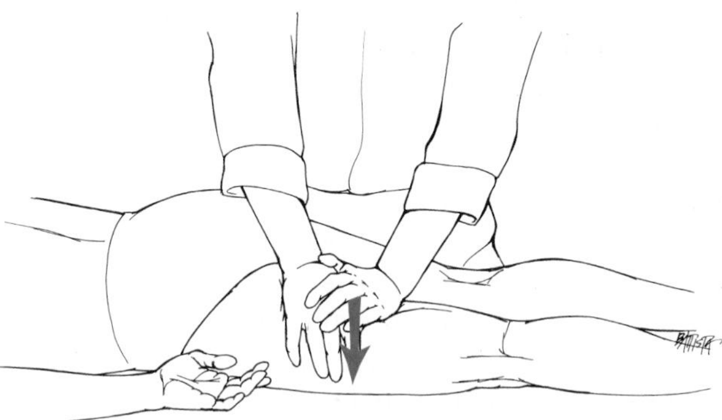

Figure 7-38. Alternate method to release the lateral side of the posterior thigh is to use a braced-thumb technique to move the soft tissue more laterally.

5. An alternative position to release the biceps femoris and lateral thigh is to stand on the opposite side, facing the table (Fig. 7-38). Place your thumbs on the midline of the thigh. Using a braced thumb, perform a series of strokes in a lateral direction. Begin just below the ischial tuberosity and continue to the lateral knee.
6. To release the hamstring attachments on the ischial tuberosity, use a braced-thumb technique or braced fingertips to perform back and forth strokes on any thickened tissue you palpate (Fig. 7-39). To "clean the bone," cover the entire area just distal to the bone and on the ischial tuberosity itself.

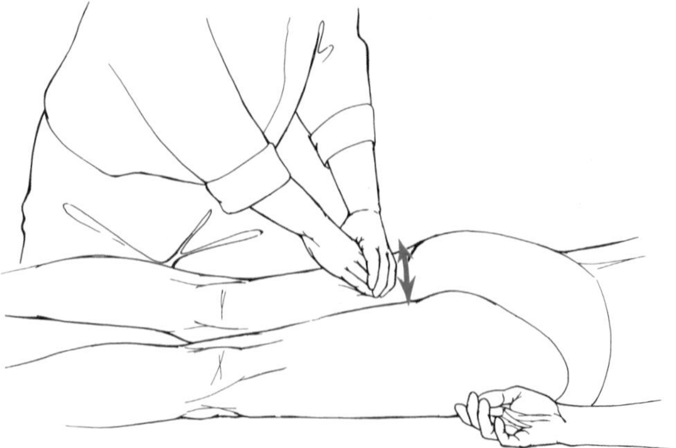

Figure 7-39. Back-and-forth strokes, with braced fingertips on the hamstrings attachment to the ischial tuberosity.

4. Unwinding the Torsion of the Thigh and Release of the Quadriceps and Adductors

- ***Anatomy***: Iliopsoas; adductor magnus, longus, and brevis; quadriceps; pectineus; and sartorius (Fig. 7-40).
- ***Dysfunction***: The soft tissue tends to wind into a medial torsion, wrapping toward the midline. This winding follows the pattern of the joint capsule, which spirals in this direction from its origin to insertion and is compounded by genu valgus (knock-knees) and pronated ankles. If you are working with a client who has retroverted hips or a client whose hips are held in external rotation, you need to reverse the stroke direction, unwind the leg in the opposite direction as described, and perform PIR on the external rotators.

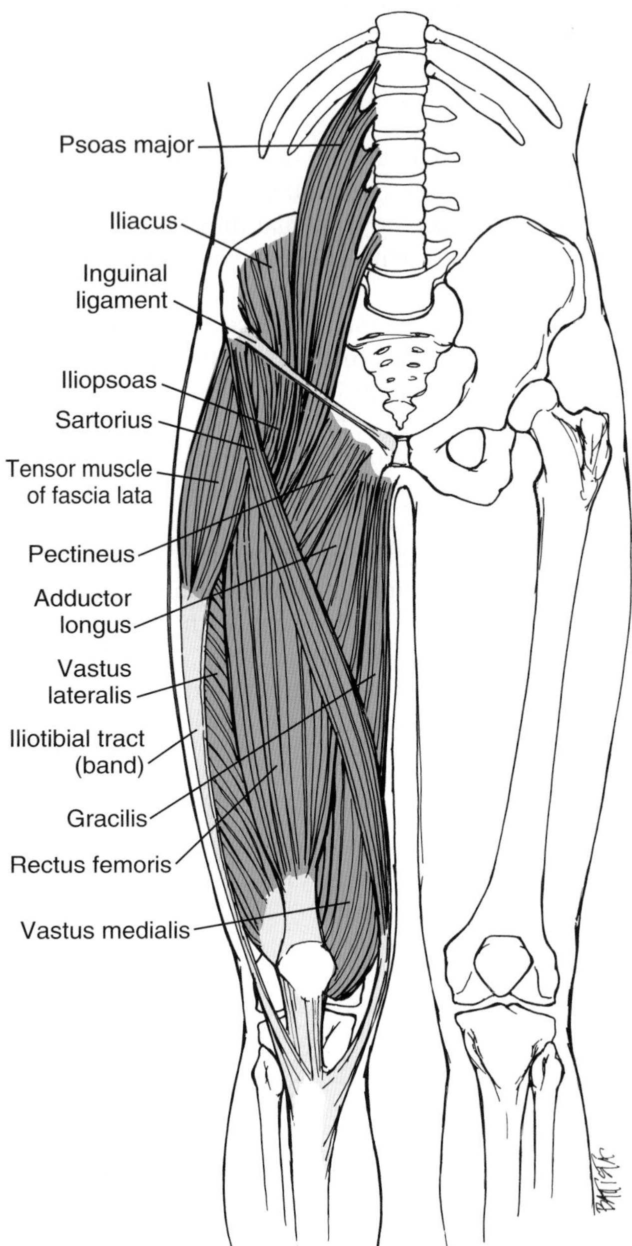

Figure 7-40. Muscles of the anterior and medial thigh.

Position

- TP—standing, facing patient, with inferior leg bent at the knee and resting on the table
- CP—supine; begin your strokes with the leg extended or a pillow under the knee, and proceed to greater flexion of the hip and knee to allow for deeper work

Strokes

This series of strokes helps to accomplish two main intentions: one, to unwind the torsion of the soft tissue of the thigh; and two, to reset specific muscles.

1. With the client's leg extended or with a pillow under his or her knee, wrap both hands around the proximal thigh, and use broad strokes to unwind the muscles and joint capsule around the femur in a counterclockwise direction on the right leg and clockwise on the left (Fig. 7-41). Begin a few inches below the inguinal ligament. Work down the entire thigh to a few inches above the patella.
2. Place your flexed knee on the table and rest the client's leg on your thigh, or you may place more pillows under the client's knee. This modified "figure-four" position helps relax the area by bringing the joint toward its open position, unwinding the joint capsule. Perform the same series of strokes as described above, rocking your body into each stroke.

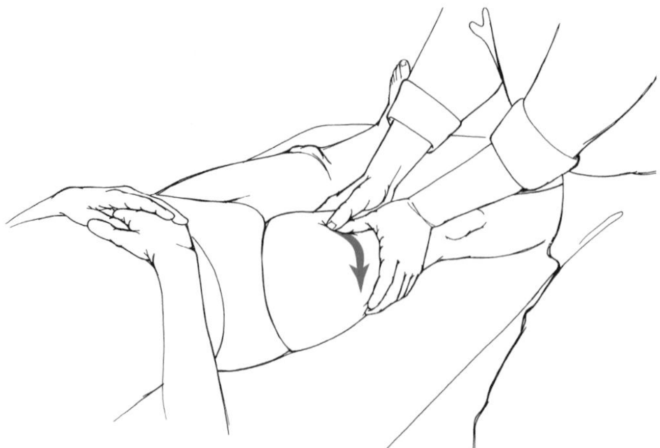

Figure 7-41. Unwinding the muscles of the anterior thigh.

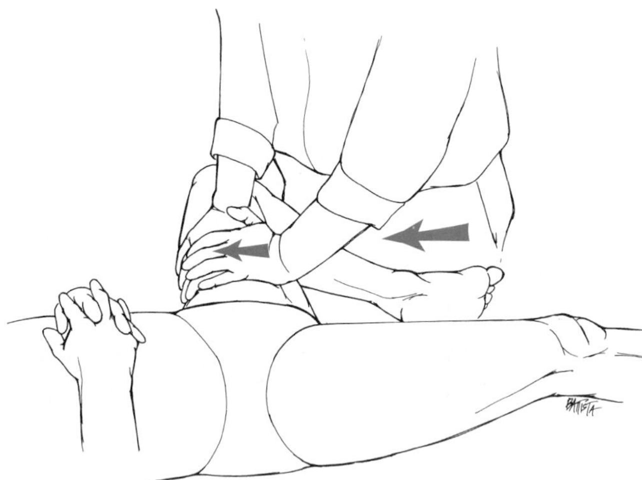

Figure 7-42. Release of the adductors in the figure-four position. The therapist's body rocks the client's hip into flexion (headward) with each stroke.

3. Rest the client's hip in a figure-four position by resting his or her thigh and leg on the table in an abducted and externally-rotated position. If this is uncomfortable, place a pillow between the table and the client's thigh. Using a braced-thumb technique, begin at the midline of the medial thigh and perform a series of scooping strokes in an M–L, P–A direction on the adductors (Fig. 7-42). Place your thigh against the client's shin just below the knee, and press the leg headward as you stroke. Cover the entire medial thigh.

5. Release of the Soft Tissue Below the Inguinal Ligament

- *Anatomy*: Sartorius, pectineus, rectus femoris, and iliopsoas (Fig. 7-43).
- *Dysfunction*: The soft tissue of the proximal thigh typically rolls into a medial torsion. The joint capsule is tightened in internal rotation and extension and slackened in external rotation and abduction.

Position

- TP—standing, facing 45° headward
- CP—supine

Strokes

Find the pulse of the femoral artery by placing your fingertips just below the inguinal ligament approximately midway between the ASIS and the pubic symphysis (see Fig. 7-6). Keep this spot in mind as you work, as you never want to put strong pressure directly on an artery.

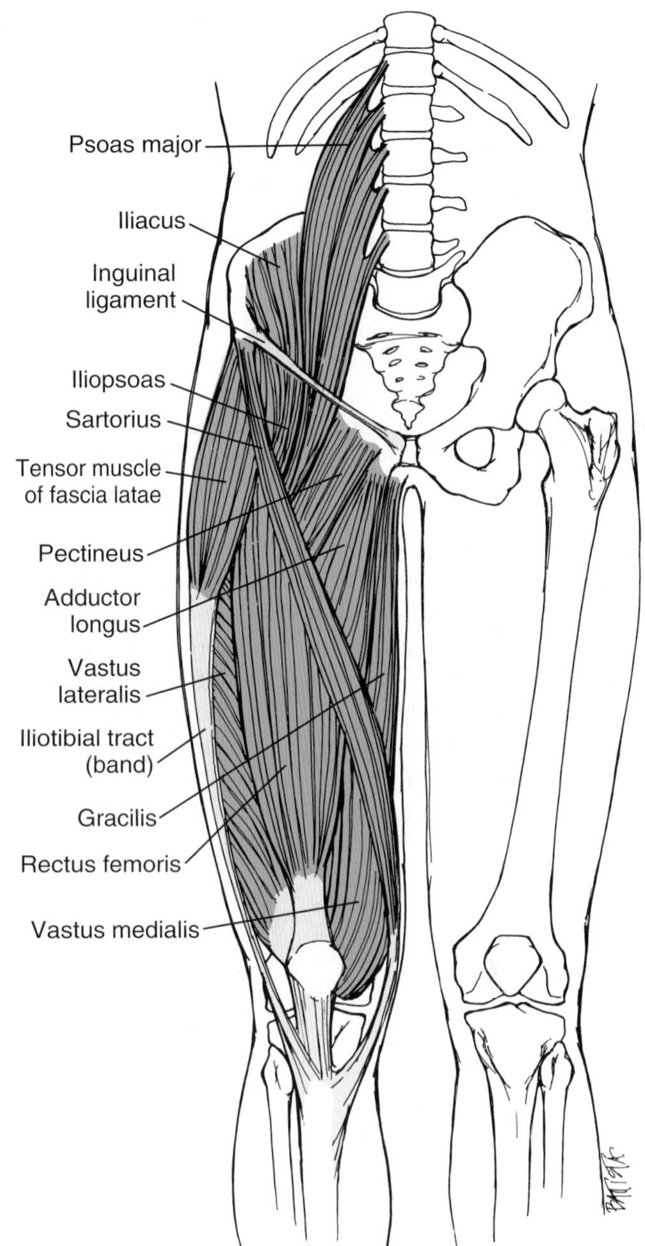

Figure 7-43. Sartorius, rectus femoris, iliopsoas, and pectineus.

1. Perform CR MET on the pectineus and rectus femoris (see Figs. 7-19 and 7-20, p. 268–269).
2. To release the myotendinous junctions of the muscles below the inguinal ligament, keep the client's flexed knee resting on your thigh or on a pillow. With fingertips, braced fingertips, or fingertips next to thumb, perform short, scooping strokes in an M–L direction (Fig. 7-44). Begin your first stroke below the ASIS and each new stroke begins a little more medially, continuing to the adductor longus.

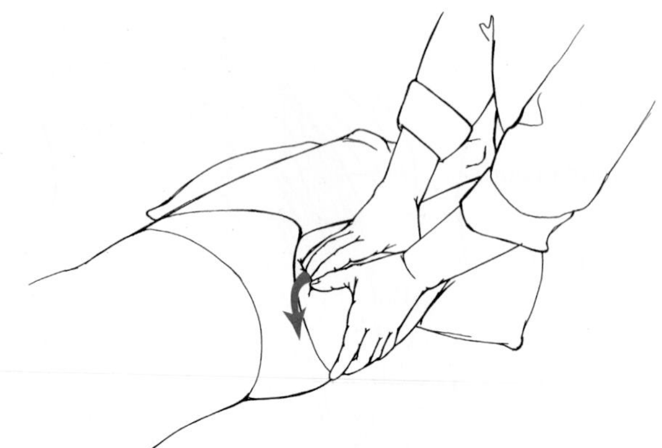

Figure 7-44. Using thumb and fingertips, perform M–L scooping strokes to the soft tissue below the inguinal ligament.

3. Bring the hip to 90° of flexion and perform CR MET on the iliopsoas by having the client resist as you attempt to pull his or her thigh footward. Next, using the fingertips of your superior hand, perform short, scooping strokes in an M–L direction inferior to the inguinal ligament (Fig. 7-45). Your inferior hand holds the knee and rocks the leg in small circles of circumduction with each stroke. We move the hip counterclockwise on the right and clockwise on the left.

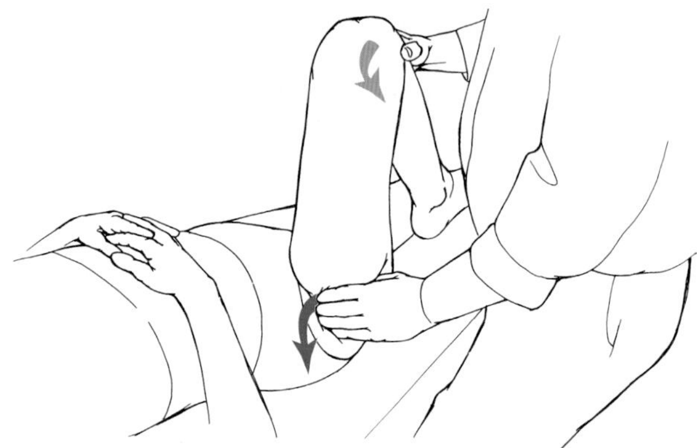

Figure 7-45. Fingertips release of the soft tissue below the inguinal ligament. With each stroke, rock the leg in the direction of the stroke.

6. Release of the Tensor Fascia Lata, Iliotibial Band, and Trochanteric Bursa

- *Anatomy*: TFL, vastus lateralis, ITB (Fig. 7-46), and trochanteric bursa (See Fig. 7-5).
- *Dysfunction*: The anterior aspect of the TFL and the anterior band of the fascia lata tend to roll anteriorly and must be reset posteriorly. This is one cause of "snapping hip syndrome." If the TFL is held in a sustained contraction, the fibrous ITB thickens. The muscle belly of the TFL shortens and tightens. The trochanteric bursa swells with acute conditions and develops adhesions in chronic conditions.

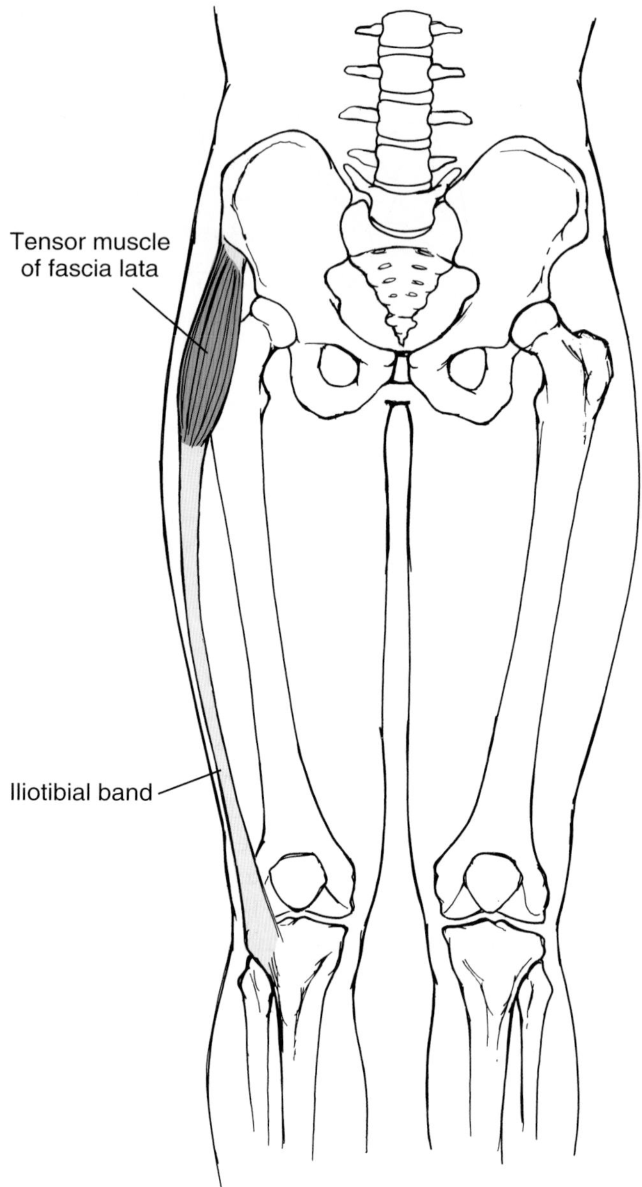

Figure 7-46. Tensor fascia lata and iliotibial band of the lateral thigh.

Position

- TP—standing, facing head ward
- CP—supine or side-lying

Strokes

1. Release the TFL by use of CR MET (see Fig. 7-28, p. 272). For chronic conditions perform PIR MET on the ITB (see Fig. 7-29, p. 273).

2. Use your thumb, fingertips, or fingertips next to thumb to roll the TFL and the fascial bands between the ASIS and the greater trochanter posteriorly in brisk, short, scooping motions (Fig. 7-47). If the area is fibrous, rock the leg into external rotation with each stroke. With less fibrous tissue, your lower hand holds distal to the knee, and you use a shearing stroke by rocking the leg medially as you stroke with the superior hand laterally and posteriorly.

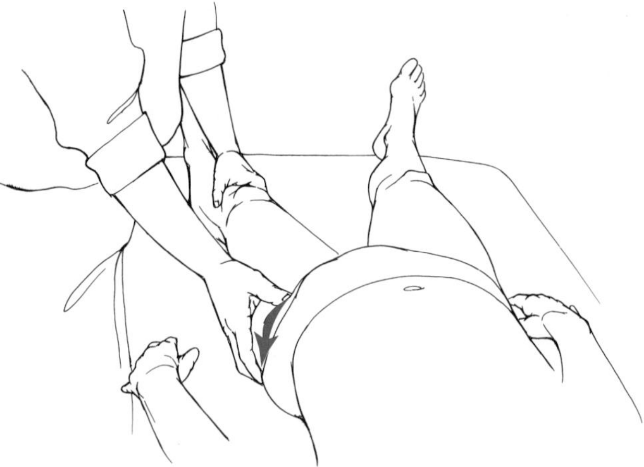

Figure 7-47. Rolling the TFL and the anterior portion of the ITB from A–P.

3. An alternate method is to bring the hip into 90° of flexion and hold the leg at the knee with your inferior hand as shown in Figure 7-45. Use the fingertips or thumb of your superior hand to scoop the TFL and ITB in an M–L and A–P direction. Rock the leg laterally with each stroke.
4. If the ITB is fibrous, place the client in a side-lying, fetal position and stand on the side of the table facing the front of the client's body (Fig. 7-48). Using a double-thumb technique, perform a series of scooping strokes in an A–P direction on the ITB of the top leg to a few inches above the knee.

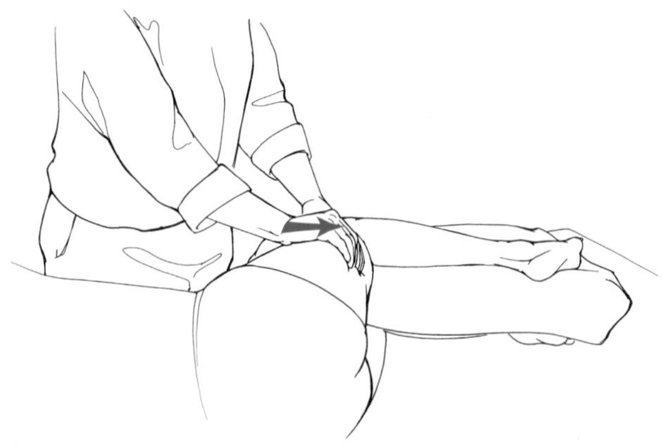

Figure 7-48. Alternate position to release the ITB. Using double-thumb or braced-thumb technique, stroke the ITB from A–P.

5. To help normalize the trochanteric bursa, face the leg as described in the previous stroke. Apply a little lotion to the lateral thigh. Using the webspace between the thumb and the index finger of one or both hands, begin several inches below the greater trochanter and lightly stroke up the lateral and posterior shaft of the femur in one continuous stroke (Fig. 7-49). Continue to the top of the trochanter. For acute bursitis, these strokes must be extremely gentle. Begin at the most superior aspect of the bursa first, and slowly stroke in 1-inch strokes, milking the fluid out. Proceed in 1-inch segments more distally.

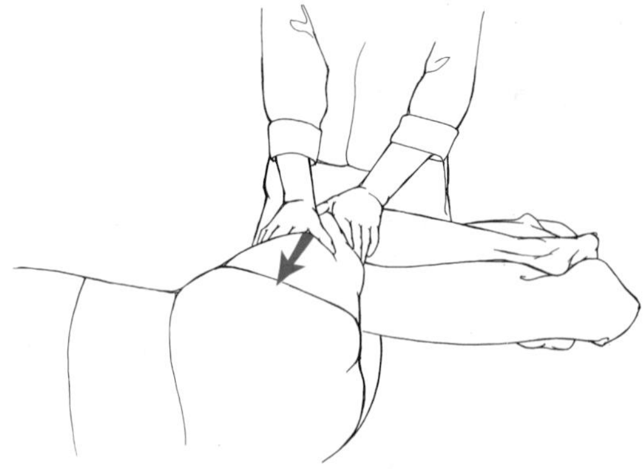

Figure 7-49. To release the trochanteric bursa, use the webspace between the thumb and the index finger and slowly stroke up the shaft of the femur.

Level II—Hip

1. Release of the Sciatic Nerve at the Greater Sciatic Notch

- *Anatomy*: The superior border of the sacrospinous ligament and the medial border of the ischium form the sciatic notch. The sciatic nerve leaves the pelvis through the greater sciatic notch. The nerve passes over the notch in the form of a thick ribbon but quickly takes its more rounded shape (Fig. 7-50).
- *Dysfunction*: A sustained hip flexion posture tightens the sciatic nerve against the notch. Hypertonicity of the hip rotators can also contribute to this entrapment syndrome.

Position

- TP—standing
- CP—side-lying, fetal position; additional pillows may be placed between the knees to bring the superficial tissue in the gluteal region into more slack

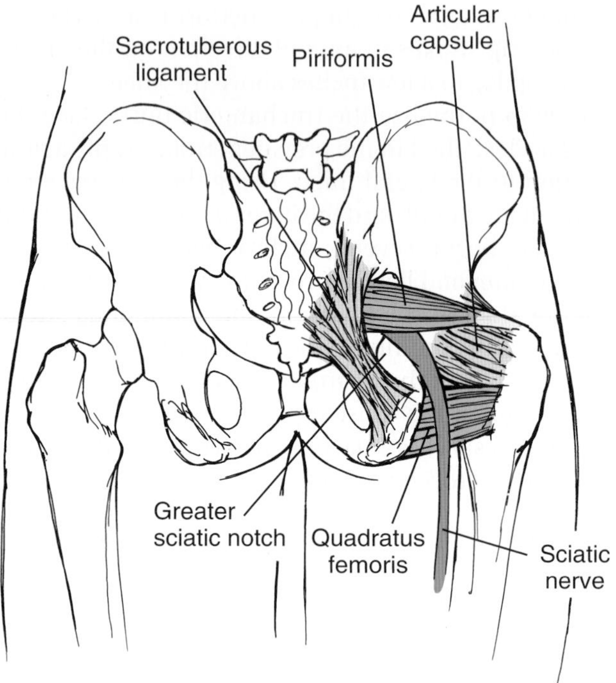

Figure 7-50. Sciatic nerve as it exits from the greater sciatic notch.

Strokes

Palpate the lowest aspect of the sciatic notch in the intersection of two lines: one, running slightly lateral to the posterior superior iliac spine (PSIS) in the inferior to superior plane, and two, running M–L at the level of the most superior aspect of the greater trochanter.

CAUTION: **Do not perform these strokes if your client has a positive SLR test. These strokes are for a client who has chronic, mild, diffuse numbing and tingling in the thigh.**

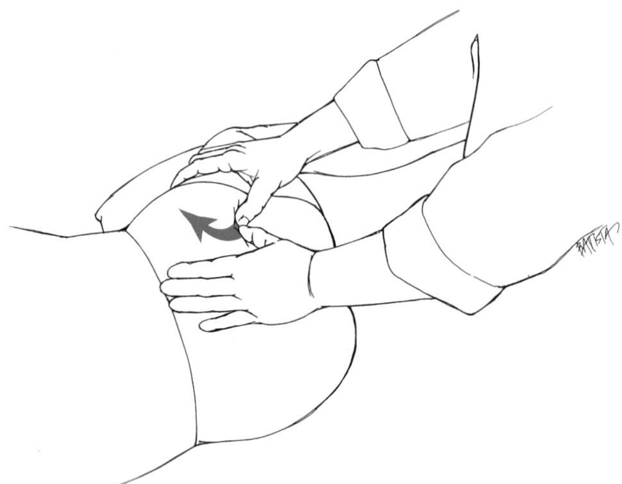

Figure 7-51. Double-thumb release of the sciatic nerve at the greater sciatic notch.

1. Perform a series of deep, lifting, scooping strokes in a superior-lateral direction (toward the shoulder) to release the sciatic nerve at the greater sciatic notch (Fig. 7-51). The notch feels fibrous if the nerve has been previously inflamed. If the nerve is entrapped, it is normal for the client to feel a slight tingling down the leg as you are working. Do not proceed if pain refers back up toward the spine, as this may indicate a nerveroot problem such as an inflamed disc. Only perform this stroke for about one minute, covering the entire area of the greater sciatic notch.

2. Release of the Muscle Attachments and Posterior Joint Capsule on the Posterior and Medial Femur

- *Anatomy:* Vastus lateralis, adductor longus, gluteus maximus, pectineus, adductor magnus, vastus medialis, posterior joint capsule (Fig. 7-52).
- *Dysfunction*: Attachment points usually become fibrotic. This fibrosis inhibits the normal extensibility of the myofascia, preventing normal muscle function. The posterior capsule can shorten, pulling the hip into a sustained external rotation. The muscles of the posterior thigh thicken if they are held in an eccentric contraction trying to counterbalance anterior pelvic tilt (increased lordosis).

Position

- TP—standing
- CP—prone; place a pillow under the client's ankle to relax the hamstrings, or place your flexed knee on the table and rest the client's leg on your thigh

Strokes

Work three lines of strokes down the entire shaft of the femur, using either short, scooping strokes; brisker, transverse strokes with fingertips over thumb, or fingertips over fingertips. Keeping your hands relaxed, rock your fingertips back and forth in the M–L plane to allow the muscle fibers to move out of your way so you can get to the bone.

1. To release the posterior joint capsule, have the client lay prone with a pillow under the ankles. Face 45° headward and place double thumbs or fingertips next to thumb approximately 2 inches medial to the lateral aspect of the greater trochanter. Perform back-and-forth strokes in a superior to inferior plane in the area between the medial side of the trochanter and the hip bone, approximately 2 inches more medially.
2. To release the vastus lateralis and the intermedius on the lateral aspect of the posterior surface of the femur, place your flexed knee on the table and rest the client's leg on your thigh (Fig. 7-53). Begin just below the

greater trochanter, and using fingertips over thumb or fingertips over fingertips, perform 1-inch, back-and-forth strokes in the M–L plane. Proceed down the entire femur to just above the knee (these techniques will be discussed in Chapter 8, "The Knee").

3. Begin a second line of strokes just below the greater trochanter in the middle of the posterior femur. Perform 1-inch, back-and-forth strokes on the attachments of the biceps femoris, adductor magnus, and gluteus maximus.
4. Beginning just below the gluteal crease, release the third line on the most medial aspect of the posterior femur for the pectineus, vastus medialis, and adductor longus.

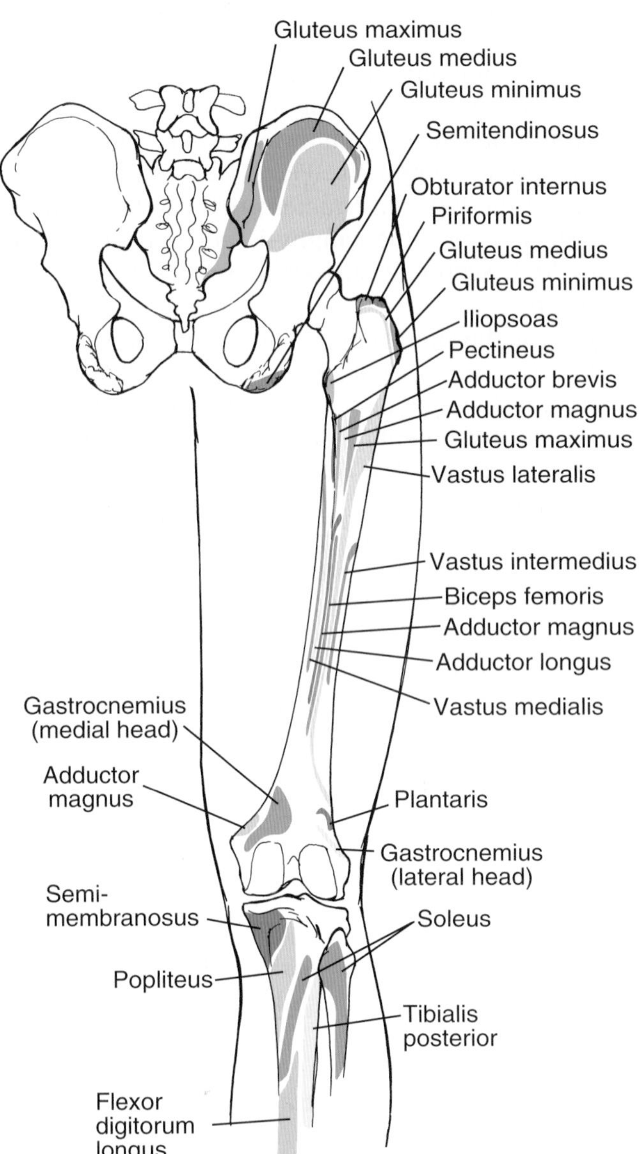

Figure 7-52. Attachments to the posterior hip, femur, and knee.

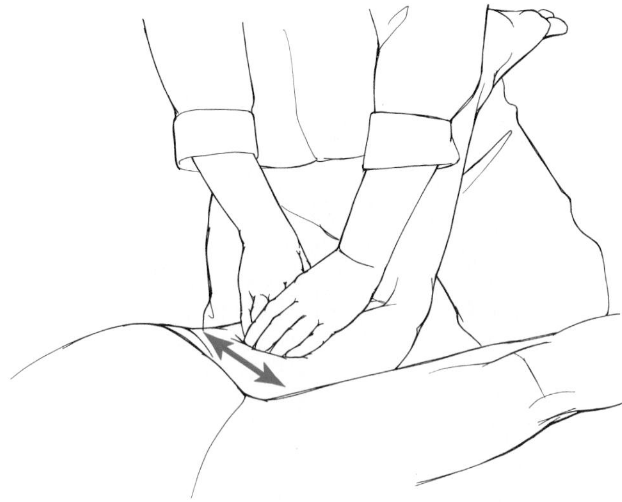

Figure 7-53. Prone release of the attachments to the posterior and medial femur.

5. To release the attachments on the medial femur, put the client in the side-lying position, with the lower leg extended and with the top leg flexed, resting on a pillow. Either face the table, or stand 45° headward. Using the same hand position described above, perform back-and-forth strokes in the M–L plane from the proximal femur to just above the knee.

3. Release of the Nerves of the Anterior Hip Above the Inguinal Ligament

- *Anatomy*: Femoral, genitofemoral, lateral femoral cutaneous, obturator nerves (Fig. 7-54), and iliopectineal bursa (see Fig. 7-5).
- *Dysfunction*: A sustained contracture in the psoas or fibrosis in the fascia of the iliacus may compress the femoral, lateral femoral, genitofemoral, and obturator nerves, leading to numbing, tingling, and pain in the anterior and medial pelvic region. Sustained contraction may also cause adhesions in the myofascia through which the nerves travel.

Position

- TP—standing, inferior knee flexed and resting on the table with the client's flexed knee resting on your thigh
- CP—supine, hip flexed and slightly abducted

Strokes

1. To release the fascia that interweaves with the inguinal ligament, stand in a 45° headward position. Using the fingertips of one or both hands, perform back-and-forth strokes along the superior border of the inguinal ligament, first from A–P and then in the M–L plane.

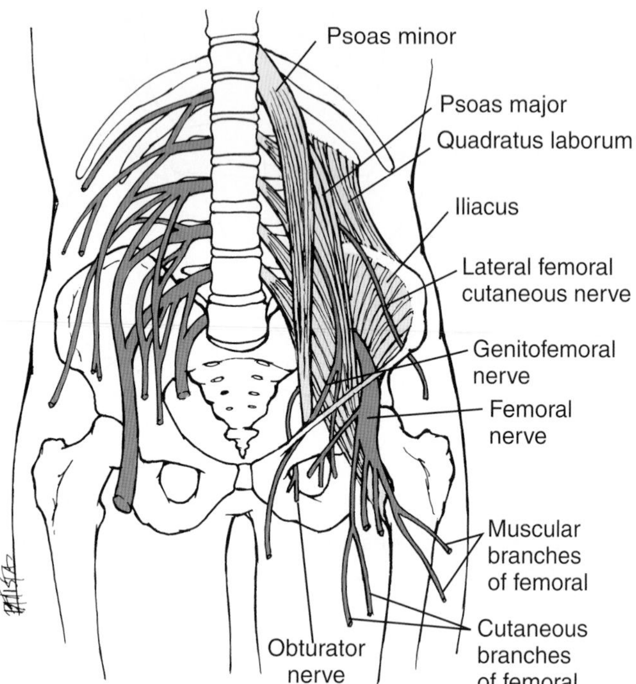

Figure 7-54. Anterior hip region nerves.

2. To release the obturator nerve above the inguinal ligament, stand in the 45° headward position, and place the fingertips of one hand over the fingertips of the other hand above the inguinal ligament, just lateral to the midline of the body (Fig. 7-55). Gently sink your hands into the client's abdomen, and perform a series of short, scooping strokes in the M–L direction. To release the genitofemoral nerve, move your hands 1 inch more laterally, and perform another series of M–L scooping strokes, just medial to the psoas.

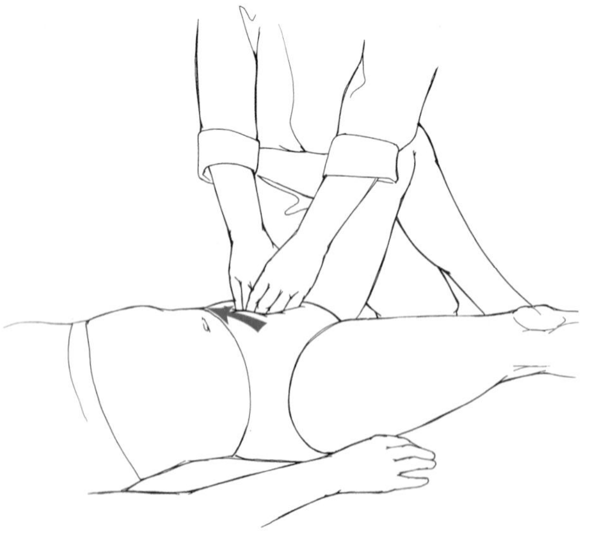

Figure 7-55. Release of the obturator, genitofemoral, and femoral nerves.

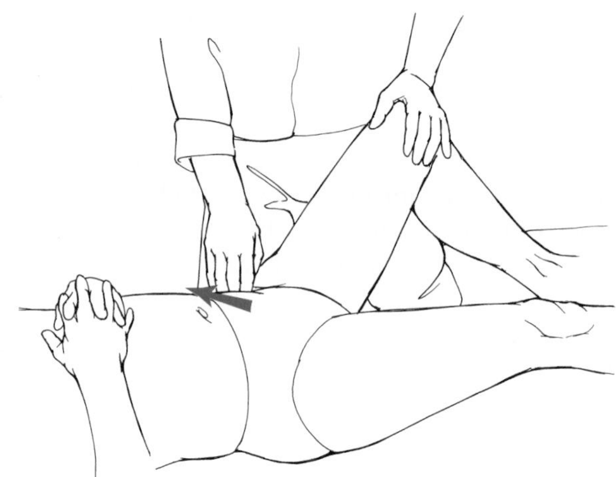

Figure 7-56. Release of the lateral femoral cutaneous nerve. Flex your fingertips over the ASIS and perform M–L strokes.

3. The femoral nerve lies in a trough between the iliacus and the psoas, superior to the inguinal ligament, approximately midway between the ASIS and the pubic symphysis. Place your fingertips just above the inguinal ligament midway between the ASIS and the pubic symphysis, and perform a series of M–L scooping strokes to release the femoral nerve.
4. Release the lateral femoral cutaneous nerve by performing short, scooping strokes in an M–L direction, in the area just superior to the inguinal ligament's attachment to the ASIS (Fig. 7-56). Flex your fingertips and allow them to follow the contour of the bone.

   Note: Strokes 1 to 4 can also be done with the hip flexed to 90° and by scooping medially to laterally with one hand as the hip is being circumducted with the other hand, as shown in Fig. 7-45.
5. Iliopectineal bursae: Place a flat thumb parallel to the inguinal ligament and several inches inferior to it. Perform a series of strokes in the superior direction while gently pumping the hip toward the opposite shoulder with each stroke.
6. To help release the inguinal lymphatics, first place some lotion on the proximal thigh. With the leg in extension, gently perform a series of long, continuous strokes from the upper thigh to the inguinal ligament. As your hand is just below the inguinal ligament, add a gentle impulse at the end of your stroke.

4. Release of the Muscle Attachments to the Pubic and Ischial Ramus

- *Anatomy:* From inferior to superior—adductor magnus, adductor longus, gracilis, pectineus, adductor brevis, obturator nerve (Fig. 7-57).

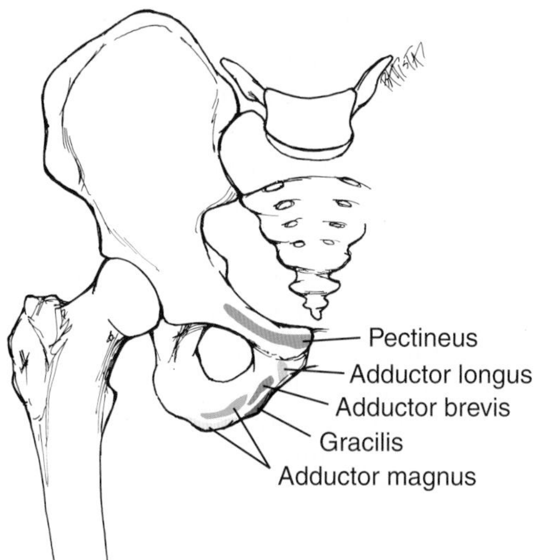

Figure 7-57. Muscle attachments to the ramus of the pubic bone and ischium.

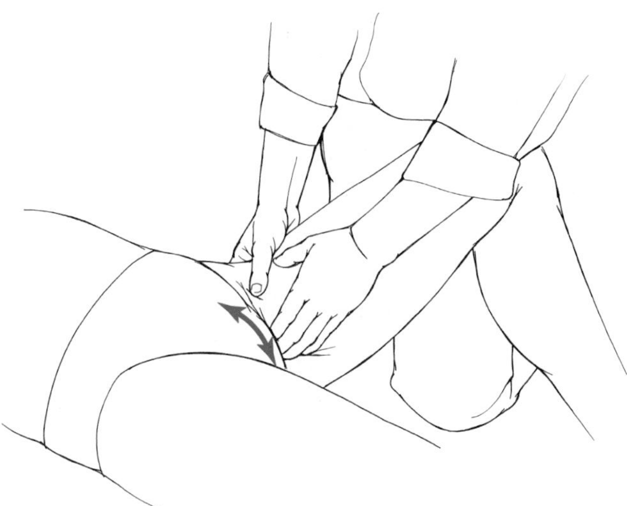

Figure 7-58. Release of the attachment of the adductor longus.

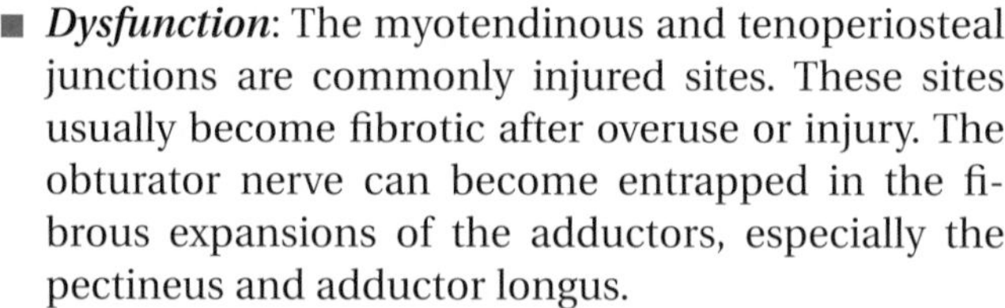

- *Dysfunction*: The myotendinous and tenoperiosteal junctions are commonly injured sites. These sites usually become fibrotic after overuse or injury. The obturator nerve can become entrapped in the fibrous expansions of the adductors, especially the pectineus and adductor longus.

Position

- TP—standing, with knee of inferior leg flexed and resting on table
- CP—supine, with hip flexed and abducted and knee flexed and resting on your thigh or on a pillow; rock the entire leg with each stroke

Strokes

To assist palpation, have the client's hip abducted and flexed. The adductor longus typically becomes prominent on the medial thigh. If it does not become prominent, have the client resist as you press at the knee toward further abduction, bringing up the adductor longus. The pectineus lies immediately lateral to the adductor longus; the adductor brevis lies deep to the longus; and adductor magnus lies posteriorly to the adductor longus. Flexing the knee emphasizes the gracilis; have the client pull his or her heel into table as you palpate the pubic ramus.

1. Place your flexed knee on the table, and rest the client's leg on your thigh (Fig. 7-58). With your forearm contacting the client's thigh to stabilize it, place your fingertips or braced fingertips on the attachment of the adductor longus at the superior pubic ramus. Perform short, back-and-forth strokes on the adductor longus as you rock your entire body with each stroke.
2. Using the same technique described above, release the gracilis and adductor brevis from the inferior ramus of the pubis, just inferior to adductor longus attachment.
3. Use fingertips or braced fingertips and perform short, back-and-forth strokes to release the adductor magnus from the lower portion of the inferior pubic ramus and the ischial tuberosity.
4. Release the pectineus from the superior pubic ramus with the same technique.
5. To release the obturator nerve, place your fingertips just lateral to the proximal part of the adductor longus. The obturator nerve enters the thigh under the pectineus. Perform a series of back-and-forth scooping strokes in the M–L plane, through the pectineus. Then, perform back-and-forth strokes on the medial side of the adductor longus and under the longus to release the branches of the nerve.

5. Release of the Muscle Attachments to the Medial and Anterior Femur and the Anterior Joint Capsule

- ***Anatomy:*** From M–L on the proximal femur—iliopsoas, vastus medialis, vastus intermedius, vastus lateralis, and gluteus minimus; from M–L on the anterior ilium—sartorius, TFL, and rectus femoris (Fig. 7-59).
- *Dysfunction*: Attachment points thicken due to chronic overuse, postural asymmetry, sustained hip flexion from back pain, or after an acute injury. The reflected head of the rectus femoris and the gluteus minimus interweave with the joint capsule. Injury to these muscles and the joint capsule can lead to prob-

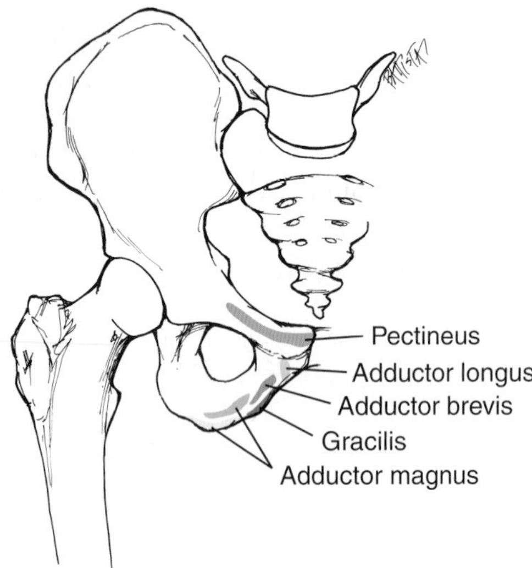

Figure 7-59. Muscle attachments to the pubic ramus and ischium.

lems of coordination and balance because of the high population of proprioceptors in the capsule.

Position

- TP—standing
- CP—supine, with the hip and knee flexed for the work on the lesser trochanter, the joint capsule, and the attachment points. Strokes 1 to 5 can also be done with the hip flexed to approximately 90° and by scooping medially to laterally with one hand as the hip is being circumducted or rocked M–L with the other hand, as shown in Fig. 7-45.

Strokes

1. To release the attachments of the sartorius on the ASIS, we use short, back-and-forth strokes with fingertips, braced fingertips, or double thumbs (Fig. 7-60). Move your hands just lateral and posterior to the sartorius attachment to release the TFL using the same back-and-forth strokes.
2. Using the same hand positions described above, release the rectus femoris from the AIIS. The AIIS can be located 1 inch inferior and 1 inch medial to the ASIS.
3. To release the anterior joint capsule, flex the hip to approximately 90°. Hold the knee with one hand and place the fingertips of your superior hand just inferior to the previous stroke, deep into the tissue. Rock the thigh back-and-forth in the M–L plane as you perform back and forth strokes with your fingertips in the M–L plane. Cover the area between the AIIS and the intertrochanteric line.
4. Using the fingertips technique, release the gluteus minimus attachment from the anterior-superior trochanter and the vastus lateralis immediately distal and medial to it. You may rock the leg with your stroke or in the opposite direction of your stroke.
5. Using fingertips, braced fingertips, or thumbs, perform a series of back-and-forth strokes in the M–L plane to release the vastus intermedius on the anterior shaft of the femur.
6. Release the iliopsoas attachment at the lesser trochanter (Fig. 7-61). With the thigh flexed and abducted and resting on your thigh, the iliopsoas is located by first grasping the adductor longus in one hand and the sartorius and rectus in the other. The psoas lies between your hands. The lesser trochanter is on the medial-posterior shaft of the femur in a line that is formed from the greater trochanter 45° inferiorly. Using fingertips, perform a series of back-and-forth strokes in the M–L plane. Rock your entire body with your strokes. Do not work on a pulse; the pulse is medial to the lesser trochanter.

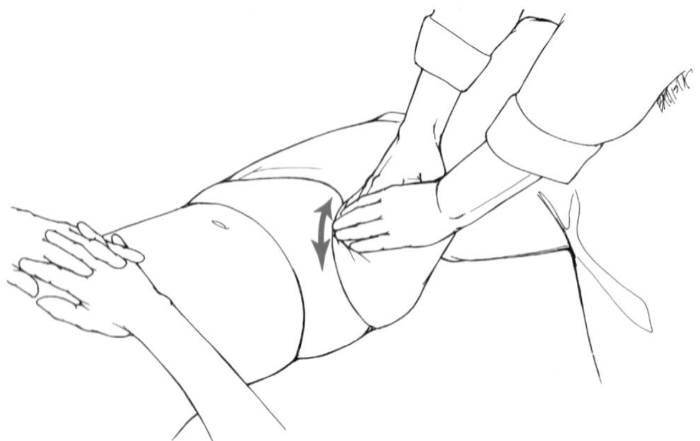

Figure 7-60. Braced-fingertips release of the ASIS and the AIIS.

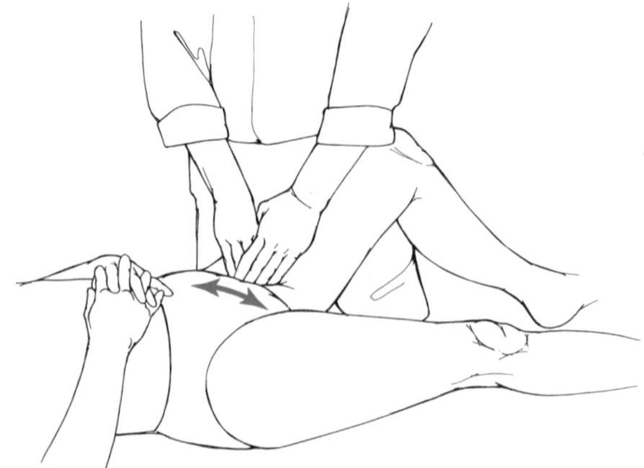

Figure 7-61. Release of the iliopsoas attachment at the lesser trochanter.

CASE STUDY

KP is a 48-year-old, 5'9", 150-lb, male psychotherapist who presented to my office with pain in the right groin. He described the pain as a diffuse, deep ache that could increase to a moderate sharp pain after a long hike. He stated that the pain began a few weeks prior to his visit, without any particular incident. His history included a minor car accident approximately 10 years previously. He stated that he did not have any prior symptoms in his groin and denied any history of back pain or injury to his hip or low back.

Examination revealed an unlevelling of the pelvis, with the ilium high on the right side. Active ROM was full and pain-free in all motions, except medial rotation. Passive ROM testing showed approximately a 50% loss of medial rotation, eliciting tenderness in the groin and a capsular end-feel. Length testing revealed shortness in the iliopsoas, rectus femoris, and TFL, but they were painless with CR MET.

A diagnosis was made of capsular fibrosis. I recommended weekly treatments for 4 weeks, with a reevaluation at that time. Treatment began with CR MET for the iliopsoas, rectus femoris (RF), and TFL. OM was then performed on each of these muscles, and the MET to increase medial rotation was performed for approximately five cycles.

KP returned in a week reporting that the pain was a little less in the groin and that the pain was more localized in the "crease," that is, the area under the inguinal ligament. The patient pointed to the AIIS. Examination showed a slight increase in passive medial rotation. CR MET was performed on the RF, TFL, and adductors. The client was then asked to sit on the end of the table, and PIR MET was performed on the iliopsoas and RF. KP was returned to the supine position, and PIR MET was performed on the adductors. MET was performed to increase medial rotation for approximately 10 cycles.

The patient returned a week later, stating that the pain was slightly better. Examination showed that there was approximately a 50% improvement in passive medial rotation. The same treatment of MET and OM was applied as in the previous visit.

On his fourth visit, examination showed that the patient had maintained his 50% improvement in medial rotation. The same treatment described above was applied. I recommended two additional treatments at weekly intervals. On his sixth visit he stated that he had taken a long hike without any discomfort. Examination showed that the ROM was normal in medial rotation. The patient elected to schedule two additional treatments. He had maintained normal ROM and was pain free. The patient was discharged from ongoing treatments and was encouraged to make a follow-up appointment in approximately 3 months to assess whether he maintained full ROM.

STUDY GUIDE

Level I

1. Describe the origin, insertion, and action of the following muscles: psoas, gluteus medius, adductor longus, hamstrings, TFL, and rectus femoris.
2. Describe the signs and symptoms of tendinitis of the gluteus medius, adductors, quadriceps, hamstrings, and iliopsoas.
3. Describe the positional dysfunction of the psoas, TFL, and adductors and describe the stroke direction to correct them.
4. Describe an MET for acute hip pain and the MET to increase medial rotation of the hip.
5. Describe the first motion to be lost in capsulitis and in arthritis of the hip.
6. Describe the MET for the following muscles: gluteus maximus, medius, and minimus; medial and lateral rotators; hamstrings; adductors; and TFL.
7. Describe which muscles of the hip are typically tight and short and which muscles are typically weak, as described in pelvic crossed syndrome.
8. Describe the symptoms of capsulitis and arthritis of the hip.
9. Describe anteverted and retroverted hips and how the ROM of the hip is affected in each condition.
10. Describe the signs and symptoms of trochanteric bursitis, iliopectineal bursitis, entrapment of the lateral cutaneous nerve of the thigh, entrapment of the obturator nerve, and entrapment of the femoral nerve.

Level II

1. Describe the origin and insertion of the pectineus, sartorius, and gracilis.
2. Describe the stroke direction to release the sciatic nerve in the gluteal region.
3. List three common sites of entrapment of the sciatic nerve in the hip region.

4. Describe the difference in symptoms among an iliopsoas tendinitis, an iliopectineal bursitis, and an entrapment of the femoral nerve.
5. Describe the typical ranges of motion of the hip.
6. Describe the MET for capsulitis or arthritis of the hip.
7. List the muscle attachments on the pubic ramus and ischial ramus.
8. Describe the sites of entrapment of the obturator, femoral, and lateral femoral cutaneous nerves and the stroke direction to release them.
9. List three factors that contribute to hip pain.
10. Describe Trendelenburg's test. Describe a positive test.

REFERENCES

1. Beattie P. The hip. In: Malone T, McPoil T, Nitz A, eds. Orthopedic and Sports Physical Therapy. St. Louis: Mosby, 1997:459–508.
2. Hertling D, Kessler R. The hip. In: Hertling D, Kessler R, eds. Management of Common Musculoskeletal Disorders. Baltimore: Lippincott Williams & Wilkins, 1996: 285–314.
3. Grieve G. The hip. Physiotherapy 1983;69:196–204.
4. Norris CM. The hip. In: Norris CM, ed. Sports Injuries: Diagnosis and Management for Physiotherapists. Oxford: Butterworth-Heinemann, 1993:160–163.

4a. Janda V. Evaluation of muscular imbalance. In: Lieberson C, ed. Rehabilitation of the Spine. Baltimore: Williams & Wilkins, 1996:97–112.

5. Garaci MC. Rehabilitation of the hip, pelvis, and thigh. In: Kibler WB, Herring SA, Press JM, eds. Functional Rehabilitation of Sports and Musculoskeletal Injuries. Gaithersburg: Aspen, 1998:216–243.
6. Kendall F, McCreary E, Provance P. Muscles: Testing and Function. 4th Ed. Baltimore: Williams & Wilkins, 1993.
7. Grofton JP. Studies in osteoarthritis of the hip: part IV. Biomechanics and clinical considerations. CMAJ 1971; 104:1007–1011.
8. Hammer W. The hip. In: Hammer W, ed. Functional Soft Tissue Examination and Treatment by Manual Methods. Gaithersburg: Aspen, 1999.

SUGGESTED READINGS

Chaitow L. Muscle Energy Techniques. New York: Churchill Livingstone, 1996.

Corrigan B, Maitland GD. Practical Orthopaedic Medicine. London: Butterworths, 1983.

Cyriax J, Cyriax P. Illustrated Manual of Orthopedic Medicine. London: Butterworths, 1983.

Garrick J, Webb D. Sports Injuries. 2nd Ed. Philadelphia: WB Saunders, 1999.

Greenman PE. Principles of Manual Medicine. 2nd Ed. Baltimore: Williams & Wilkins, 1996.

Hoppenfeld S. Physical Examination of the Spine and Extremities. New York: Appleton-Century-Crofts, 1976.

Kendall F, McCreary E, Provance P. Muscles: Testing and Function. 4th Ed. Baltimore: Williams & Wilkins, 1993.

Kessler R, Hertling D. Management of Common Musculoskeletal Disorders. 3rd Ed. Baltimore: Lippincott Williams & Wilkins, 1996.

Magee D. Orthopedic Physical Assessment. 3rd Ed. Philadelphia: WB Saunders,1997.

Norkin C, Levangie P. Joint Structure and Function. 2nd Ed. Philadelphia: FA Davis, 1992.

Platzer W. Locomotor System, vol 1. 4th Ed. New York: Thieme Medical, 1992.

Reid DC. Sports Injury and Assessment. New York: Churchill Livingstone, 1992.

The Knee

The knee is one of the most commonly injured joints in the body and represents nearly 50% of sports-related physician visits.[1] Acute injuries typically affect the ligaments and the menisci, fibrocartilage discs inside the knee. The knee also includes the joint between the knee cap or patella and the femur, and patellofemoral dysfunction is one of the most common overuse injuries to the athlete.[2] Chronic knee pain is typically caused by degeneration of the joint. It is a common complaint in the elderly and represents a significant source of disability.

Anatomy, Function, and Dysfunction of the Knee

GENERAL OVERVIEW

The distal end of the femur, the proximal end of the tibia, and the patella, or knee cap, form the knee joint (Fig. 8-1). Two separate articulations comprise the knee joint: the **tibiofemoral joint** and the **patellofemoral joint.** The tibiofemoral joint is the articulation between the distal femur and the proximal tibia. The patellofemoral joint is the articulation between the patella and the femur. The knee is a synovial joint with two fibrocartilage **menisci,** a **patella,** a **joint capsule,** numerous **ligaments, bursae, nerves** and is surrounded by **muscles.**

KNEE BONES AND JOINTS

Femur

- *Structure*: The distal end of the femur has two cartilage-covered expansions, the **medial** and **lateral epicondyles.** At the anterior surface is the cartilage-covered patellar surface (trochlear groove) upon which the patella glides. A small bony protuberance above the medial epicondyle is called the adductor tubercle, which serves as the attachment for the adductor magnus.
- *Function*: The distal end of the femur serves as a weight-bearing surface and for attachment sites of the soft tissue.
- ***Dysfunction and injury:*** Discussed below after the description of the tibia.

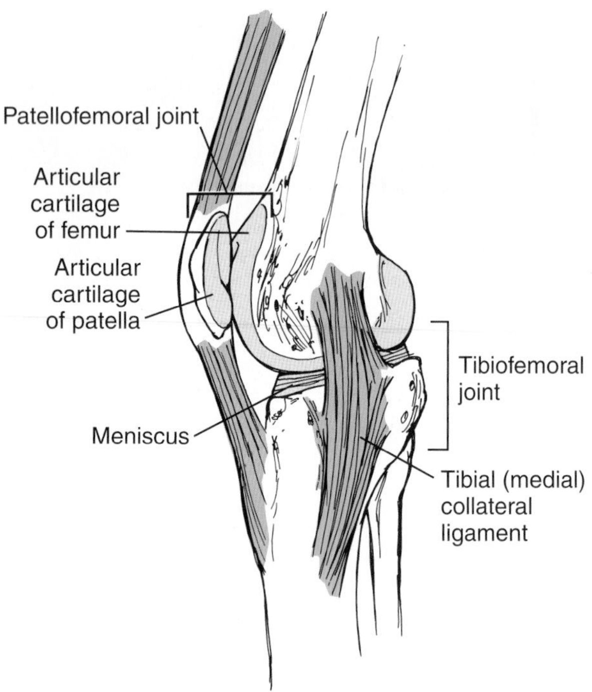

Figure 8-1. Knee consists of two joints. The tibiofemoral joint is the articulation of the distal end of the femur and the proximal tibia. The patellofemoral joint is the articulation of the femur and patella.

Tibia

- *Structure*: The proximal tibia contains the tibial plateau for articulation with the femur, the medial and lateral condyles, the intercondylar eminence, and the tibial tuberosity. The **medial** and **lateral condyles** have two cartilage-covered articular surfaces. In between these articulating surfaces are two bony prominences, the **intercondylar eminences,** which serve as attachment sites for the cruciate ligaments. On the anterior surface of the tibia is a bony projection, the **tibial tubercle,** where the quadriceps attaches.
- *Function*: The proximal tibia serves as a weight-bearing surface and for attachment sites of the soft tissue.

Patella and the Patellofemoral Joint

- *Structure:* The patella, or knee cap, is the largest sesamoid bone in the body. A **sesamoid bone** is a cartilage-covered bone that grows in tendons that cross the ends of bones. The posterior surface of the patella has a central, vertical ridge that divides it into medial and lateral facets. This surface is covered with hyaline cartilage, which articulates with the patellar surface (trochlear groove) on the distal femur, forming the **patellofemoral joint.** This cartilage is the thickest in the human body.[3]
- *Function*: The function of the patella is to protect the knee; to help distribute the compressive forces of the quadriceps tendon to prevent the tendon fibers from digging into the articular cartilage of the femur; and to lengthen the quadriceps, increasing its leverage and therefore allowing the quadriceps to develop greater force. During flexion and extension the patella slides on the femur. To function normally the patella must have adequate mobility to accept the contractile forces in different positions of the knee, and it must have adequate stability to ensure that the cartilage surfaces are not overly stressed. During extension of the knee, the patella is designed to move upward in line with the central groove of the femur. The line of movement is determined by the combined actions of the vastus medialis obliquus (VMO) and the vastus lateralis. In standing, with normal alignment the patella should face straight forward.[4]
- *Dysfunction and injury:* There are two common dysfunctions of the patellofemoral joint: one, becoming too compressed; and two, moving too far laterally in the intercondylar groove. Both conditions cause abrasion of the cartilage, leading to inflammation and degeneration.
  - It becomes too compressed due to increased flexion of the knee, which is caused by sustained tension in the hamstrings, iliotibial band (ITB), and gastrocnemius or by a shortened joint capsule. This compressive force is dramatically increased when a person climbs stairs or gets up from a chair.
  - If the patella is compressed laterally in the trochlear groove it is called patellar tracking dysfunction. Two potential causes are (1) genu valgus, which is associated with an anteverted hip, lateral tibial torsion, and pronated ankle; and (2) a weakening of the VMO and an overdevelopment of the vastus lateralis, lateral retinaculum, and tensor fascia lata (TFL). The weakening of the VMO may be caused by two mechanisms. The first is a previous knee injury. When the knee has been injured it is often difficult to extend it fully because any swelling causes the knee to assume some flexion. Because the VMO functions primarily during the last 15° of extension, the loss of terminal extension causes an atrophy of the VMO. The second cause is

the knee's arthrokinetic reflex. With this reflex, any irritation of the joint leads to neurologic inhibition and weakening of the VMO.

- *Treatment implications*: Muscle energy technique (MET) is performed to reduce the hypertonicity of the TFL, ITB, hamstrings, and gastrocnemius and to facilitate or strengthen the VMO and adductors. Orthopedic massage (OM) is used to reduce the fibrosis that typically develops around the periphery and underneath the surface of the patella.

Knee Joint (Tibiofemoral Joint)

- *Structure:* The distal end of the femur and the proximal end of the tibia form the tibiofemoral joint (See Fig. 8-1). The fibula does not form part of the knee and will be considered in Chapter 9, "The Leg, Ankle, and Foot." The knee joint is the largest joint in the body, formed by the two largest bones in the body. The knee is a synovial joint with two fibrocartilage **menisci;** a **joint capsule;** and numerous **ligaments, bursae, nerves** and is surrounded by **muscles.** The knee also contains an **infrapatellar fat pad,** which causes the skin to bulge on both sides of the infrapatellar ligament.
- *Function*: The knee is considered a modified hinge joint, because in addition to the primary motions of flexion and extension, the joint has the ability to rotate. Also, some degree of adduction and abduction is present. The key motion of the tibiofemoral joint is a spiral (i.e., a winding and an unwinding of the tibia relative to the femur). The open (most relaxed) position of the knee is slight flexion, a position in which the joint capsule, quadriceps, and hamstrings are most relaxed. The closed-packed position is extension.
- *Dysfunction and injury:* The articular cartilage of the femur and tibia are common sites for degeneration, leading to arthritis. This degeneration could result from a specific traumatic episode or from cumulative stress. Dysfunctions and injuries of the specific soft tissue structures are discussed separately below.
- *Treatment implications:* Arthritis of the knee usually manifests as decreased flexion. During assessment, passive flexion has a reduced range of motion (ROM) and a capsular end feel, representing fibrosis or thickening of the joint capsule. MET is used to increase flexion and to increase the joint capsule length. OM is performed to dissolve fibrosis in the capsule and surrounding soft tissue.

KNEE ALIGNMENT

- *Structure*: The alignment of the femoral shaft to the center of the knee is normally approximately 10° lateral to the mechanical axis and is called the normal valgus angle or the **Q-angle** (quadriceps angle). This is because the femoral head and the hip joint are medial to the shaft. The mechanical axis describes the normal line of force that travels from the center of the hip joint, through the center of the knee, to the center of the ankle.[5]
- *Dysfunction:* Increases in the normal valgus angle is called **genu valgus** (knock-knees) and causes compressive forces on the lateral side of the joint, including the lateral side of the patella, and tensile forces on the medial side. It can be caused by ITB tightness, femoral anteversion, and pronation of the foot. **Genu varus** or bow legs describes a decrease in the normal valgus angle and causes compression on the medial side of the knee and tensile stresses on the lateral side.
- *Treatment implications:* To assess the alignment of the knee is complex and involves assessment and treatment of the feet, hips, and lumbopelvic region, as well as structures in the knee itself. For the massage therapist, the goals are to reduce the muscle hypertonicity and to perform MET to facilitate the weak muscles. All clients who have chronic knee pain or signs of knee misalignment need to be referred to a chiropractor, osteopath, or podiatrist.

KNEE SOFT-TISSUE STRUCTURES

Menisci

- *Structure*: The knee contains the **medial** and the **lateral menisci.** The menisci are C-shaped fibrocartilage discs. They are wedge-shaped, and the outer margin is thicker than the inner margin. Both menisci are firmly attached to bony protuberances called the intercondylar tubercles in the middle portion of the tibial plateau. They are also attached along the periphery of the tibia by expansions of the joint capsule called the coronary ligaments.
  - The **medial meniscus** is far less mobile than the lateral meniscus because it is firmly attached to the tibial plateau. It is interwoven with the medial (tibial) collateral ligament, the joint capsule, the coronary ligament, and the anterior cruciate ligament (ACL). It is also attached to the semimem-

branosus muscle, which pulls the meniscus posteriorly during knee flexion.[3]

- The **lateral meniscus** has much more mobility than the medial meniscus and is therefore much less susceptible to injury. The lateral meniscus has attachments to the posterior cruciate ligament (PCL), the joint capsule, the coronary ligaments, and the popliteus muscle, but it is not attached to the lateral (fibular) collateral ligament. The popliteus assists in drawing the meniscus posteriorly during knee flexion.[4]

- ***Function***: The medial and the lateral menisci form joint sockets for the femoral condyles. This adds stability to the articulation of the asymmetric, concave tibial plateau and the asymmetric, convex femoral condyles. They increase lubrication and nutrition and reduce friction. The menisci are weight-bearing structures, designed to be shock absorbers. They help carry as much as 50% of the load, which increases with knee flexion. The menisci also play a role in proprioception.[6] The anterior portion of the menisci are somewhat mobile. As the knee extends, the anterior aspects of the menisci glide forward, and as the knee flexes, the menisci are drawn back.
- ***Dysfunction and injury:*** Any injury to the meniscus increases the amount of weight carried by the articular cartilage and increases the risk of degeneration (arthritis). The medial meniscus is much more susceptible to injury than the lateral meniscus because it is far less mobile. As with all fibrocartilage, the menisci are susceptible to cumulative stresses and to an acute traumatic episode. Acute injury usually involves a twisting motion to a weight-bearing knee; a blow to the side of the knee, called traumatic valgus stress; or full flexion combined with external rotation. The cartilage injury can range from a bruise to a complete tear.
- ***Treatment implications:*** Injury causes swelling and potential subluxation. Assessment reveals a loss of active and passive extension. Lauren Berry, RPT, taught that if the torn tissue in the meniscus could maintain contact with each other and not separate, there was an increased likelihood of repair. A mobilization in the OM protocol was taught by Berry and has proved remarkably effective in normalizing the menisci position to allow proper healing.

Joint Capsule

- ***Structure***: The joint capsule of the knee encloses the tibiofemoral and the patellofemoral joints (Fig. 8-2). It is attached to the femur approximately two finger-widths above the patella and to the proximal tibia. The anterior part of the joint capsule may be divided into superficial and deep portions. The superficial portion is wide and loose, is thin in the front and sides, and is reinforced by the fascial expansion of the quadriceps muscle, called the **patellar retinaculum** and the **patellar ligament** (infrapatellar tendon). The retinaculum has several thickenings that are called the **patellofemoral and the patellotibial ligaments.**[3] The deep portion of the joint capsule has two parts. One, a deep transverse thickening of the retinaculum from the medial and lateral epicondyles to the patella, and two, the **meniscofemoral** and **meniscotibial ligaments,** also called the **coronary ligaments,** that help stabilize the meniscus to the tibial plateau. The posterior capsule is strengthened by the tendinous expansions of the semimembranosus, popliteus, and gastrocnemius. The oblique popliteal ligament, an expansion of the semimembranosus, interweaves with the arcuate popliteal ligament, a thickening in the posterior wall of the capsule.

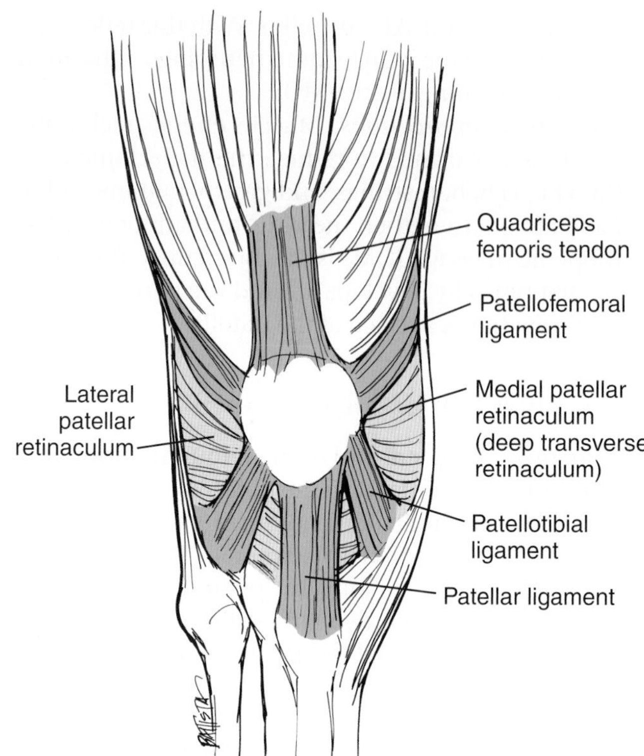

Figure 8-2. Anterior knee showing the patellar retinaculum. The superficial portion of the joint capsule interweaves with the retinaculum. The retinaculum has distinct thickenings, the patellofemoral and patellotibial ligaments.

- *Function*: The joint capsule provides stability to the joint and menisci, serves to lubricate the articulating surfaces, and provides a neurosensory role. Tension is placed on the menisci when the quadriceps, semimembranosus, and popliteus contract through the ligaments that form part of the joint capsule. During knee flexion and extension, the synovial fluid lubricates the articulating surfaces by moving from one recess to another.[4]
- *Dysfunction and injury:* In an acute injury, the knee assumes a slightly flexed position, as the capsule becomes relaxed and allows more fluid. Joint capsule dysfunction and injury has two possible outcomes that have connective tissue, muscular, and neurologic consequences. One, the capsule and associated bursae can develop fibrosis, which thickens and dehydrates the structures. The knee loses some extension, and flexion is often restricted to only 90° to 100°. Restricted flexion leads to articular nerve dysfunction, which decreases sensory input from the mechanoreceptors and leads to arthrokinetic reflexes. Arthrokinetic reflexes typically inhibit (weaken) the quadriceps and lead to joint dysfunction and potential degeneration. Two, the capsule and associated ligaments can become too slack due to injury, losing their stabilizing function and allowing for excessive joint movement, potential inflammation, and early joint degeneration resulting from the associated muscular inhibition caused by the arthrokinetic reflex.
- *Treatment implications:* As full knee extension is essential to normal gait and as decreased flexion interferes with many daily activities, the therapist's primary intention in any acute knee injury is to normalize the ROM. This normalization is accomplished through contract-relax MET. The CR cycle pumps excess fluid out of the joint, reduces muscle hypertonicity, and helps reestablish normal neurologic communication to the surrounding muscles. For chronic thickening in the joint capsule, the therapist's intention is to increase the joint capsule extensibility. Perform MET to increase knee flexion and perform OM to reduce sustained hypermobility in the hamstrings, quadriceps, ITB, gastrocnemius, and popliteus.

Ligaments

- *Structure*: The supporting structures classified by function are divided into the **static** and **dynamic stabilizers.** The static stabilizers are the superficial fascia, called the crural fascia; the joint capsule; and the ligaments. The dynamic stabilizers are the muscles and their fascial expansions.

As mentioned, many thickenings of the joint capsule may also be classified as ligaments. Classification of the ligaments by location divides the structures into the anterior, posterior, medial, lateral, and internal. The **anterior ligaments** include the patellar ligament (infrapatellar tendon), which is the portion of the quadriceps that attaches to the tibial tuberosity; the medial and lateral patellofemoral and patellotibial ligaments (patellar retinaculum), which are broad tendinous (ligamentous) bands that connect the VMO and the vastus lateralis to the patella and tibia; and the medial and lateral coronary ligaments (meniscotibial and meniscofemoral ligaments). The **posterior ligaments** include the posterior oblique popliteal ligament and the arcuate popliteal ligament. The **medial ligament** is the medial collateral ligament (MCL). **The lateral ligament** is the lateral collateral ligament (LCL). The **internal ligaments** include the anterior cruciate ligament (ACL) and the posterior cruciate ligament(PCL).

- Medial patellofemoral and patellotibial ligaments (medial patellar retinaculum) (Fig. 8-3).
    - ***Origin:*** VMO superficial fibers and medial epicondyle deep (transverse) fibers form these ligaments.
    - ***Insertion:*** The medial patellofemoral and patellotibial ligaments insert on the superior portion of the medial patella and continue to insert on the tibial tuberosity.
- Lateral patellofemoral and patellotibial ligaments (lateral patellar retinaculum) (Fig. 8-4)
    - ***Origin:*** Superficial fibers of the vastus lateralis, some fibers from the rectus femoris (RF), and deep fibers from the lateral epicondyle of the femur form these ligaments. Fibers from the ITB insert into and strengthen it.
    - ***Insertion:*** The lateral patellofemoral and patellotibial ligaments insert on the superior portion of the lateral patella and continue to insert on the tibial tuberosity.
- Posterior oblique popliteal ligament (Fig. 8-5)
    - ***Origin:*** A tendinous expansion of the semimembranosus muscle forms this ligament.
    - ***Insertion:*** The posterior oblique popliteal ligament attaches to the posterior aspect of the medial tibial condyle and the joint capsule and to the central part of the posterior aspect of the joint capsule. Contraction of the semimembranosus

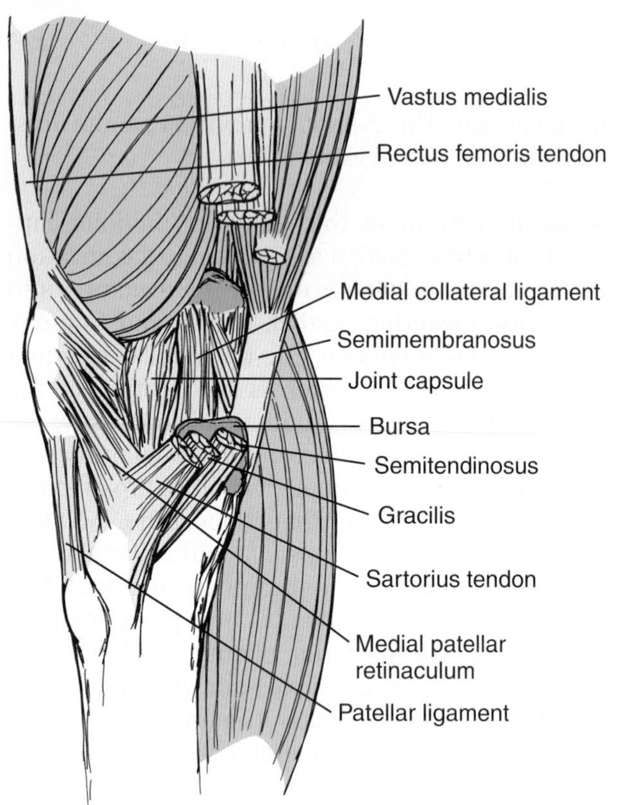

Figure 8-3. Medial knee showing the ligaments, joint capsule, retinaculum, interweaving tendons, and pes anserinus bursa.

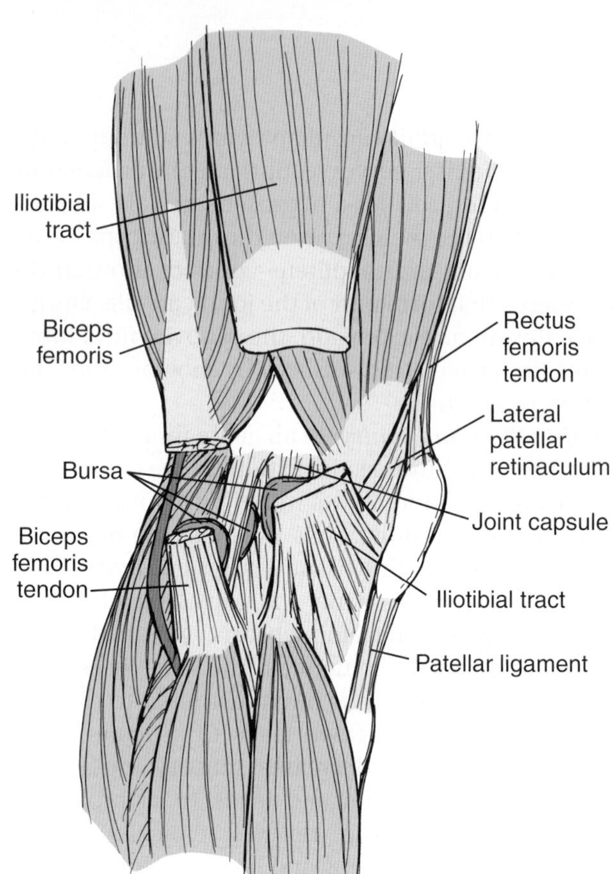

Figure 8-4. Lateral knee showing the ligaments, joint capsule, retinaculum, interweaving tendons, and the bursae under the iliotibial tract, and biceps femoris.

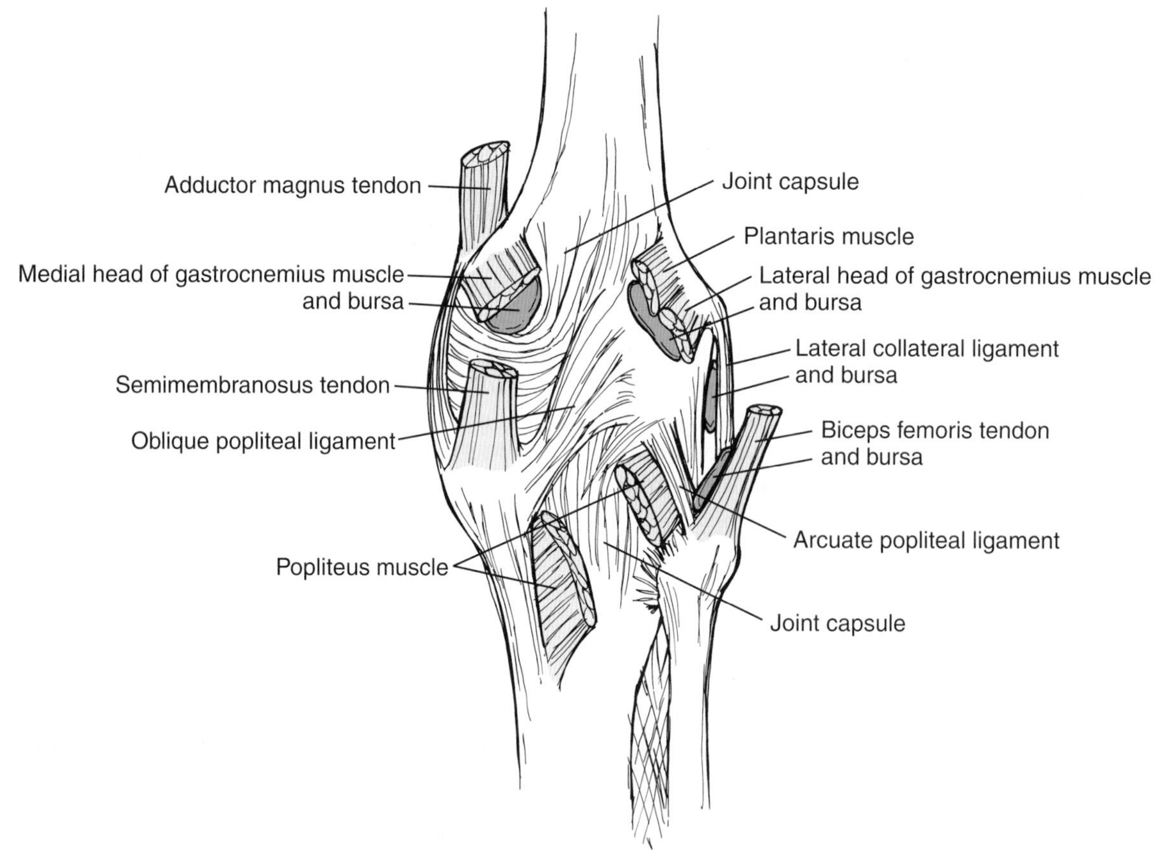

Figure 8-5. Joint capsule, ligaments, bursae, and muscles of the posterior knee.

pulls the medial meniscus posteriorly during knee flexion.

- Arcuate popliteal ligament (see Fig. 8-5)
  - ***Origin:*** Considered a thickening of the joint capsule, the arcuate popliteal ligament arises from the posterior aspect of the head of the fibula.
  - ***Insertion:*** The arcuate popliteal ligament attaches to the intercondylar area of the tibia, the lateral epicondyle of femur, the posterior-lateral capsule, and the lateral meniscus.
- MCL (See Fig. 8-3)
  - ***Origin:*** A flat and triangular ligament, the MCL blends into the fibrous membrane of the capsule and fuses with the medial meniscus. It originates at the medial aspect of the medial femoral condyle and has superficial and deep fibers.
  - ***Insertion:*** The MCL inserts into the medial tibia approximately 4 inches below the joint line.
- LCL (See Fig. 8-4)
  - ***Origin:*** From the lateral epicondyle of the femur, this round, cordlike structure (the LCL) is neither fused with the capsule nor attached to the lateral meniscus.
  - ***Insertion:*** The LCL inserts into the fibular head, traveling underneath the biceps femoris tendon.
- Coronary (meniscotibial and meniscofemoral) ligaments (Fig. 8-6)
  - Coronary ligaments are deep portions of the joint capsule that attach the menisci to the tibia. This deep part of the joint capsule helps bind the periphery of the medial and lateral menisci to the tibia.
- ACL (See Fig. 8-6)
  - ***Origin:*** The ACL originates from the anterior tibial plateau.
  - ***Insertion:*** The ACL inserts on the inner portion of the lateral condyle of the femur. It primarily restricts forward movement of the tibia relative to the femur and internal rotation of the tibia.
- PCL (see Fig. 8-6)
  - ***Origin:*** The PCL originates on the lateral surface of the medial condyle of the femur.
  - ***Insertion:*** The PCL inserts into the posterior tibial plateau and primarily restricts posterior movement of the tibia relative to the femur and internal rotation of the tibia on the femur.
- ***Function***: The knee ligaments control joint movement more than any other joint in the body.[5] The ligaments are extremely dense, and dislocations are rare. As with all other synovial joints, the ligaments play an important neurosensory role. Ligaments provide vital information about joint position, movement, pressure, and pain and have reflex connections to the surrounding muscles.
- ***Dysfunction and injury:*** Knee ligaments are some of the most commonly injured structures in the body. The ACL and the MCL are the most frequently injured. Ligament injuries are graded 1 to 3, based on the amount of laxity in the joint. Lauren Berry discovered that the collateral ligaments develop a posterior misalignment or positional dysfunction after any injury to the knee that involves swelling. The knee takes a position of sustained flexion after injury, as flexion allows for more fluid in the knee. As mentioned, the knee also maintains a sustained flexion after a meniscus injury.
- ***Treatment implications:*** The collateral ligaments need to be lifted in a posterior to anterior direction. The other ligaments do not have a positional dysfunction and need to be released transverse to the line of the fiber. As with the joint capsule, injury and

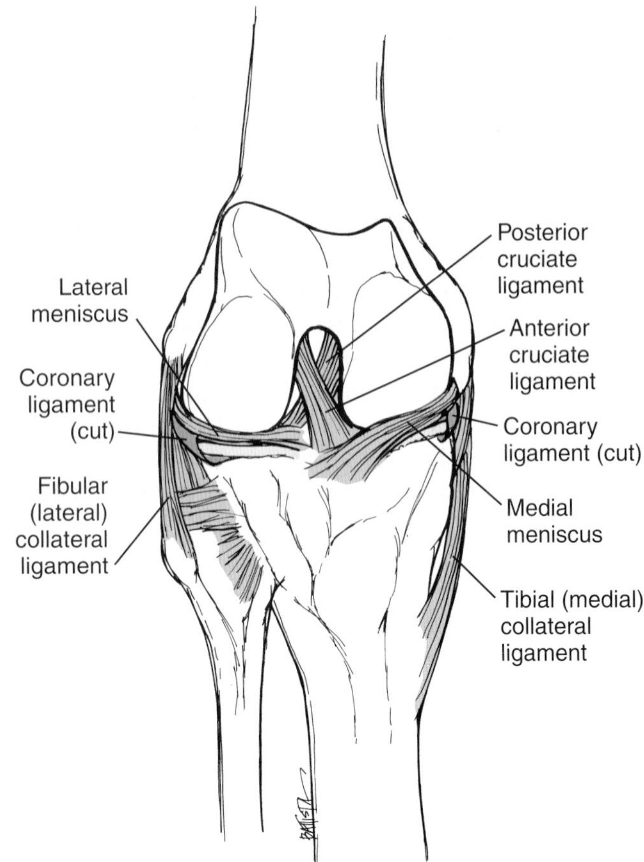

Figure 8-6. Internal structures of the knee, showing the anterior cruciate ligament; the posterior cruciate ligament; the medial and lateral menisci; and the coronary ligament, a part of the deep joint capsule.

dysfunction to the ligaments have two possible outcomes. One, the ligaments become too slack, leading to instability, irritation, and degeneration. These ligaments are treated with exercise rehabilitation. Two, the ligaments can become too tight and fibrotic, decreasing joint movement and leading to degeneration. If the ligaments are external, they are treated with OM to dissolve the fibrosis and to rehydrate the tissue and with MET to help normalize the neurologic function.

Bursae

- *Structure*: A bursa is a synovial-lined sac filled with synovial fluid (see Figs. 8-2 to 8-5). More than 24 bursae are located in the knee area. Three are recesses in the joint capsule that form the suprapatellar, semimembranosus, and gastrocnemius bursae.

Bursae are also under the muscles of the knee, including the biceps femoris, the semimembranosus, the ITB, and the pes anserinus tendons (see below).

- *Function*: Bursa function is to decrease friction.
- ***Dysfunction and injury:*** Three areas are commonly involved clinically: the bursae of the anterior knee, including the prepatellar, infrapatellar, and suprapatellar bursae; the pes anserine bursae of the medial knee; and the semimembranosus and the medial gastrocnemius bursae in the posterior knee. Joint swelling of the posterior knee is also called a "**Baker's cyst.**" The bursae of the anterior knee are susceptible to direct impact and to prolonged kneeling, called "housemaid's knee." The bursae under the ITB and the pes anserinus tendons are commonly irritated because of excessive friction, such as running.
- *Treatment implications*: Bursae may be manually drained. The treatment involves gentle, slow, broad strokes toward the heart. Active or passive knee flexion and extension also assists in reducing the swelling by pumping the fluid out of the joint.

Nerves

- *Structure*: Innervation of the knee is from **the tibial, common peroneal, and saphenous nerves** (Figs. 8-7 and 8-8). The sciatic nerve divides into the tibial and common peroneal nerves in the distal third of the posterior thigh. The tibial nerve travels through the center of the popliteal fossa of the posterior knee, and the common peroneal nerve travels posterior to the fibular head between the biceps femoris and the lateral head of the gastrocnemius (see Fig. 8-3). The saphenous nerve is the terminal branch of the femoral nerve and gives off the infrapatellar branch that travels superficially in the medial knee between the tendons of the sartorius and the gracilis.
- *Function*: The tibial and common peroneal nerves have articular, muscular, and cutaneous branches

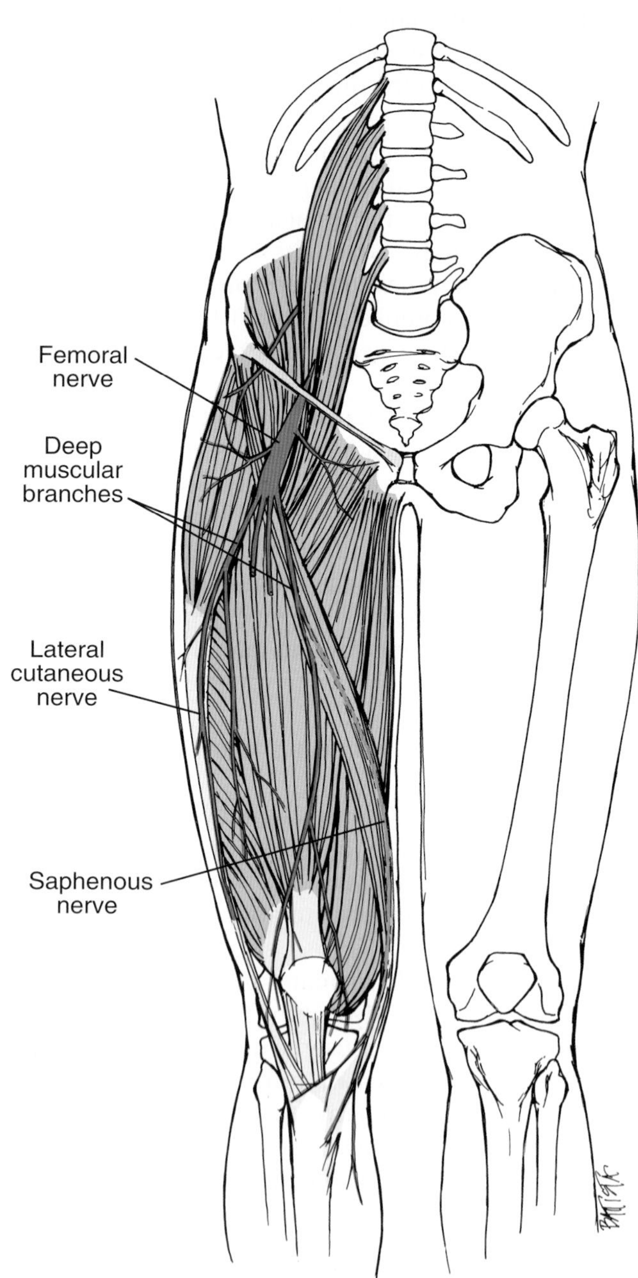

Figure 8-7. Nerves of the anterior and medial thigh and knee.

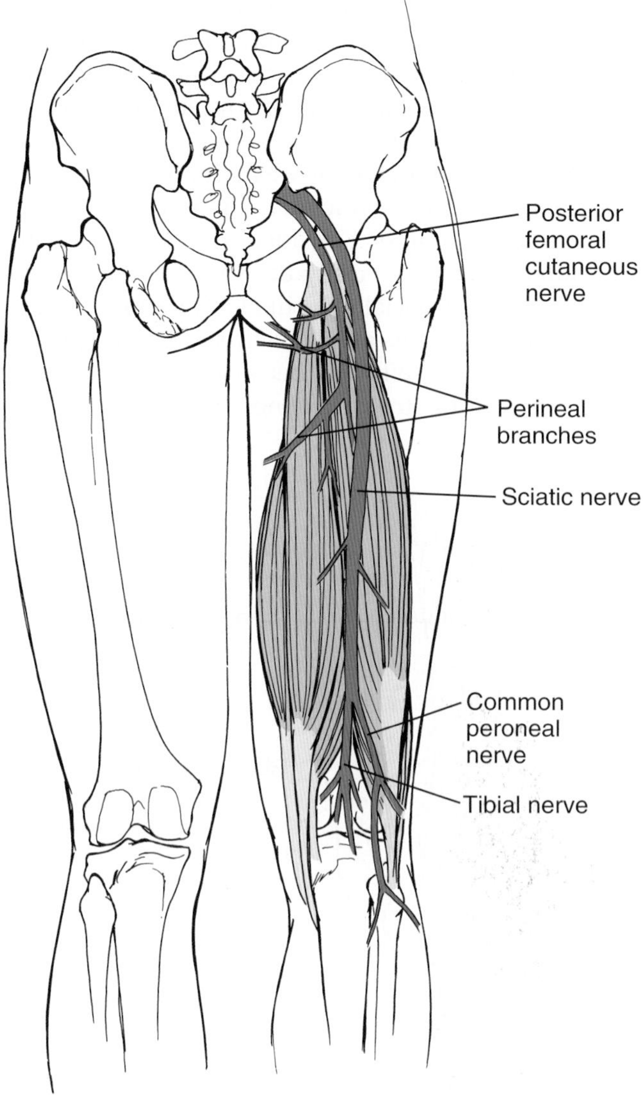

Figure 8-8. Nerves of the posterior thigh and knee.

(the sural nerve). The saphenous nerve is a cutaneous nerve innervating the skin in front of the patella and the skin of the leg and foot.

- *Dysfunction and injury:* The common peroneal and saphenous nerves are susceptible to irritation because of the friction of the contracting muscles through which they travel. Excessive running or jumping creates vigorous flexion, compressing the nerves. The common peroneal nerve is susceptible to trauma because it is exposed at the neck of the fibula. Impact injuries from falls or kicks, as in soccer, can injure the nerve. Irritation of this nerve can cause a sharp, local pain, numbing, or tingling that starts at the fibular head and travels down the lateral leg to the dorsum of the foot. Irritation of the saphenous nerve can create anterior and medial knee pain, numbing, or tingling.
- *Treatment*: Treat peripheral nerves, as with all other body areas, by stroking transverse to the nerve line. These are gentle scooping strokes, not transverse friction strokes.

Muscles

- *Structure*: The muscles that move the knee are located in the thigh and in the leg. The thigh muscles that move the knee can be divided into the anterior and posterior groups. The **anterior muscle group** extends the knee and includes the sartorius and the four muscles of the quadriceps, which are the rectus femoris, vastus lateralis, intermedius, and medialis (see Fig. 7-9, p. 252). The **posterior group** consists of knee flexors and medial and lateral rotators of the tibia. It includes the three hamstrings (biceps femoris, semimembranosus and semitendinosus) and popliteus and gastrocnemius (See Fig. 7-12). The muscles may also be classified by location into the medial and lateral compartments. The **medial compartment** includes the medial head of the gastrocnemius; the sartorius, gracilis, and semitendinosus tendons, collectively called the **pes anserinus;** the semimembranosus and the quadriceps retinaculum from the vastus medialis (see Fig. 8-9). The pes anserinus muscles are the longest muscles in the anterior, medial, and posterior regions and act like a tripod to stabilize the knee. The **lateral compartment** includes the ITB, biceps femoris, popliteus, and quadriceps expansion from the vastus lateralis (Fig. 8-10).
- *Function*: Muscles and their fascial expansions are the **dynamic stabilizers** of the knee. The hamstrings cross two joints and not only flex the knee but rotate the tibia and pelvis. The semimembranosus muscle attaches to the medial meniscus and retracts it during knee flexion.
- *Dysfunction and injury:* Muscle injury has two categories: acute trauma and cumulative stress. As with the hip, the most commonly injured knee muscles are the two-joint muscles, especially the quadriceps and the hamstrings. One of the main functions of these muscles is eccentric contraction (i.e., to contract while the muscle is lengthening), during which muscles are much more prone to injury. The quadriceps must eccentrically contract to decelerate the hip and knee, and the hamstrings eccentrically contract as the knee comes to full extension at heel

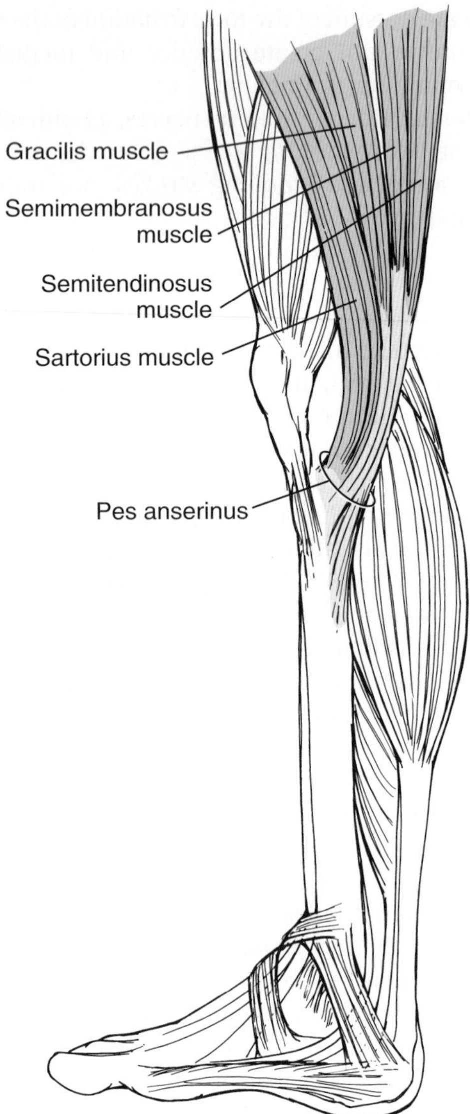

Figure 8-9. Muscles and fascia of the medial knee. The tendons of the sartorius, gracilis, and semitendinosus interweave at their insertion to form the pes anserinus ("goose's foot").

strike.[7] The ITB is often irritated due to repetitive friction of the ITB against the lateral femoral condyle.

Muscle dysfunction has two categories, muscle imbalance and positional dysfunction. Muscle imbalance describes a condition in which certain muscles are weak, and others are short and tight. Muscle imbalance alters movement patterns and therefore add a continuing stress to the joint system.

Muscle Imbalances of the Knee

- **Muscles that tend to be tight and short:** Iliopsoas, TFL and the ITB, RF, quadratus lumborum, pectineus, gracilis, adductors, hamstrings (biceps femoris more than semitendinosus or semimembranosus), soleus and gastrocnemius (plantar flexors of the ankle), piriformis, and other external rotators of the hip.
- **Muscles that tend to be weak (inhibited):** Gluteus maximus; hip abductors; hip internal rotators (gluteus minimus and medius); vastus lateralis; intermedius, especially the VMO; dorsiflexors of the ankle, especially the tibialis anterior.
  - The adductors are typically short and tight, but they are often weak because of the phenomenon of tightness weakness in which a muscle

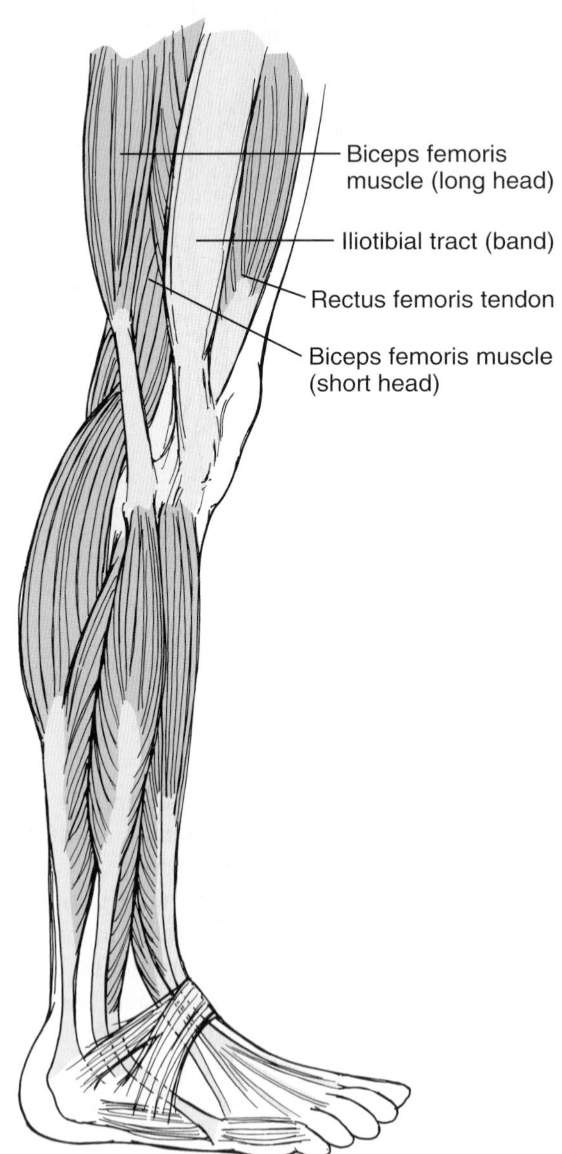

Figure 8-10. Muscles and fascia of the lateral knee.

that is habitually in its shortened position is weak (see Ch. 2). The VMO attaches to the adductor magnus; it is important to facilitate the adductors to create a stable base from which the VMO contracts.[8]

Positional Dysfunction of Knee Muscles

- Gracilis, sartorius, and semitendinosus (pes anserinus tendons) at their attachments on the tibia tend to roll into a posterior torsion along with the MCL.
- ITB at the knee tends to roll into a posterior torsion along with the LCL.
- Hamstrings, gastrocnemius, and soleus tend to shorten and roll toward the midline.

The classic postural dysfunction of the lower extremity is a genu valgus deformity, with an internally rotated femur, externally rotated tibia, pronated ankles, and the patella sitting laterally on the femur. This is a collapsed position and expresses gravity's toll on the body.

Anatomy of the Knee Muscles

See Muscle Table 8.1.

Muscular Actions of the Knee

See Table 8.2.

Knee Dysfunction and Injury

FACTORS PREDISPOSING TO KNEE PAIN

- Abnormal position of the patella
- Instability caused by weakness in the static or dynamic stabilizers
- Muscle imbalances (tight flexors, including the hamstrings, ITB, and gastrocnemius; and weak extensors, especially the VMO)
- Altered gait
- Soft-tissue fibrosis (adhesions), especially in the joint capsule or lateral retinaculum
- Abnormal alignment, including knock-knees (genu valgus), bow legs (genu varus), or hyperextended knees (genu recurvatum)
- Femoral anteversion
- Internal tibial torsion
- Pronation or an unstable ankle
- Rigid foot, which decreases shock-absorbing capacity[8]
- Immobilization, previous surgery
- Recent change in exercise. A change of more than 10% in an exercise routine is associated with greater injuries[10]
- Fatigue. Most knee injuries happen at the end of the day, at the end of a performance, at the end of a ski run, etc.
- Previous injury

DIFFERENTIATION OF KNEE PAIN

- It is important to realize that knee pain can come from structures other than the neuromusculoskeletal system. See the section "Contraindications to Massage Therapy: Red Flags" in Chapter 2, "Assessments & Technique" for guidelines on when massage is contraindicated and when referral is necessary. Assuming that knee pain is not pathological, differentiation may be categorized according to structures involved.
- The knee joint is innervated from L3 to S2 nerves, and pain in the knee area may be referred from irritation of the nerve roots from the lumbosacral spine. Typically, the pain is described as a deep ache, numbing, or tingling in the anterior or medial knee. The straight–leg-raising (SLR) test or passive hip extension increases the pain with nerve root involvement (See Chapters 3, "Lumbosacral Spine," and 7, "The Hip" for those tests.)
- The hip and the knee joints have common innervation, and knee pain may be referred from the hip. Painful, decreased passive flexion and medial rotation of the hip suggests hip degenerative joint disease (DJD).
- Myofascial pain of acute onset is described as a sharp, localized pain that is often associated with swelling, heat, and redness. It is increased with isometric contraction, performed during CR MET, and is better with rest.
- Acute knee pain is typically the result of trauma. The most commonly injured structures are the ACL and the MCL or the medial meniscus. With a severe injury, the knee swells immediately. With a less severe injury the swelling takes 6 to12 hours.[4] The pain is typically localized at the medial joint line, and usually the client is unable to straighten the knee fully.
- Chronic pain caused by degeneration is usually diffuse. Outside of injury, the most common area of

TABLE 8-1 ANATOMY OF THE KNEE MUSCLES

Quadriceps

Muscle	*Origin*	*Insertion*
Rectus femoris (the only quadriceps that crosses two joints)	Arises by two tendinous heads—a straight head from the anterior inferior iliac spine and a reflected head that arises from a groove above the acetabulum and from the fibrous capsule of the hip.	Ends in a broad, thick aponeurosis and flattened tendon attached to the upper surface of the patella; central, superficial part of the quadriceps tendon.
Vastus lateralis	From the lateral surface of the greater trochanter and the lateral lip of the linea aspera.	Quadriceps tendon, which forms the lateral patellar retinaculum attaching to the lateral pole of the patella and the tibial tuberosity.
Vastus intermedius	Anterior and lateral surfaces of the femur shaft.	Quadriceps tendon; it covers the articular muscle of the knee (genu articularis), which inserts into the capsule of the knee.
Vastus medialis	Medial aspect of the linea aspera and intertrochanteric line.	Quadriceps tendon, forming the medial patellar retinaculum; consists of two parts, separated by a fascial plane: the vastus medialis longus and the VMO; whereas the fibers of the longus portion are directed vertically, the fibers of the oblique portion are directed almost horizontally.
Popliteus	On the posterior aspect of the lateral femoral condyle and the lateral meniscus.	Attaches to the medial portion of the tibia.

See also Hamstrings, sartorius, and gracilis in Chapter 7 and the gastrocnemius and plantaris in Chapter 9.

pain is the anterior knee, usually as a result of tracking disorders of the patellofemoral joint. The pain arises or is worsened with prolonged sitting or going down stairs. In chronic knee dysfunction, the knee may buckle or give way, indicating joint instability. This instability is caused by loose ligaments, muscle inhibition, or a torn meniscus. In the elderly, complaints of stiffness and diffuse pain implicate osteoarthritis.

- Many older patients report that they have been told that their knee pain is just caused by getting older, when in fact in most of those patients, the pain is in one knee only—obviously their other knee is just as old. The pain is often caused by a previous injury or cumulative stress that resulted in imbalances in knee alignment and function. Proper alignment of the pelvis, feet, and ankles is critical to healthy knees.

COMMON TYPES OF KNEE DYSFUNCTION AND INJURY

Medial Collateral Ligament Sprain

- *Cause:* The most common injury is a blow to the lateral knee when the foot is planted. The MCL is the primary stabilizer to valgus stress.
- *Symptoms:* MCL sprain is the most common ligament disorder in the body. It usually accompanies a history of trauma, leading to well-localized pain at the medial or posteromedial knee. With chronic MCL injuries, clients may experience an ache or a feeling of the ligament giving way during exertion.
- *Sign:* Pain at the medial knee on valgus stress test at 30° of knee flexion is a sign of MCL sprain.
- *Site:* MCL sprains occur at three sites. The ligament may tear at the femoral or the tibial insertions or at

Action	*Dysfunction*
Extends the leg and assists in flexion of the hip.	RF is tight and short, contributing to an anterior pelvic tilt. Tightness of the RF and the other hip flexors inhibits the gluteus max. Vasti are weak, inhibited by hamstring tightness. The weakness causes difficulty in climbing stairs and in getting up and down from a seated position.[9] The VMO is the only primary dynamic stabilizer of the medial patella and is weak, allowing lateral displacement of the patella, called patellar tracking dysfunction.
Medially rotates the tibia on the femur when the foot is not fixed (open kinetic chain) and laterally rotates the femur on the tibia in a closed kinetic chain; assists the posterior movement of the meniscus in knee flexion.	

the joint line in the ligament midbody, developing interbody adhesions, or adhesions to the femur or tibia.

- *Treatment:* Perform transverse release of the ligament. Gentle, pain-free, transverse strokes to an acute injury help realign the healing fibers. Deep transverse friction strokes on a chronic MCL injury help dissolve adhesions.

Lateral Collateral Ligament Sprain

- *Cause:* Typically, a blow to the medial knee causes LCL sprain, which is much less common than MCL injuries.
- *Symptoms:* LCL sprains usually involve a history of trauma, leading to well-localized pain at the lateral knee. With chronic LCL sprains, clients may experience an ache or a feeling of the ligament giving way during exertion.
- *Sign:* Pain at ligament on varus stress test at 30° of knee flexion is a sign of LCL sprain.
- *Sites:* LCL sprains occur at the femoral or fibular attachments or at the joint line.
- *Treatment:* Perform transverse release of the LCL. See MCL treatment.

Anterior Cruciate Ligament Lesion

- *Cause:* An ACL injury usually results from a twisting motion combined with hyperextension and a varus or a valgus stress.[7]
- *Symptoms:* Pain and swelling in the anterior knee are symptoms of ACL lesion. With chronic ACL lesions, clients experience a feeling of the knee giving way.
- *Sign:* A positive anterior drawer test is a sign of an ACL lesion.

TABLE 8-2 KNEE MUSCULAR ACTIONS

Twelve muscles contribute to knee flexion and extension and to leg rotation.

- Flexion
  - Semimembranosus
  - Semitendinosus
  - Biceps femoris
  - Gracilis
  - Sartorius
  - Popliteus—also medially rotates the lower leg
  - Gastrocnemius—also plantar flexes the ankle
  - Plantaris—also plantar flexes the ankle
- Extension
  - RF
  - Vastus medialis
  - Vastus intermedius
  - Vastus lateralis
- Lower Leg Rotation
- Medial Rotation
  - Semimembranosus
  - Gracilis
  - Popliteus
  - Semitendinosus
  - Sartorius
- Lateral Rotation
  - Biceps femoris

- *Sites:* ACL injuries occur at the tibial or femoral attachments internal to the knee.
- *Treatment:* Maintain good functional balance between flexors and extensors of the knee. Treatment usually involves release of the ITB and facilitation (strengthening) of the VMO.

Posterior Cruciate Ligament Sprain

- *Cause:* PCL strain can be caused by vigorous whip kick in the breaststroke ("breast stroker's knee") or by a direct blow to a flexed knee.
- *Symptoms:* Clients experience pain and swelling around the knee. With chronic PCL strain, clients experience a feeling of the knee giving way.
- *Sign:* A positive posterior sag test is a sign of PCL strain.
- *Sites:* PCL strain occurs at the tibial or the femoral attachments internal to the knee.
- *Treatment:* Maintain good functional balance between flexors and extensors of the knee. Treatment usually involves release of the ITB and facilitation (strengthening) of the VMO.

Coronary (Meniscotibial) Ligament Sprain

- *Cause:* Repetitive twisting, such as when playing tennis or dancing, or prolonged walking downhill can cause coronary ligament sprain.
- *Symptoms:* Clients experience well-localized pain, usually medially at the tibial plateau.
- *Sign:* Pain at the medial tibial plateau to palpation, pain with full passive flexion of the knee, during the anterior drawer test, or passive lateral rotation are signs of meniscotibial ligament sprain.
- *Treatment:* Perform transverse massage to the ligament with the strokes directed down onto the tibial plateau.

Joint Capsule Fibrosis

- *Cause:* Any inflammatory condition, whether it is caused by a chronic microinflammatory environment as a result of chronic irritation or by a frank inflammation with the usual signs of redness, heat, and swelling can result in capsular fibrosis.
- *Symptoms:* Clients experience pain on either side of the superior portion of the patella after exertion. The knee feels stiff, especially after the client sits for long periods.
- *Sign:* The palpation of a thickened, tender tissue at the sites described above is a sign of joint capsule fibrosis.
- *Treatment:* Perform MET to increase knee flexion by lengthening the joint capsule, and perform OM to the capsule, which broadens the fibers and helps dissolve the adhesions within the substance of the capsule and between the bone.

Quadriceps Tendinitis at the Knee

- *Causes:* Repetitive or excessive running, dancing, or hiking are causes of quadriceps tendinitis at the knee.
- *Symptoms:* Clients experience pain on the front of the knee after exertion. This pain is well localized to one of three common sites: (1) tenoperiosteal insertion at the superior portion of patella; (2) infrapatellar tendon (jumper's knee); (3) medial and lateral quadriceps expansion (patellar retinaculum).
- *Signs:* Pain on resisted knee extension at site of injury; possible pain on full passive knee flexion are signs of quadriceps tendinitis at the knee.
- *Treatment:* Perform MET to reduce hypertonicity, to lengthen shortened connective tissue, or to facilitate

weakness, and perform OM to release adhesions in the soft tissue.

Hamstrings Tendinitis at the Knee

- *Causes:* Hamstrings tendinitis at the knee is common in runners and is associated with pronation of the ankles and anteverted hips. The hamstrings eccentrically contract as the knee comes to full extension at heel strike, making it vulnerable to injury.
- *Symptoms:* With biceps femoris injury, clients experience pain at the posterolateral aspect of the knee at the tenoperiosteal insertion at the fibular head. With semimembranosus involvement, clients experience pain at posteromedial surface of the tibia.
- *Signs:* With hamstrings tendinitis at the knee, clients exhibit the following signs: for biceps femoris injury, pain elicited on resisted knee flexion when performed with lateral rotation of the thigh and leg, and for semimembranosus involvement, pain elicited on resisted knee flexion with medial rotation of thigh and leg.
- *Treatment:* For acute conditions, perform CR MET or reciprocal inhibition (RI) on the hamstrings by contracting the quadriceps, and for chronic conditions, perform CR-antagonist-contract (CRAC) MET to lengthen the muscles and then OM to release the muscles.

Arthritis of the Knee

- *Causes:* Arthritis of the knee results from cumulative trauma or from the sequela of a specific traumatic event, such as a fall on the knee or injury to the ACL, MCL, etc.
- *Symptoms:* Clients experience a dull ache that increases with activity and stiffness in the morning and after long periods of sitting.
- *Sign:* A decrease in passive flexion with capsular or hard end feel is a sign of arthritis of the knee.
- *Treatment:* Perform MET to increase knee flexion and OM to release the joint capsule.

Plica Syndrome

- *Causes:* The plica is a vestigial remnant of the synovial lining and is normally found in approximately 60% of the population.[11] Repetitive stress to the anteromedial knee, such as prolonged running, biking, etc., can cause a friction irritation.
- *Symptoms:* Clients experience pain approximately 1 inch proximal to the inferior pole of the medial patella.
- *Signs:* The presence of a cordlike structure medial to the patella and revealed with palpation is a sign of plica syndrome.
- *Treatment:* Perform OM to release the fibrosis in the area of the capsule near the plica.

Popliteus Tendinitis or Tenosynovitis

- *Causes:* Popliteus tendinitis is often associated with pronated ankles and excessive running or hiking.
- *Symptoms:* Clients experience pain at the posterolateral corner of the knee at the femoral attachment, especially after walking or running downhill or sitting cross-legged.
- *Signs:* Pain with resisted medial rotation of the tibia with knee flexed 20° and pain at the posterior aspect of the knee with passive knee flexion are signs of popliteus tenosynovitis.
- *Site:* Tenosynovitis or tendinitis occurs in the belly, centrally in the popliteal space, or at posterolateral femur at the tenoperiosteal junction.
- *Treatment:* Perform MET to release a sustained contracture in the muscle or to facilitate an inhibited muscle. Perform OM to release any adhesions in the muscle.

Iliotibial Band Syndrome

- *Cause:* Repetitive friction of the ITB against the lateral femoral condyle, which is common in cyclists and runners.
- *Symptoms:* Clients experience pain at the lateral aspect of the knee at the lateral femoral condyle.
- *Sign:* Pain reproduced while the client extends the knee from 90° flexion to approximately 30° flexion at lateral femoral condyle.
- *Treatment:* Perform MET for the TFL and ITB (see Chapter 7). Perform OM to release the ITB and the associated fascia of the lateral knee.

Bursitis

- *Cause:* Repetitive contraction of the muscles of the respective bursae irritate the bursae and causes swelling and pain. The prepatellar bursa is irritated with prolonged kneeling or from a direct blow to the anterior knee. Any swelling in the joint may cause a swelling of the semimembranosus and gastrocnemius bursae. If chronic, the bursae may dry out because of lack of movement to the painful area and develop adhesions within the bursae.

- *Symptoms:* Clients experience local swelling and achy, throbbing, burning pain. There are three common areas of knee involvement (see Signs).
- *Signs:* With bursitis, signs are particular to the area involved.
  - **Prepatellar ("housemaid's knee"):** Swelling superficial to the patella.
  - **Pes Anserinus:** Lies between the tibial collateral ligament and the tendinous insertions of gracilis, sartorius, and semitendinosus; well-localized swelling approximately 2 inches below medial joint line.
  - **Semimembranosus ("Baker's cyst"):** Swelling in the posterior knee; lies between medial head of gastrocnemius and semimembranosus tendon; best seen with knee in extension.
- *Treatment:* The bursae of the body respond to lymphatic massage, which is part of the OM protocol.

Patellar Tracking Dysfunction (Patellofemoral Joint Dysfunction)

- *Cause:* Anteversion of the femur, external tibial torsion, pronation, weakness of the VMO, and tightness of the ITB create a bowstring effect, pulling the patella laterally.
- *Symptoms:* Clients experience anterior knee pain and pain behind the patella, especially after prolonged sitting or going down stairs, and cracking and popping noises (crepitation).
- *Signs:* Pain behind the patella on resisted knee extension and while performing the squat test and pain on patellar compression, weak VMO, tight ITB, and fibrosis of the lateral patellar retinaculum to palpation are signs of patellar tracking dysfunction.
- *Treatment:* Perform postisometric relaxation (PIR) MET for the TFL and ITB. Facilitate the VMO, and perform manual release of the ITB and the soft tissue of the lateral knee.

Chondromalacia Patella

- *Cause:* Chondromalacia patella is usually the result of a fall onto the flexed knee, creating inflammation and releasing enzymes that cause a softening of the hyaline cartilage of the patella, with loosening of the fiber matrix (fibrillation), and consequent calcium deposits. This condition often leads to arthrosis of the patellofemoral joint.
- *Symptoms:* Clients experience a deep-seated ache under the patella, especially going up and down stairs or after sitting for long periods.
- *Sign:* Pain reproduced by compressing the patella against the femur, called the patellar grinding test.
- *Treatment:* Perform MET to release quadriceps hypertonicity, and perform OM to release any fibrosis in the patellar retinaculum. Perform conservative mobilization of the patella.

Menisci Dysfunctions and Injuries

- *Cause:* Twisting on a weight-bearing leg is a frequent cause of menisci dysfunction and injury.
- *Symptoms:* Clients experience an acute tear that involves a sudden onset of pain that is usually severe, "somewhere inside the knee." If chronic, clients usually have a history of knee locking and of a painful snapping or catching sensation inside the knee. Or clients have a history of the knee suddenly giving way.
- *Signs:* Loss of normal knee movement, usually lost at the end range of either full flexion or full extension, and an inability to extend the knee fully.
- *Treatment:* Perform pain-free, figure-eight mobilization of the knee.

Saphenous Nerve Entrapment

- *Causes:* Excessive knee extensions and contracted adductors.
- *Symptoms:* Clients experience medial and anterior knee pain, and pressure over the adductor canal may radiate pain to the medial knee and down to the ankle.
- *Sign:* Medial knee pain with digital compression in adductor canal area.
- *Treatment:* Perform OM stroking transverse to the nerve at the medial thigh and knee.

Entrapment of the Common Peroneal Nerve at the Fibula

- *Causes:* Entrapment of the common peroneal nerve at the fibula is caused by repetitive running or jumping, especially if there is foot inversion with plantar flexion, because the nerve passes through an arcade or opening in the fibers of the peroneus longus. The nerve is also susceptible to direct trauma from impact to the nerve as it travels around the fibular head.[11]
- *Symptoms:* Clients experience sharp, localized pain, numbing, or tingling at the lateral fibular head. This pain radiates distally down the lateral leg and creates pain on the dorsum of the foot. Loss of dorsi-

flexion and eversion of the foot and dorsiflexion of the toes occur, resulting in "foot drop." Also, clients experience a usually temporary loss of sensation over the dorsum of the foot.

- *Sign:* Pain reproduced by digital stroking of the nerve at the fibula and a positive SLR with the foot inverted and plantar flexed, are signs of this type of nerve entrapment.
- *Treatment:* Perform transverse release of the nerve at the posterolateral fibular head and medial to the bicipital tendon in the popliteal space.

Knee Assessment

HISTORY QUESTION FOR THE CLIENT WHO HAS KNEE PAIN

- Have you had an injury recently?

The first task for the therapist is to differentiate acute from chronic problems. In acute problems your intention is to reduce muscle spasms, increase the joint ROM, and stimulate normal muscle firing in cases in which the muscle may be inhibited. For the client who has chronic knee pain or stiffness, your goal is to restore proper alignment and muscle function to reduce cumulative stresses to the knees. Carefully observe the alignment of the pelvis, hip, knees, ankles, and feet and assess the length of the ITB, hamstrings, adductors, and gastrocnemius and the strength of the VMO, TFL, and abductors.

OBSERVATION AND INSPECTION

Gait

- Observe the client walk around the treatment room. Indications that there may be a knee problem are a limp and an inability to straighten the knee at toe-off phase. Are the knees in a genu valgus or varus alignment in walking? Note if the ankles are pronated or supinated and whether the feet are inverted or everted.

Alignment (for Chronic Conditions Only)

- *Position:* Client is standing, facing the therapist, with the knees and ankles as close together as possible.
- *Action:* First observe the alignment of the knees, including the distance between the knees, and the facing of the patellae (Fig. 8-11). Place your thumb and index finger on one patella at a time to help determine the direction it faces. Next, ask the client to tighten the quadriceps to lift the knee cap, and observe the medial part of the distal thigh to see if the VMO contracts and creates a bulge just above and medial to the superior pole of the patella when it contracts.
- *Observation:* If the knees touch and the ankles do not, the client has genu valgum (knock-knees). If the ankles touch and there is more than two finger-widths between the knees at the joint line, the client has genu varum (bow legs). The facing of the patella is primarily dictated by the rotation in the femur. With the ankles and knees as close together as possible, the patella should face forward. With femoral anteversion, the femur is rotated internally and the patella faces inwardly ("squinting patella"). The VMO is often atrophied after a knee injury or chronic knee dysfunction, caused by an arthrokinetic re-

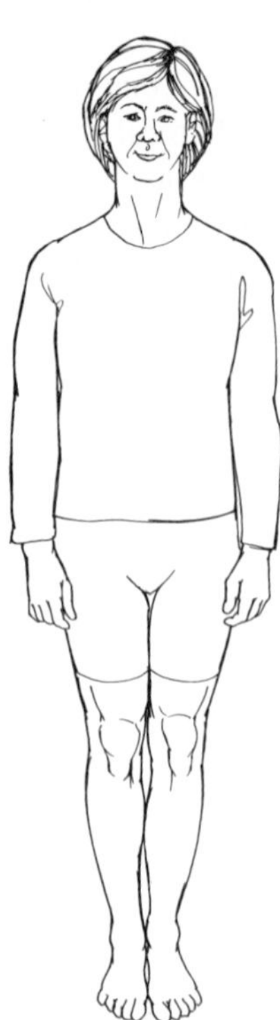

Figure 8-11. Observe the alignment of the knees by having the client bring the feet together. The patellae should point straightforward.

flex from irritation in the joint. Atrophy also occurs because of the loss of full extension for a time after an injury. As the VMO is a key muscle to terminal extension of the knee, it often atrophies after a knee injury.

Observation for Swelling

- *Position:* Client is sitting, with the knees over the edge of the table.
- *Action:* Observe for swelling.
- *Observation:* Check for the normal concavity at the anteromedial joint line that is obliterated with swelling.

ACTIVE MOVEMENTS

Extension

- *Position:* Client is sitting, with knees over the edge of the table.
- *Action:* Have the client extend the knee from the 90° flexed position (Fig. 8-12). Repeat extension as you place your hand on the patella.
- *Observation:* Observe and feel how the patella moves. Normally, the patella moves straight upward until the end of extension, when it is pulled slightly laterally. Lateral deviation early in knee extension indicates a patellar tracking dysfunction. Crepitus or pain in the anterior knee indicates patellofemoral joint degeneration. If there is a jump or jog in the patella as the client moves from flexion to extension, it indicates a potential mediopatellar plica. Loss of full extension often indicates a meniscal injury.

Squat Test (For Chronic Conditions Only)

- *Position:* Client is standing, with one hand on the table for support.
- *Action:* Have the client perform a squat to the comfortable limit and then come to standing again. Ask the client to keep his or her feet parallel and shoulder-width apart (Fig. 8-13).
- *Observation:* Observe the ROM and ask if there is any pain. This procedure is a quick screening test for chronic knee pain and stiffness. There is often pain behind the knee cap and crepitus with patellofemoral joint dysfunction and a loss of motion and pain with tibiofemoral joint problems.

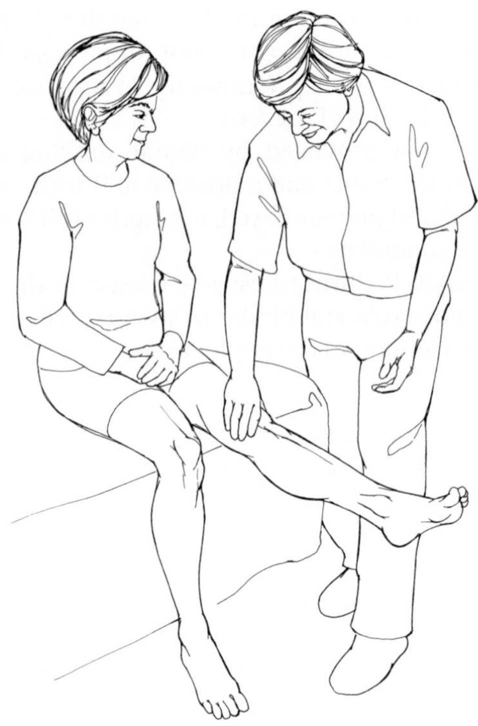

Figure 8-12. Active extension. First, observe the movement of the patella. Next, place one hand on the patella and have the client repeat knee extension. Feel for noise (crepitus) and whether the movement of the patella is smooth.

Flexion

- *Position:* Client is supine, with a pillow under the knee if condition is acute.
- *Action:* Have the client lift his or her thigh toward the chest, pulling the heel toward the buttock as far as possible (Fig. 8-14).
- *Observation:* The normal ROM is approximately 140°. There is a loss of flexion in acute and in chronic knee problems. In the acute knee, the loss of motion is caused by swelling, and in the chronic knee, it is caused by fibrosis of the joint capsule or loss of joint space resulting from cartilage degeneration.

PASSIVE MOVEMENTS

Flexion

- *Position:* Client is supine, with a pillow under the knee if the injury is acute.
- *Action:* First, bring the knee into flexion and place the foot on the table. Next, place one hand on the

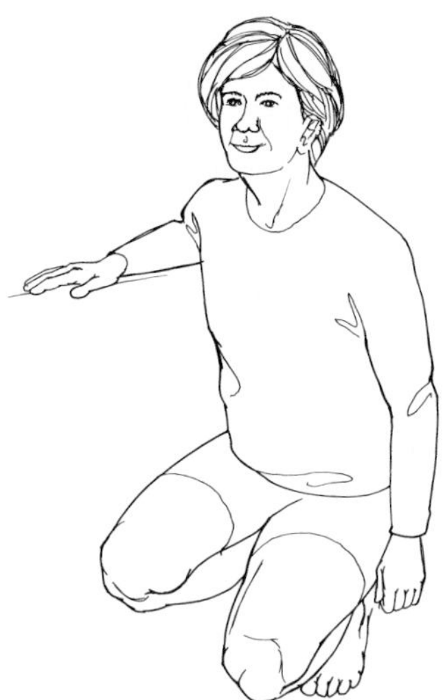

Figure 8-13. Squat test. This is for chronic conditions only.

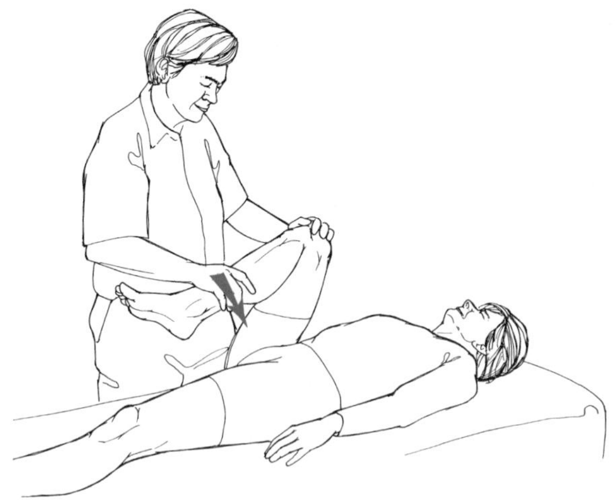

Figure 8-15. Passive flexion. The intention is to assess the ROM and the end feel, the quality of resistance at the end of the passive ROM.

knee and hold the distal leg with the other hand. Slowly bring the hip to 90° of flexion, with the hip in neutral and not internally or externally rotated. Slowly press the knee into the comfortable limit of flexion. If there is no pain, you may press further to assess the end feel (Fig. 8-15).

- ***Observation:*** The heel should touch the buttock with overpressure. Flexion is the first motion lost in capsular fibrosis (leathery end feel) and in degenerative joint problems (hard end feel). Acute injuries of the menisci or cruciates present with loss of full passive flexion with an empty end-feel. Tight quadriceps have a tissue stretch end-feel.

Extension

- ***Position:*** Client is supine.
- ***Action:*** Perform passive flexion (see Fig. 8-15), and then move your superior hand and place it behind the knee. Slowly lower the knee into extension. If you can achieve full painless extension, flex the knee approximately 10°, and let the knee fall into the last 10° of extension (Fig. 8-16).
- ***Observation:*** Normally, the knee has a solid, bony end feel if it drops into full passive extension. Loss of motion in passive extension is a key finding in meniscus injuries, although any acute injury to the knee causes a loss of full extension. An injury to the meniscus presents as a springy block to full extension.

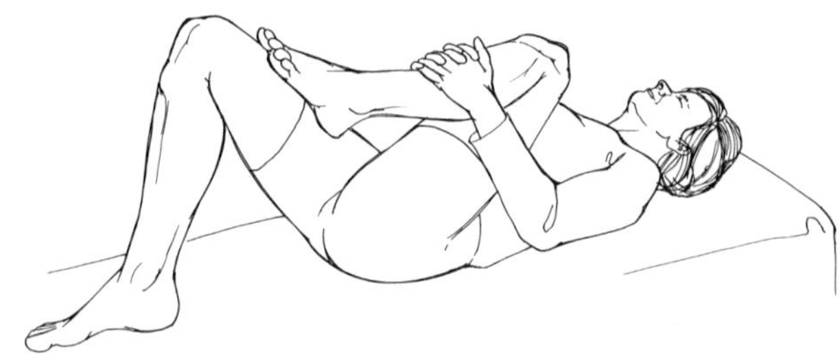

Figure 8-14. Active flexion. This test is for acute conditions to determine the knee ROM.

McMurray Test

- ***Intention:*** To assess the medial meniscus (Fig. 8-17).
- ***Position:*** Client is supine.

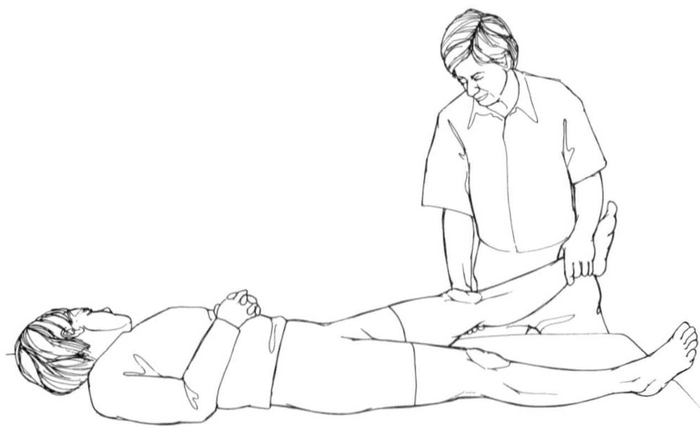

Figure 8-16. Passive extension. Loss of extension with pain and a springy-block end feel is often indicative of a meniscus injury.

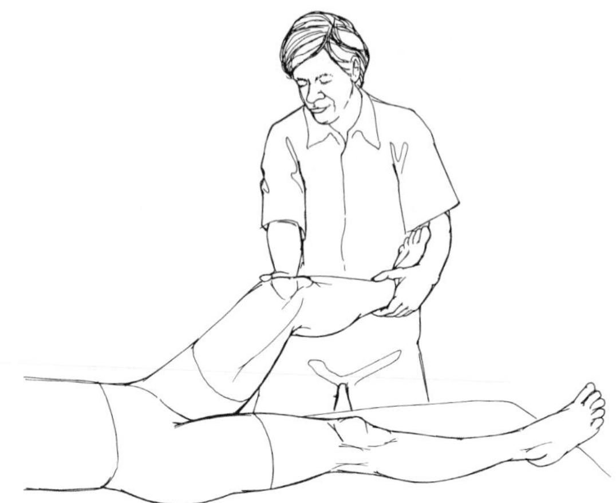

Figure 8-17. McMurray's test to assess the medial meniscus.

- ***Action:*** Place one hand over the knee and hold the distal leg with the other hand. Slowly flex the knee as far as possible; then exert a lateral to medial pressure on the knee (valgus stress) as you externally rotate the foot and tibia and extend the knee.
- ***Observation:*** This is a screening test for injuries to the medial meniscus. With a meniscus injury, the client may experience a painful pop or click along the joint line.

Valgus Stress Test

- ***Intention:*** To assess the MCL (Fig. 8-18).
- ***Position:*** Client is supine. Two positions are used to assess the MCL in flexion and then in extension. First, bring the knee into approximately 20° to 30° of flexion and place the client's leg in your axilla, with both of your hands around the knee. The second position is to keep the client's leg on the table, and place one hand on his or her lateral knee, with the other hand holding the medial ankle. Keep the hip in neutral; do not allow internal or external rotation.
- ***Action:*** Attempt to pull the lower leg laterally by rotating your body and pressing the outside of the knee with the superior hand. The same action is performed with the knee in full extension, whether with the client's leg in your axilla or resting on the table. Compare both sides.
- ***Observation:*** Pain at the medial knee typically indicates an MCL injury. An increased gapping compared with that of the uninjured knee indicates a tear of the MCL. There should be no gapping at all with the knee in full extension, as the PCL is stabilizing the knee in full extension. Any lateral movement in knee extension indicates a much worse injury.

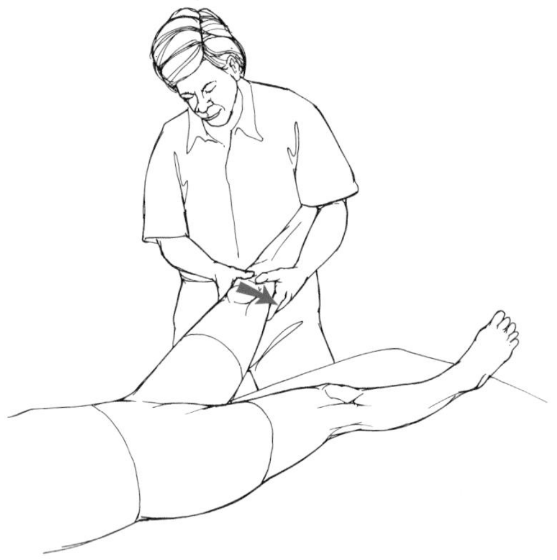

Figure 8-18. Valgus stress test to assess the MCL.

Posterior Sag Sign

- ***Intention:*** To assess the integrity of the PCL.
- ***Position:*** Client is supine, with the hip and knee flexed, feet on the table.
- ***Action:*** Observe from the side to see if the tibia drops posteriorly relative to the femur. Compare both sides.
- ***Observation:*** Normally, the tibia extends slightly anterior to the femoral condyles. If the tibia drops posteriorly relative to the femur, it indicates an injury to the PCL. It is important to perform this test prior to the anterior drawer test described in the next section, because if the tibia is sagging posteriorly, you may get a false-positive anterior drawer test.

Anterior Drawer Test

- ***Intention:*** To assess the ACL (Fig. 8-19).
- ***Position:*** Client is supine, feet on the table, with the hip flexed 45° and the knee flexed 90° and the tibia in neutral (i.e., with the feet pointed straight ahead). Therapist sits on the table, facing headward.
- ***Action:*** Stabilize the foot by sitting gently on the toes. Wrap both hands around the proximal tibia with your thumbs on either side of the infrapatellar tendon. Your fingers can sense if the hamstrings are relaxed, which is necessary for this test

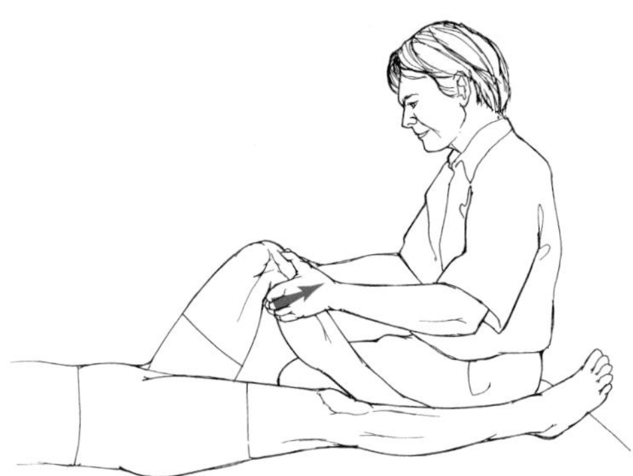

Figure 8-19. Anterior drawer test to assess the integrity of the ACL.

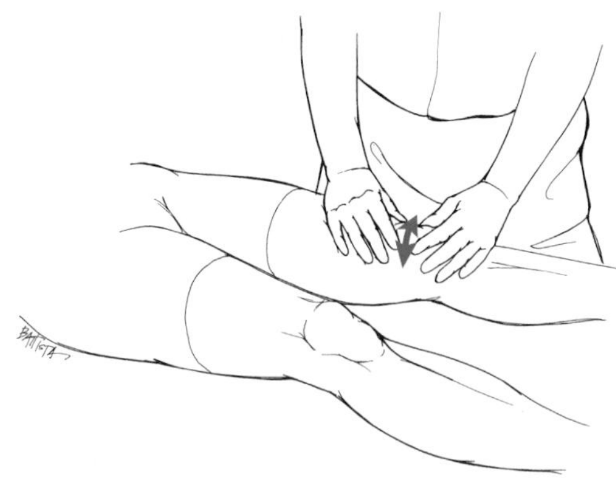

Figure 8-20. Patellar mobility test. Loss of patellar glide is a common clinical finding and is a sign of adhesions in the retinaculum.

to be accurate. Pull the tibia anteriorly. Repeat several times.

- *Observation:* Compare both sides. An increased movement of the tibia relative to the femur compared with that of the uninjured knee is one indication that there may be a tear in the ACL.

Patella Lateral Pull Test

- *Intention:* To assess patellar tracking dysfunction.
- *Position:* Client is supine, with knee extended.
- *Action:* Have the client contract the quadriceps.
- *Observation:* Normally, the patella moves straight headward (superiorly) in the initial phase of quadriceps contraction, or it moves superiorly and laterally in equal proportions. Patellar movement in a primarily lateral direction indicates patellofemoral dysfunction and typically a weakness of the VMO. A simple, yet effective, exercise to retrain the VMO is to have the client sit up with the legs on the table. Have him or her place an index finger on the superior-medial border of the patella. Instruct the client to contract the VMO by trying to press his or her index finger medially. Repeat 50 times a day until this action is recovered. It is also important to release the TFL and ITB, as they are typically tight and short.

Patellar Mobility Test

- *Intention:* To assess adhesions in the patellar retinaculum.
- *Position:* Client is supine, with the knee extended.
- *Action:* Hold the patella with your thumb and index finger, and move the patella medially and laterally and then proximally and distally (Fig. 8-20).
- *Observation:* The patella should move one-half the width of the patella medially to laterally; check for a decrease or an increase in movement. Be cautious pushing laterally. With a history of subluxation or dislocation, there may by apprehension, as nearly all dislocations are lateral.

Patellar Grinding Test

- *Intention:* To assess calcium depositions in the patellofemoral joint.
- *Position:* Client is supine, with the knee extended.
- *Action:* Stabilize the leg in neutral, so that the femur is not internally or externally rotated. Stabilize the patella with the thumb and index finger of your superior hand, and place the palm of the inferior hand over the patella. Press the patella into the femur, and move the patella superiorly and inferiorly several times to feel and listen for calcium deposits (Fig. 8-21).

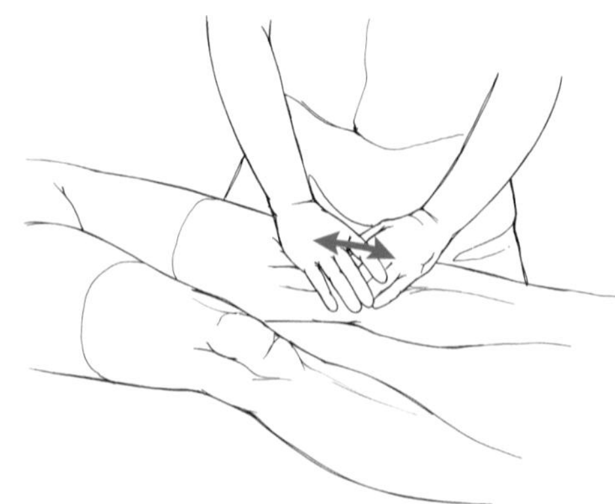

Figure 8-21. Patellar grinding test.

- Observation—Crepitation or pain suggests patellofemoral joint degeneration, also called chondromalacia patella.

PALPATION

- Most palpation for the massage therapist is done in the context of performing the strokes. However, before you begin your massage, feel for heat in the knee by placing your hands on the same areas on both knees to compare the temperature. Obviously, heat is an indication of inflammation and requires much less pressure in your strokes.

Techniques

MUSCLE ENERGY TECHNIQUE

MET and length assessment for the hamstrings and quadriceps were also addressed in Chapter 7.

Muscle Energy Techniques for Acute Pain

1. Contract-Relax Muscle Energy Technique for Acute Knee Injury

- *Intention:* The first intention is to attempt to increase flexion. If the knee is capable of weight bearing, you may perform gentle MET to help disperse the swelling, to increase the ROM, and to help normalize neurologic function.
- *Position:* Client is supine. Place one hand under the knee and the other hand at the ankle.
- *Action:* Gently flex the knee to its comfortable limit. If it is too painful to lift the foot off the table, place a pillow under the knee. Have the client resist as you use light pressure to attempt to flex the knee. Have the client relax; then slowly move the client's knee into greater flexion until it is painful or until you encounter the next resistance barrier. Remember, it should not be painful. Repeat several more times. Have the client relax; then gently flex and extend the client's knee in 1-inch movements to pump the excess fluid out. Next, have the client resist as you gently attempt to extend the knee. Alternate, performing resisted flexion and extension for several cycles. After each cycle, move the knee into greater flexion. Keep moving the knee to the end ranges of flexion and extension within comfortable limits (Fig. 8-22).

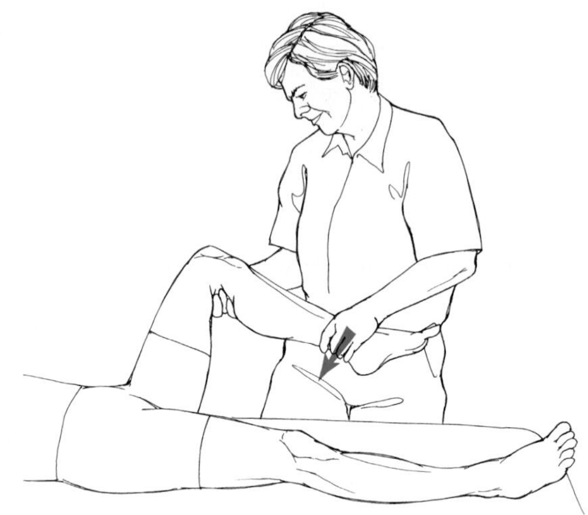

Figure 8-22. CR MET for acute knee injury.

Length Assessment and Muscle Energy Techniques for Hypertonicity

2. Length Assessment of the Gastrocnemius

- *Intention:* The gastrocnemius is typically short and tight.
- *Position:* Client is supine, with knee extended. Place one hand on the client's knee to keep it extended and the other hand on the ball of the foot.
- *Action:* Pull the ball of the foot toward client's head (Fig. 8-23).
- *Observation:* The normal length of these muscles should allow the foot to reach 90° (i.e., perpendicular to the leg).

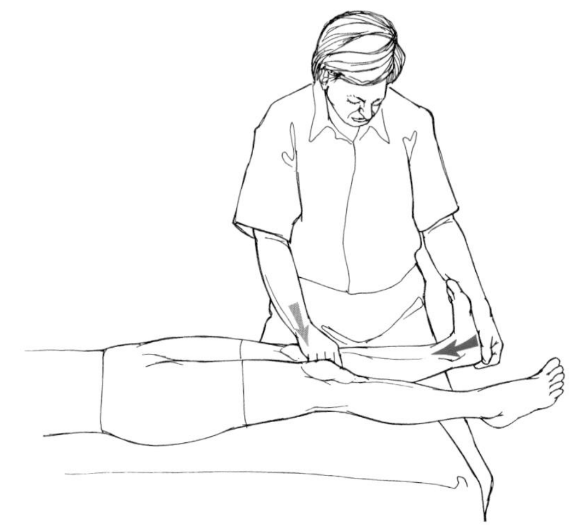

Figure 8-23. Length assessment of the gastrocnemius.

3. Contract-Relax-Antagonist-Contract Muscle Energy Technique for the Gastrocnemius

- ***Intention:*** As this muscle is usually short and tight, we typically want to lengthen it.
- ***Position:*** Client is supine, with the knee extended. Place one hand on the client's knee with the other hand holding the heel and the forearm resting on the ball of the foot.
- ***Action:*** Have the client pull the foot into dorsiflexion, relax in this position, and then resist as you attempt to pull the foot further into dorsiflexion. Hold for 5 seconds. Have the client relax and then move the foot headward. Repeat CR antagonist-contract (CRAC) cycle several times. Repeat on the other side (See Fig. 8-23).

4. Contract-Relax and Reciprocal Inhibition Muscle Energy Technique for the Hamstrings

- ***Intention:*** The position for this MET is easily incorporated into the massage sequence.
- ***Position:*** Client is prone. Place one hand on the client's hamstrings to stabilize the femur and for sensory cueing, the other hand holding the client's distal leg.
- ***Action:*** Flex client's knee to 50° to 70° and have the client resist as you attempt to extend the knee (i.e., pull the leg back to the table). Hold for 5 seconds and repeat several times. RI for the hamstrings is to have the client resist as you attempt to press the foot to the buttock. The knee should not be flexed more than 90°, as the leg may cramp. Stabilizing hand holds down posterior femur (Fig. 8-24).
- ***Variations:*** To emphasize the medial hamstrings, rotate the hip medially, dorsiflex the ankle to lock the foot to the ankle, and rotate the leg medially on the thigh by turning the foot medially. To emphasize biceps femoris, rotate the hip laterally and rotate the leg slightly by turning the foot laterally.

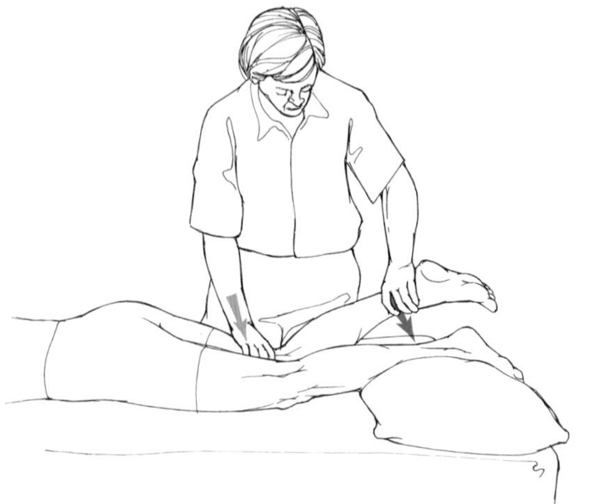

Figure 8-24. CR and RI MET for the hamstrings.

5. Postisometric Relaxation Muscle Energy Technique for the Hamstrings Lower Attachments

- ***Intention:*** This position is different from the MET shown in the chapter, "The Hip," in that it emphasizes the contraction at hamstrings attachments to the posterior knee.
- ***Position:*** Client is supine
- ***Action:*** Bring the hip to 90° of flexion, and slowly extend the knee to the tension barrier. Have the client resist as you attempt to push the knee into greater extension (i.e., by pushing at the foot for approximately 5 seconds). Relax, wait a few seconds, and while the client is relaxed, extend the knee to a new resistance barrier. Repeat the CR–lengthen cycle several times (Fig. 8-25).
- ***Observation:*** Normally, the range of knee extension is approximately 70° with the hip flexed to 90°.

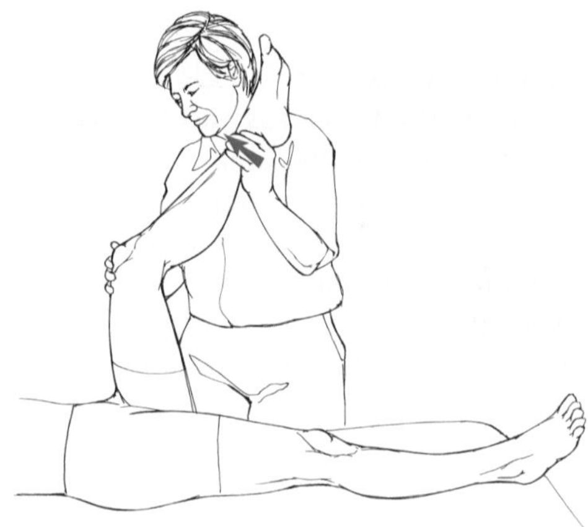

Figure 8-25. PIR MET for the hamstrings lower attachments.

6. Length Assessment (Ely's Test) and Postisometric Relaxation Muscle Energy Technique for the Quadriceps

- ***Intention:*** The intention is to assess passive flexion and restore normal passive flexion of the knee if the heel does not touch the buttock with overpressure.
- ***Position:*** Client is prone. Place one hand on the sacrum to stabilize it and the other hand on the ankle.
- ***Action:*** Do not allow medial or lateral rotation or abduction or adduction of the hip. If the client is hyperlordotic or has low-back discomfort, place a pillow under the abdomen to flex the lumbar spine. Flex the client's knee by pressing the foot toward the buttock until the resistance barrier is

felt. If heel does not touch the buttock, have the client resist as you attempt to press the heel further toward the buttock. Have the client relax, and as client relaxes, flex the knee until new resistance barrier is encountered. Have the client relax. Repeat this cycle several times (Fig. 8-26).

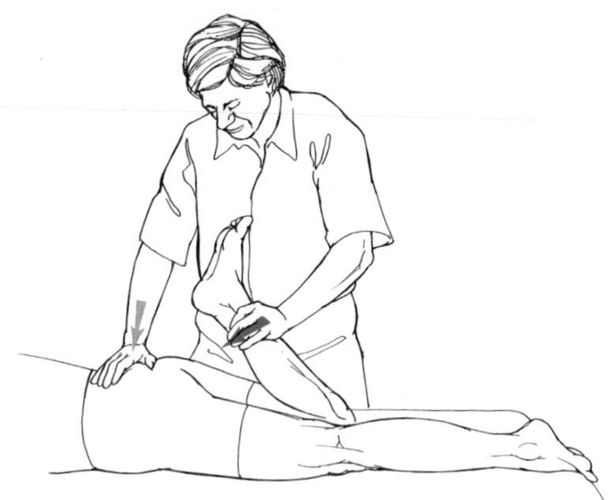

Figure 8-26. Length assessment (Ely's test) and PIR MET for the quadriceps.

7. Postisometric Relaxation Muscle Energy Technique for the Popliteus and to Increase External Rotation of the Tibia

- ☐ ***Intention:*** The intention is to help restore normal external rotation of the tibia. Normal knee extension requires external rotation of the tibia during the last 10° to 15°. A short or tight popliteus or a short posteromedial capsule often causes decreased external rotation. Resisted medial rotation helps release popliteus hypertonicity and increase tibial external rotation.
- ☐ ***Position:*** Client is prone, with the knee flexed approximately 20°. Place one hand on the back of the knee to stabilize it and the other hand on the medial arch of the foot.
- ☐ ***Action:*** To release the popliteus medially rotate the tibia by first dorsiflexing the ankle to lock the foot to the ankle and then by cocking the foot medially (toward the other leg). Have the client resist as you attempt to laterally rotate the tibia by pulling the foot laterally. Instruct the client to relax, and then move the client's tibia more laterally. Have the client relax. Repeat the cycle several times (Fig. 8-27).

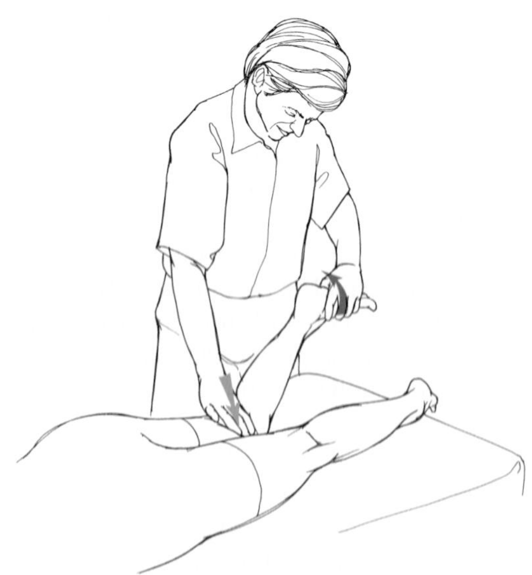

Figure 8-27. PIR MET for the popliteus and to increase external rotation of the tibia.

Muscle Energy Technique for Chronic Capsular Fibrosis and Loss of Knee Motion

8. Muscle Energy Technique to Increase Knee Flexion

- ☐ ***Intention:*** Chronic loss of flexion is a sign of capsular fibrosis or cartilage degeneration. The end feel of fibrosis is thick, leathery. Degeneration has a hard end feel.
- ☐ ***Position:*** Client is supine. Place one hand on the knee and the other hand on the distal leg.
- ☐ ***Action:*** Lift the client's leg to the comfortable limit of knee flexion. Have the client resist as you attempt to flex it further. Instruct the client to relax, and as the client relaxes, move the knee into greater flexion. Repeat several times (Fig. 8-28).
- ☐ ***Observation:*** When performing this MET, ensure that the client's hip is in neutral (i.e., no internal or external rotation, abduction, or adduction).

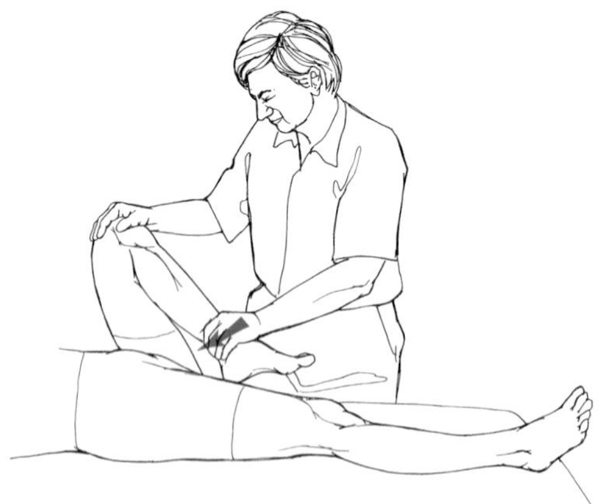

Figure 8-28. MET to increase knee flexion.

ORTHOPEDIC MASSAGE

Level 1—Knee

1. Transverse Release of the Distal Thigh

- *Anatomy*: Gracilis, sartorius, adductor magnus; saphenous nerve, quadriceps expansion of vastus medialis, intermedius, and lateralis; and suprapatellar tendon of the RF (Fig. 8-29).

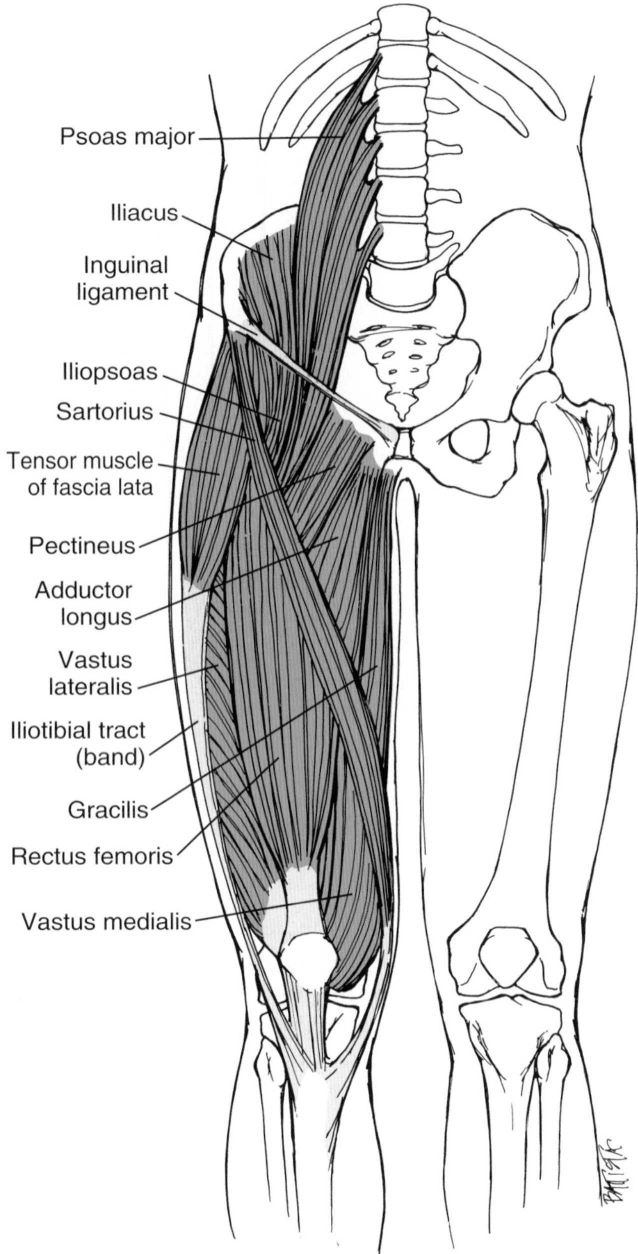

Figure 8-29. Muscles and fascia of the anterior thigh and knee.

- *Dysfunction*: The fascial expansions of the quadriceps can become fibrous because of previous inflammation as a result of a knee injury or because of chronic irritation caused by the cumulative stresses of weight-bearing dysfunctions, such as pronated ankles or genu valgus (knock-knees). The saphenous nerve can become entrapped in the area of the adductor canal in the distal third of the medial thigh. As mentioned in Chapter 7, "The Hip," if you are working with a client who has retroverted hips, you need to reverse the direction of your strokes and roll the thigh inward from the externally rotated position.

Position

- TP—standing, either 45° headward or facing table
- CP—supine; if the client has an acute knee injury, place a pillow under the knee

Strokes

1. Facing 45° headward, place the femur in neutral or in approximately 10° to 15° of external rotation. Hold the distal one-third of the thigh with both hands (Fig. 8-30). Your thumbs should be on the anterior thigh, and your fingertips are on the medial and lateral thigh. Perform short scooping strokes, in a medial to lateral direction, to unwind the entire soft tissue around the bone. These strokes are brisk, 1-inch strokes to release the adhesions in the soft tissue of the thigh and not to rotate the femur externally. You can brace the leg with your thigh to prevent it from rotating. Cover the entire distal thigh and continue to the patella.
2. Using the same hand positions, now focus attention on the fingertips of both hands for specific release of the medial and lateral thigh. Use the fingertips of both hands to perform two types of strokes. The first type of stroke is a 1-inch, scooping stroke. The fin-

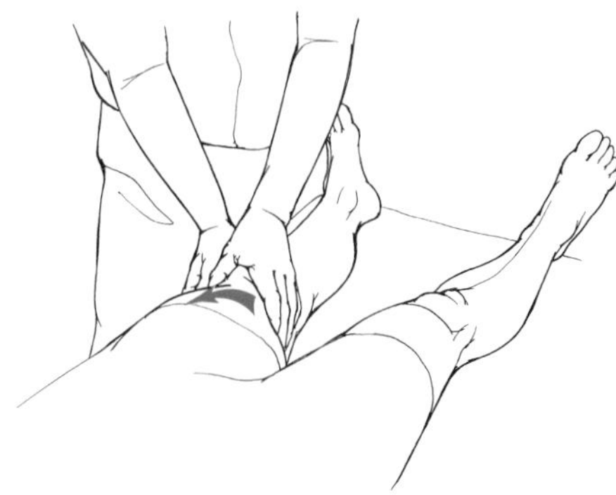

Figure 8-30. Transverse release of the distal thigh by unwinding the soft tissue around the bone in a medial to lateral direction.

gertips on the medial thigh are lifting anteriorly, while the fingertips on the lateral thigh are scooping posteriorly. The second type of stroke is a brisk, back-and-forth stroke in the anterior to posterior (A–P) plane with the hands moving in the opposite directions. Cover the area from the distal third of the thigh to the patella to release the saphenous nerve, vastus medialis, and quadriceps expansion on the medial side and the ITB, vastus lateralis, and lateral quadriceps expansion on the lateral side.

3. Using a double-thumb technique, perform brisk, back-and-forth strokes in the medial to lateral plane, on the suprapatellar tendon of the RF and the vastus intermedius underneath (Fig. 8-31). Begin approximately 6 inches above the patella and continue to the superior pole of the patella.

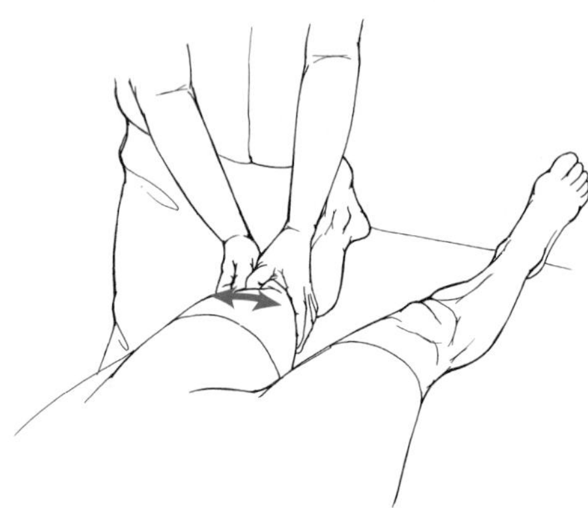

Figure 8-31. Double-thumb technique to release the suprapatellar tendon.

2. Lifting Medial Soft Tissue Anteriorly

- *Anatomy*: Vastus medialis and pes anserinus tendons, which are, from A–P, the sartorius, gracilis, and semitendinosus (Fig. 8-32).
- *Dysfunction*: This soft tissue tends to misalign posteriorly and needs to be lifted anteriorly. In most injuries and dysfunctions of the knee, there is an inability to extend the knee fully, thus keeping the soft tissue in a sustained posterior position relative to the joint. Adhesions can develop within the body of the muscles or between the soft tissue and the bone.

Position

- TP—standing, facing perpendicular to the table
- CP—supine, usually with the knee extended; if injury is acute, place a pillow under the knee

Strokes

The first intention is to reset the soft tissue from posterior to anterior; the second is to dissolve any fibrosis that may have developed in response to injury or overuse. The area of the medial knee is divided into three lines from A–P. Begin your strokes on the first line at the distal thigh a few inches proximal to the patella and proceed to the proximal tibia. The second line is approximately 1 inch posterior to the first line, and the third line is approximately 1 inch posterior to the second. Cover the entire medial knee.

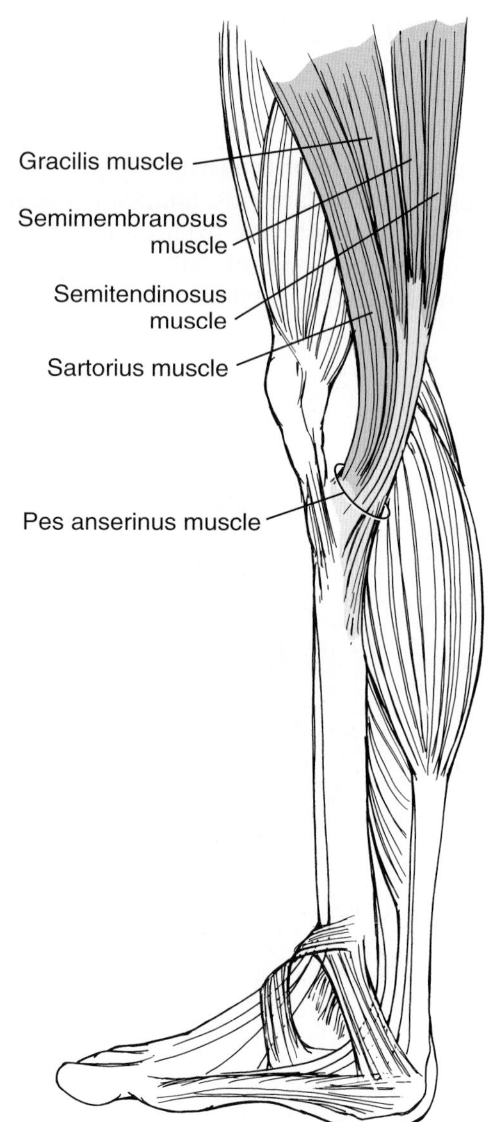

Figure 8-32. Muscles and fascia of the medial knee. The tendons of the sartorius, gracilis, and semitendinosus interweave at their insertion to form the pes anserinus ("goose's foot").

1. Use the fingertips of both hands to perform broad, 1-inch, scooping strokes in a posterior to anterior direction on the first line for the vastus medialis and medial retinaculum (Fig. 8-33). Begin at the distal thigh and continue to the proximal tibia. Stabilize the leg with your thumbs and the base of your

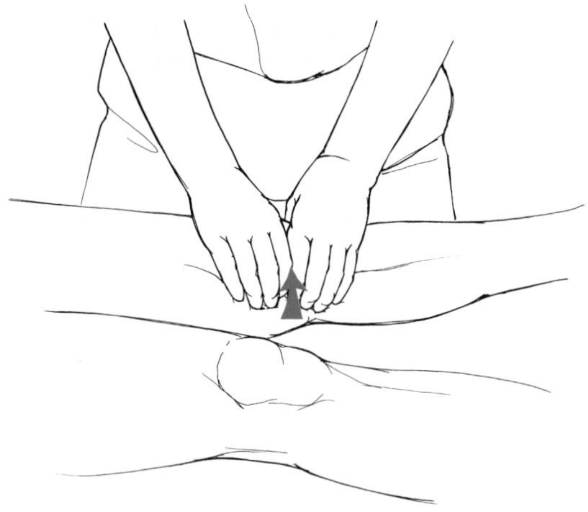

Figure 8-33. Lifting the soft tissue of the medial knee anteriorly.

hands to limit the amount of external rotation of the femur.

2. Perform the same series of strokes (as described in stroke 1) on the second line of the thigh, 1 inch posterior to the first line, for the sartorius. Begin your strokes at the distal thigh and continue to the proximal knee.
3. Perform the same strokes (as described in stroke 1) on the third line for the gracilis, semimembranosus, and semitendinosus.
4. To assist the realignment of the tissue mechanically, place the flexed knee of your superior leg on the table and by resting the client's leg on your thigh (Fig. 8-34). With your inferior hand holding the client's ankle, keep the leg in neutral, and lift the foot to extend the knee as you use the fingertips of your superior hand to lift the soft tissue anteriorly.

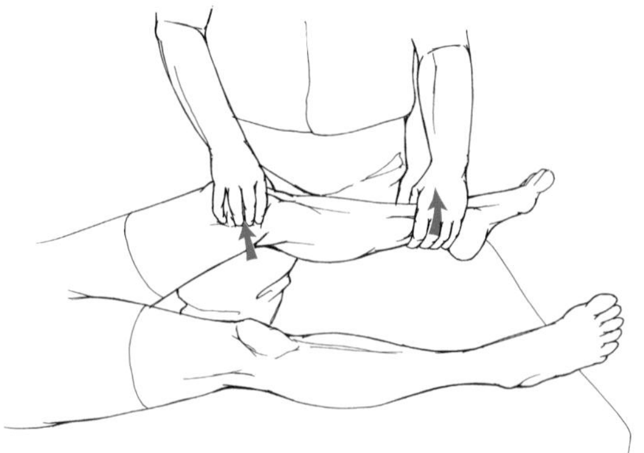

Figure 8-34. Using the fingertips of one hand to lift the soft tissue anteriorly; the other hand lifts the knee into extension with each stroke.

3. Lifting Lateral Soft Tissue Anteriorly

- *Anatomy*: ITB, vastus lateralis and lateral patellar retinaculum, and biceps femoris (Fig. 8-35).
- *Dysfunction*: As mentioned in the previous stroke, the soft tissue of the knee tends to misalign posteriorly. The ITB usually becomes taut, and the lateral retinaculum usually becomes thick, anchoring the lateral patella against the lateral femur. This condition may be as a response to a knee injury, because the VMO becomes inhibited and the vastus lateralis and ITB get short and tight. Or it may be in response to cumulative tension through weight distribution dysfunction, such as genu valgus and pronated ankles.

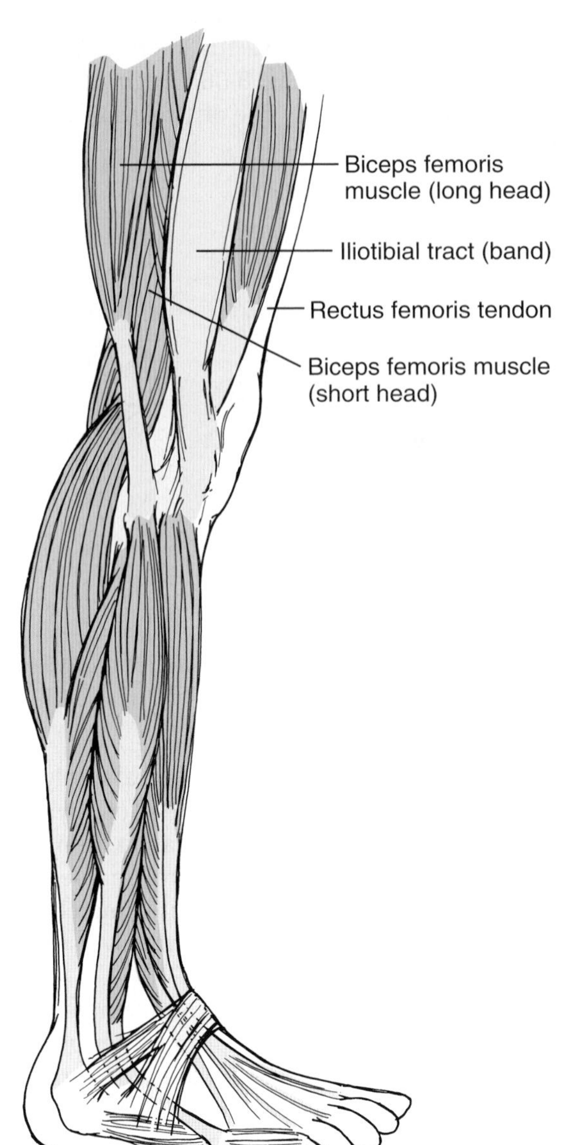

Figure 8-35. Muscles and fascia of the lateral knee.

Position

- TP—standing, facing the table
- CP—supine; place a pillow under an acute knee

Strokes

As in the previous stroke, divide the lateral knee into three lines from A–P. The first line is just lateral to the patella. Begin strokes on the first line at the distal thigh a few inches proximal to the patella and proceed to the proximal fibula. Roll the thigh into neutral if it is in external rotation, and stabilize it in neutral with the base of your hands. These strokes move the soft tissue relative to the bone, rather than externally or internally rotating the thigh or leg.

1. Facing the table and using both thumbs, perform short, scooping strokes from posterior to anterior on the first line for the vastus lateralis and lateral patellar retinaculum (Fig. 8-36). Begin at the distal thigh and continue this line of strokes to the proximal leg.

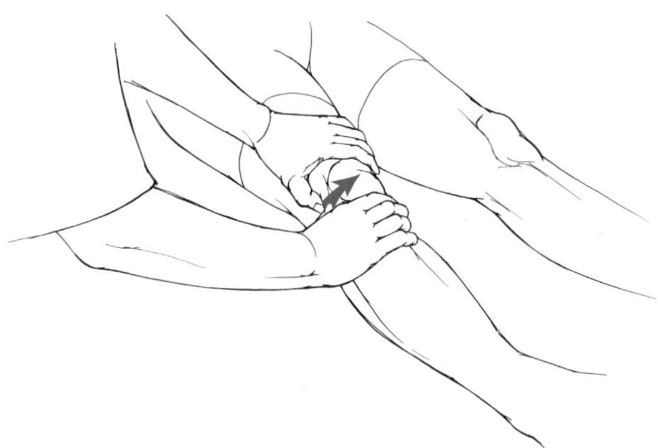

Figure 8-36. Double-thumb technique to lift the lateral soft tissue anteriorly.

2. Begin a second line of strokes approximately 1 inch posterior to the first line at the lateral condyle of the femur to release the ITB and the fascia from the ITB to the patella. Continue to the proximal leg. Begin with broad, scooping strokes approximately 1 inch long and proceed to more brisk, transverse strokes as you work closer to the bone.
3. Perform a third line of strokes approximately 1 inch posterior to the second line for the anterior portion of the biceps femoris and from the anterior ligament to the fibular head. As in the previous strokes, begin at the distal thigh and continue your strokes to fibular head and the proximal leg.
4. You can mechanically assist realigning the tissue by placing the flexed knee of your superior leg on the table and by resting the client's leg on your thigh (Fig. 8-37). With your inferior hand holding the client's ankle, keep his or her leg in neutral, and lift the foot to extend the knee, as you use the thumb of your superior hand to lift the soft tissue anteriorly.

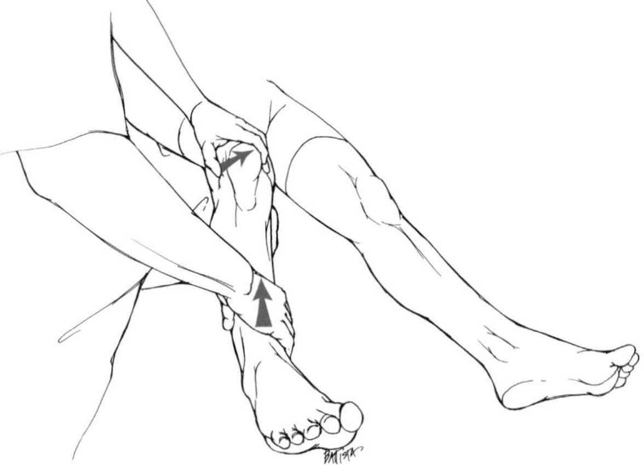

Figure 8-37. To mechanically assist the realigning of the soft tissue, lift the tissue with the thumb of one hand while the other hand lifts the knee into extension with each stroke.

4. Release of the Patellar Retinaculum

- *Anatomy*: The patellar retinacula, which is an expansion of the quadriceps fascia and the thickenings of the superficial joint capsule, attaches at four major points to the superior and inferior margins of the patella. If twelve o'clock is headward, the approximate points of attachment are at 2, 4, 8, and 10 o'clock. The retinacula also attaches to the under surface of the patella. (Fig. 8-38).
- *Dysfunction*: The quadriceps expansion often develops fibrosis at its attachment to the patella, constricting the normal glide of the patella and increasing the pressure of the patellofemoral joint. Typically, the lateral retinaculum is thickest.

Position

- TP—standing
- CP—supine; place a pillow under the knee if it has been injured

Strokes

1. Release the superior portion of the medial patella by facing the table and stabilizing the patella with your inferior hand. Perform back-and-forth strokes with the fingertips of your superior hand on the superior aspect of the medial side of the

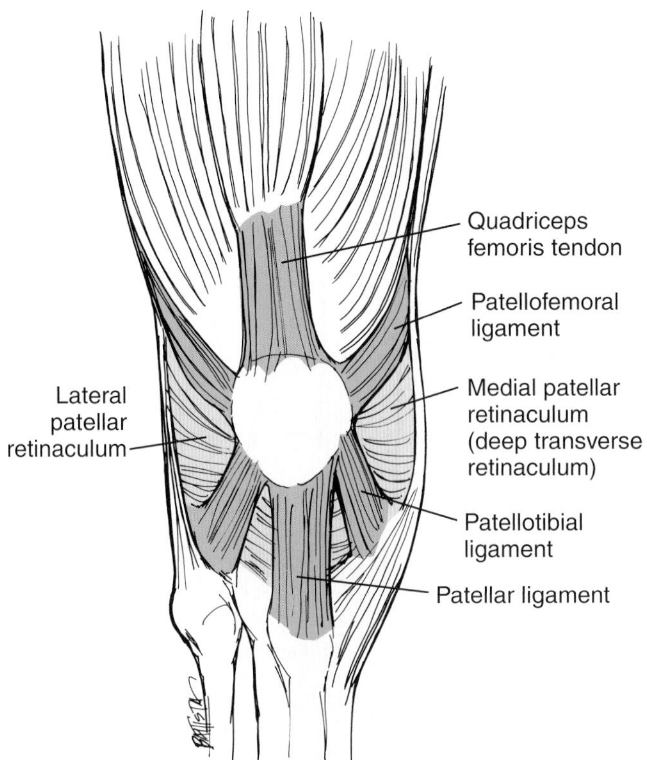

Figure 8-38. Anterior knee showing the patellar retinaculum. The superficial portion of the joint capsule interweaves with the retinaculum and has distinct thickenings, the patellofemoral and patellotibial ligaments.

patella (Fig. 8-39). To release the inferior aspect of the medial patella, switch hands, stabilize with your superior hand, and use the fingertips of your inferior hand. To release the lateral patella, perform back-and-forth strokes with the thumb while stabilizing the medial patella with your fingertips.

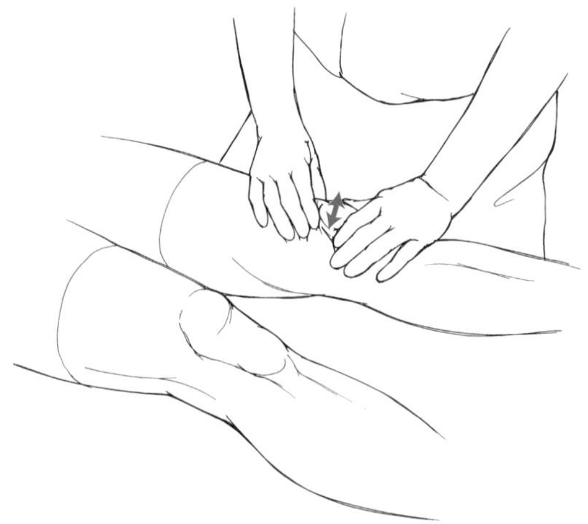

Figure 8-39. Fingertips release of the superior portion of the patellar retinaculum with back-and-forth transverse strokes.

2. Dissolve adhesions in the deeper aspect of the tissue by applying a shearing motion. Assume the same stance and hand position as described in stroke 1. To release the medial tissue, push the patella with your thumb as you pull the medial tissue with your fingertips. For the lateral retinacula, reverse your hands and pull the patella toward you with your fingertips as you scoop into the lateral retinacula with your thumb. Repeat this stroke many times in an oscillating motion. **This is for chronic conditions only.**
3. Release the under surface of the lateral pole of the patella by facing headward and using the fingertips of one hand to stabilize the medial patella (Fig. 8-40). Move it slightly laterally, and use the fingertips of your other hand to perform brisk strokes in the inferior to superior plane, on the edge, and underneath surface of the patella.

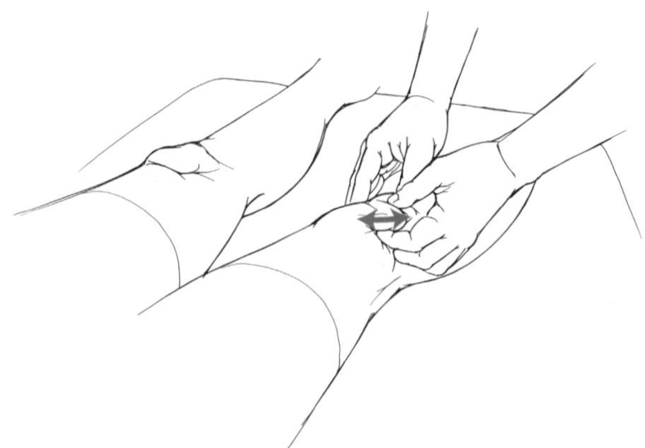

Figure 8-40. Fingertips perform back-and-forth strokes to the under surface of the lateral patella.

4. Release the under surface of the medial superior pole by turning your body to face the table and by pushing the patella medially with your superior hand. Use the fingertips of your inferior hand to perform brisk, back-and-forth strokes in the inferior to superior plane, on the edge, and underneath surface of the medial patella.
5. Perform transverse strokes in the medial to lateral plane on the infrapatellar tendon with fingertips or with a double-thumb or a single-thumb technique (Fig. 8-41). Stabilize the knee cap if the leg is in extension, or put the knee in flexion if it has been injured, is in pain, or has a history of subluxation. The most clinically involved areas are the medial and lateral borders of the tendon.

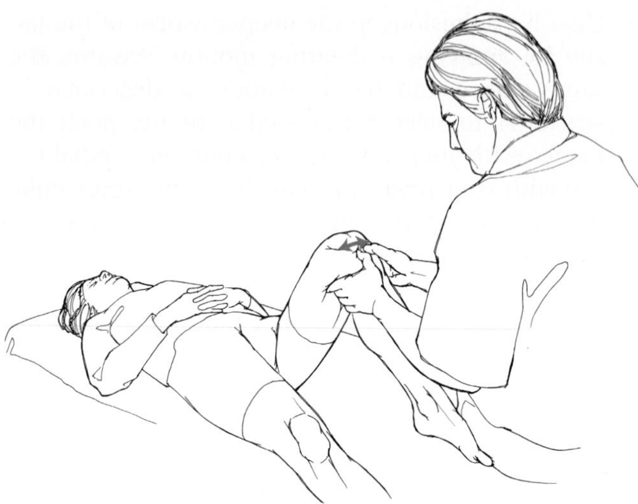

Figure 8-41. Transverse release of the infrapatellar tendon by use of the double-thumb technique.

5. Release of the Hamstrings and Bursae at the Popliteal Fossa

- *Anatomy*: Biceps femoris, semimembranosus, and semitendinosus (Fig. 8-42); and semimembranosus and medial gastrocnemius bursae (see Fig. 8-5).
- *Dysfunction*: The flexors of the knee are typically short and tight, inhibiting the quadriceps. Attachment points usually thicken and become fibrotic with overuse or injury. Sustained flexion due to injury or degeneration shortens and thickens the hamstrings and gastrocnemius attachments. The semimembranosus and medial gastrocnemius bursae communicate with the articular cavity and are often swollen after a knee injury.

Position

- TP—standing, facing headward
- CP—prone, with a pillow under the ankle to keep the knee in slight flexion or with your flexed thigh under his or her flexed leg

Strokes

1. Face headward, and place your flexed knee on the table (Fig. 8-43). Flex the client's knee, and rest his or her shin on your thigh. Using a double-thumb technique, roll the biceps femoris laterally and the semimembranosus and semitendinosus medially. As you approach the attachment points, the tissue changes from muscle to tendon and naturally becomes more cordlike. The intention is to release any fibrosis on the body of the tendons. Keep your hands soft and make your strokes more brisk and of shorter amplitude.

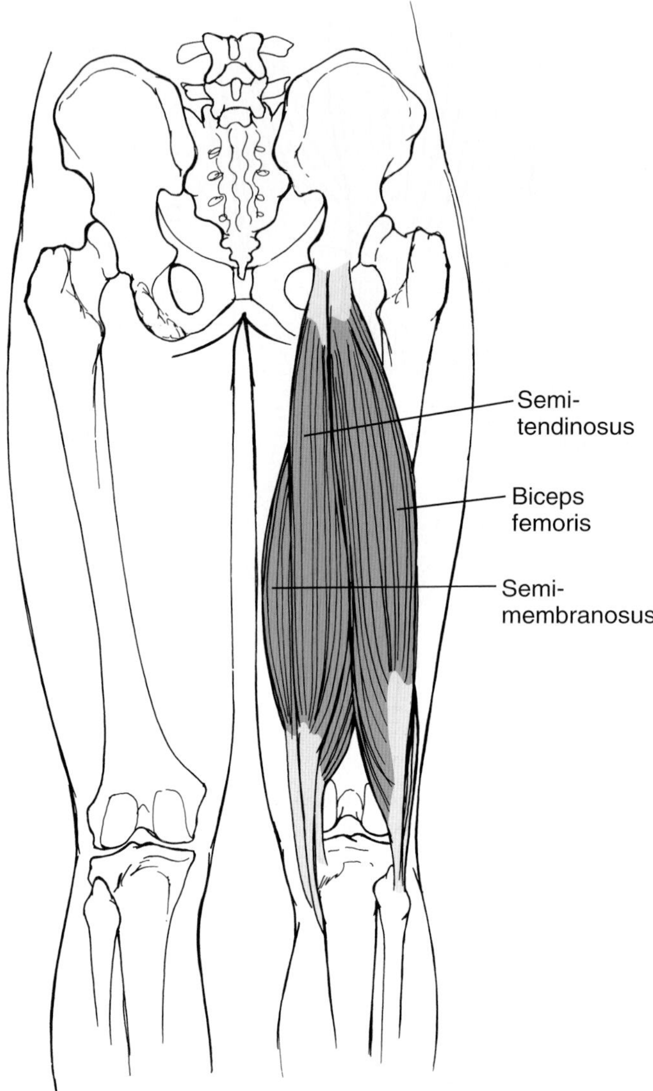

Figure 8-42. Posterior thigh and knee showing the hamstrings.

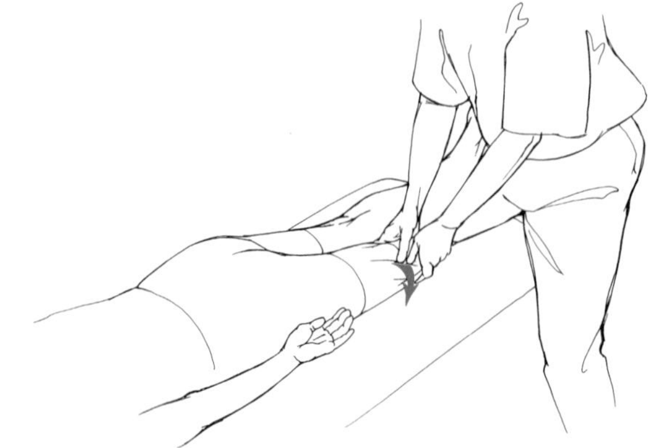

Figure 8-43. Double-thumb technique performing medial to lateral strokes on the biceps femoris.

2. An alternate method is to stand facing the table. Flex the client's knee to 90° (Fig. 8-44). Place your fingertips on the medial tendons with one hand, and hold the client's distal leg or foot with the other hand. Next, move the leg toward and away from you, massaging the tendons under your working hand. You may use a shearing motion and move your fingertips in the opposite or in the same direction as the leg. Next, place your thumb on the lateral tendons and perform the same strokes described in stroke 1.

CAUTION: **Do not work the center of the popliteal fossa in this manner, as the neurovascular bundle runs through this region and could be bruised with deep work on it.**

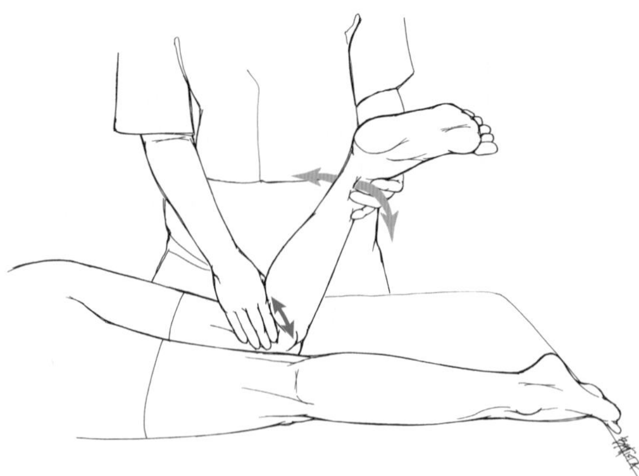

Figure 8-44. Technique to assist the release of distal hamstrings mechanically. Move the client's leg medially and laterally with one hand, while the fingertips or thumb of the other hand strokes the tendons.

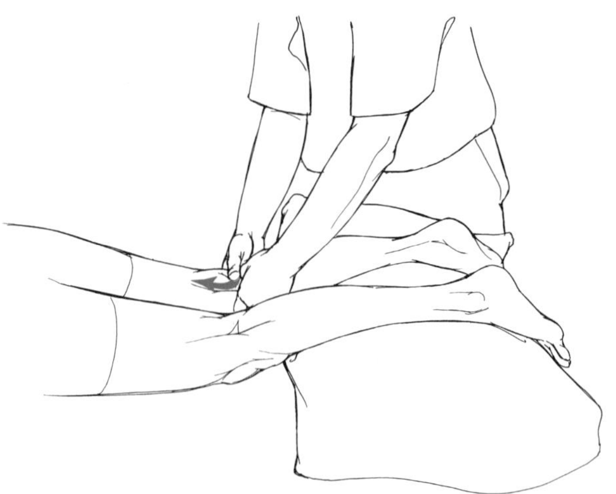

Figure 8-45. Massage of the bursae of the posterior knee with flat thumbs.

3. Release the bursae and lymphatics of the popliteal fossa by placing a pillow under the client's ankle. Apply some lotion or oil on the back of the knee. Face 45° headward. Wrap your hands around the proximal leg just below the knee, using a parallel-thumb technique in the midline of the fossa. Perform a series of long, slow continuous stokes in a headward direction (Fig. 8-45).

Level II—Knee

1. Release of the Coronary and Medial Collateral Ligaments and of the Pes Anserinus Bursa

- ***Anatomy***: Coronary ligament (Fig. 8-46), MCL (see Fig. 8-1), and pes anserinus bursa (see Fig. 8-3).
- ***Dysfunction***: The coronary and MCL ligaments are often involved in knee injuries. Fibrosis of the coronary ligament gives local pain, typically at the medial joint line, and prevents the normal movement of the joint capsule during knee flexion. The MCL is either thick and fibrotic or slack and weak in the chronic phase after an injury. Deep transverse mas-

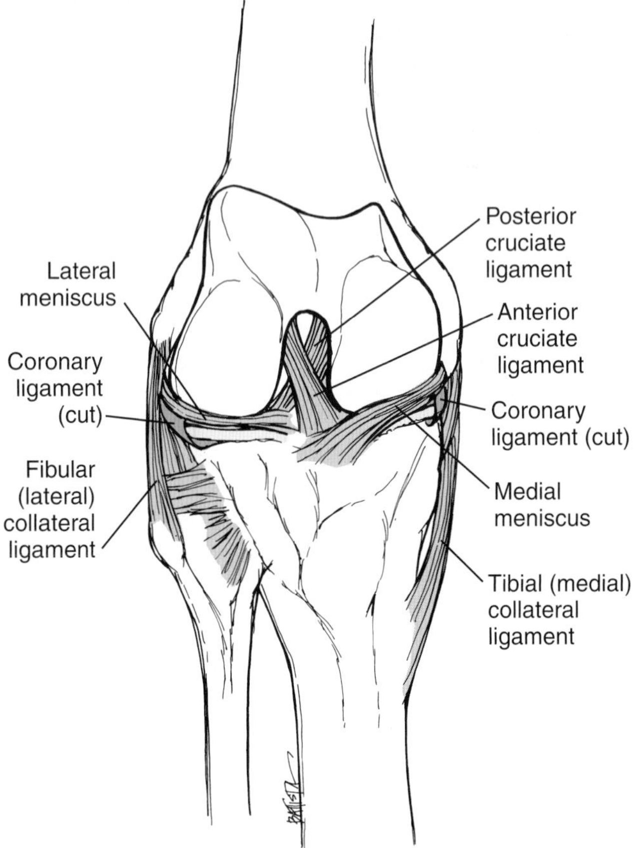

Figure 8-46. Anterior knee showing the coronary ligaments.

sage is applied only to thickened ligaments. Rehabilitation for ligaments that are too loose is through exercise. The pes anserinus bursa swells after acute or overuse injuries, with sustained genu valgus posture, or with a pronated foot.

Position

- TP—standing, facing work
- CP—supine

Strokes

1. Release the medial aspects of the coronary ligament by bringing the client's knee into flexion and placing the foot on the table (Fig. 8-47). Turn the foot laterally, which places the tibia into slight external rotation and exposes the medial plateau of the tibia. Using a single-thumb technique, perform brisk, back-and-forth strokes in the medial to lateral plane on the tibial plateau and the tibial rim for the attachment points of the ligament. Most of the work must be directed inferiorly onto the superior portion of the tibial plateau. To release the lateral portion of the coronary ligament, internally rotate the tibia by turning the foot inward and repeat the same strokes as described in stroke 1 on the lateral plateau of the tibia.

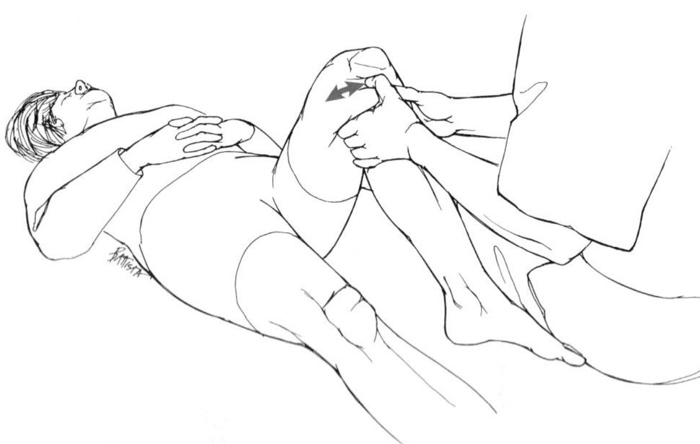

Figure 8-47. Single-thumb technique to release the medial coronary ligament.

2. Place your flexed knee on the table, and rest the client's leg on your thigh. The MCL is attached to the femur medial condyle of the femur just inferior to the adductor tubercle and on the tibia 2 to 4 inches below the joint line, posterior and deep to the pes anserinus tendons. Using a fingertips technique, perform short, back-and-forth strokes in the posterior to anterior plane from the proximal to the distal attachment sites (Fig. 8-48).

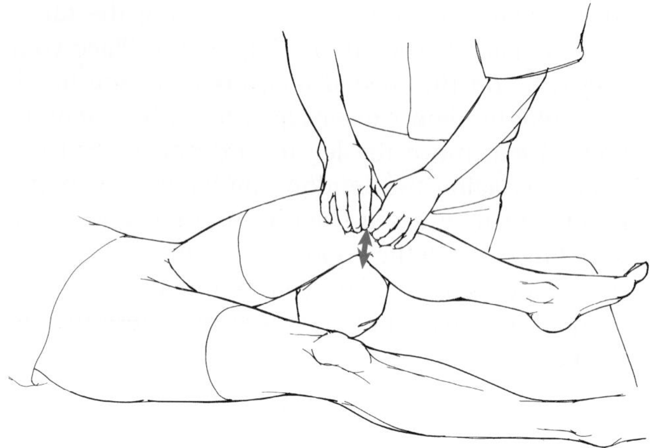

Figure 8-48. Fingertips performing transverse strokes on the MCL.

3. Bring the client's leg to rest on the table again. Place a little lotion on the medial knee and use a flat index finger to stroke the pes anserinus bursa gently in long, continuous strokes in a superior direction (Fig. 8-49). Begin on the medial leg at the level of the tibial tuberosity and continue to the distal thigh.

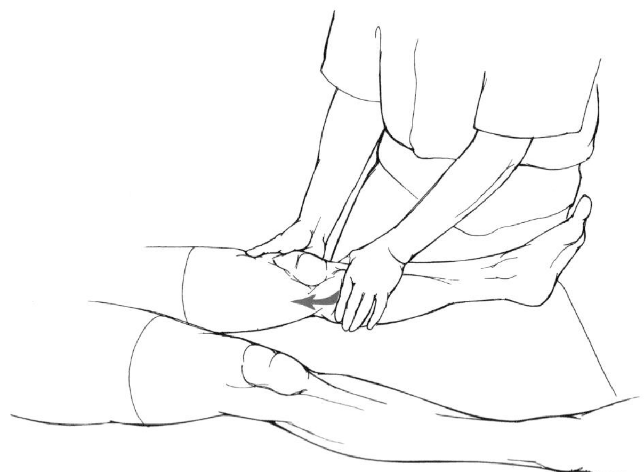

Figure 8-49. Massage of the pes anserinus bursa head ward with the flat surface of the fingers.

2. Release of the Soft-Tissue Attachments on the Lateral Aspect of the Knee

- *Anatomy*: ITB, lateral joint capsule, and fibular collateral ligament (Fig. 8-50).
- *Dysfunction*: Attachment points thicken with overuse or after injury. Previous work in this area was designed for the superficial tissue (see p. 315). This series of strokes releases the deep portion of the joint capsule and the soft tissue attachments to the periosteum covering the bone.

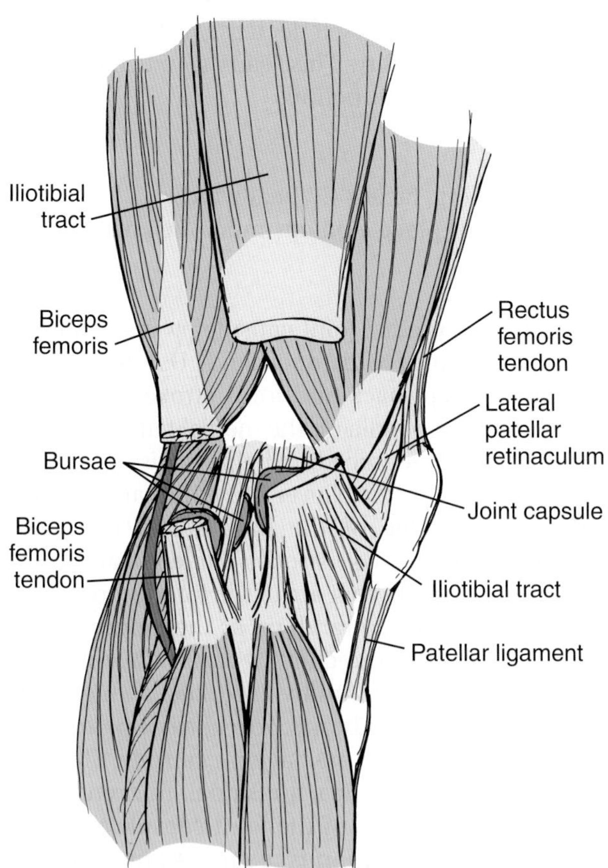

Figure 8-50. Lateral knee showing the ligaments, joint capsule, retinaculum, interweaving tendons, and the bursae under the iliotibial tract, and biceps femoris.

Position

- TP—standing
- CP— supine, knee extended

Strokes

1. Perform CR and PIR MET for the TFL and the ITB (see Figs. 7-28 and 7-29, p. 272). if the ITB palpates as hypertonic.
2. Release the attachment sites of the ITB at the femur and the tibia. The ITB inserts on the femoral supracondylar tubercle, the lateral tubercle of the tibia (Gerdy's tubercle), the patella, and the patellar tendon. To assist palpation, place your fingertips at the lateral knee approximately two finger-widths lateral to the patella. With the knee extended, have your client lift his or her leg off the table slightly. Feel the ITB come into tension. Using double thumbs or fingertips, perform deep, back-and-forth strokes in the posterior to anterior plane, starting from the lateral condyle of the femur to the lateral tibia (Fig. 8-51). If the area feels fibrotic, use brisk, transverse friction strokes.

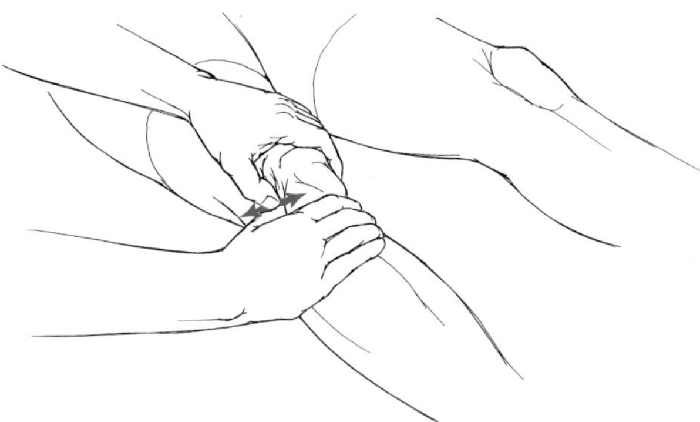

Figure 8-51. Double-thumb technique performing transverse strokes to release the attachment sites of the ITB at the femur and tibia.

3. Face 45° headward, and use a double-thumb or a fingertips technique to release the fascial expansion of the ITB and the lateral patellar retinaculum underneath it (Fig. 8-52). Perform these strokes in the A–P and the inferior to superior plane, because the retinaculum and ITB is at various angles. Feel for thick, fibrous, "thready" tissue. Cover the entire area between the ITB and lateral patella.

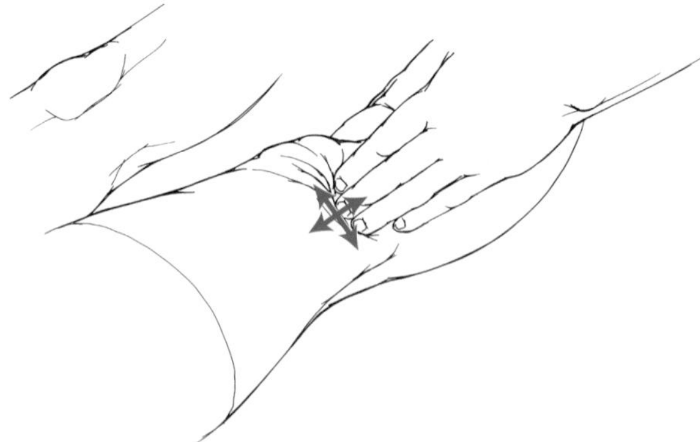

Figure 8-52. Fingertip release of the lateral retinaculum and ITB between the fibula and the lateral pole of the patella.

4. Palpate the fibular collateral ligament by first placing the knee in a figure-four position (flexed knee, abducted, and externally rotated hip). The ligament palpates as a taut cord at the joint line. Bring the leg back onto the table, placing a pillow under the knee. Using a fingertips or a double-thumb technique, perform deep, back-and-forth strokes transverse to the line of its fiber, from the lateral epicondyle of the femur to the fibular head (Fig. 8-53). Perform brisk, transverse friction strokes if it feels fibrotic.

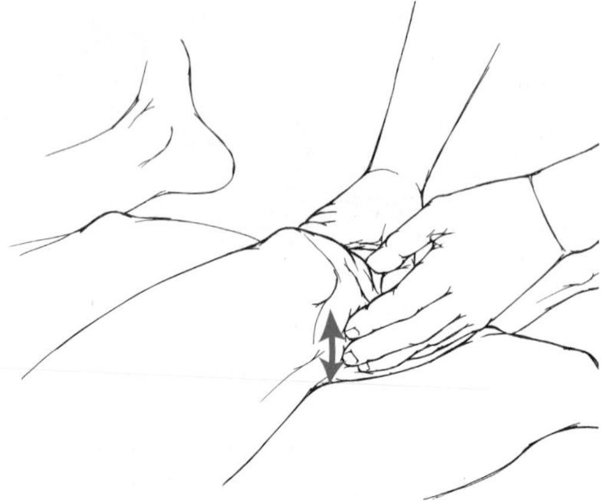

Figure 8-53. Fingertips performing transverse release of the fibular (lateral) collateral ligament.

3. Release of the Anterior Joint Capsule

- *Anatomy*: The joint capsule of the knee is attached to the femur below the superior margin of the condyles, and on the tibia it is attached immediately below the margin of the articular cartilage. (Fig. 8-54).
- *Dysfunction*: The joint capsule thickens in response to overuse or injury. The medial side of the capsule is more commonly involved clinically than the lateral side. The joint capsule can also form redundant folds in which adjacent parts of the capsule adhere to each other. These adhesions to the periosteum or within the capsule itself decrease its lubrication and normal extensibility. This leads to mechanical and neurosensory dysfunctions.

Position

- TP—standing, facing 45° headward
- CP—supine; place a pillow under the knee

Strokes

1. Release the medial joint capsule by first stabilizing the lateral knee with one hand. Use fingertips to perform deep, back-and-forth strokes in the area medial to the patella on the medial femoral condyle (Fig. 8-55). This procedure helps to dissolve fibrosis in the joint capsule. Cover the entire area between the medial edge of the patella and the medial femoral condyle. Use strokes that are transverse to the femoral shaft, that are in the inferior to superior plane, and that are random, as the joint capsule is interwoven in all directions. Feel for any thickening compared with the uninvolved knee, which might indicate capsular fibrosis. You may palpate a cord-like structure in the medial joint capsule. This cord-like structure is a plica, a residual, thickened seam in the two portions of the joint capsule that fused together. The intention is to cross transverse to the plica and clean any potential fibrosis adhesions to the underlying bone or any other aspects of the capsule.

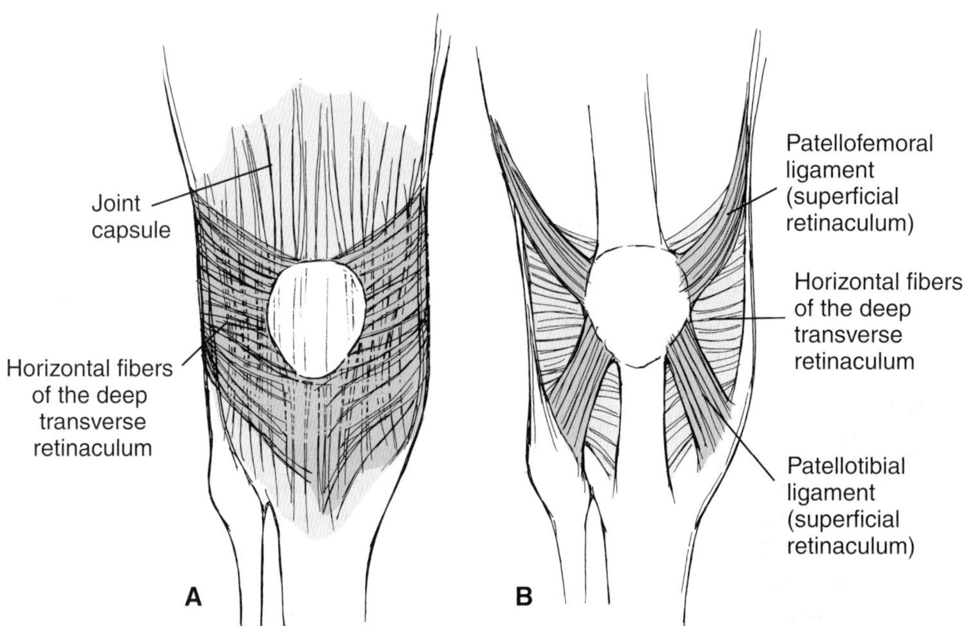

Figure 8-54. A. The anterior joint capsule and the horizontal fibers of the deep transverse retinaculum. **B.** Patellofemoral and patellotibial ligaments are distinct thickenings in the superficial fibers of the retinaculum (quadriceps extension).

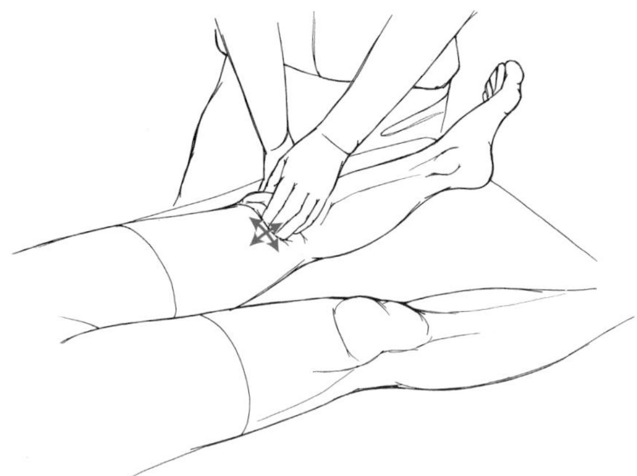

Figure 8-55. Fingertip release of the anterior joint capsule.

2. Release the lateral joint capsule of the knee by performing the same strokes (as described in stroke 1) on the lateral femoral condyle. Cover the entire area between the lateral aspect of the patella and the ITB.
3. Release the attachments of the joint capsule on the tibia just below the tibial plateau. Work on either side of the infrapatellar tendon. Use fingertips and perform deep, back-and-forth strokes on the bone. The bone should feel glistening and smooth. **These strokes are for chronic conditions only.**

4. Release of the Attachments in the Posterior Aspect of the Knee

- *Anatomy*: Medial femur—medial head of the gastrocnemius (Fig. 8-56); lateral femur—plantaris, lateral head of the gastrocnemius, and popliteus; posterior tibia—semimembranosus and popliteus; and posterior fibula—soleus (see Fig. 9-7).
- *Dysfunction*: The semimembranosus attaches to the medial meniscus. Sustained contraction can create a dysfunction in the position of the medial meniscus. The popliteus attaches to the lateral meniscus, and sustained tension creates a dysfunction in the position of the lateral meniscus. The posterior attachment points are often strained in hyperextension injuries of the knee, or they shorten owing to a sustained contraction after an injury to the knee ligaments or cartilage.

Position

- TP—standing, facing 45° headward
- CP—prone, placing his or her shin on your thigh

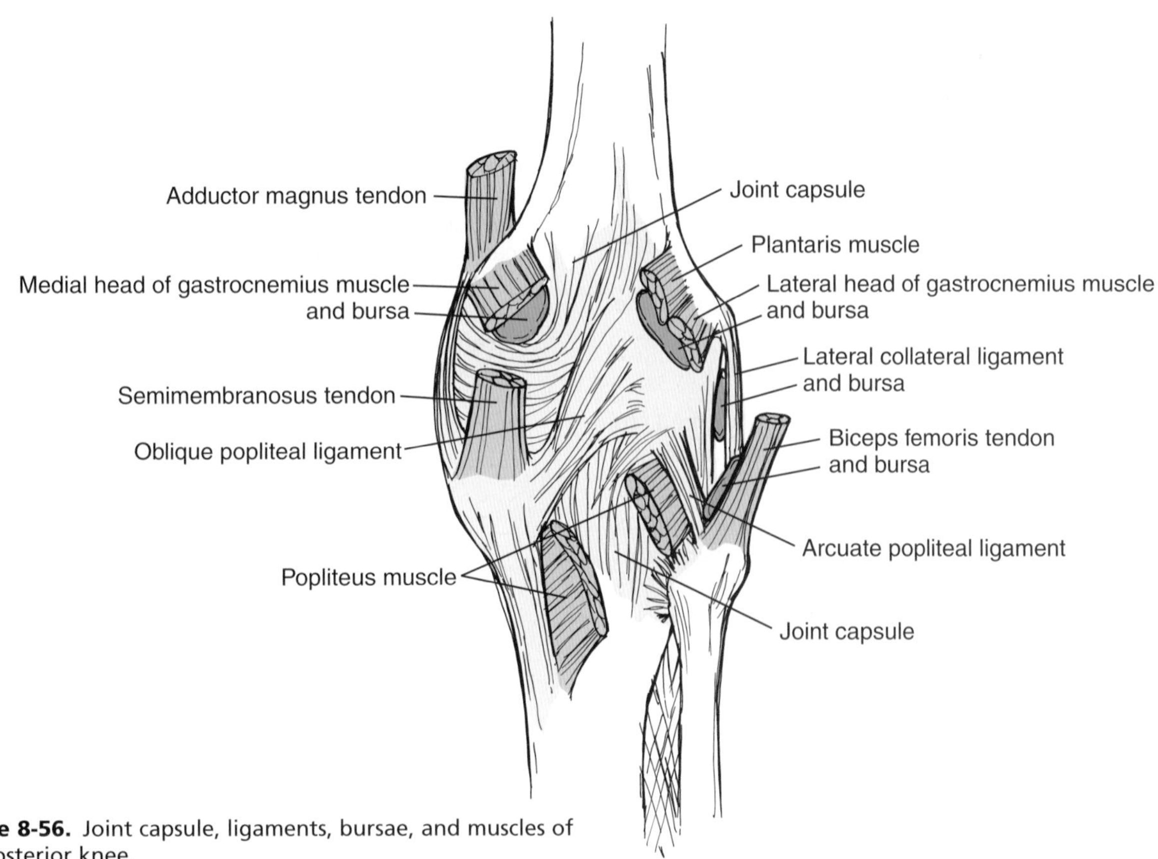

Figure 8-56. Joint capsule, ligaments, bursae, and muscles of the posterior knee.

Strokes

1. Release the plantaris, lateral head of the gastrocnemius, and popliteus from the lateral femur by standing, facing 45° headward. Place the flexed knee of your inferior leg on the table, and rest the client's shin on your thigh. Use a double-thumb technique, wrapping your hands around the distal femur (Fig. 8-57). Medially rotate the femur by moving the leg laterally, and place your thumbs on the medial side of the biceps tendons. Press laterally and deeply until your thumbs are in the area of the posterior surface of the lateral femoral condyle. Next, rock the client's entire leg medially and laterally, as you perform small, back-and-forth strokes in the medial to lateral plane. It is difficult to touch these attachments unless these areas have had a great deal of preparation. Next, perform a series of back and forth strokes in the inferior to superior plane on the popliteus, from the lateral femur to the medial tibia. Be careful not to work over an area in which you feel the pulse of the artery.

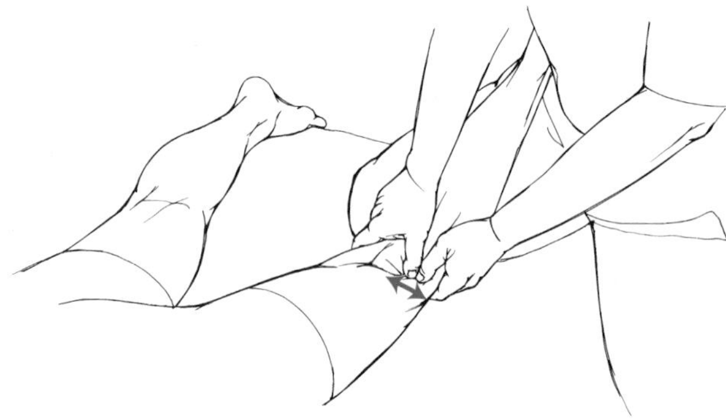

Figure 8-57. Double-thumb release of the attachments to the lateral aspect of the posterior knee.

2. Use the same technique (as described in stroke 1) to release the medial aspects of the posterior femur and tibia (Fig. 8-58). First, laterally rotate the femur by moving the leg medially, and place your thumbs on the lateral side of the semimembranosus and semitendinosus tendons. Press medially and deeply until your thumbs are on the gastrocnemius, moving toward its attachment on the posterior surface of the medial femoral condyle. Next, rock the client's leg into medial and lateral rotation, and perform small, back-and-forth strokes in the medial to lateral plane. Continue to the medial aspect of the proximal tibia to release the semimembranosus and popliteus attachments.

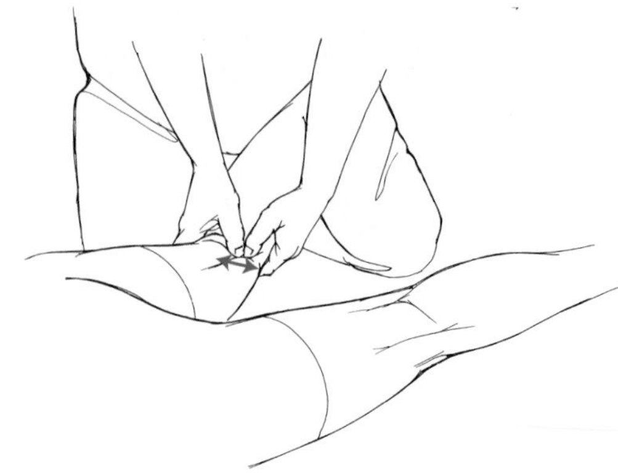

Figure 8-58. Double-thumb release of the attachments to the medial aspect of the posterior knee.

5. Mobilization of the Knee

■ *Anatomy*: Patellofemoral joint and tibiofemoral joint (Fig. 8-59) and the medial and lateral meniscus (see Fig. 8-6). Normally, a slight negative pressure exists in the joint cavity, which is lowered even further with joint distraction.[12] Lauren Berry taught that a decrease in knee joint pressure would draw the meniscus into the joint slightly and help normalize their position. The figure-eight mobilization would then help seat the cartilage properly. This is an extremely effective mobilization.

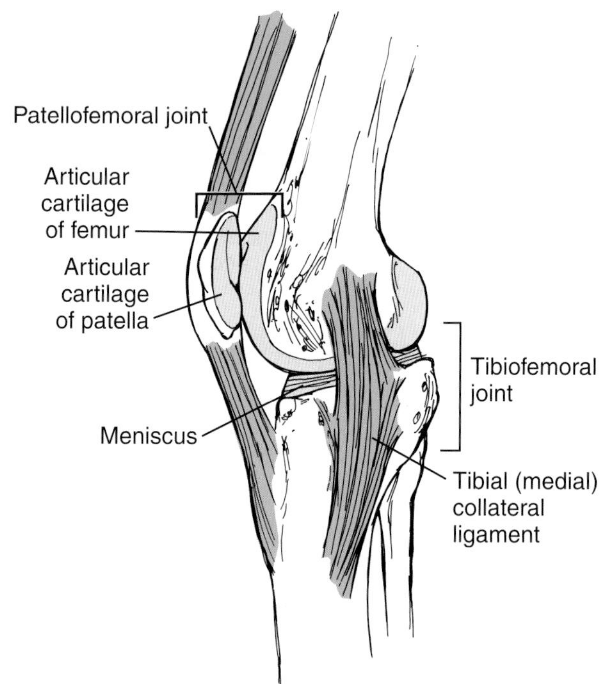

Figure 8-59. Knee consists of two joints. The articulation of the distal end of the femur and the proximal tibia is called the tibiofemoral joint. The articulation of the femur and patella is called the patellofemoral joint.

- ***Dysfunction***: The patella can develop a roughened surface from either acute injury or chronic irritation. The inflammation digests the cartilage surface, pitting it, and the cartilage heals with a roughened surface. The menisci are susceptible to adhesions, malposition, abrasion, and tearing, which inhibit their normal gliding characteristics.

Position

- TP—standing
- CP—supine

Strokes

1. Place the patella in the palm of your superior hand. Your inferior hand stabilizes the inferior aspect of the patella (Fig. 8-60). Gently push the patella into the joint and mobilize in all planes of motion with back-and-forth oscillations. If a high-pitched grinding is heard or felt, perform the grinding for no more than 1 minute per session, as too much treatment may irritate the joint. This gentle grinding helps resolve the pain and dysfunction of this joint. A low-toned grinding may indicate a pedunculated calcification (rounded), and it is not the intention to dissolve these protuberances but to clean around them with great care. This technique can be safely performed for approximately 1 minute.
2. Help normalize the function of the menisci by bringing the client's hip into approximately 90° of flexion and by placing your forearm in the popliteal space (Fig. 8-61). Hold the client's distal leg with your other hand and bring the knee into passive flexion until tension; then exert an overpressure. This gaps the joint. This passive flexion should be painless. Next, perform a figure-eight motion. Place the lower leg under your axilla and hold the leg next to your body. Place your thumbs on either side of the patellar tendon at the joint line, with fingertips holding the posterior surface of the knee (Fig. 8-62). Take the knee into a circular motion, first up and laterally, while you increase the pressure of the thumb on the lateral side. Then bring the knee down and back to the center, placing traction on the knee by leaning back with your body. Repeat the circle and traction to the medial side. Perform this circle, traction, and circle medially and laterally (figure eight) several times, making the circle smaller each time and extending the knee. End with the knee resting on the table in full extension and externally rotated approximately 15°. Place the webspace between your thumb and index finger at the joint space of the client's knee, and press posteriorly as you passively extend the knee.

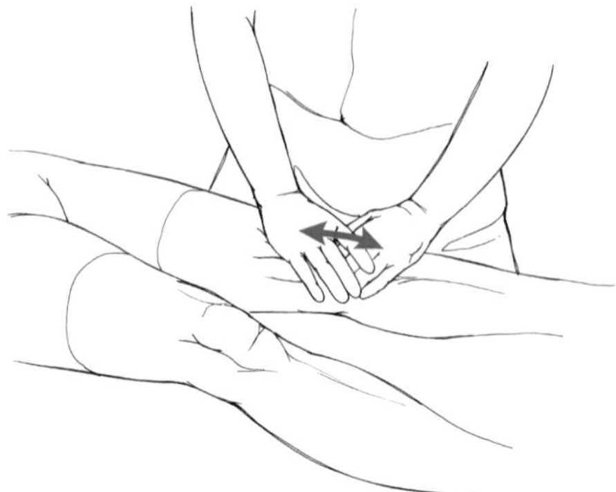

Figure 8-60. Mobilization of the patellofemoral joint.

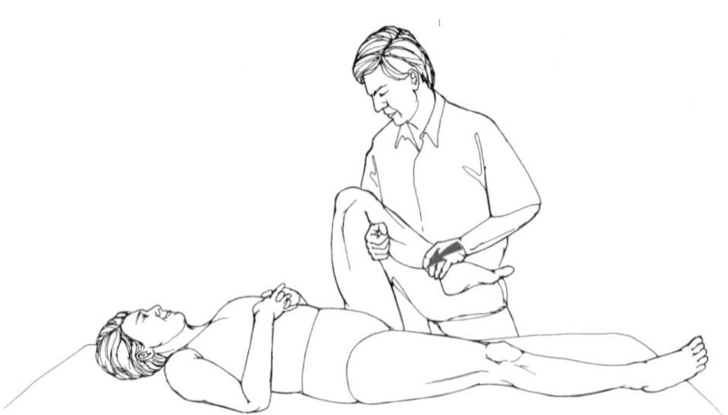

Figure 8-61. Passive flexion of the knee with the forearm in the popliteal fossa decreases the pressure in the joint cavity and draws the menisci toward their resting position.

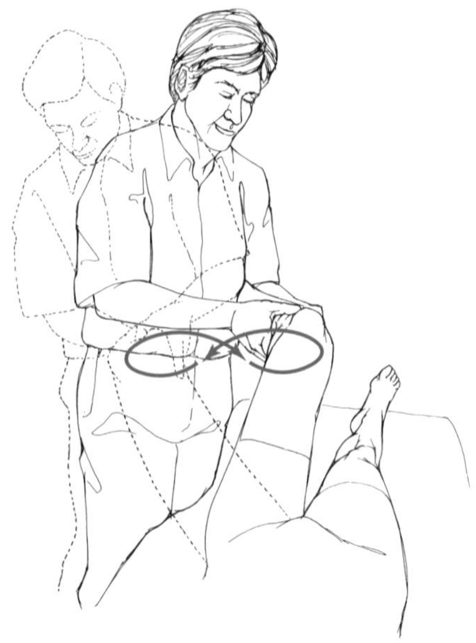

Figure 8-62. Figure-eight mobilization of the knee.

CASE STUDY

HG is a 22-year-old, 5'8", 150-lb, female college student who presented to my office with a painful and swollen left knee. She stated that the knee felt weak and unstable and had a "gravelly, popping" sound. She described the pain as an ache that worsened when she climbed stairs and that improved with rest. Her history includes several patellar dislocations since she was 13 years old. She became a competitive diver at an early age, but the dislocations became so frequent that she had to stop. Eight months previously, she had had surgery that involved a tibial tubercle transfer and a lateral release. She had received physical therapy and massage and was working with an athletic trainer.

Examination revealed an inward facing patella, the right greater than the left, and a pronated ankle on the right. Active ROM and the squat test were normal. She showed inadequate recruitment of the VMO on the lateral pull test of the patella, indicating a slight weakness of the VMO. Decreased passive glide of the patella was also found. Palpation revealed thick, fibrotic tissue at the medial patellar retinaculum, at the medial coronary ligament, at the medial joint capsule, and the underneath surface of the patella.

A diagnosis was made of capsular fibrosis. Recommendations were made for four treatments on a weekly basis. Treatment began with the client supine. A pillow was placed under the left knee, and CR MET was performed on the quadriceps and the hamstrings to release the hypertonicity and to increase the extensibility of the quadriceps attachments to the patella. OM was performed on the retinaculum, on the medial coronary ligament, on the medial joint capsule, and the underneath the surface of the patella.

HG returned to the office 1 week later reporting that the knee had been sore to the touch after the treatment. Examination findings were essentially unchanged. The same treatment was applied as on the previous visit, but I emphasized the MET and applied less depth with the OM.

She received weekly treatments for 2 additional weeks. On her fourth visit she reported that she was feeling slightly better. Examination revealed less fibrosis and better tracking of the patella on the lateral pull test. Recommendations were made for two additional treatments. The same MET and OM were applied.

After the fifth treatment she stated that she was feeling much better. Palpation revealed that the fibrosis was substantially reduced and that the patella was tracking normally. HG returned for follow-up visits on two occasions, the latter approximately 1 year after her first visit. She stated that she had returned to diving with only slight, occasional pain. Two years later the patient was seen for a midback complaint, and she stated that the knee felt completely normal and that she continued to dive.

STUDY GUIDE

Level I—Knee

1. Describe the MET for an acute knee.
2. Describe genu valgus and three factors that cause it.
3. Describe why the medial meniscus is more commonly injured than the lateral.
4. Describe the signs and symptoms of sprains of the MCL and the LCL, the coronary ligament, fibrosis of the joint capsule, and arthritis of the knee.
5. Describe the stroke direction to release the soft tissue of the medial and lateral knee, and describe why that direction is used.
6. List four factors predisposing to knee pain.
7. Describe the structure and function of the coronary ligaments and the stroke direction to release them.
8. List which knee muscles tend to be tight and which tend to be weak.
9. Describe the medial and lateral patellar retinaculum and their attachments.
10. Describe the two possible outcomes of injury to the ligaments and the implications for the massage therapist.

Level II—Knee

1. Describe the MET for the popliteus, quadriceps, and lower attachments of the hamstrings.
2. Describe the signs and symptoms of the following conditions: popliteal tendinitis, chondromalacia patella, and injuries of the menisci.
3. List the structures that are released on the medial and lateral aspect of the knee.
4. List the structures that attach onto the posterior aspect of the femur and onto the tibia and fibula at the knee.
5. Describe the knee muscle most commonly atrophied after an injury, and explain why.
6. Describe the intention of performing figure-eight mobilization of the knee.
7. Describe patellar tracking dysfunction, and list two causes.

8. Describe the stroke direction to release the joint capsule.
9. Describe the assessment findings of an injury to the meniscus.
10. Describe the test to assess patellar tracking dysfunction.

REFERENCES

1. Garrick J, Webb D. Sports Injuries. 2nd Ed. Philadelphia: WB Saunders, 1999.
2. Shelbourne KD, Rask B, Hunt S. Knee injuries. In: Schenck R, ed. Athletic Training and Sports Medicine. 3rd Ed. Rosemont, Il: American Academy of Orthopedic Surgeons, 1999: 435–488.
3. Wallace L, Mangine R, Malone T. The knee. In: Malone T, McPoil T, Nitz A, eds. Orthopedic and Sports Physical Therapy. St. Louis: Mosby, 1997:295–325.
4. Hertling D, Kessler R. The knee. In: Hertling D, Kessler R, eds. Management of Common Musculoskeletal Disorders. Baltimore: Lippincott Williams & Wilkins, 1996: 315–378.
5. Norkin C, Levangie P. The knee complex. In: Joint Structure and Function. Philadelphia: FA Davis, 1992:337–378.
6. Frick H, Leonhardt H, Starck D. Human Anatomy, vol. 1. New York: Thieme Medical, 1991.
7. Press J, Young J. Rehabilitation of the patellofemoral pain syndrome. In: Kibler WB, Herring SA, Press JM, eds. Functional Rehabilitation of Sports and Musculoskeletal Injuries. Gaithersburg: Aspen, 1998:254–264.
8. Richards D, Kibler WB. Rehabilitation of knee injuries. In: Kibler WB, Herring SA, Press JM, eds. Functional Rehabilitation of Sports and Musculoskeletal Injuries. Gaithersburg: Aspen, 1998:244–253.
9. Kendall F, McCreary E, Provance P. Muscles: Testing and Function. 4th Ed. Baltimore: Williams & Wilkins, 1993.
10. Henning C, Lynch M, Glick K. Physical examination of the knee. In: Nicholas J, Hershman E, eds. The Lower Extremity and Spine in Sports Medicine. St. Louis: CV Mosby, 1986:765–800.
11. Hammer W. Functional Soft Tissue Examination and Treatment by Manual Methods. 2nd Ed. Gaithersburg: Aspen, 1999.
12. Grieve G. Common Vertebral Joint Problems. Edinburgh: Churchill Livingstone, 1981.

SUGGESTED READINGS

Corrigan B, Maitland GD. Practical Orthopaedic Medicine. London: Butterworths, 1983.

Cyriax J, Cyriax P. Illustrated Manual of Orthopedic Medicine. London: Butterworths, 1983.

Hammer W. Functional Soft Tissue Examination and Treatment by Manual Methods. 2nd Ed. Gaithersburg: Aspen, 1999.

Hertling D, Kessler R. The knee. In: Hertling D, Kessler R, eds. Management of Common Musculoskeletal Disorders. Baltimore: Lippincott Williams & Wilkins, 1996:315–378.

Hoppenfeld S. Physical Examination of the Spine and Extremities. New York: Appleton-Century-Crofts, 1976.

Kendall F, McCreary E, Provance P. Muscles: Testing and Function. 4th Ed. Baltimore: Williams & Wilkins, 1993.

Magee D. Orthopedic Physical Assessment. 3rd Ed. Philadelphia: WB Saunders, 1997.

Norkin C, Levangie P. The knee complex. In: Joint Structure and Function. Philadelphia: FA Davis, 1992:337–378.

Reid DC. Sports Injury and Assessment. New York: Churchill Livingstone, 1992.

Wallace L, Mangine R, Malone T. The knee. In: Malone T, McPoil T, Nitz A, eds. Orthopedic and Sports Physical Therapy. St. Louis: Mosby, 1997:295–325.

The Leg, Ankle, and Foot

The leg is the fourth most frequently involved region in athletic injuries.[1] Most of these injuries involve a strain of the gastrocnemius and the Achilles tendon. The Achilles tendon is the most common site of overuse injury in the lower extremity and the most frequently ruptured tendon in the body.[2] The ankle sprain is probably the most common injury in sports and perhaps the most commonly injured ligament in the body.[3] The foot is more susceptible to degenerative problems rather than to acute injuries. Most painful conditions in the foot originate in the soft tissue.[4]

General Overview of the Leg, Ankle, and Foot

The leg consists of those structures between the knee and ankle. Leg bones are the **tibia** and the **fibula.** The distal ends of the tibia and fibula, called the medial and the lateral malleolus respectively, form part of the ankle with the talus bone. The 12 muscles of the leg contribute to foot and ankle movements; 3 of these 12 contribute to knee flexion. The foot contains 26 bones, 30 joints, and 20 intrinsic muscles. The top of the foot is called the **dorsum,** and the bottom of the foot is called the **plantar** surface. To bend the foot toward the ground is called foot and ankle flexion or **plantar flexion,** and to bring the top of the foot and ankle toward the anterior leg is called extension of the foot and ankle, also referred to as **dorsiflexion.**

Anatomy, Function, and Dysfunction of the Leg

BONES AND JOINTS OF THE LEG

See Figure 9-1.

Tibia

- *Structure*: The tibia, or shin bone, is a strong, triangular bone, which connects the distal femur and the bones of the ankle and foot. The sharp anterior sur-

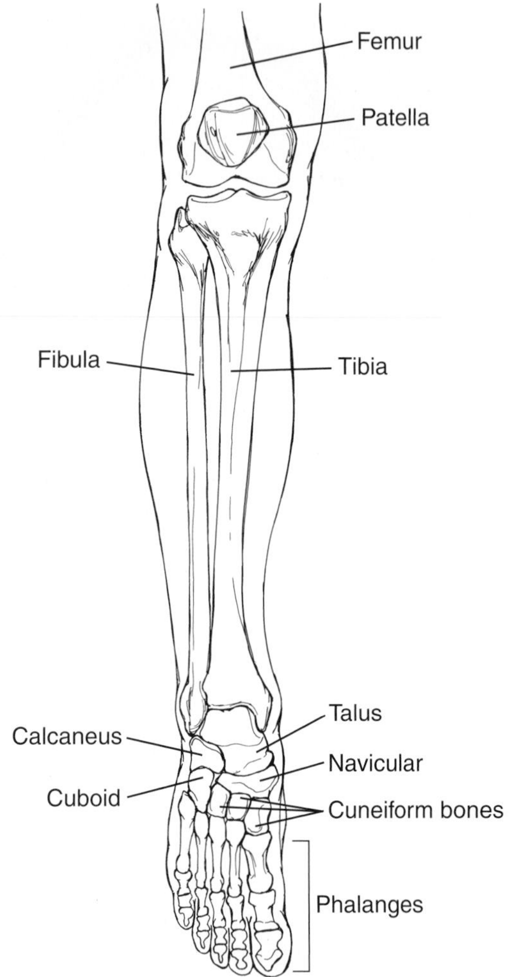

Figure 9-1. Bones of the leg, ankle, and foot.

face has a protrusion on its proximal portion called the **tibial tuberosity** where the quadriceps tendon attaches. The proximal portion of the tibia was discussed in Chapter 8, "The Knee." The distal end of the tibia has an expansion on the medial side called the medial malleolus, and the inferior part of the tibia articulates with the talus, a part of the ankle discussed below. The tibia is rotated externally approximately 15° between its proximal and distal ends and is called the **normal tibial torsion.**

- *Function*: The tibia bears nearly all the weight from the thigh to the foot. As mentioned, only the tibia forms the articulation with the femur at the knee, and the tibia is the major weight-bearing surface at the ankle. Along the medial side of the distal tibia is a groove for the tibialis posterior tendon.

Fibula

- *Structure*: The fibula is a thin bone, composed of a triangular shaft and proximal and distal ends. The distal end has an expansion on its lateral surface called the lateral malleolus, which articulates with the talus. A groove is in the posterior aspect of the lateral malleolus for the peroneus brevis tendon.
- *Function*: The fibula is an attachment site for muscles of the foot and ankle and forms part of the ankle joint. It carries approximately one-sixth of the static weight of the leg.[5]

Tibiofibular Joints

- *Structure*: The tibia and fibula form three joints. The first and second are the **proximal** and the **distal tibiofibular joints;** the third is a **fibrous joint** formed by the **interosseous membrane** connecting the first and the second joints. The proximal tibiofibular joint is a synovial joint, with a joint capsule and anterior and posterior ligaments of the fibular head. The distal tibiofibular joint is a fibrous joint, without a synovial membrane, supported by the anterior and the posterior tibiofibular ligaments. A strong interosseous membrane reinforces both joints.
- *Function*: Although slight, there is some movement between the proximal and the distal tibiofibular joints. With foot dorsiflexion, the distal tibiofibular joint widens slightly to accommodate the talus, and the proximal fibula has a corresponding superior glide. The interosseous membrane functions to connect the two bones and serves as an extensive area for muscular attachments. Unlike the radius and ulna of the forearm that allow forearm pronation and supination, the interosseous membrane of the leg is so dense that a similar motion cannot be performed.
- ***Dysfunction and injury:*** The distal ends of the tibia and fibula are frequent sites of fractures. The bootstrap fracture of the fibula is common in the skier, and fatigue or stress fractures in the tibia can occur with excessive or unusual stress, such as long-distance running. The client often walks with a limp and has acute tenderness at the fracture site, usually localized to an area less than 1.5 inches in diameter.[1] The ligaments, retinacula, and fascia thicken after a fracture. The tibiofibular joint consequently has limited dorsiflexion, and the fibula loses its normal gliding characteristics at the proximal joint.

SOFT-TISSUE STRUCTURES OF THE LEG

Fascia and Retinaculum

See Figure 9-2.

- *Structure*: The fascia of the leg is called the **crural fascia** and is a continuation of the fascia lata of the thigh. It is interwoven to the periosteum of the medial surface of the tibia. The anterior and lateral portions are extremely dense and have little ability to expand, whereas the posterior portion is loose and relaxed. The deep crural fascia forms three **intermuscular septa.** With the addition of the interosseous membrane between the tibia and the fibula, there are four compartments of the leg that contain the muscles primarily concerned with movement of the foot and ankle. The **anterior compartment** contains the extensor muscles; the **lateral compartment** contains the evertors; and the **superficial** and **deep posterior compartments** contain the flexor muscles. The fascia is reinforced by transverse thickenings called **retinaculum.** The retinaculum acts like a strap to prevent the muscles and tendons running under it from lifting off the bone during contraction.

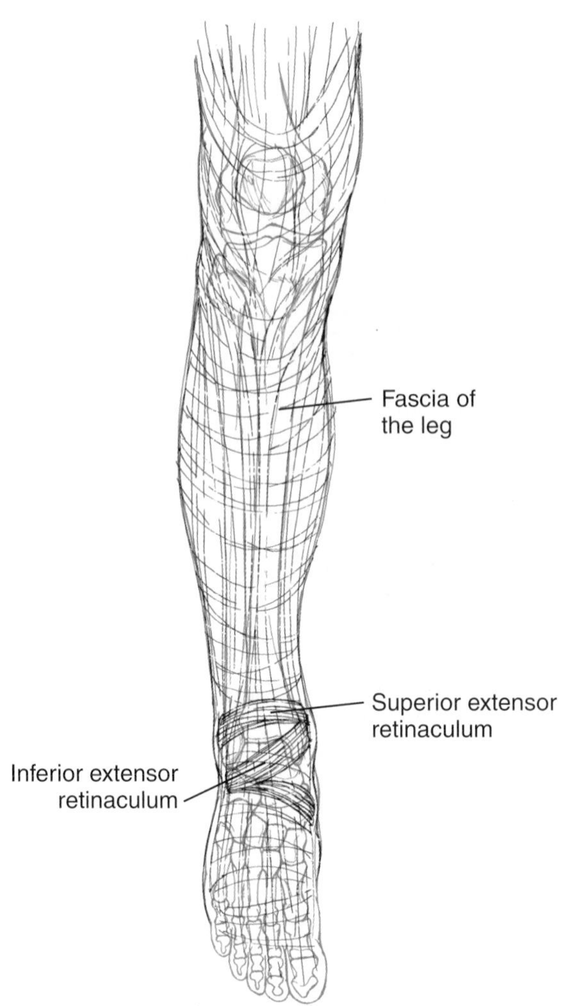

Figure 9-2. Fascia of the leg, ankle, and foot and the superior and inferior retinaculum.

  - On the distal aspect of the anterior leg is the **superior** and **inferior extensor retinaculum.** The superficial layer of this fascia stabilizes the tendons that extend (dorsiflex) the foot, including the tibialis anterior, extensor hallucis longus (EHL), and the extensor digitorum longus.
  - Between the medial malleolus and the calcaneus is the **flexor retinaculum** or **laciniate ligament,** which has a superficial and deep layer. The deep layer stabilizes the tendons that flex (plantar flex) the foot, including the tibialis posterior, flexor hallucis longus, and the flexor digitorum longus. The area between the superficial and deep layers of the flexor retinaculum is called the **tarsal tunnel,** and it contains the **posterior tibial nerve** that innervates the sole of the foot.
  - The lateral ankle has expansions of the fascia called the **superior** and **inferior peroneal retinaculum** and stabilizes the peroneus longus and brevis.
- *Function*: The fascia of the anterior and lateral compartments is extremely dense to contain the hydrostatic pressure from carrying the body weight. The fascial compartments guide muscle contraction. Each of the muscles within these fascial compartments normally can slide relative to each other and relative to the fascial envelope. The compartments also contain the major arteries and nerves of the leg. During vigorous exercise, there may be a 20-fold increase in the blood flow in the leg.[5]
- *Dysfunction and injury*: Many factors predispose to fascial stress. Leg-length inequality, muscle imbalances, and pronation are three common factors.[6] Injuries to the fascia of the leg are described with various names by different authors. The basic categories of injury include the acute and chronic compartment syndromes and the shin splint. Chronic compartment syndrome is similar to a shin splint.
  - **Acute compartment syndrome** is often caused by a fracture, or a tear in the muscle or fascia. It

causes extreme swelling within the dense anterior and lateral compartments of the leg, and since this fascia expands only slightly, it may compress the arteries, veins, and nerves and cut off the blood supply and sensation to the foot.

- **Chronic compartment syndrome** describes a swelling of the muscle fibers that can be caused by either static or dynamic stresses. A static stress describes an occupation that requires standing most of the day. A dynamic stress is typically exercise induced. In the chronic condition, the stress on the fascia causes an eventual thickening in the superficial and the deep layers and a loss of the normal gliding characteristics of the muscles.
- A **shin splint** is a tenoperiosteal tear of the muscle's fascia where it interweaves with the periosteum, called the tenoperiosteal junction. This is the acute manifestation of a chronic condition. Excessive stress to the fascia is typically the result of the cumulative stresses of vigorous activity, such as running.

- ***Treatment implications***: Perform muscle energy technique (MET) to reduce the hypertonicity of the muscles within the compartments and orthopedic massage (OM) to stretch the superficial and deep layers of the fascia and to dissolve the fibrosis at the tenoperiosteal junction. Postisometric relaxation (PIR) MET is used to lengthen short muscles and their fascia. Identify the weak muscles with the isometric contractions of contract-relax (CR) MET, and strengthen those muscles with MET, or refer the client for exercise rehabilitation. With acute compartment syndrome the client presents with extreme pain in the leg and a cold foot. Refer to an emergency room (ER) because the loss of blood supply to the foot can cause permanent damage.

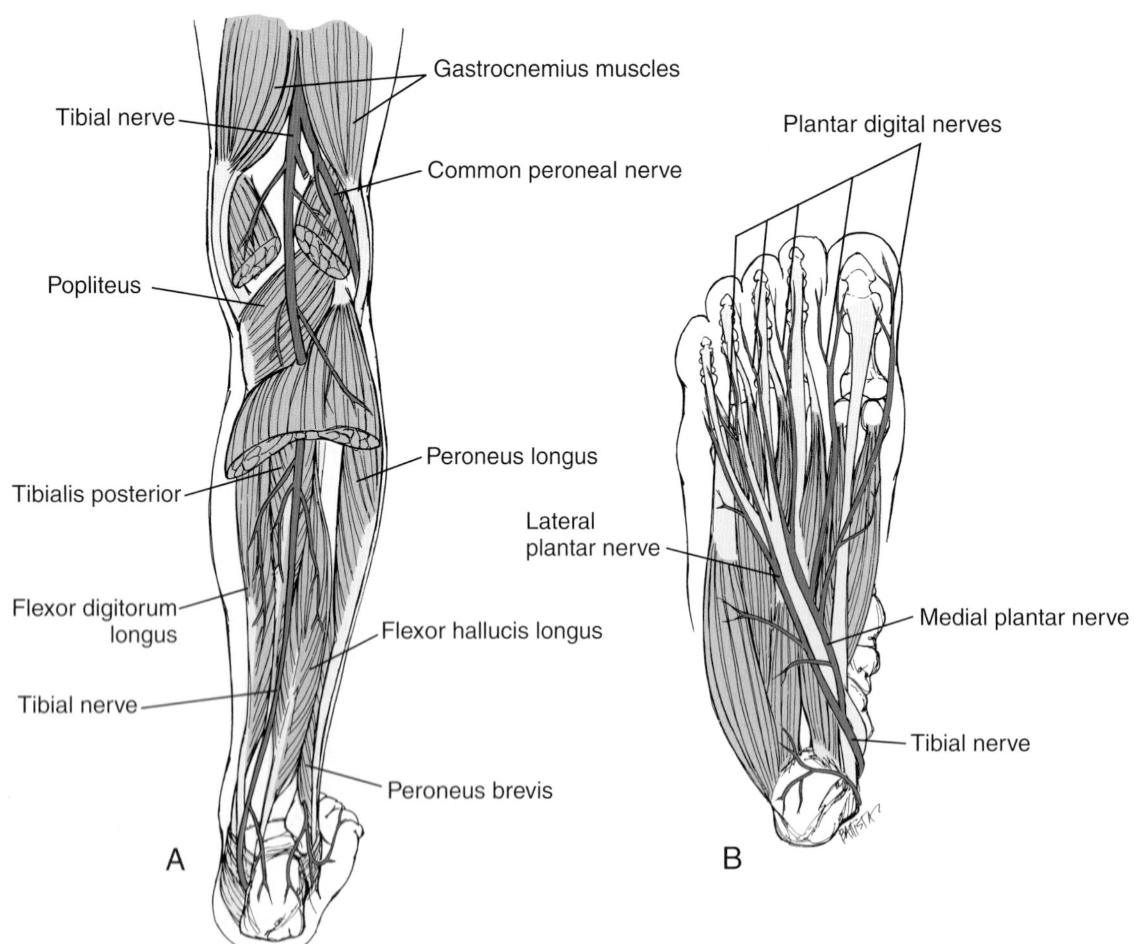

Figure 9-3. A. Tibial nerve and the muscles innervated by the tibial nerve. **B.** Tibial nerve continues into the bottom of the foot as the medial and lateral plantar nerves.

Nerves

See Figures 9-3**A** and **B** and 9-4.

- *Structure*: The major nerves of the leg are branches of the sciatic nerve. They are the **superficial** and **deep peroneal, tibial, saphenous,** and **sural nerves.** The superficial and deep peroneal nerves travel through an arcade or opening in the peroneus longus, just distal to the fibular head.[5] The tibial nerve becomes the posterior tibial nerve as it travels through a fibrous arch in the soleus muscle in the proximal calf. It continues as the medial and lateral plantar nerves in the foot. The saphenous nerve is a terminal branch of the femoral nerve and becomes superficial at the medial thigh and knee. The sural nerve is a cutaneous nerve from branches of the tibial and peroneal nerves.
- *Function*: The deep peroneal nerve innervates the muscles in the anterior compartment and gives sensation to the webspace between the first and the second toes on the dorsum (top) of the foot. The superficial peroneal nerve innervates the lateral compartment and gives sensation to most of the dorsum of the foot. The posterior tibial nerve innervates the deep posterior compartments and gives sensation to the plantar (bottom) aspect of the foot. The saphenous nerve supplies sensation to the medial leg and foot. The sural nerve supplies sensation to the lateral and posterior distal third of the leg.
- *Dysfunction and injury*: The nerves can become entrapped in the leg, ankle, or foot. The common peroneal nerve can become entrapped just distal to the head of the fibula and approximately 4 to 5 inches proximal to the lateral ankle, and the posterior tibial nerve can become entrapped in the proximal leg as it passes under the soleus. The sural nerve can become entrapped proximal to the lateral ankle, and the saphenous nerve can become entrapped in the medial thigh.
- *Treatment implications*: The nerves of the leg are treated with gentle transverse scooping strokes to reduce the tension in the fascia suspending the nerve, and to dissolve the adhesions restricting the normal gliding characteristics of the nerves.

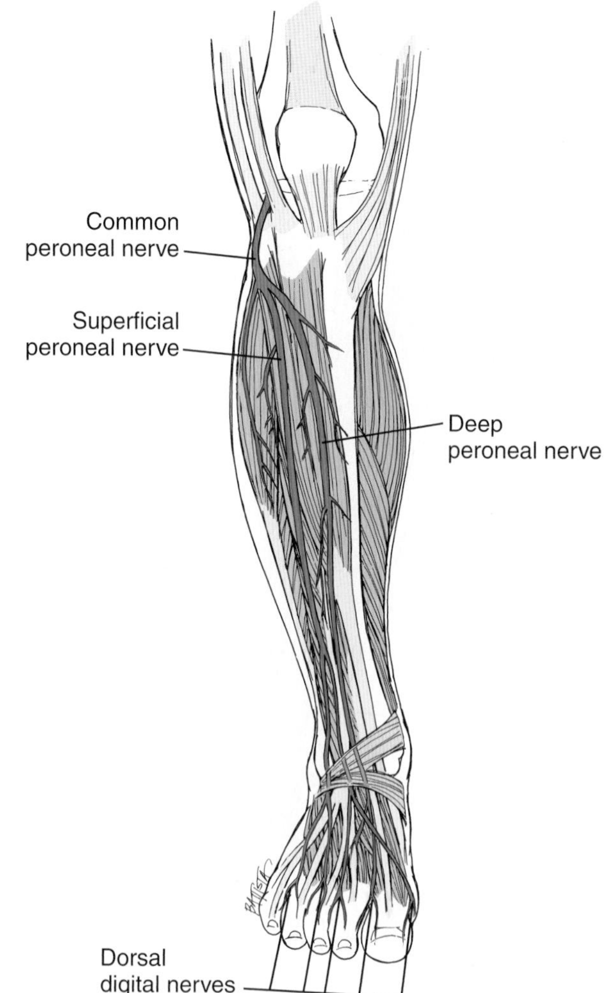

Figure 9-4. Common, superficial, and deep peroneal nerves.

Muscles

- *Structure*: Leg muscles are broadly categorized by location. The extensor muscles of the ankle and foot lie in the anterior and lateral leg (Fig. 9-5; see Fig. 8-10). The flexors of the ankle and foot lie in the posterior leg, and the tendons travel around the medial ankle (Figs. 9-6 and 9-7; see Fig. 8-9). Leg muscles are classified by **fascial compartments** also. Four compartments—the anterior, lateral, superficial posterior, and deep posterior—contain 12 muscles, all of which attach to bones in the foot, except the popliteus.
  - The **anterior compartment** contains the extensor muscles of the ankle and foot (dorsiflexors) and includes the tibialis anterior, EHL, extensor digitorum longus, and peroneus tertius, a variant of the extensor digitorum longus extending to the fifth toe (see Fig. 9-5). The common peroneal nerve serves the anterior compartment.
  - The **lateral compartment** contains the evertors of the ankle and foot and includes the peroneus

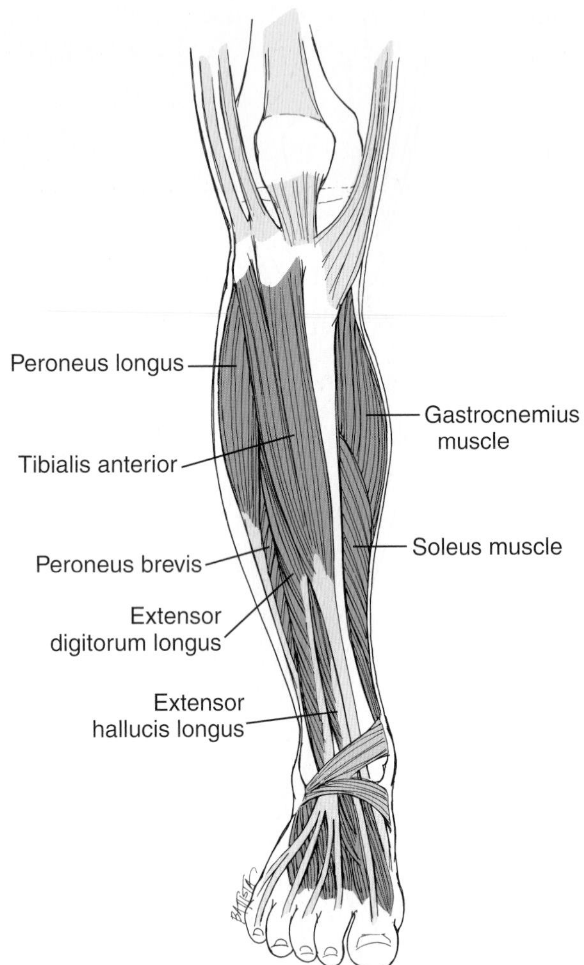

Figure 9-5. Muscles of the anterior compartment of the leg include the tibialis anterior, the extensor digitorum longus, and the EHL.

longus and the peroneus brevis. The common peroneal nerve serves this compartment as well (see Fig. 8-10).

- The **superficial posterior compartment** contains the two heads of the gastrocnemius, the soleus, and the plantaris. The superficial and deep compartments contain the foot and ankle flexors (plantar flexors) and are served by the tibial nerve. The gastrocnemius and soleus form the Achilles tendon, the main plantar flexor of the ankle (see Fig. 9-6).
- The **deep posterior compartment** contains the popliteus, flexor hallucis longus, flexor digitorum longus, and tibialis posterior (see Fig. 9-7).

- ***Function***: The gastrocnemius and soleus must maintain some contraction during relaxed standing posture so the body does not fall forward, as the center of gravity is in front of the ankle.[4] The muscles of the leg provide dynamic support to the knee, ankle, and foot and are responsible for fine postural control, movement of the body, and dynamic stability to the foot and ankle. As with all muscles, they contain muscle spindles and Golgi tendon organs that have reflexive connections to the mechanoreceptors in the soft tissue surrounding the joints, including the ligaments and the joint capsule. The other muscles have functions for the foot and ankle and are discussed in the section "Muscles of the Ankle and Foot," p. 339.
- ***Dysfunction and injury:*** The most commonly injured muscle of the leg is the gastrocnemius. This muscle is called a two-joint muscle because it crosses the knee and the ankle. The gastrocnemius is more commonly injured because one of the main functions of this muscle is eccentric contraction (i.e., to contract while the muscle is lengthening). Muscles are much more prone to injury during eccentric contraction. Achilles tendinitis is the most common tendinitis of the leg.

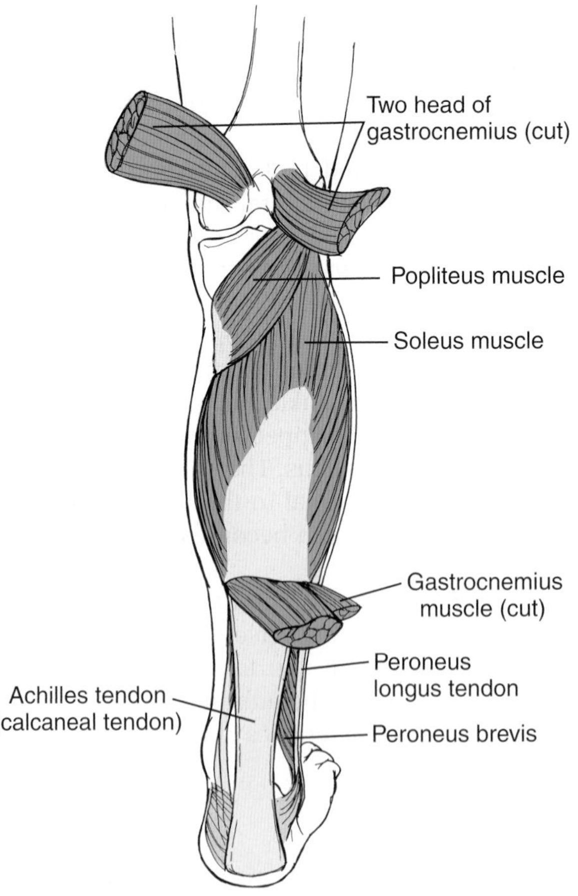

Figure 9-6. Superficial posterior compartment showing the gastrocnemius cut away to reveal the underlying soleus.

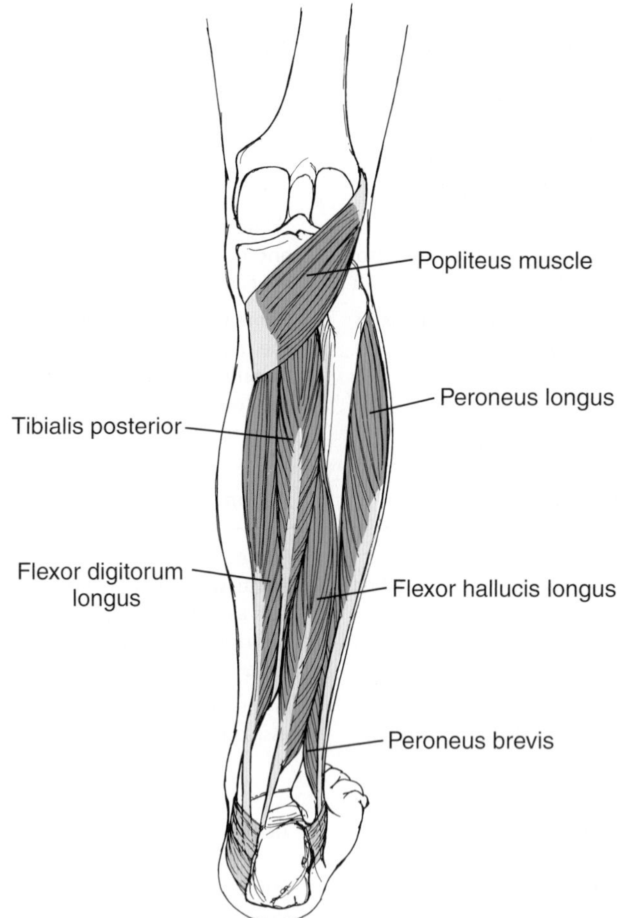

Figure 9-7. Deep posterior compartment showing the tibialis posterior, flexor digitorum longus, and the flexor hallucis longus.

Muscle cramps in the gastrocnemius and soleus are also common. The cramps typically occur as a result of salt depletion and after prolonged activity.[5] The exact cause is not clearly understood, and low calcium is also implicated.

Muscle Imbalances of the Leg

Two basic categories of muscle dysfunction are muscle imbalance and positional dysfunction. Muscle imbalance describes a condition in which certain muscles tend to be weak, and others tend to be short and tight. Muscle imbalances alter movement patterns and therefore add a continuing stress to the joint system. In the leg, Janda[16] has described certain predictable patterns of muscle imbalance.

- **Muscles that tend to be tight and short:** Triceps surae (gastrocnemius and soleus) and the tibialis posterior are tight, short muscles.
- **Muscles that tend to be inhibited and weak:** Tibialis anterior and the peroneals are inhibited, weak muscles.

Positional Dysfunction of the Leg Muscles

- The gastrocnemius tends to develop a torsion that pulls it to the midline. With a pronated ankle the triceps surae (gastrocnemius and soleus) is pulled laterally. The other muscles are contained so tightly within their fascial compartments that no other positional dysfunctions occur.

- *Treatment implications:* Muscle cramps are treated with passive stretching. The other muscles' dysfunctions and injuries are treated with MET and OM as described in the "Technique" section.

Muscles of the Leg (Extrinsic Muscles of the Ankle and Foot)

See Muscle Table 9-1.

Anatomy, Function, and Dysfunction of the Leg

BONES AND JOINTS OF THE ANKLE

See Fig. 9-1.

- *Structure*: The ankle is the articulation between the talus and the tibia and fibula and is referred to as the **talotibial joint.** The body weight is transferred from the femur, through the tibia to the talus, and then to the calcaneus, the main contact point with the ground. The ankle joint is referred to as a mortice, as the distal ends of the tibia and fibula, called malleoli, form a socket that holds the talus in between them. On the medial side of the talus is a groove for the flexor hallucis longus tendon.
- *Function*: The ankle is a synovial joint with two possible motions, flexion and extension. At the ankle, flexion and extension are called plantar flexion and dorsiflexion, respectively. The foot moves within the ankle due to the contraction of the gastrocnemius–soleus muscles that create plantar flexion and the muscles of the anterior leg that cause dorsiflexion. The ankle joint faces approximately 15° laterally in its neutral position, since the medial malleolus is anterior to the lateral malleolus. It produces a normal toe-out stance, which is referred to as the **Fick**

TABLE 9-1 MUSCLES OF THE LEG (EXTRINSIC MUSCLES OF THE ANKLE AND FOOT)

Anterior Compartment

Muscle	*Origin*	*Insertion*	*Action*
Tibialis anterior	Upper two thirds of the lateral surface of the tibia.	Medial and plantar surface of the medial cuneiform bone and the base of the first metatarsal.	Prime mover for dorsiflexion and inversion of the foot.
Extensor digitorum longus	Lateral condyle of the tibia, the upper three-fourths of the anterior surface of the fibula.	Dorsal aspects of the four lesser toes and their extensor expansions.	Prime mover for toe extension and dorsiflexion and for eversion of the foot.
Extensor hallucis longus	Anterior surface of the fibula and of the interosseous membrane, at the middle half of the leg.	Base of the distal phalanx of the great toe.	Prime mover for extension of the great toe; assists with dorsiflexion and inversion of the foot.

Lateral Compartment

Muscle	*Origin*	*Insertion*	*Action*
Peroneus longus	Lateral condyle of the tibia and the upper two thirds of the lateral aspect of the fibula.	Lateral side of the first cuneiform bone and the first metatarsal.	Prime mover for eversion; assists with plantar flexion; acts as a bowstring, bracing the transverse arch of the foot.
Peroneus brevis	Lower two thirds of the lateral surface of the fibula.	Tuberosity at the proximal end of the fifth metatarsal.	Prime mover for eversion; assists with plantar flexion.

Posterior or Superficial (Triceps Surae) Compartment

Muscle	*Origin*	*Insertion*	*Action*
Gastrocnemius	By two tendons from the posterior aspect of the condyles of the femur; some fibers also arise from the capsule of the knee.	Posterior surface of the calcaneus as the Achilles tendon.	Prime mover for plantar flexion; assists with knee flexion; stabilizes the femur on the tibia.
Soleus	Upper part of the posterior surfaces of the tibia, fibula, and interosseous membrane.	By the Achilles tendon into the calcaneus.	Prime mover for plantar flexion; stabilizes the lower leg on the tarsus.
Plantaris	Posterior, lateral femoral condyle proximal to gastrocnemius; joint capsule.	Blends with the medial edge of the Achilles tendon.	Weak assistant for knee and plantar flexion.

Posterior or Deep Compartment

Muscle	*Origin*	*Insertion*	*Action*
Popliteus	Lateral condyle of the femur.	Posterior surface of the tibia.	Flexes leg; rotates femur medially.
Flexor hallucis longus	Inferior two thirds of the posterior surface of the fibula and from the lowest part of the interosseous membrane.	Under surface of the base of the last phalanx of the great toe.	Prime mover for flexion of the great toe; assists with plantar flexion and inversion of the foot.
Flexor digitorum longus	Posterior surface of the body of the tibia from just below the popliteal line and from the fascia covering the tibialis posterior.	Bases of the distal phalanges of the four small toes; each tendon passes through an opening in the corresponding tendon of the flexor digitorum brevis.	Prime mover for flexion of the second through fifth toes; assists with plantar flexion and inversion.
Tibialis posterior	Upper half of the posterior surface of the interosseous membrane and the adjacent parts of the tibia and fibula.	Tuberosity on the inferior surface of the navicular and the three cuneiform bones.	Prime mover for inversion; assists with plantar flexion.

angle. Because of this angle, dorsiflexion elicits an up and out movement of the foot, and plantar flexion results in the foot moving down and medially.

- *Dysfunction and injury:* If the ankle is in its neutral position, there is a vertical alignment through the tibia, talus, and calcaneus (heel bone). **Pronation** is a common weight-bearing dysfunction in which the talus is positioned anteriorly and medially, and the bottom of the heel angles laterally (everts). **Hallux valgus,** or lateral deviation of the great toe, and pain in the great toe may develop as a result of pronation. Leg pain can also develop from pronation caused by excessive tension of the anterior and posterior tibialis, and knee pain is common because of lateral tracking of the patella from the genu valgus position of the knee associated with pronation.[7] Traumatic injuries to the ankle bones or joints often leave the area fibrotic, decreasing the normal range of motion (ROM) in the joint, typically causing a loss of dorsiflexion.
- *Treatment implications*: Loss of joint motion in the ankle is treated initially with MET. OM is performed on the periarticular soft tissue (i.e., the soft tissue surrounding the joint) to dissolve adhesions and to allow for greater extensibility. PIR MET is performed on the short and tight muscles, especially the gastrocnemius and soleus, which may be inhibiting the normal ROM of the joint. And finally, mobilization is performed to stimulate the nutritional exchange in the cartilage and to help dissolve calcium deposits on the articular surfaces. Perform CR MET to help strengthen the intrinsic muscles of the feet and the anterior and posterior tibialis muscles.

SOFT-TISSUE STRUCTURES OF THE ANKLE

Joint Capsule and Ligaments

- *Structure*: The joint capsule of the ankle joint is thin and provides little support. The ligaments and muscles provide passive and dynamic stability, respectively. The ligaments on the medial and lateral sides can be grouped together as the medial and lateral collateral ligaments.
    - The **medial collateral ligament** is also called the **deltoid ligament** and consists of fibers that run from the medial malleolus to the navicular, talus, and calcaneus. These ligament fibers blend into one another, unlike the lateral collateral ligament, which is formed from separate bands (Fig. 9-8).

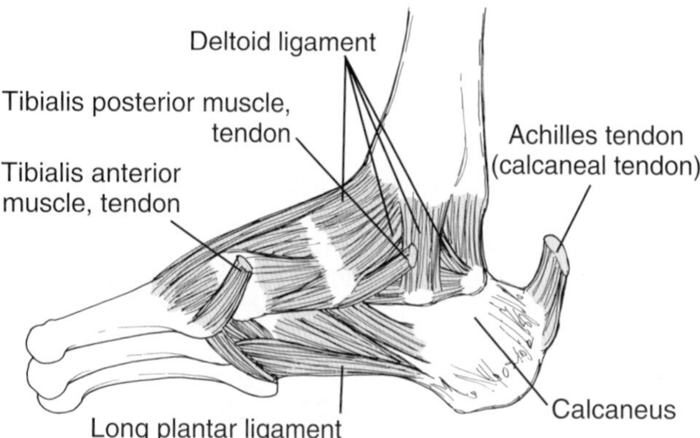

Figure 9-8. Ligaments and tendons of the medial ankle.

    - The **lateral collateral ligament** consists of the anterior and posterior talofibular ligaments and the calcaneofibular ligaments (Fig. 9-9).
- *Function*: The joint capsule and ligaments of the ankle provide passive stability to the ankle and foot. In plantar flexion, the anterior talofibular ligament restricts inversion of the talus. The ligaments also have a dense population of mechanoreceptors that function in the control of posture and movement. Arthrokinetic and arthrostatic reflexes exist between these mechanoreceptors and the muscles of the leg that function to provide instantaneous and precise contractions for control of the foot and ankle in movement and fine postural control.[8]
- *Dysfunction and injury*: Ankle sprains are injuries to the ligaments. The **anterior talofibular** is the weakest ligament of the ankle, the first ligament to be affected in an inversion stress, and the most commonly injured ligament of the ankle.[8] Injury occurs as a result of either acute or cumulative inversion stress for two anatomic reasons: one, the distal end of the fibula extends further than the tibia and helps provide lateral stability and two, the deltoid ligament is much stronger than the lateral collateral ligaments. After an ankle sprain, two outcomes are possible. One, the ankle becomes fibrous and stiff with a decreased ROM. Two, the ankle becomes unstable. Studies show that approximately 40% of injuries to the lateral ligament of the ankle lead to the feeling that the foot tends to "give way."[2] Freeman et al.[2] suggest that the ankle becomes unstable because of a partial loss of the normal reflex activity between the mechanoreceptors of the capsule and ligaments and the calf muscles.
- *Treatment implications*: If the ankle ligaments have become fibrous and thickened due to the deposit of excessive collagen after an injury, perform CR MET

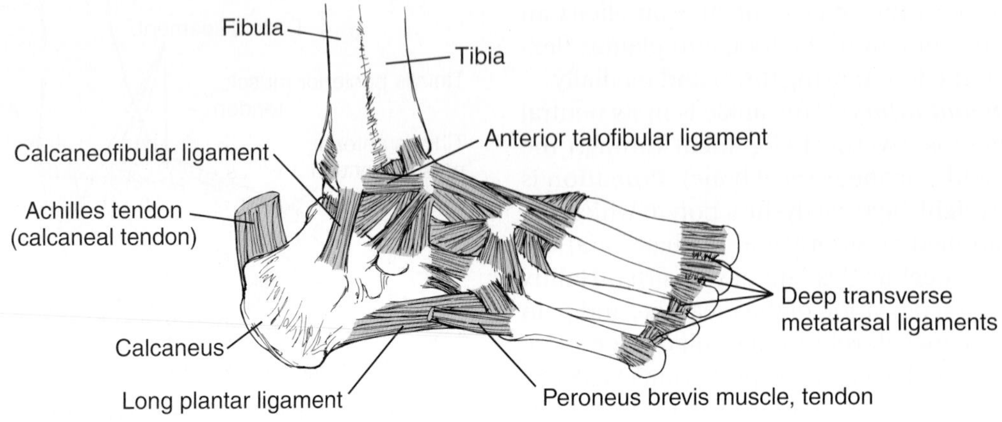

Figure 9-9. Ligaments and tendons of the lateral ankle.

to the muscles that cross the ankle, as this increases the extensibility to the ligaments. Next, perform OM, including transverse friction massage, to the body and attachment points of the ligaments. This combined treatment helps dissolve the adhesions and restore the normal extensibility. Decreased passive glide of the ankle is treated with mobilization. If the ligaments have become too slack and the ankle is unstable, exercise rehabilitation is recommended, including balance and proprioception exercises to restore normal neurologic function.

Ligaments of the Ankle

See Table 9-2.

Nerves of the Ankle

See Figures 9-3**A** and **B** and 9-4.

- *Structure*: The deep peroneal nerve passes under the extensor retinaculum of the ankle to the dorsum of the foot. The superficial peroneal nerve travels under the skin on the anterolateral ankle and foot. The posterior tibial nerve travels behind the medial malleolus between the superficial and the deep layers of the flexor retinaculum, in what is called the **tarsal tunnel.**
- *Function*: The deep peroneal nerve supplies the anterior compartment and provides sensation to the webspace between the first and the second toes. The

TABLE 9-2 LIGAMENTS OF THE ANKLE

The tibiofibular-talar joint, or ankle joint, is stabilized medially by the medial collateral ligament complex and laterally by the lateral collateral ligament complex. The following ligaments are listed in the order of frequency of injury.

Ligament	*Origin*	*Insertion*
Anterior talofibular ligament (part of lateral collateral ligament)	Lateral malleolus (fibula)	Neck of the talus
Calcaneofibular (part of lateral collateral ligament)	Distal fibula	Calcaneus
Calcaneocuboid	Distal aspect of the lateral calcaneus	Lateral surface of the cuboid
Anterior tibiofibular	Distal aspect of the lateral tibia	Distal aspect of the medial fibula
Deltoid ligament (medial collateral ligament)	Comprises the tibionavicular, tibiocalcaneal, and the anterior and posterior tibiotalar ligaments; originates at the distal tibia	Inserts on the navicular, talus, and calcaneus

superficial peroneal nerve supplies the skin to the dorsum of the foot. The posterior tibial nerve supplies the intrinsic muscles of the foot and provides sensation to the bottom of the foot through its branches, the medial and lateral plantar nerves (see the section "Nerves of the Foot").

- *Dysfunction and injury*: Entrapment of the nerves that cross the ankle is common. The posterior tibial nerve can become compressed in the tarsal tunnel owing to injury to the ankle or to pronation. The deep peroneal nerve can become compressed under the extensor retinaculum because of ankle injury, tight-laced boots, or high heels.
- *Treatment implications*: As in the other areas of the body, the nerves are released by gentle scooping strokes, transverse to the line of the nerve. This treatment releases the adhesions and takes the nerve out of tension.

Muscles of the Ankle and Foot

- *Structure*: Thirty-one muscles contribute to foot and ankle movements. Of these 31 muscles, 11 originate in the leg and are called extrinsic muscles of the foot, and 20 originate in the foot and are called intrinsic. All the muscles of the calf cross the ankle as tendons and insert on the foot. They are held in place by the retinaculum described above. These tendons have tendon sheaths as they cross the ankle and are therefore susceptible to tenosynovitis and stenosing tenosynovitis in this region. The muscles and tendons may be divided into four categories, depending on function and location.

    - The **flexors** pass behind the medial malleolus and under the flexor retinaculum, and each is contained within its own synovial sheath. The flexors from anterior to posterior (A–P) are the tibialis posterior, the flexor digitorum longus, and the flexor hallucis longus (see Fig. 8-9).
    - The **extensors** cross on the dorsum of the foot under the superior and inferior extensor retinaculum, each within its own synovial sheath. The extensors include the tibialis anterior, the EHL, and the extensor digitorum longus (see Fig. 9-5).
    - The **evertors** pass behind the lateral malleolus under the superior and inferior peroneal retinaculum through a common peroneal sheath. The peroneals exit the common sheath distal to the inferior retinaculum (see Fig. 8-10).
    - The **invertors** are the anterior and posterior tibialis.

- *Function*: Ankle muscles provide dynamic stability to the ankle and foot. The muscles are responsible for postural control, balance, coordination, and movement.
- *Dysfunction and injury*: With excessive or repetitive ankle stress, such as running, dancing, and hiking or with chronic postural stress, such as from pronation, the synovial lining in the tendon sheaths can become irritated and inflamed where they cross the ankle. In the acute stage it manifests as local pain and swelling at the involved tendon. In the chronic phase, thickening may develop on the sheath due to the fibrous deposition from the inflammation and leads to a narrowing of the sheath, called a **stenosing tenosynovitis.**
- *Treatment implications*: The tendons of the ankle are treated with OM, stroking transverse to the line of the tendon. Adhesions around or in the tendon sheath are treated with transverse friction massage. To reduce the hypertonicity in the muscle–tendon unit, perform CR MET. To lengthen a shortened muscle–tendon unit, perform PIR MET.

Muscular Actions of the Ankle

See Table 9-3.

Anatomy, Function, and Dysfunction of the Foot

BONES AND JOINTS OF THE FOOT

See Figure 9-1.

- *Structure*: The foot contains 26 bones and 30 joints, and it may be divided into the hindfoot, midfoot, and forefoot. The **hindfoot** consists of the talus and calcaneus. The **midfoot** consists of the navicular, the cuboid, and the three cuneiforms. The **forefoot** consists of the 5 metatarsals and the 14 phalanges that make up the 5 toes.
- *Function*: The motions of the foot are dorsiflexion, plantar flexion, inversion, and eversion. Inversion is the combination of adduction, supination (elevation of the medial margin), and plantar flexion. Eversion is abduction, pronation (lowering of the medial margin of the foot), and dorsiflexion. The toes may flex, extend, abduct, and adduct. Normal function of the foot is essential for fine postural control. It must

TABLE 9-3 MUSCULAR ACTIONS OF THE ANKLE

The ankle is the articulation of the talus bone with the tibia and fibula. It is a hinge-type joint capable of two movements: flexion (plantarflexion) and extension (dorsiflexion).

Plantarflexion

Eight muscles contribute to plantar flexion; seven of these muscles span two joints.

- Gastrocnemius
- Soleus
- Peroneus longus—also causes eversion of the foot and helps maintain the arch of the foot
- Peroneus brevis—also causes eversion of the foot
- Flexor digitorum longus—also inverts the foot and flexes the toes
- Tibialis posterior—also assists in inversion
- Flexor hallucis longus—flexes the big toe, inverts the foot, plantar flexes the ankle
- Plantaris

Dorsiflexion

Four muscles contribute to dorsiflexion.

- Tibialis anterior—also inverts the foot
- Extensor digitorum longus—also extends the toes, and everts the foot
- EHL—also extends the great toe
- Peroneus tertius—also everts the foot

---

have adequate mobility for proper gait and to accommodate uneven surfaces. It must also have stability for sustained weight bearing and strength for dynamic movement of the body. In the following section, the joints are described individually for clarification.

Subtalar (Talocalcaneal) Joint

- *Structure*: The **subtalar or talocalcaneal** joint is the articulation between the calcaneus (heel) and the talus.
- *Function*: The subtalar joint has two possible motions, inversion and eversion. In the normal standing posture, the tibia, talus, and calcaneus are in vertical alignment.
- *Dysfunction and injury*: If the calcaneus angles laterally into a valgus position, it is associated with **pronation,** and if it angles medially into a varus position, it is associated with supination. A valgus heel creates an eversion of the forefoot, is associated with the lateral deviation of the great toe (hallux valgus), and causes the Achilles tendon to deviate laterally and to shorten.[4]

Pronation may result from weak supination muscles (e.g., the triceps surae, tibialis posterior, flexor hallucis longus, flexor digitorum longus, and tibialis anterior). It may also be caused by a shortness of the peroneus longus, the strongest pronator. If pronation becomes chronic, fibrous deposition at the anterior mortice and a loss of full dorsiflexion of the ankle occur.

Pes varus or clubfoot is the condition in which the heel angles medially and contributes to supination. This angulation may be caused by weakness in the pronators, including the peroneals, extensor digitorum longus, and EHL, or it may be caused by a shortness of the supinators, including the triceps surae and flexor digitorum longus.[10]

Metatarsophalangeal Joints

- *Structure*: The metatarsophalangeal (MTP) joints are the articulation of the metatarsals and phalanges (toes). They are synovial joints with a joint capsule and three ligaments: the plantar, transverse metatarsal, and collateral (see the section, "Ligaments of the Foot"). On the plantar surface of the head of the first metatarsal are two **sesamoid bones,** the medial and the lateral, which lie in the plantar ligament, the joint capsule, and the tendons of the flexor hallucis brevis. The medial sesamoid is also the attachment site for the abductor hallucis, and the lateral sesamoid is also the attachment site of the oblique and transverse heads of the adductor hallucis.
- *Function*: The MTP joint has four possible motions: flexion, extension, adduction, and abduction. When a person stands on one leg, 100% of the body weight comes through the talus, then 50% of the weight moves posteriorly to the heel, and 50% forward. The first MTP joint carries 25% of that forward-moving weight, and the lateral four toes carry the other 25%.[9,11]

The great toe stabilizes the foot and assists in the push-off phase during gait. The great toe extends (dorsiflexes) with every step, some 900 times a day.[4] The first MTP must be capable of 45° to 60° of extension at toe-off phase, or the gait is altered, leading to compensation and potential degeneration in the foot, ankle, knee, and hip. As in other areas of the body, the sesamoids function to help distribute pressure and reduce friction.

- *Dysfunction and injury*: The first MTP joint is a common site of degeneration and dysfunction. Functional **hallux limitus** is the inability of the proximal phalanx to extend on the first metatarsal head during the push-off phase of gait. Through either acute or repetitive stress to this joint, inflammation degenerates the cartilage and thickens the joint capsule and causes **hallux rigidus,** a fusion of the first MTP joint. With weight distribution imbalances, such as pronation, the great toe migrates laterally, called **hallux valgus.** The toe-out position improves balance and may also compensate for lower-back dysfunction or injury or for decreased dorsiflexion of the ankle. With a loss of the arches, the foot loses its soft-tissue shock absorbers, and the weight falls on the metatarsal heads, irritating the MTP joints and potentially causing pain at the metatarsal heads or MTP joints, a condition called **metatarsalgia.** Pain under the great toe may be inflammation of the sesamoids, a condition called **sesamoiditis.** Sesamoiditis may develop because of a high arch, or the wearing high heels, or of a hallus valgus. Lateral deviation of the great toe (hallus valgus) creates a subluxation of the sesamoids laterally.
- *Treatment implications*: Acute irritation or inflammation of the great toe is best treated with CR MET of the flexors and extensors of the great toe. Chronic conditions need to be assessed for weight distribution problems, such as pronation, genu valgus, or leg-length imbalances. As always, the primary intention in performing treatment is to reduce the hypertonicity in the tight or short muscles and then to facilitate (strengthen) the weak muscles. OM is performed on the joint capsule, and mobilization is performed on the joints. Chronic imbalances often require a referral to a physical therapist or to a personal trainer for proper instruction in developing the strength to maintain proper alignment. The sesamoids are mobilized in a medial direction to help correct the positional dysfunction.

Interphalangeal Joints

- *Structure*: The interphalangeal (IP) joints of the toes are synovial joints with an articular capsule and two collateral ligaments. Two joints, called the proximal interphalangeal (PIP) joints and the distal interphalangeal (DIP) joints, exist between the phalanges of all the toes except for the great toe.
- *Function*: The IP joints serve to balance, stabilize, and coordinate the motions of the foot. They have two possible motions, flexion and extension.
- *Dysfunction and injury*: The toes can become inflamed through injury or from the cumulative stress of weight-bearing dysfunction in the foot. One result of acute or chronic inflammation is fibrosis of the joint capsule of the IP joints, leading to a condition called **hammer toes.** Hammer toes are hyperextension of MTP joints and flexion contracture of PIP. **Claw toes** describes a condition in which the PIP and the DIP are held in a sustained flexion, combined with hyperextension of MTP joints. Both hammer toe and claw toe can develop if the intrinsic muscles of the foot are weak and if the extrinsic toe extensors are in a sustained contraction.
- *Treatment implications*: Perform PIR MET on the toe extensors and suggest exercises for the intrinsics of the toes, such as picking up a sock with the toes. Hammer toes and claw toes are often caused by a complex combination of factors. These conditions typically require a referral to a physical therapist for proper instruction in a strengthening and stretching program.

SOFT-TISSUE STRUCTURES OF THE FOOT

Ligaments of the Foot

The clinically important ligaments of the foot may be described by location (Fig. 9-10).

Ligaments of the Metatarsophalangeal Joints

- The **plantar ligaments (plantar plate)** are thick, dense, and fibrous or fibrocartilaginous structures firmly attached to the bases of the proximal phalanges but loosely attached to the heads of the metatarsal bones. They are grooved for the flexor tendons.
- The **transverse metatarsal ligaments** consist of four short bands that have both superficial and deep layers. The heads of all the metatarsals are connected together by the deep layer. The plantar digital nerve travels between the superficial and the deep layers.
- The **collateral ligaments** are two strong, rounded cords, located on the medial and lateral sides of the MTP joints. These ligaments connect the head of the metatarsal to the base of the phalanx.

Ligaments of the Interphalangeal Joints

- The **collateral ligaments** wrap around the IP joints like a sleeve. The fibers are oriented in a proximal to distal direction following the shaft of the bone. They help guide the flexion and extension movements of the IP joints.

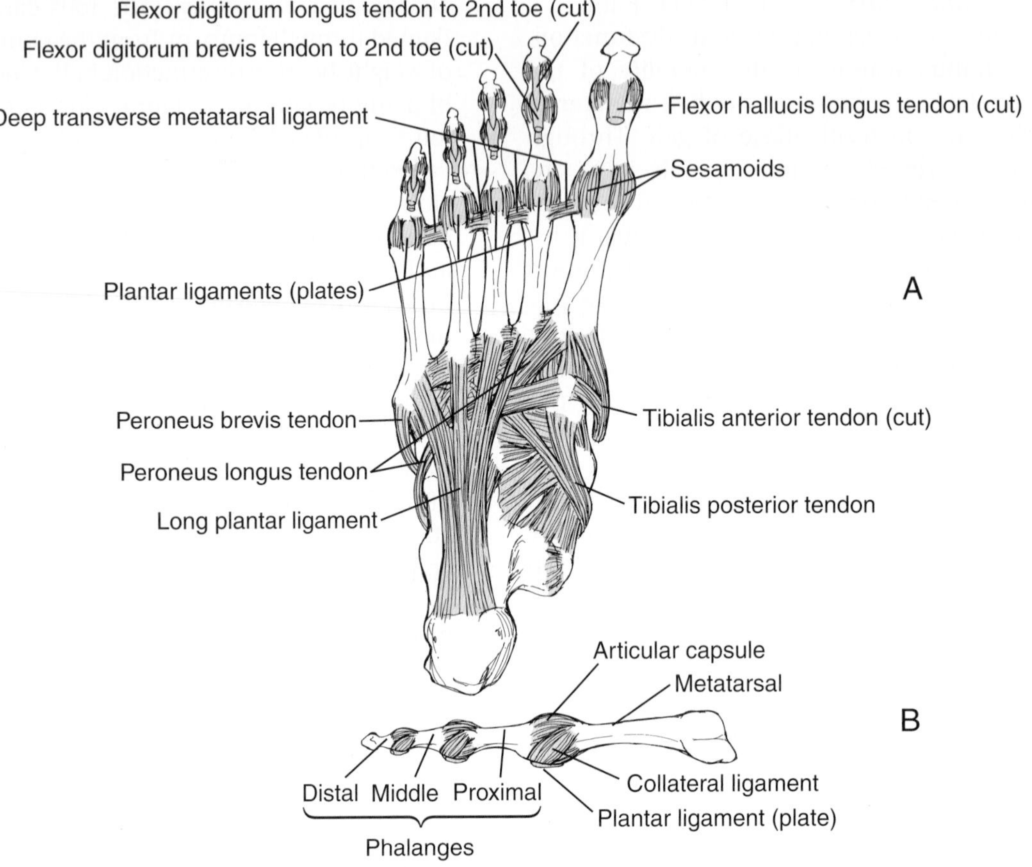

Figure 9-10. A. Ligaments and tendon insertions on the plantar aspect (bottom) of the foot. **B.** Joint capsule and collateral ligaments of the MTP and IP joints. Note that the fibers of the joint capsule are aligned parallel to the shaft of the bone and that the collateral ligaments are angled in a dorsal to plantar direction.

- The **plantar ligament** is a fibrocartilaginous thickening of the joint capsule at the plantar surface of the joint. Sesamoids may be part of the plantar ligament.

- *Function*: As in each joint of the body, the joint capsule and associated ligaments provide passive stability to the joint and play a role in muscle function, coordination, and balance through reflexes between the mechanoreceptors of the ligaments and the surrounding muscles.
- *Dysfunction and injury*: The transverse metatarsal ligament is important clinically because it tends to thicken caused by static or dynamic stresses. This thickening pulls the metatarsal heads closer together and causes an irritation of the joints. The thickening also can lead to an entrapment in the plantar digital nerve that travels through the superficial and deep layers and can potentially lead to a fibrous deposit, called a **neuroma,** on the nerve. The collateral ligaments of the IP joints thicken because of fibrosis and contribute to loss of IP joint motion and to hammer toe and claw toes (see above).
- *Treatment implications*: The ligaments of the foot are treated with two different strokes. Either deep, back-and-forth scooping strokes transverse to the line of the fiber or brisk transverse friction strokes.

Plantar Fascia

See Figure 9-11.

- *Structure*: By interweaving with the deep transverse metatarsal ligament, the plantar fascia thickens in the middle of the foot into an aponeurosis that is a dense band of fascia from the calcaneus to the proximal phalanx of each toe.[11] The plantar aponeurosis splits at the MTP joints to allow for the passage of the flexor tendons.
- *Function*: The plantar fascia contributes significantly to the longitudinal arch. The plantar fascia extends into four deep septa or connective tissue spaces that contain the muscles of the sole of the foot.
- *Dysfunction and injury*: Irritation of the **plantar fascia** is called plantar fasciitis and may be caused by

excessive dynamic loading, such as running, or by cumulative static stresses such as excessive standing. Irritation causes a pain on the heel, usually on the anterior medial surface, that is often worse in the morning. The attachment of the fascia interweaves with the periosteum of the heel, and excessive pulling on the fascia and periosteum can cause a traction spur, called a **heel spur.** Heel spurs are also found in approximately 10% of the nonsymptomatic population.[4]

- ***Treatment implications***: To treat plantar fasciitis and heel pain perform transverse massage on the fascia, relieve the tension on the crural fascia, and reduce the hypertonicity of the muscles of the foot. Lauren Berry, RPT, taught a method of using a blunt tool, such as the knuckle of the second MTP joint or a T-bar, to treat heel spurs. Deep, brisk strokes are performed in all directions on the heel to dissolve small calcium spicules and fibrous depositions on the heel.

Arches of the Foot

- ***Structure***: The **longitudinal (medial) arch** describes the area from the calcaneus to the first metatarsal head. The **transverse arch** describes the area of the midtarsal region, with the middle cuneiform as the highest point. The shape of the foot bones forms the longitudinal and transverse plantar arches, which are maintained by ligamentous and muscular support. Genetic factors influence the height of the longitudinal arch.
    - **Ligamentous support:** The order of importance for ligamentous support for the arches is as follows: the spring ligament (plantar calcaneonavicular), the long plantar ligament, the plantar aponeurosis, and the short plantar ligament (plantar calcaneocuboid).[11]
    - **Muscular support:** The anterior and posterior tibialis muscles and the intrinsic plantar muscles support the medial arch.
- ***Function***: The arches are designed as shock absorbers and provide mobility to accommodate uneven surfaces.
- ***Dysfunction and injury:*** The loss of the arches is referred to as **pes planus** or **flat foot.** This loss may be caused by femoral anteversion, pronation, weakness of the intrinsic plantar muscles, weakness of the anterior and posterior tibialis, or loss of plantar ligament integrity resulting from static stress, such as standing on the feet all day. Loss of the arch places much more stress on the plantar fascia, and the fascia tends to thicken. In a person who has flat feet, much more muscle action is required, which makes the muscles more susceptible to fatigue and pain.[7] A high arch is referred to as **pes cavus** and may involve short plantar ligaments, tight intrinsics of the sole of the foot, or tight anterior and posterior tibialis muscles.
- ***Treatment implications***: To treat a flat foot, perform MET on the anterior and the posterior tibialis muscles and provide manual release of the tight intrinsics with OM. A low arch is treated with exercise rehabilitation.

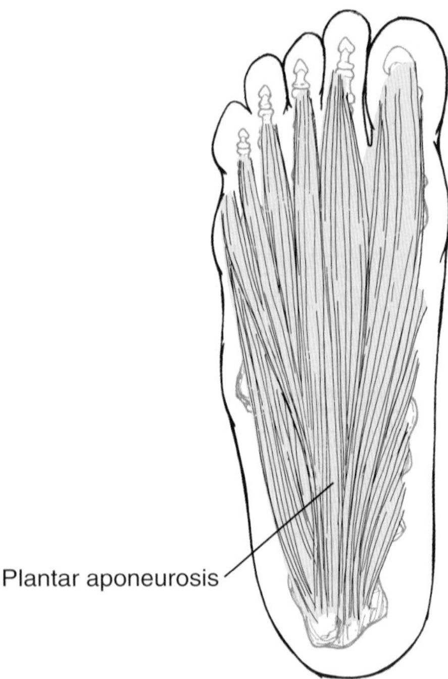

Figure 9-11. Plantar aponeurosis is a thickening of the deep fascia on the sole of the foot.

Nerves of the Foot

See Figures 9-3 and 9-4.

- ***Structure***: The posterior tibial nerve branches into the medial and lateral plantar nerves. They continue as the interdigital nerves, traveling between the superficial and the deep layers of the transverse metatarsal ligament. The deep peroneal nerve travels under the extensor retinaculum at the ankle. The superficial peroneal nerve travels under the skin into the dorsum of the foot. The sural nerve travels to the lateral heel.
- ***Function***: The medial and lateral plantar nerves supply the intrinsic muscles on the plantar aspect of the foot and give sensation to the bottom of the foot. The interdigital nerves receive sensory information from the toes. The deep peroneal nerve supplies the extensor digitorum brevis and the extensor hallucis

brevis and provides sensation to the webspace between the first and the second toes. The superficial peroneal nerve supplies the skin to the dorsum of the foot. The sural nerve supplies sensation to the lateral heel and side of foot.

- *Dysfunction and injury*: Entrapment of the interdigital nerve is a frequent cause of metatarsal head pain.[4] Morton's neuroma is a chronic irritation of the interdigital nerve that results in a fibrous deposition on the nerve.
- *Treatment implications*: Release the interdigital nerves by first releasing the transverse metatarsal ligament. Stroke the nerves transverse to the line of the nerve.

Muscles

- *Structure:* Intrinsic muscles of the feet consist of 20 muscles that have origins and insertions in the foot. Of these 20, 18 are on the sole of the foot and may be divided into 4 layers by their fascia.

  Extrinsic foot muscles consist of 11 muscles that have origins in the leg and insertions in the foot. Three tendons form a sling by crossing from one side of the foot to the opposite side. These three muscles assist in holding the foot in a neutral position and are the tibialis anterior and the peroneus longus (these attach to the base of the first metatarsal) and the tibialis posterior (this attaches to the navicular, cuboid, and base of the second, third, and fourth metatarsals).

- *Function*: The extrinsic muscles help support the arches, act as shock absorbers for the foot, and provide dynamic stability to the ankle and foot. The intrinsic muscles of the foot provide fine adjustments for coordination and balance, help provide dynamic stability, and help maintain the arch. The muscles of the foot have nerves that communicate with the surrounding joints through the joint capsules and ligaments. The mechanoreceptors in the capsules and ligaments sense position, movement, and irritation and stimulate muscle contraction or weakness (inhibition). Also, instantaneous righting reflexes occur from the foot to the muscles of the leg.
- *Dysfunction and injury*: Muscles of the feet are susceptible to cumulative stresses caused by dynamic activity and to the static stress of standing for prolonged periods. Strain of the foot muscles is associated with running, hiking, dancing, basketball, and other such activity. However, muscular activity offers dynamic stability. With disuse, injury, pronation, or inadequate footwear, the muscles weaken, and the ligaments and capsules are excessively loaded, leading to collapse of the arches of the foot and creating pain in the soft tissue.

Muscle Imbalances of the Leg, Ankle, and Foot

- **Muscles that tend to be tight and short:** The extrinsic plantar flexors and the extensors of the toes are usually tight, short muscles. The intrinsic muscles are usually tight but functionally weak because of the phenomenon of tightness weakness. The adductor hallucis is typically tight, contributing to hallux valgus.
- **Muscles that tend to be inhibited and weak:** The extrinsic dorsiflexors are usually tight but functionally weak because of the phenomenon of tightness weakness. The abductor hallucis and the intrinsic muscles, including the lumbricals and interossei, are usually functionally weak, except for the adductor hallucis.

Positional Dysfunction of the Muscles of the Leg, Ankle, and Foot

- The gastrocnemius and soleus (Achilles tendon) and the flexor hallucis brevis tend to be pulled laterally.

Intrinsic Muscles of the Foot

See Muscle Table 9-4 and Figures 9-12, 9-13, 9-14, 9-15.

Muscles of the Dorsum of the Foot

See Figure 9-16 and Muscle Table 9-5.

Muscular Actions of the Foot

See Table 9-6.

Dysfunction and Injury of the Leg, Ankle, and Foot

FACTORS PREDISPOSING TO PAIN IN THE LEG, ANKLE, AND FOOT

- Leg-length inequality
- Pelvic unlevelling
- Femoral anteversion
- Genu valgus or genu varus
- Pronation (valgus position of the talus or calcaneus) or supination (varus position of the talus or calcaneus)

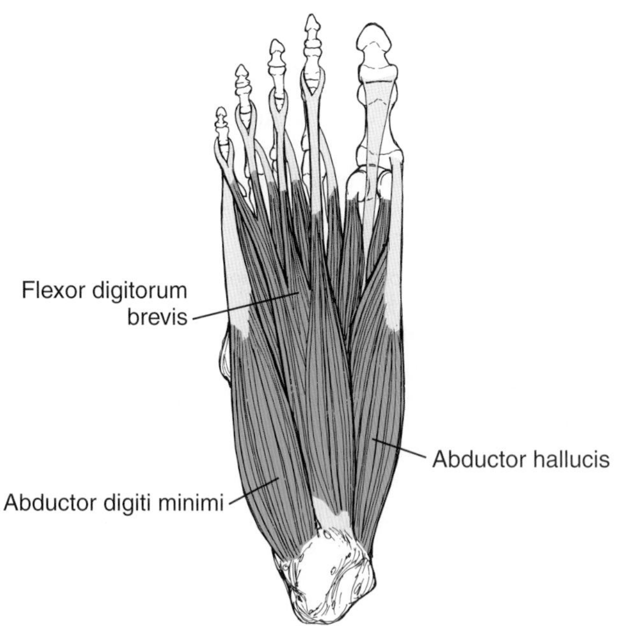

Figure 9-12. First layer of muscles on the plantar aspect of the foot includes the abductor hallucis, flexor digitorum brevis, and the abductor digiti minimi.

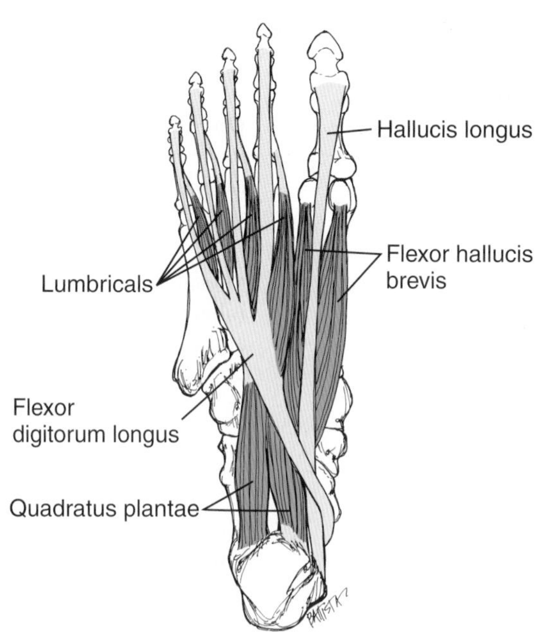

Figure 9-13. Second layer of plantar muscles includes the quadratus plantae and the four lumbrical muscles.

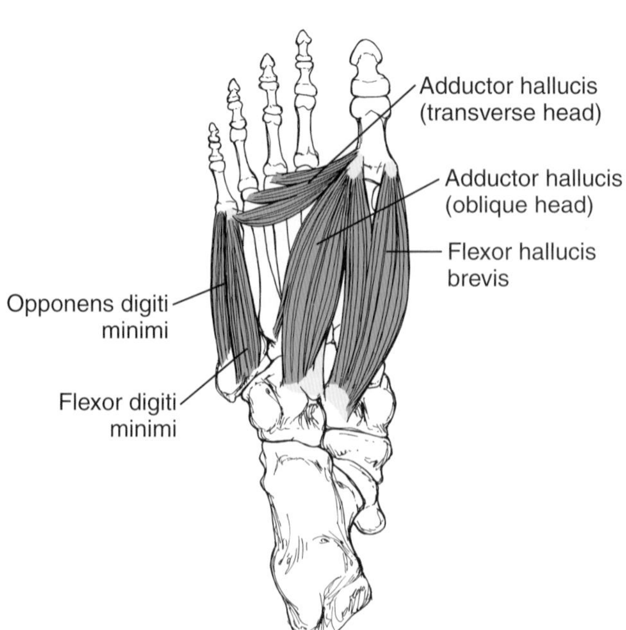

Figure 9-14. Third layer of muscles on the bottom of the foot includes the flexor hallucis brevis, flexor digiti minimi, opponens digiti minimi, and oblique and transverse heads of the adductor hallucis.

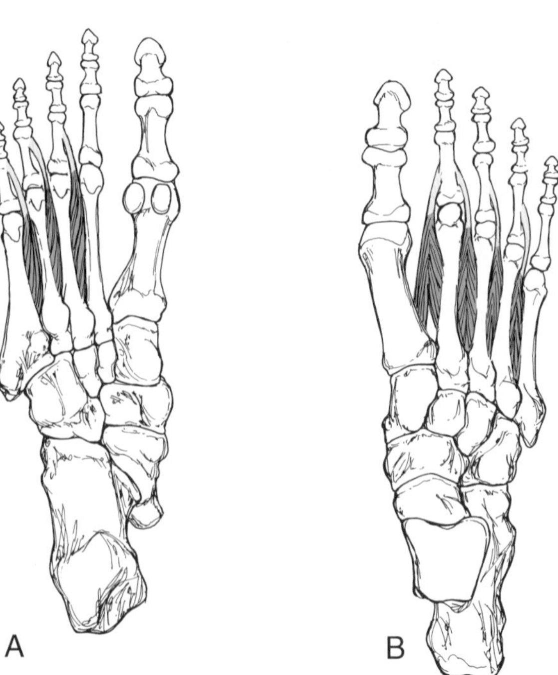

Figure 9-15. A. Plantar interossei are one part of the fourth layer of muscles on the plantar aspect of the foot. **B.** Dorsal interossei are also part of the fourth layer of muscles on the plantar aspect of the foot.

TABLE 9-4 INTRINSIC MUSCLES OF THE FOOT

First Layer

Muscle	*Origin*	*Insertion*	*Action*
Abductor hallucis	Medial process of the tuberosity of the calcaneus.	Base of proximal phalanx of the great toe and the medial sesamoid bone.	Abducts the great toe.
Flexor digitorum brevis	Medial process of the tuberosity of the calcaneus and the medial part of the plantar aponeurosis.	By four thin tendons on the middle phalanges of the four lateral toes; at the base of the corresponding phalange, the tendon divides into two slips perforated by the tendon of the flexor digitorum longus.	Flexes the proximal IP joint.
Abductor digiti minimi	Medial and lateral tuberosity of calcaneus; plantar aponeurosis.	Lateral side of the proximal phalanx of small toe.	Abducts small toe.

Second Layer

Muscle	*Origin*	*Insertion*	*Action*
Quadratus plantae (flexor digitorum accessorius)	Arises by two heads from the plantar surface of the calcaneus separated by the long plantar ligament.	Lateral margin of the tendon of the flexor digitorum longus muscle.	Contracts simultaneously with the flexor digitorum longus, stabilizing the pull of the tendon by decreasing the obliquity of the pull relative to the axis of the foot.
Lumbricals I–IV	Arises from the tendons of the flexor digitorum longus.	End on the medial sides of the four lateral toes, attached to the dorsal digital expansions of the proximal phalanges, just as in the hand.	Flex proximal phalanges, as in the hand.

Third Layer

Muscle	*Origin*	*Insertion*	*Action*
Flexor hallucis brevis	From the plantar surface of the cuboid and the lateral cuneiform and the tendon of the tibialis posterior.	By two heads that contain the sesamoid bones of the great toe and to the medial and lateral sides of the base of the proximal phalanx of the great toe.	Flexes the great toe.
Flexor digiti minimi brevis	Base of the fifth metatarsal and the sheath of the peroneus longus.	Proximal phalanx of small toe.	Flexes the small toe.
Adductor hallucis—oblique head	Bases of metatarsals 2–4, sheath of tendon of peroneus longus muscle.	Lateral side of the base of the proximal phalanx of the great toe; lateral sesemoid bone.	Adducts the great toe.
Adductor hallucis—transverse head	MTP ligaments of the three lateral toes; deep transverse metatarsal ligament.	Lateral side of the base of the proximal phalanx of the great toe; lateral sesamoid bone.	Adducts the great toe.

TABLE 9-4	INTRINSIC MUSCLES OF THE FOOT—cont'd		

Fourth Layer

Muscle	*Origin*	*Insertion*	*Action*
Dorsal interossei I–IV	Each arises by two heads from adjacent sides of two metatarsal bones (i.e., they are between the metatarsals).	Attach to the bases of the proximal phalanges and to the dorsal digital expansions.	Abduct the toes from the midline of the foot.
Plantar interossei I–III	Three muscles below, rather than between, the interossei; arise from the bases and medial sides of the third to the fifth metatarsals.	Attached to the medial sides of the bases of the proximal phalanx of the same toes and into the dorsal digital expansion.	Adduct the lateral three toes to the midline.

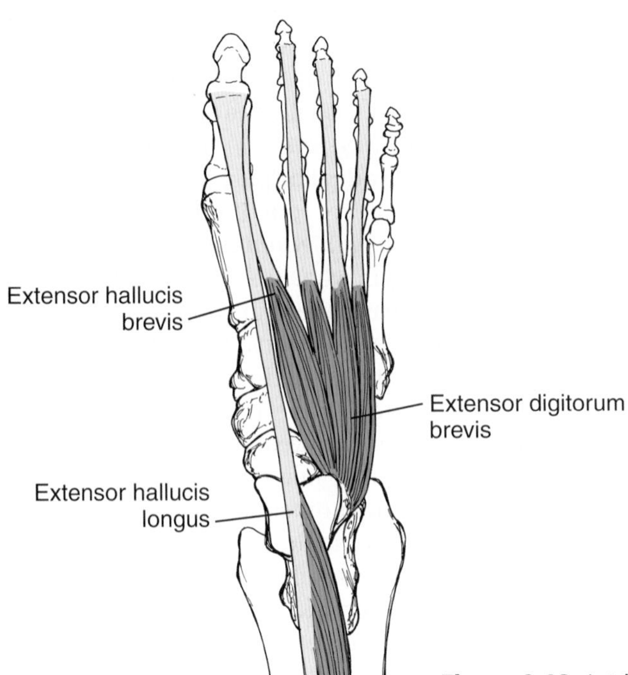

Figure 9-16. Intrinsic muscles on the dorsum of the foot include the extensor hallucis brevis and the extensor digitorum brevis.

TABLE 9-5	MUSCLES OF THE DORSUM OF THE FOOT		
Muscle	***Origin***	***Insertion***	***Action***
Extensor digitorum brevis	Lateral and dorsal surface of the calcaneus	Dorsal aponeurosis of three middle toes	Extension of the toes; assist in dorsiflexion of the ankle
Extensor hallucis brevis	Dorsal surface of the calcaneus	Base of first phalanx of great toe	Extension of the great toe and dorsiflexion of the ankle

TABLE 9-6 MUSCULAR ACTIONS OF THE FOOT

The foot is capable of inversion, eversion, plantarflexion, dorsiflexion, and circumduction. Inversion is the combination of adduction (moving the forefoot toward the midline), supination (elevation of the medial margin), and plantarflexion. Eversion is abduction (moving toes away from the midline of the foot), pronation (lowering of the medial margin of the foot), and dorsiflexion. The toes may be flexed, extended, abducted, or adducted. For simplification, I have followed Platzer[9] and equate inversion with supination and eversion with pronation.

Supination and Inversion

- Triceps surae
- Tibialis posterior
- Flexor hallucis longus
- Flexor digitorum longus
- Tibialis anterior

Toe Flexion

- Flexor digitorum longus
- Flexor hallucis longus
- Flexor digitorum brevis
- Flexor hallucis brevis
- Adductor hallucis—also adducts
- Lumbricals
- Quadratus plantae

Toe Extension

- Extensor digitorum longus and brevis
- EHL and brevis

Pronation and Eversion

- Peroneus longus
- Peroneus brevis
- Extensor digitorum longus
- Peroneus tertius

Abduction

- Abductor hallucis
- Abductor digiti minimi
- Dorsal interossei

Adduction

- Adductor hallucis
- Plantar interossei

- Flat feet (foot pronation) or abnormally high arch
- Abnormal gait
- Loss of extension of the great toe (less than 45° to 60° of extension is problematic)
- Fatigue from static or dynamic stress, such as prolonged standing (static) or running (dynamic)
- Immobilization, which weakens the tissue
- Previous injury

DIFFERENTIATION OF LEG, ANKLE, AND FOOT PAIN

It is important to realize that pain in the leg, ankle, and foot can come from disease processes rather than from injuries or dysfunctions of the neuromusculoskeletal system. See the section "Contraindications to Massage Therapy: Red Flags" in Chapter 2, "Assessments & Technique" for guidelines on when massage is contraindicated and when to refer the client to a doctor.

The leg, ankle, and foot are common areas where pain, numbing, or tingling is referred from the lumbosacral spine. As mentioned in Chapter 3, "Lumbosacral Spine," one type of referred pain is caused by muscle, ligament, joint capsule, disc, or dura mater. These tissues elicit what is called **sclerotomal** pain when they are injured. Usually the sclerotomal pain is described as *deep, aching, and diffuse.* A second type of referred pain, called **radicular** pain, is caused by an irritation of the spinal nerve root. If the sensory (dorsal) root is irritated, *sharp pain, numbing, or tingling that is well-localized* occurs in what are called dermatomes. A dermatome is an area of the skin supplied by the sensory root of a single spinal nerve (see Chapter 3 for a figure of the dermatomes). If, in addition to the pain, numbing, and tingling, there is compression of the motor (ventral) nerve root, weakness may occur in the muscles supplied by that nerve root, called the myotome. The relevant myotomes of the leg, ankle, and foot are as follows: L4 is ankle dorsiflexion; L5 is great-toe extension; and S1 is ankle eversion. The entrapment of a peripheral nerve in the region of the leg, ankle, and foot may also lead to pain, numbing, or weakness. In peripheral entrapment, manual pressure over the entrapped nerve typically increases the symptoms temporarily. This increase in symptoms is an indication for treatment. The OM treatment to release the peripheral nerves is so effective that if your treatment does not resolve the symptoms in several sessions, refer the client to a chiropractor or an osteopath for spinal evaluation.

Differentiation of other conditions may be categorized according to the region involved. Sudden, severe pain in the mid-calf is often a gastrocnemius strain. Isometric challenge to plantar flexion or raising of the toes is painful. A dull aching in the leg that increases with activity is often a chronic compartment syndrome that progresses to a shin splint.

An ankle sprain usually results from an acute episode, leading to well-localized pain, most commonly at the anterior portion of the distal fibula. A ligament sprain is painless with isometric challenge and is painful with passive stretching. Pain in the ankle region may also be a tendinitis or a tenosynovitis of the extrinsic muscles of the foot. The pain is increased with isometric challenge.

Pain on the bottom of the feet is usually plantar fasciitis, although pain on the heel may be a heel spur. Pain on the bottom of the great toe is often sesamoiditis (application of manual pressure to the painful sesamoid confirms this condition). Chronic diffuse aching pain and stiffness in the region of the first MTP joint is often a degeneration of the cartilage of the great toe, a sign of osteoarthritis.

COMMON DYSFUNCTIONS AND INJURIES IN THE LEG, ANKLE, AND FOOT

Gastrocnemius Strain (Tennis Leg)

- *Causes:* Gastrocnemius strain is the most common muscle injury to the leg. It involves a strain of the musculotendinous junction of the medial head of the gastrocnemius. Increased intensity or duration of running or activities that involve quick movements of plantar flexion, such as tennis, racquet sports, basketball, and dance, cause this strain.
- *Symptoms:* Gastrocnemius strain symptoms are often described as a sudden, severe pain in mid-calf, followed by muscle spasms in the calf and pain in walking. The injury site is nearly always at the musculotendinous junction of the medial gastrocnemius in the midcalf.
- *Signs:* Clients experience muscle spasm in the calf, painful knots in the medial aspect of midcalf, pain on toe raises, and pain with passive dorsiflexion.
- *Treatment:* Perform PIR MET to lengthen the gastrocnemius and OM to dissolve the adhesions.

Achilles Tendinitis

- *Causes:* Achilles tendinitis is the most common tendinitis of the foot and ankle, and the Achilles tendon is the most commonly ruptured tendon in the body. It involves a tearing of the tendon caused by prolonged or excessive activity that fatigues the tissue. Common activities that cause this condition are running, hiking, skiing, and dancing.
- *Symptoms:* Achilles tendinitis symptoms are pain in the Achilles tendon where it inserts into the calcaneus at the medial, lateral, and anterior borders or pain just proximal to this insertion site. The pain worsens with activity. The area feels stiff, especially when the client first gets out of bed in the morning.
- *Signs:* Clients experience pain on resisted plantar flexion or when standing on tiptoes. The area is tender to palpation and is swollen.
- *Treatment:* Acute tendinitis is treated with CR MET. Chronic conditions are treated with PIR MET to lengthen the tissue and OM to dissolve the adhesions.

Ankle Sprain

- *Causes:* Ankle sprain is usually an incident of a sudden plantar flexion and inversion twist to the ankle or of repetitive inversion stress. The anterior talofibular ligament is the most commonly injured ligament in the body.
- *Symptom:* An ankle sprain symptom is pain at the anterolateral ankle, occurring anterior to the distal fibula.
- *Signs:* Clients experience localized swelling within several days of the injury, and the swelling may progress to diffuse bruising. They may also experience pain with passive inversion during plantar flexion.
- *Treatment:* Acute sprains are treated with CR MET to the plantar flexors and dorsiflexors of the ankle. Chronic sprains are treated with OM, including transverse friction massage.

Plantar Fasciitis and Heel Spurs

- *Causes:* Static stress of prolonged standing or excessive walking, running, hiking, and dancing cause plantar fasciitis and heel spurs. An irritation of the fascia can cause a traction spur on the heel.
- *Symptom:* Plantar fasciitis and heel spur symptoms are pain that is usually well-localized over the anteromedial calcaneus but that may radiate distally. These conditions are often painful when the foot hits the ground, especially when the client gets out of bed in the morning.
- *Signs:* Clients experience pain that may be reproduced by full passive dorsiflexion of the ankle and all the toes. Also, palpation of the fascia on the anteromedial heel is painful.
- *Treatment:* Perform OM, transverse to the line of the fascia. Heel spurs are treated with brisk, deep friction strokes on the heel.

Posteromedial Shin Splint

- ***Introduction***: Much confusion exists in the literature regarding the terms **shin splint** and **chronic compartment syndrome.** Following Hertling and Kessler,[7] I use the term shin splint to mean exercise-induced pain caused by repetitive stress of any musculotendinous unit originating in the lower leg. Shin splints then describe a condition similar to chronic compartment syndrome. A chronic compartment syndrome describes exercise-induced swelling of the muscle fibers, whereas shin splint describes the irritation of muscle attachments with the periosteum. An **acute compartment syndrome,** on the other hand, is a rare medical emergency that is caused by rapid swelling, venous stasis, ischemia resulting from bone fracture, muscle rupture, or severe overuse of the muscles.
- ***Cause:*** A shin splint is a tenoperiosteal or fascial tear of the soleus or tibialis posterior induced by a sudden increase in the duration or intensity of an exercise, usually running. Predisposing factors include leg-length differences, muscles imbalances, excessive valgus heel, excessive pronation, inadequate or worn-out shoes, or running on hard surfaces or on uneven terrain.[6]
- ***Symptoms:*** Dull, aching pain over the distal third of the medial leg is a symptom of shin splint. An acute compartment syndrome manifests as severe pain, numbing, tingling and swelling in the leg and foot.
- ***Sign:*** Pain with resisted plantar flexion and inversion implicates the tibialis posterior, or pain with passive dorsiflexion and eversion of foot implicates the soleus.
- ***Treatment:*** Chronic shin splints are treated with CR MET to reduce the hypertonicity of the soleus and tibialis posterior. OM is performed to help dissolve the adhesions that result from the chronic inflammation.

Anterolateral Shin Splint or Chronic Anterior Compartment Syndrome

- ***Causes:*** Sudden and vigorous running, dancing, or jumping can lead to anterolateral shin splint or chronic anterior compartment syndrome. The muscles in the anterior compartment are usually weak compared with the short, tight gastrocnemius and soleus. Anterolateral shin splint or chronic anterior compartment syndrome is considered a periosteal or fascial tear of the tibialis anterior, extensor hallucis longus, or extensor digitorum longus; these conditions must be differentiated from a stress fracture. A fracture is a local, pointed pain, not more than 1.5 inches in diameter over the tibia or fibula, and an inflammation of the periosteum (periostitis) is a more diffuse pain.[1]
- ***Symptoms:*** Exercise-induced tightness and diffuse, dull aching in middle-third of anterior leg that comes on gradually are symptoms of anterolateral shin splint. Occasionally, a sharp pain occurs with activity.
- ***Signs:*** Clients experience pain with resisted dorsiflexion and passive plantar flexion, and the overlying skin may be edematous.
- ***Treatment:*** Perform MET to release the sustained hypertonicity in the involved muscles and OM to dissolve the fibrosis.

Pronation

- ***Causes:*** Pronation may be a result of weakness of the anterior and posterior tibialis, which dynamically support the arch, or it may be caused by a local structural dysfunction, such as a medial subluxation of the talus. Genetic factors are also a cause.
- ***Symptoms:*** Pronation may be painful. If painful, it is usually along the medial arch, between the anterior heel to the great toe, due to the excessive tensile stress to the plantar aponeurosis, short and long plantar ligaments, and the excessive loading of the intrinsic flexors.
- ***Signs:*** Clients experience a flattening of the medial arch, a valgus position of the heel, decreased dorsiflexion caused by a tight Achilles tendon, and a tenderness along the medial arch.
- ***Treatment:*** Stretch the gastrocnemius and soleus with PIR and CR MET. To help facilitate (strengthen) the intrinsic feet muscles and the anterior and posterior tibialis muscles, instruct the client to rise up on the toes while externally rotating the leg and keeping the great toe planted on the floor. Another exercise for the client to perform is to use the toes to pick up a sock; this exercise strengthens the intrinsic flexors of the feet. Repeat 50 times or until fatigue, whichever comes first. Refer the client to a chiropractor, podiatrist, or physical therapist for evaluation of the alignment of the foot bones and for assessment of the need for an orthotic.

Metatarsalgia

- ***Cause:*** Metatarsalgia results from weight-bearing imbalance such as pronation, tight Achilles tendons, and weak intrinsic toe flexors. Weak intrinsic toe flexors decrease the arch, which causes the weight to fall excessively on the heads of the metatarsals rather than through the passive and dynamic supporters of the arch.

- *Symptom:* Pain at the metatarsal heads or at the MTP joints.
- *Signs:* Digital pressure on the metatarsal heads is painful. Squeezing all the MTP joints together is painful.
- *Treatment:* Perform PIR MET for the gastrocnemius and soleus to stretch the Achilles tendon; perform manual release of the muscles attaching to the heads of the metatarsals and the transverse metatarsal ligament; and instruct the client on exercises to correct pronation (see above, "Pronation").

LESS COMMON DYSFUNCTIONS AND INJURIES

Lateral Shin Splint or Chronic Lateral Compartment Syndrome

- *Causes:* Lateral shin splint or chronic lateral compartment syndrome is associated with pronation and inversion sprains of the ankle. These conditions are common in dancers who have repetitive eversion of the foot.
- *Symptom:* Pain in the lateral leg at the tenoperiosteal junction of the peroneal muscle attachments to the fibula is a symptom of lateral shin splint or chronic lateral compartment syndrome.
- *Sign:* Clients experience pain at the site of injury with resisted eversion or passive inversion.
- *Treatment:* Perform MET and OM for the peroneals.

Tibialis Anterior Tendinitis and Tenosynovitis

- *Cause:* The tibialis anterior is typically weak, often inhibited by a short and tight gastrocnemius and soleus or a pronated foot. It is the principal decelerator of the foot at heel strike.[12]
- *Symptom:* Pain, usually well-localized to the musculotendinous junction, approximately 6 inches above the ankle or just below the superior extensor retinaculum and at tendon insertion near the medial cuneiform is a symptom of tibialis anterior tendonitis and tenosynovitis.
- *Signs:* Clients experience localized pain with resisted dorsiflexion and inversion and pain with passive plantar flexion and foot eversion. Active dorsiflexion is difficult or painful.
- *Treatment:* Perform MET and OM for the tibialis anterior.

Tibialis Posterior Tendinitis and Tenosynovitis

- *Cause:* The tibialis posterior usually is in a lengthened contraction because of foot pronation, and therefore it is eccentrically loaded, predisposing it to irritation.
- *Symptoms:* Tibialis posterior tendinitis and tenosynovitis manifest in three common sites of pain: on the tendon proximal to the medial malleolus, on the tendon posterior to the ankle, and on the tenoperiosteal junction on the navicular.
- *Sign:* Clients experience pain on resisted inversion and plantar flexion or on full passive eversion and dorsiflexion. These movements may be done with the client standing. Ask the client to invert the foot and raise up on the toes.[13]
- *Treatment:* Perform OM and MET to the tibialis posterior.

Peroneus Longus and Brevis Tendinitis and Tenosynovitis

- *Causes:* The peroneal tendons pass immediately behind the lateral malleolus and are held next to the bone by a retinaculum. They are surrounded by synovium, and when irritated, can cause a tenosynovitis. If the tunnel narrows because of scarring, a stenosing synovitis may develop. Excessive eversion and an inversion strain are predisposing factors.[14]
- *Symptoms:* Pain at the base of the fifth metatarsal for brevis and pain in the bony groove of the cuboid for the longus tendon are tendinitis symptoms. A symptom of tenosynovitis is pain behind the lateral malleolus.
- *Sign:* Clients experience pain on resisted eversion and plantar flexion or pain on full passive dorsiflexion and inversion of foot.
- *Treatment:* Perform MET and OM to the peroneus longus and brevis.

Hallux Limitus or Hallus Rigidus Syndrome

- *Cause:* Hallux limitus is a shortening of the joint capsule of the great toe. Hallus rigidus is the end-stage degeneration of the joint. The cause of a shortened capsule is a repetitive trauma that creates inflammation or an acute event involving stubbing, or catching of the great toe ("turf toe"). The trauma or stubbing can lead to inflammatory joint degeneration.

- *Symptom:* Pain in the great toe, and first MTP joint, especially in the push-off phase of walking is a symptom of hallux limitus or hallus rigidus syndrome.
- *Sign:* It is essential to have 45° to 60° of passive extension of the great toe for normal gait; therefore, limited extension of the great toe caused by degenerative joint disease (DJD) of the first MTP is a sign of this syndrome, which is manifest in acute (younger patients) and chronic types (older patients).
- *Treatment:* Release of the intrinsic and extrinsic muscles that attach to the great toe, release of the collateral ligaments and joint capsule, and mobilization of the first MTP joint in (A–P) and medial to lateral (M–L) glide.

Hallux Valgus Syndrome

- *Causes:* Heredity or weight distribution problems such as pelvic obliquity, genu valgus, and pronated ankles cause hallux valgus syndrome.
- *Symptom:* Pain at the first MTP joint of the foot, often caused by pronation and sustained contracture of adductor hallucis is a symptom of hallux valgus syndrome.
- *Signs:* Lateral deviation of the great toe and medial deviation of the head of the first metatarsal are signs of this syndrome. Often a bunion develops over the medial side of the head of the first metatarsal. A bunion is a combination of a callus, thickened bursa, and excessive bone (exostosis).
- *Treatment:* Establish correct posture, and normalize the function of the hips, knees, ankles, and foot. Release the adductor hallucis, and show the client MET for the abductor hallucis. If the condition is moderate to severe, refer the client to a chiropractor or a podiatrist for a foot orthotic.

Sesamoiditis

- *Causes:* Sesamoiditis is inflammation of the capsule surrounding the sesamoids. A high arch, the wearing of high-heel shoes, or the lateral deviation of the sesamoids from hallux valgus are often causes of this condition.
- *Symptom:* Pain under the great toe is a symptom of sesamoiditis.
- *Sign:* Clients experience pain with passive extension of the great toe.
- *Treatment:* Perform CR MET for the flexor hallucis brevis and the adductor hallucis, and perform OM to help dissolve adhesions and normalize the position of the sesamoids.

Hammer Toes and Claw Toes

- *Causes:* Hammer toes and claw toes are often associated with a high arch (pes cavus), weak lumbricals and interossei, and sustained contraction of extensor digitorum longus, which increases the passive tension on the extrinsic toe flexors.[11] Hammer toes are also the result of fibrosis of the joint capsules of the IP joints.
- *Symptom:* Pain or cramping in the toes is a symptom of these conditions.
- *Signs:* Hammer toes involve hyperextension of the MTP joints and flexion contracture of the PIP joints. Claw toes involve hyperextensions of the MTP joints and flexion of the PIP and the DIP joints.
- *Treatment:* Strengthen the lumbricals and interossei; perform PIR MET to extensor digitorum longus; and release the joint capsule of the MTP and the IP joints.

Superficial Peroneal Nerve Entrapment

- *Cause:* Inversion sprains can cause an irritation of the nerve in runners due to repetitive inversion and plantar flexion.
- *Symptoms:* Pain, burning, numbness, or tingling at the lateral border of the distal calf or at the lateral aspect of the dorsum of the foot and ankle are symptoms of entrapment.
- *Signs:* With superficial peroneal nerve entrapment, there are no reproducible signs.
- *Treatment:* Perform gentle transverse release of the lateral leg with attention to the two entrapment sites described above. Feel for fascial thickening.

Deep Peroneal Nerve Entrapment (Anterior Tarsal Tunnel Syndrome)

- *Causes:* Tight-fitting boots, ankle sprains, and excessive running are causes of deep peroneal nerve entrapment.
- *Symptoms:* Pain, tingling, or numbing between the first and the second toes. The nerve can become entrapped under the superior and inferior extensor retinaculum at the ankle. The medial branch can be compressed as it travels under the extensor hallucis brevis and the lateral branch as it travels under the extensor digitorum longus tendons.[15]
- *Signs:* Deep peroneal nerve entrapment is primarily a motor condition and can lead to weak dorsiflexion. Digital pressure on the dorsum of the foot at the extensor retinaculum can cause symptoms.

- *Treatment:* Perform gentle transverse release of the dorsum of the foot and ankle.

Posterior Tibial Nerve Entrapment (Tarsal Tunnel Syndrome)

- *Causes:* The neurovascular bundle containing the posterior tibial nerve or its two terminal branches, the medial and lateral plantar nerves, can become compressed under the flexor retinaculum (laciniate ligament), the abductor hallucis, or the quadratus plantae. Tarsal tunnel is associated with pronated ankles.
- *Symptoms:* Burning pain and a pins-and-needles sensation in the plantar aspect of foot or toes are symptoms of tarsal tunnel syndrome.
- *Sign:* For tarsal tunnel, perform the hyperpronation test. Hold the ankle in hyperpronation for 60 seconds and the burning, or pins-and-needles sensation, may be reproduced.
- *Treatment:* Perform gentle, transverse scooping strokes at the tarsal tunnel.

Plantar Digital Nerve Entrapment (Morton's Neuroma)

- *Causes:* Plantar digital nerve entrapment causes are as follows: the wearing of high heels or tight-fitting shoes, the presence of weak intrinsic foot muscles, and the cumulative stress of running, hiking, dancing, and other such activity.
- *Symptoms:* Morton's neuroma has many symptoms, such as a burning or throbbing in the metatarsal head region that moves to the toes. The nerve is entrapped in the transverse metatarsal ligament, usually between the third and the fourth toes. Pain related to walking is another symptom. This pain can persist at night, and if the foot is chronically inflamed, a fibrous enlargement around the nerve, called a Morton's neuroma, may develop.
- *Signs:* Pain reproduced by squeezing the metatarsal heads together or by passively extending the toes are signs of digital nerve entrapment.
- *Treatment:* Release any sustained contracture in the foot, and release the transverse metatarsal ligament and plantar nerve.

Sural Nerve Entrapment

- *Causes:* The sural nerve can be entrapped and irritated by tight fitting boots or by a tight crural fascia.
- *Symptoms:* Sural nerve entrapment symptoms are pain and burning along the posterior lateral leg, the lateral ankle, and the foot.
- *Signs:* For this condition, there are no reproducible tests.
- *Treatment:* Perform transverse release of the posterior leg, the ankle, and the lateral foot.

Assessment of the Leg, Ankle, and Foot

BACKGROUND

The leg, ankle, and foot are susceptible to acute and chronic conditions and commonly reflect overuse syndromes in athletes. Inability to bear weight, severe pain, and rapid swelling indicates a severe injury.[15] The leg is a common site of referral of pain, numbing, and tingling from irritation of the L4 and L5 nerve roots. If you have pain, numbing, and tingling in the leg, ankle, and foot and active, passive, and isometric testing is strong, it indicates either a peripheral entrapment of the nerve(s) or an irritation of the lumbosacral nerve roots. Perform the straight–leg-raising (SLR) and the femoral nerve stress tests (see Chapter 3). If these are negative, perform the strokes to release the peripheral nerves. If the client is unresponsive, refer him or her to a chiropractor or an osteopath. The leg is also a common site for overuse syndromes, such as shin splints and tendinitis.

The ankle is a common site of sprains, usually caused by an acute episode. The foot reflects local conditions, such as trauma, but it is much more common to have a fatigue-type pain in the feet caused by chronic weight distribution dysfunctions. This weight distribution dysfunction may be caused by obesity or by conditions such as pronation. The feet also reflect systemic conditions such as the neuritis and dermatitis of diabetes and can be a referral site from irritation of the L5, S1 to S2 nerve roots. Referral from the nerve roots would create weakness, numbing, and tingling or weakness alone, but it would not create pain.

Normal function of the leg, ankle, and foot requires proper alignment of the lumbopelvic region and lower extremity, as well as a balance of length and strength in the fascia and muscles affecting the lower extremity.

HISTORY QUESTIONS FOR THE CLIENT WHO HAS LEG, ANKLE, OR FOOT PAIN

- Is there some movement that you can do to elicit the pain?

This question is another way of asking what aggravates the pain. The client can often elicit local conditions in the leg, ankle, and foot if he or she moves in a certain way. One specific movement usually does not elicit conditions caused by chronic misalignment or weight distribution dysfunctions, such as pronation. Also, referral of pain, numbing, or tingling cannot be generated or aggravated by active motion of the lower extremity.

INSPECTION AND OBSERVATION

- Have the client put on shorts so that you can see from the thighs to the feet. Observe for swelling, which may be diffuse and bilateral or localized at the lateral ankle. Localized bruising and swelling typically indicates an ankle sprain, whereas swelling without bruising, would indicate previous injury with unresolved edema. Swelling in both feet indicates systemic problems, such as lymphatic congestion or circulatory problems.
- Notice if calluses resulting from pressure from shoes are on the top of the toes. Look for swelling over the medial side of the great toe, indicating a bunion.

Alignment of the Toes

- ***Position:*** The client is standing, facing the therapist, with feet shoulder-width apart.
- ***Observation:*** Observe the alignment of the toes; are they straight and parallel? Note whether the following conditions are present: hallux valgus, which is a lateral deviation of the big toe; hammer toes, which is a hyperextension of the metacarpophalangeal (MCP) and the DIP joints and flexion of the PIP; or claw toes, which is a hyperextension of the MCP and flexion of the PIP and DIP. The capsular pattern of the IP joints is that flexion is most limited.

Assessment of the Longitudinal Arch

- ***Position:*** The client is standing, facing the therapist, with feet shoulder-width apart.
- ***Action:*** Place your fingertips on the medial arch.
- ***Observation:*** Feel for a low arch (pes planus/flatfoot) or a high arch (pes cavus). A low arch in weight-bearing that normalizes in non-weight-bearing is a functionally low arch caused by muscle weakness or ligament laxity. To confirm your findings, have the client stand on tiptoes. A functional low arch will rise on tiptoes.

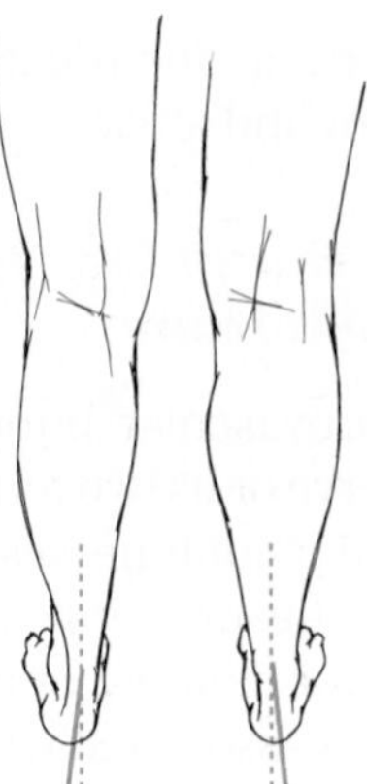

Figure 9-17. Assessment of the alignment of the Achilles tendon. Note that this client's tendons are angled medially, a sign of pronation in the ankles.

Assessment of the Achilles Tendon Alignment

- ***Position:*** The client is standing, facing away from the therapist, with feet shoulder-width apart (Fig. 9-17).
- ***Action:*** Observe the vertical alignment of the Achilles tendon.
- ***Observation:*** Note whether the Achilles tendon is in its normal vertical alignment, and the existence of any swelling of the Achilles tendon. If the tendon is bowed in, the heel is everted with weight on the heel on the medial side, called **rearfoot valgus.** The foot is also pronated, and the medial longitudinal arch is lowered, called **pes planus.** If the Achilles is bowed out, the heel is inverted, called **rearfoot varus,** bringing the weight to the lateral side; the foot is supinated; and the medial longitudinal arch is higher, called **pes cavus.**

ACTIVE MOVEMENTS

Great-Toe Extension Test

- ***Position:*** The client is standing. Place your thumb under the great toe (Fig. 9-18).
- ***Action:*** Ask the client to lift the great toe into extension. Then, continue the movement passively until pain or tissue tension.
- ***Observation:*** Extension of the great toe should be approximately 45° to 60° to maintain normal gait. Decreased extension indicates hallux limitus, an early degeneration, and capsular fibrosis of the first MTP joint or possibly hallux rigidus, an advanced degeneration of the first MTP joint. Pain under the first MTP is usually sesamoiditis.

Active Dorsiflexion

- *Position:* The client stands on one leg, next to a wall for support.
- *Action:* Ask the client to lift his or her toes and forefoot off the ground 10 times or until there is pain or fatigue.
- *Observation:* This procedure is a good functional screening test for the anterior tibialis, EHL, and extensor digitorum longus. Pain is elicited with the anterolateral leg with shin splints or tendinitis of those muscles. Generally, 10 to 15 painless repetitions is considered functionally normal.[15] Painless weakness implicates an inhibition caused by short or tight plantar flexors or involvement of the L4 to L5 and S1 nerve roots.

Active Plantar Flexion

- *Position:* The client stands on one leg, next to a wall for support.
- *Action:* Ask the client rise up on the toes 10 times or until there is pain or fatigue.
- *Observation:* This action is a good screening test for strength of plantar flexion, principally the gastrocnemius and soleus, and the function of the L4 to L5 and S1 to S2 nerve roots. Painless inability to lift up on the heels implicates a dysfunction or injury of those nerves. If client cannot lift up on the toes, ask if pain, weakness, or a lack of motion in the toes prevents this action. A client who has hallux rigidus cannot lift the heel far off the ground. Pain at the Achilles tendon indicates Achilles tendinitis; pain at the lower posteromedial border of the tibia implicates a fascial tear of the soleus; and pain in the medial aspect of the midcalf is usually a tendinitis of the gastrocnemius. Heel lifting also challenges the tibialis posterior, flexor digitorum longus, or flexor hallucis longus, which elicits pain if there is a tendinitis in those muscles.

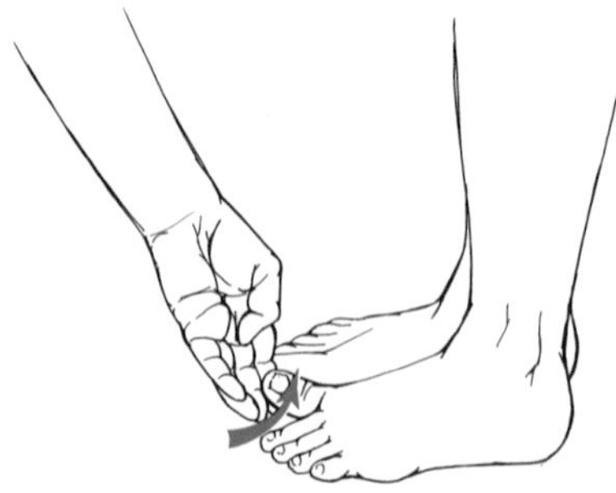

Figure 9-18. Great toe extension test. Have the client actively lift up the great toe. Continue the movement passively until pain or a resistance barrier is encountered.

Active Movements: Client Sitting

- *Position:* The client sits on the edge of the table.
- *Action:* Ask client to perform plantar flexion, dorsiflexion, inversion and eversion, toe flexion and extension, and abduction of the toes. Have him or her perform these movements on both feet at the same time.
- *Observation:* Compare the ROM, and ask the client is there is any pain.

PASSIVE MOVEMENTS

Ankle Plantar Flexion or Dorsiflexion

- *Position:* The client is supine. Hold the calcaneus with one hand and invert the forefoot with the other hand to lock it into the hindfoot.
- *Action:* First lift the foot into dorsiflexion, and then press it into plantar flexion. The range is approximately 20° of dorsiflexion and approximately 50° of plantar flexion.
- *Observation:* Painless restriction of dorsiflexion is often caused by previous ankle sprains. Pain with dorsiflexion implicates plantar fascitis, posteromedial shin splint, or gastrocnemius tendinitis, depending on pain location. Pain with passive plantar flexion implicates an anterolateral shin splint or an anterior tibialis tendinitis.

Assessment for Sprain of the Anterior Talofibular Ligament

- *Position:* The client is supine. Stabilize the ankle with one hand and place the other hand on the dorsum of the foot (Fig. 9-19).
- *Action:* Slowly plantar flex and invert the foot.
- *Observation:* Positive test is pain at the anterior, inferior aspect of the fibula. The anterior talofibular is the most commonly injured ligament in the ankle.

Assessment for Metatarsalgia and Morton's Neuroma

- *Position:* The client is supine. Stabilize the ankle with one hand and place the other hand around the toes at the MTP joints.
- *Action:* Slowly squeeze the metatarsal heads together.

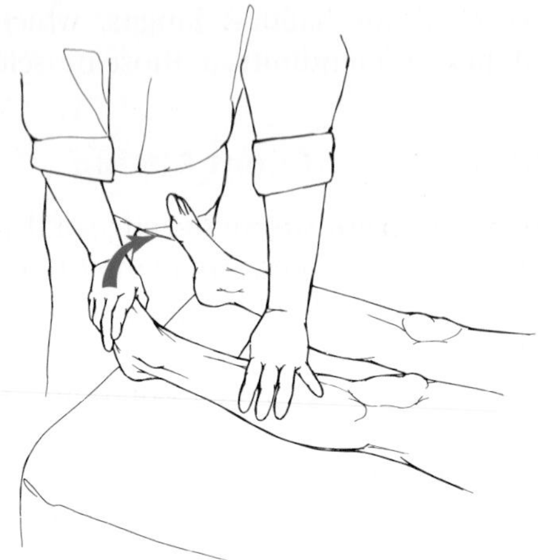

Figure 9-19. Assessment of the anterior talofibular ligament. Passively plantar flex and invert the foot.

- *Observation:* Pain in the region of the plantar aspect of the third and the fourth toes is a positive sign for Morton's neuroma (i.e., a fibrous enlargement of the plantar digital nerve). Pain in the MTP joints is a positive sign of metatarsalgia.

Techniques

MUSCLE ENERGY TECHNIQUE

As mentioned, the CR MET serve not only as therapeutic techniques but as assessment tools. It is important to realize that the muscles in the leg, ankle, and foot are often weak because of an irritation, injury, or dysfunction of the nerves in the lumbosacral spine. This statement is also true for the muscles of the elbow, wrist, and hand, which are myotomes for nerves from the cervical spine (see Chapter 10, The Elbow, Forearm, Wrist, and Hand).

Muscle Energy Technique for Acute Ankle Pain

1. Contract-Relax Muscle Energy Technique for Acute Ankle Pain

- *Intention:* The intention is to contract and relax the muscles of plantar flexion and dorsiflexion. This contract-relax cycle pumps the waste products and swelling out of the injured area, increases the nutritional exchange, and helps realign the healing fibers.

CAUTION: This type of MET is performed only within pain-free limits. Beneficial effects are achieved with only grams of pressure.

- *Position:* Client is supine with the ankle in a pain-free resting position. Place one hand on the dorsum (top) of the foot and the other hand under the ball of the foot (Fig. 9-20).
- *Action:* Have the client resist as you slowly and gently press the top of the foot toward plantar flexion for approximately 5 seconds. Relax for a few seconds. Have the client resist as you slowly and gently press up on the ball of the foot toward dorsiflexion. Relax, and repeat cycle several times.

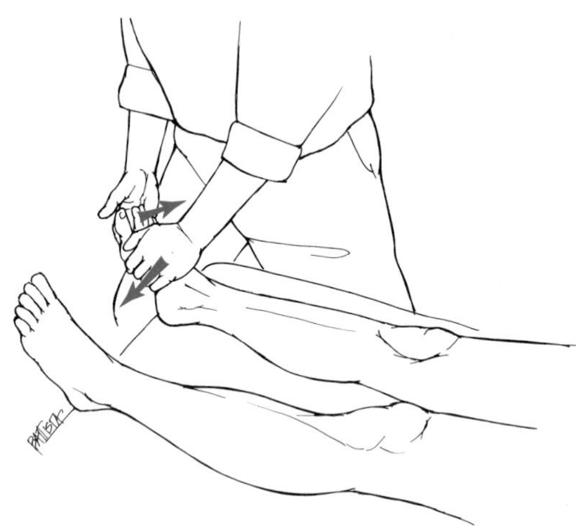

Figure 9-20. CR MET for acute ankle pain.

Muscle Energy Technique for Leg, Ankle, and Foot Muscles

1. Contract-Relax Muscle Energy Technique for the Tibialis Anterior

- *Intention:* The intention is to reduce the hypertonicity or to facilitate (strengthen) and bring sensory awareness to the tibialis anterior.
- *Position:* Client is supine. Place one hand on the dorsum of the foot and the other hand on the tibialis anterior for a sensory cue (Fig. 9-21).
- *Action:* Have the client dorsiflex the ankle, invert foot, and resist as you press toward plantar flexion and eversion.
- *Observation:* Painless weakness may be a result of L4 nerve root injury or dysfunction or of deep peroneal nerve entrapment.

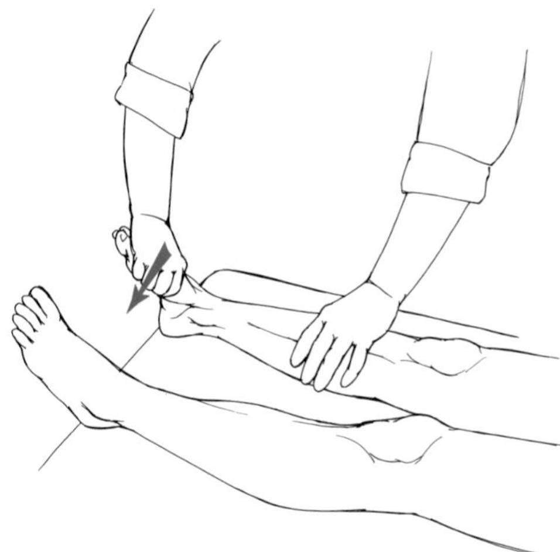

Figure 9-21. CR MET for the tibialis anterior.

2. Contract-Relax Muscle Energy Technique for the Peroneus Longus and Brevis

- ☐ ***Intention:*** The intention is to reduce the hypertonicity or to facilitate (strengthen) and bring sensory awareness to the peroneals.
- ☐ ***Position:*** Client is supine. Place one hand on the lateral foot and the other hand on the peroneals for a sensory cue (Fig. 9-22).
- ☐ ***Action:*** Have the client evert the foot with slight plantar flexion of ankle and resist as you press toward inversion and dorsiflexion.
- ☐ ***Observation:*** Painless weakness implicates a problem with the S1 nerve root. Pain at the lateral leg implicates injury to the peroneal muscles or a lateral shin splint. Pain behind the ankle indicates a tenosynovitis of the peroneals. Pain at the fifth metatarsal or cuboid indicates a tendinitis of the peroneus brevis and longus, respectively.

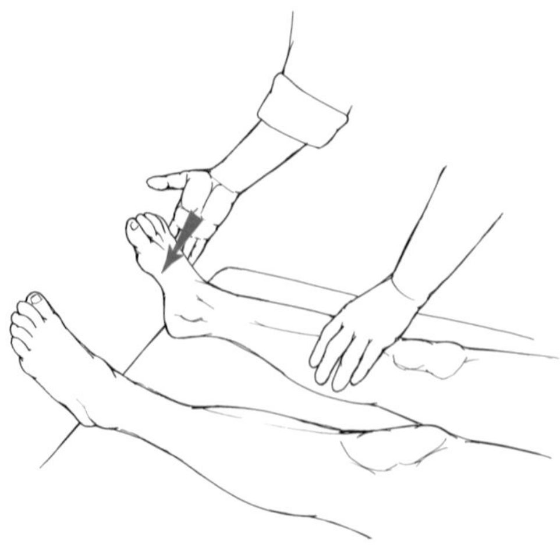

Figure 9-22. CR MET for the peroneus longus and brevis.

3. Contract-Relax Muscle Energy Technique for the Tibialis Posterior

- ☐ ***Intention***—To reduce the hypertonicity or facilitate (strengthen) and bring sensory awareness to the tibialis posterior.
- ☐ ***Position:*** Client is supine. Hold the medial arch with one hand, and place the other hand on the posterior aspect of the medial tibia (Fig. 9-23).
- ☐ ***Action:*** Have the client invert the foot with plantar flexion of the ankle and resist as you attempt to dorsiflex and evert.
- ☐ ***Observation:*** Painless weakness implicates the L5 nerve root. Pain indicates a tendinitis or tenosynovitis of the tibialis posterior or a posteromedial shin splint.

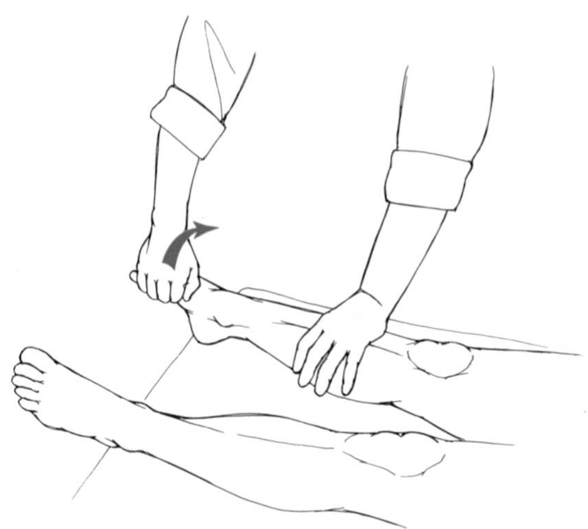

Figure 9-23. CR MET for the tibialis posterior.

4. Contract-Relax Muscle Energy Technique for the Flexor Digitorum Longus and Brevis and the Flexor Hallucis Longus and Brevis

- ☐ ***Intention:*** The intention is to use CR MET to reduce the hypertonicity or to facilitate (strengthen) and bring sensory awareness to the flexor digitorum and flexor hallucis muscles.
- ☐ ***Position:*** Client is supine. Place one hand under the toes and the other hand on the leg for stability (Fig. 9-24).
- ☐ ***Action:*** Have the client flex the toes and resist as you attempt to pull the toes into extension for approximately 5 seconds. Relax for a few seconds and repeat.

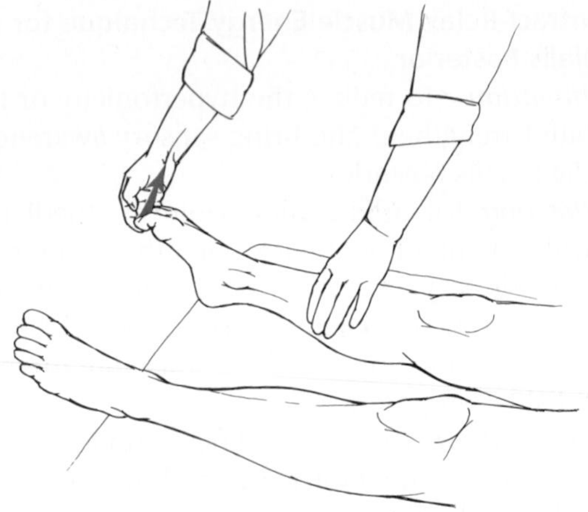

Figure 9-24. CR MET for the flexor digitorum longus and brevis and for the flexor hallucis longus and brevis.

5. Postisometric Relaxation Muscle Energy Technique for the Flexor Digitorum Longus and Brevis and the Flexor Hallucis Longus and Brevis

- ☐ ***Intention:*** The intention is to use PIR MET to lengthen the flexors to help bring normal extension to the toes.
- ☐ ***Position:*** Client is supine. Place one hand under the toes and pull the toes into extension to their comfortable limit of stretch. Place the other hand on the leg for stability (Fig. 9-25).
- ☐ ***Action:*** Have the client resist as you attempt to pull the toes into greater extension for approximately 5 seconds. Relax, and then gently stretch the toes into further extension, and have client resist again. Repeat the CR–lengthen–contract cycle several times.

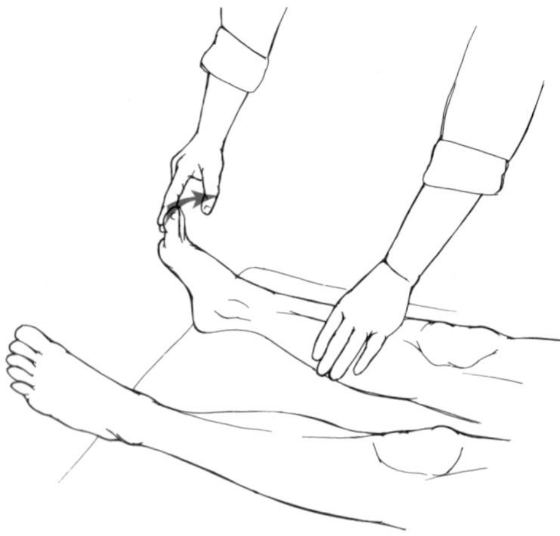

Figure 9-25. PIR MET for the flexor digitorum longus and brevis and for the flexor hallucis longus and brevis.

6. Contract-Relax Muscle Energy Technique for the Extensor Hallucis

- ☐ ***Intention:*** The extensor hallucis is often weak. This weakness may be a result of myotomal weakness from irritation or injury to the L5 nerve. Weakness may also arise from an arthrokinetic reflex from fibrosis of the capsular ligaments of the great toe or from degeneration of the first MTP joint. The intention in using this MET is to help facilitate (strengthen) and bring sensory awareness to the extensor hallucis.
- ☐ ***Position:*** Client is supine. Place one hand on the top of the great toe (Fig. 9-26).
- ☐ ***Action:*** Have the client extend the great toe to the comfortable limit and then resist as you press the toe toward flexion.
- ☐ ***Observation:*** Painless weakness implicates an irritation, injury, or dysfunction of the L5 nerve root. This muscle is often weak, as lower back dysfunction and injury is so common.

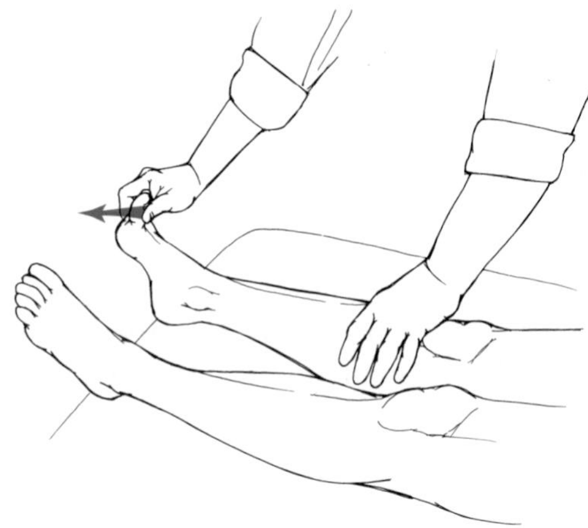

Figure 9-26. CR MET for the EHL and brevis.

7. Contract-Relax and Postisometric Muscle Energy Technique for the Extensor Digitorum Longus

- ☐ ***Intention:*** The extensor digitorum longus is often held in a sustained contraction, leading to claw toes. The intention in using this MET is to reduce the muscle hypertonicity and to lengthen the myofascia.
- ☐ ***Position:*** Client is supine. Place one hand on the top of the toes.
- ☐ ***Action:*** To perform CR MET, have the client extend the toes and resist as you press the toes toward flexion. Relax and repeat (Fig. 9-27).To perform PIR MET, after the relaxation cycle, press the toes into greater flexion and have the client resist

as you press the toes toward further flexion. Relax and repeat the CR–lengthen cycle several times.

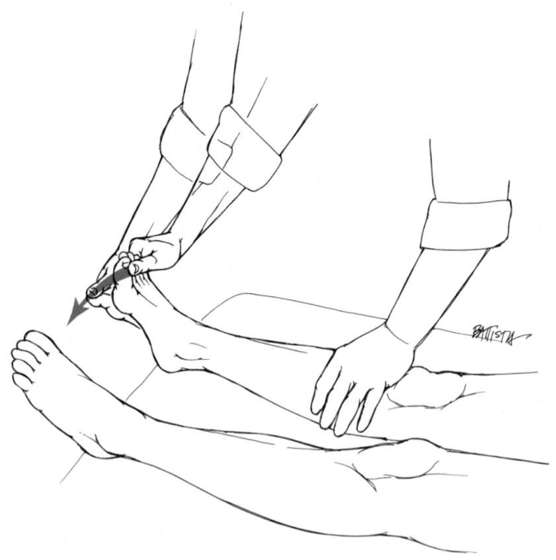

Figure 9-27. CR and PIR MET for the extensor digitorum longus and brevis.

8. Contract-Relax-Antagonist-Contract Muscle Energy Technique for the Soleus and Muscle Energy Technique to Increase Ankle Dorsiflexion

- *Intention:* The soleus is typically short and tight. This muscle forms part of the Achilles tendon with the gastrocnemius. Unlike the gastrocnemius, the soleus does not cross the knee. The intention in using this MET to increase ankle dorsiflexion, which is often decreased after an ankle injury.

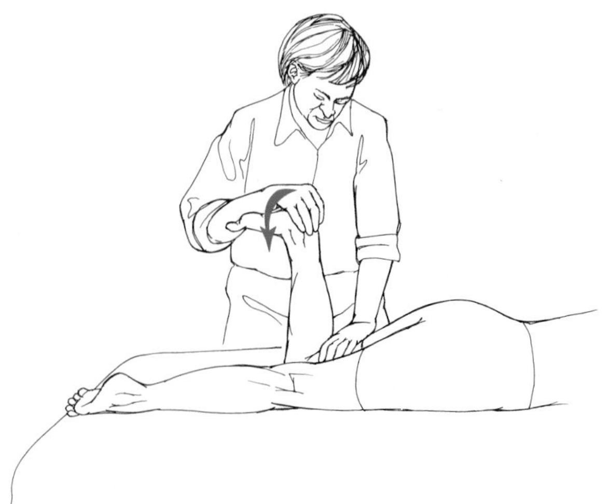

Figure 9-28. CRAC MET for the soleus and MET to increase dorsiflexion of the ankle.

- *Position:* Client is prone. Place the hand on the heel and the forearm on the ball of the foot (Fig. 9-28).
- *Action:* Have the client resist as you attempt to press the ball of the foot toward the table (i.e., to dorsiflex the ankle) for approximately 5 seconds, then instruct the client to relax. Have the client actively dorsiflex the ankle until pain or a new resistance barrier is encountered. As the client is actively dorsiflexing, press the forearm down on the ball of the foot to assist the stretch. Have client resist again at this new ROM for approximately 5 seconds, then instruct the client to relax. Repeat this CR-antagonist-contract (CRAC) cycle several times.

ORTHOPEDIC MASSAGE

Level I—Leg, Ankle, Foot

1. Release of the Anterior and Lateral Compartments

- *Anatomy:* Crural fascia, extensor digitorum longus, EHL, tibialis anterior, peroneus longus, and peroneus brevis (Fig. 9-29).
- *Dysfunction*: With overuse or injury the crural fascia is initially pulled away from the bone, but as it heals, it tends to thicken and adhere to the bone. This thickening and adhesion reduces the elasticity of the anterior and lateral compartments. The underlying muscles tend to dehydrate and lose their gliding characteristics.

Position

- Therapist position (TP)—standing
- Client position (CP)—supine

Strokes

The first three strokes are for chronic conditions only.

1. Release the anterior compartment by first stretching the crural fascia. Use some lotion to prevent skin burn. The tool is a soft fist. First, with the wrist in neutral, perform a series of long, continuous strokes from the ankle to the knee on the anterior and lateral compartments (Fig. 9-30). Second, using the soft-fist technique, place the supporting hand next to the soft fist, and hold the supporting hand's thumb to stabilize the working hand (Fig. 9-31). Beginning at the lateral border of the proximal tibia, press into the leg and while maintaining even pres-

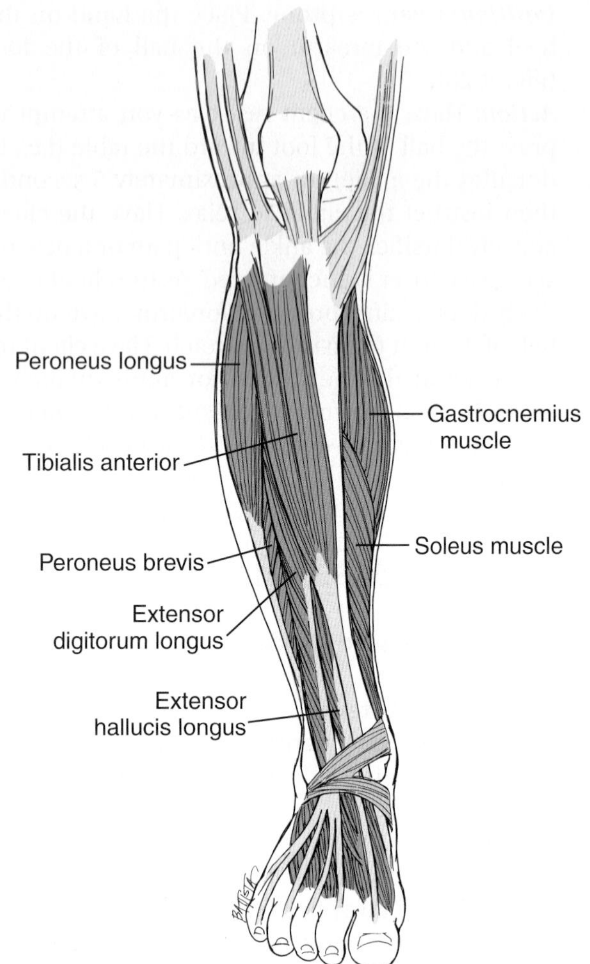

Figure 9-29. Muscles of the anterior compartment of the leg include the tibialis anterior, extensor digitorum longus, and EHL.

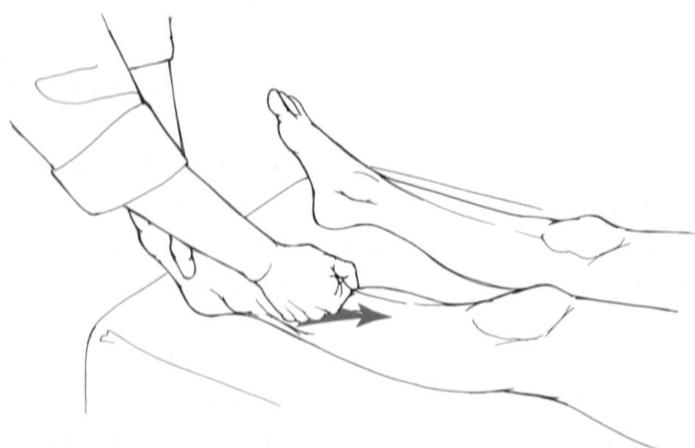

Figure 9-30. Using a soft fist, stretch the fascia of the leg with long, continuous strokes. This is for chronic conditions only.

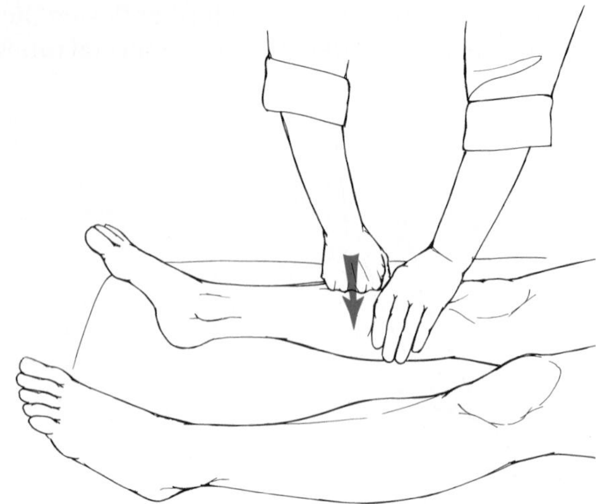

Figure 9-31. Using a soft fist, stretch the fascia of the leg in an A–P direction.

sure, and slowly slide the fist on the skin and fascia posteriorly. You may also roll the fist posteriorly by flexing the wrist in a smooth, gliding motion. For the lateral compartment, rotate the leg medially with the supporting hand and cover the lateral surface. Emphasize the index knuckle or all the knuckles in the pronated position, or emphasize the flat surface of the proximal phalanges in the neutral wrist position. Continue these strokes to the ankle.

2. Place your hands next to each other for stability, and using your fingertips, spread the fascia from the midline of the anterior tibia in slow, spreading strokes. Begin below the knee, and move inch by inch down the tibia. Release the superior and inferior extensor retinaculum at the ankle.
3. Using double-, braced-, or single-thumb technique, perform 1-inch, scooping strokes from the ankle to the knee. Work in three lines between the lateral edge of the tibia and the fibula. This procedure releases the muscles in the anterior and lateral compartments. Maintain some tension in the tissue as you finish one stroke, as this keeps the fascia in tension and allows for a greater stretch.
4. For acute conditions, place the knee in flexion, with the foot on the table (Fig. 9-32). While holding the entire leg, use double-thumb technique to perform gentle, 1-inch, scooping strokes in the M–L, A–P direction on the entire anterior and lateral compartments. These transverse scooping strokes may also be performed with the client in the fetal position, with a pillow between the knees. Face the anterior leg, perform A–P scooping strokes on the anterior and lateral compartments from the proximal leg to the lateral ankle.

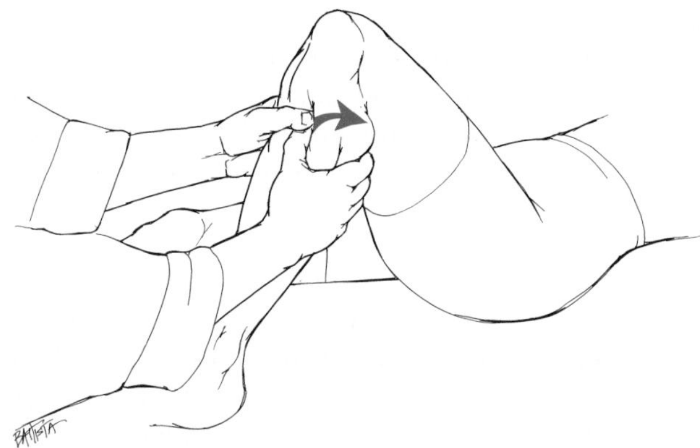

Figure 9-32. Double-thumb release of the anterior and lateral compartments for acute conditions.

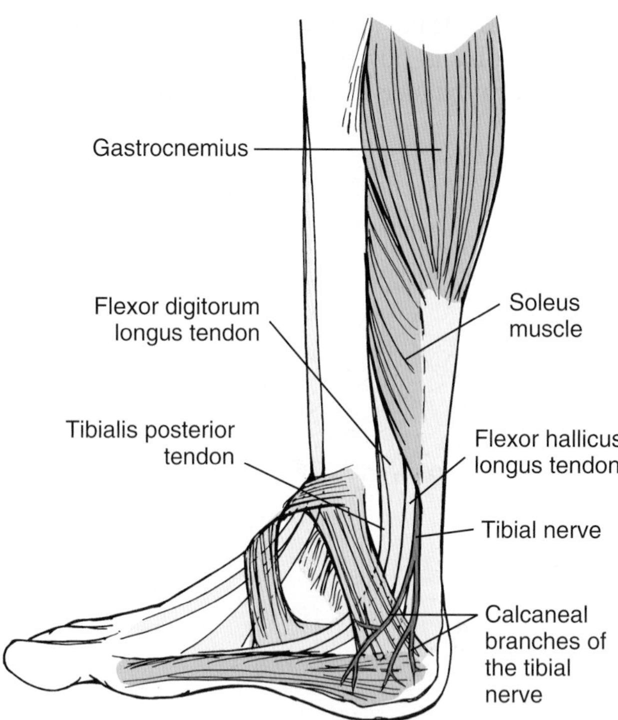

Figure 9-33. Medial leg, ankle, and foot showing the tendons of the tibialis posterior, flexor digitorum longus, and flexor hallucis longus traveling around the medial ankle.

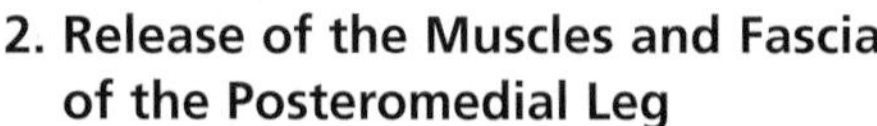

2. Release of the Muscles and Fascia of the Posteromedial Leg

- *Anatomy*: Crural fascia, tibialis posterior, soleus, flexor hallucis longus, plantaris, and flexor digitorum longus (Fig. 9-33).
- *Dysfunction*: The posteromedial leg is the most common injury site of the compartment syndromes or shin splints. It involves the tenoperiosteal or fascial tear of the soleus, the tibial origin of the flexor digitorum longus, or the tibialis posterior. The crural fascia covers the area superficially.

Position

- TP—standing
- CP—side lying, with a pillow under the knee of the top leg, with bottom leg extended

Strokes

1. Place the client onto her left side for work on the left medial aspect of the leg. Stand facing headward and perform the same series of strokes described in the previous series. First, using a soft fist, perform a series of long, slow continuous strokes from the ankle to the knee on the medial leg. Next, move to the side of the table closest to the extended leg. Place the supporting hand next to the soft fist and hold the supporting hand's thumb to stabilize the stroke. Begin at the medial border of the proximal tibia and, while maintaining even pressure, roll and slide the fist posteriorly in a smooth, gliding motion.
2. Face headward. Place your hands next to each other for stability, and using your fingertips, perform slow, spreading strokes by moving the fingertips away from each other, spreading the fascia of the medial leg (Fig. 9-34). One hand is on the soft tissue, and the other hand is on the fascia covering the bone. Begin below the knee, and move inch by inch down the tibia to the ankle.
3. Using double-, braced-, or single-thumb technique, perform 1-inch, scooping strokes from the ankle to the knee in several lines on the fascia covering the muscles and in between the muscles of the posteromedial leg.
4. Move to the opposite side of the table to face the anterior aspect of the extended leg, and ask the client to move closer to you so that you are not reaching. Using double- or braced-thumb technique, perform a series of 1-inch, scooping strokes on the medial compartment from just below the knee to the ankle

(Fig. 9-35). At the medial ankle, release the tendons of the tibialis posterior, flexor digitorum longus, and flexor hallucis longus by scooping anteriorly to posteriorly.

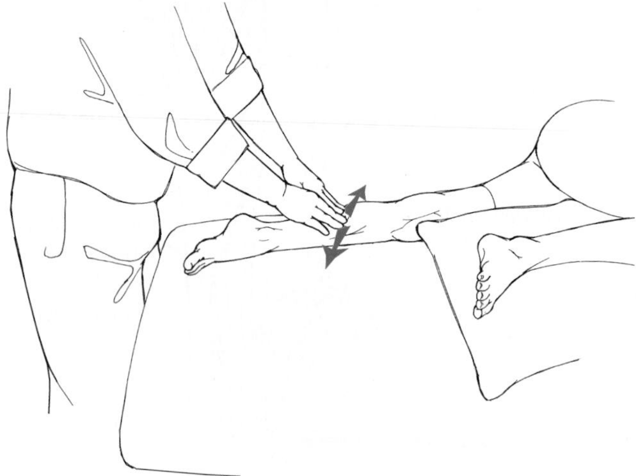

Figure 9-34. Fingertips technique used to perform a spreading motion to part the midline of the medial leg.

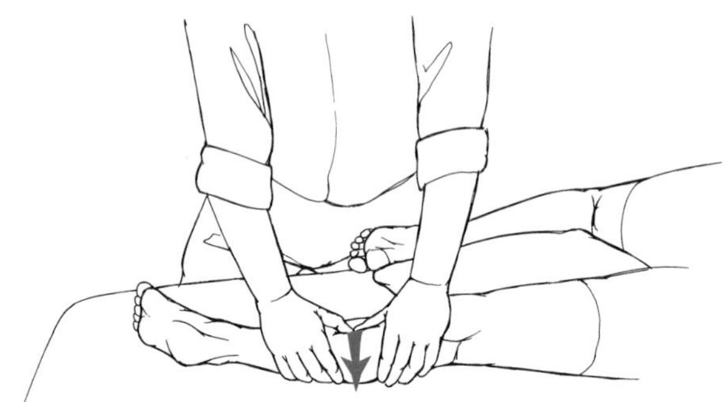

Figure 9-35. Double-thumb technique used to perform scooping strokes in an A–P direction on the medial leg.

3. Prone Release of the Posterior Compartment and the Achilles Tendon

- ***Anatomy***: Gastrocnemius, soleus, plantaris, flexor hallucis longus, and flexor digitorum longus (Fig. 9-36A and B).
- ***Dysfunction***: "Tennis leg" is a strain of the gastrocnemius and soleus. The injury normally lies near the musculotendinous junction. Achilles tendinitis is a common injury in runners and dancers. The injury site is usually at the insertion of the tendon on the posterior-superior calcaneus and 1 to 2 centimeters proximal to the insertion.

Position

- TP—standing, facing headward
- CP—prone, with the foot off the edge of the table; place a pillow under the ankle if the leg is particularly tense or sensitive as this brings the tissue into more slack

Strokes

1. Facing headward, release the posterior aspect of the crural fascia. Use a soft fist, and perform long, slow strokes from the ankle to the knee as described in the previous strokes. Follow the gastrocnemius heads to the medial and lateral aspects of the popliteal fossa. Keep your wrist in neutral, midway between pronation and supination. Do not put deep pressure in the center of the popliteal fossa.
2. To release the hypertonicity in the muscles and stretch their fascial coverings, use single-, double-, or braced-thumb technique as described in the previous strokes. Perform 1-inch, scooping strokes in an inferior to superior direction on three lines, the medial, middle, and lateral aspects of the posterior leg.
3. To release the torsion in the soft tissue, part the midline by taking the lateral tissue laterally and the medial tissue medially. Using double thumbs, perform short, scooping strokes, beginning at the midline below the knee (Fig. 9-37). These strokes may also be performed standing at the side of the table facing the client.
4. There are three strokes for the Achilles tendon. First, face headward and use double-thumb technique to perform short, back-and-forth strokes in the M–L plane on the posterior surface of the Achilles tendon (Fig. 9-38). You may stabilize the tendon by pressing your thigh against the client's foot. Second, with your fingertips slightly flexed, perform back-and-forth strokes in the A–P plane on the medial and lateral surfaces of the tendon (Fig. 9-39). Move in opposite directions with the fingers in an oscillating rhythm. Third, face the table, and place a flexed knee on the table. Rest the client's shin on your flexed thigh. Hold the Achilles tendon between your thumb and fingertips, and roll the tendon back-and-forth. In this position, you may stabilize the tendon. First stabilize with the thumb and perform back-and-forth strokes with the fingers, and then switch to use the fingers to stabilize and the thumb to perform the strokes.

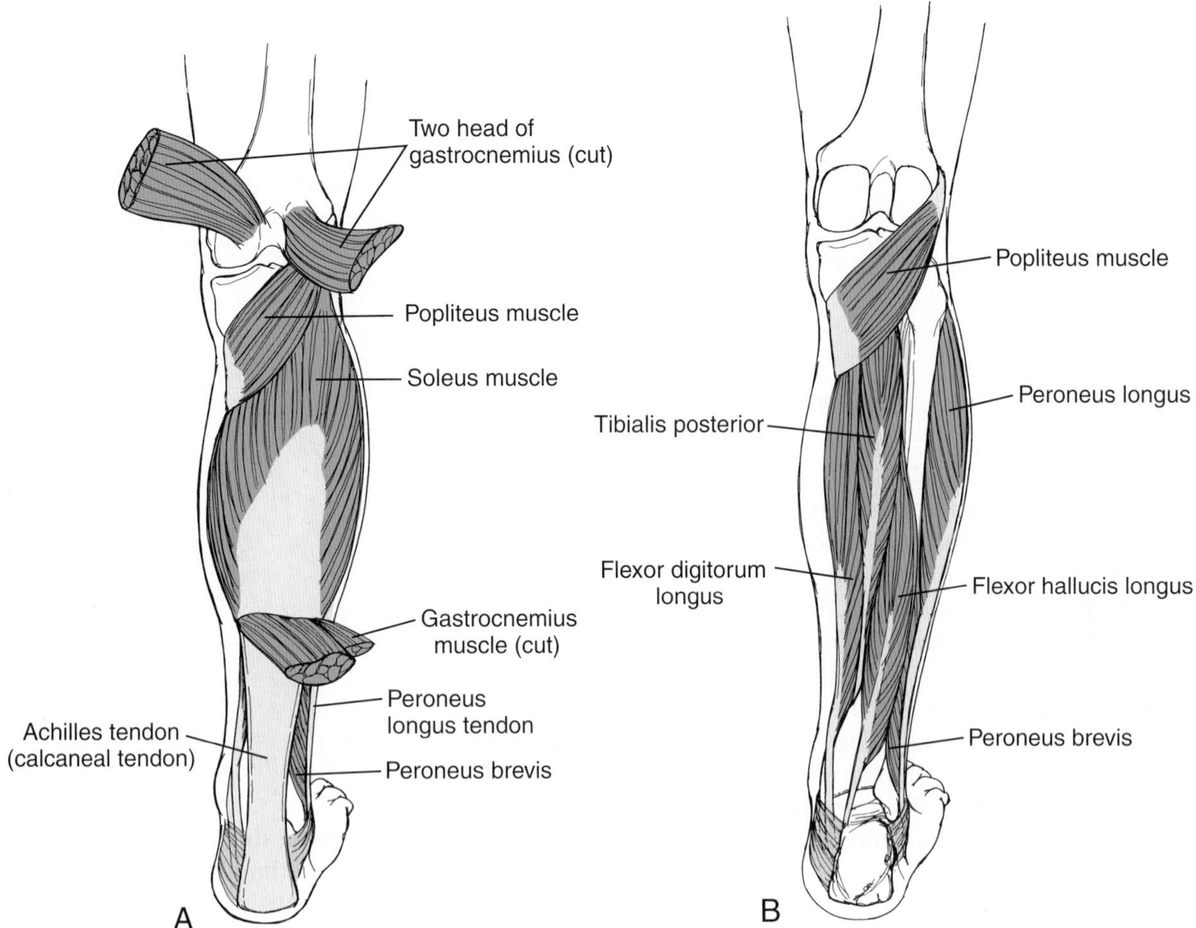

Figure 9-36. A. Superficial posterior compartment showing the gastrocnemius cut away to reveal the underlying soleus. **B.** Deep posterior compartment showing the tibialis posterior, flexor digitorum longus, and the flexor hallucis longus.

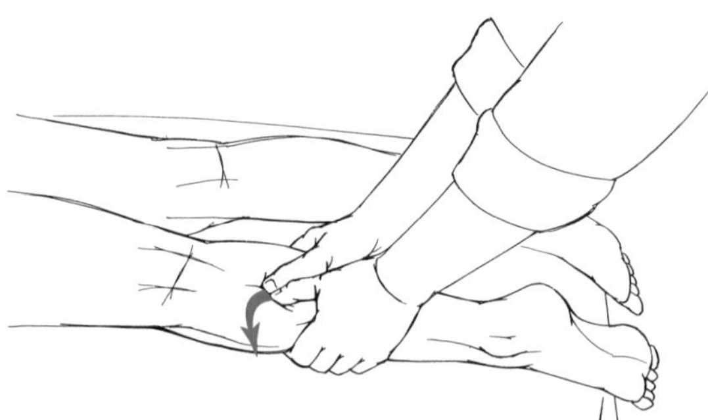

Figure 9-37. Double-thumb technique used to perform short, scooping strokes from the knee to the ankle, taking the lateral tissue more laterally and the medial tissue more medially.

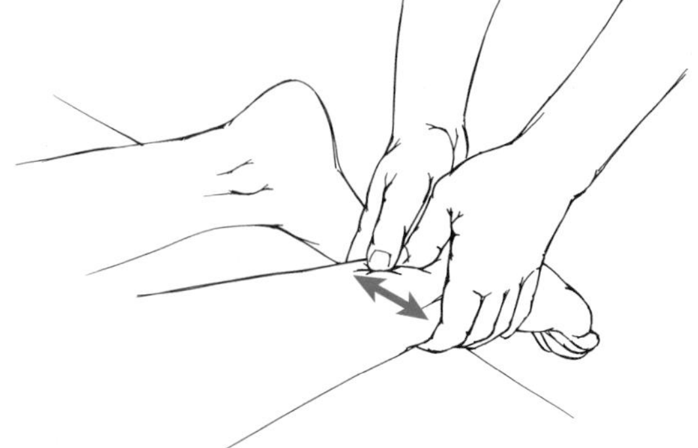

Figure 9-38. Double-thumb technique used to perform back-and-forth strokes in the M–L plane on the Achilles tendon.

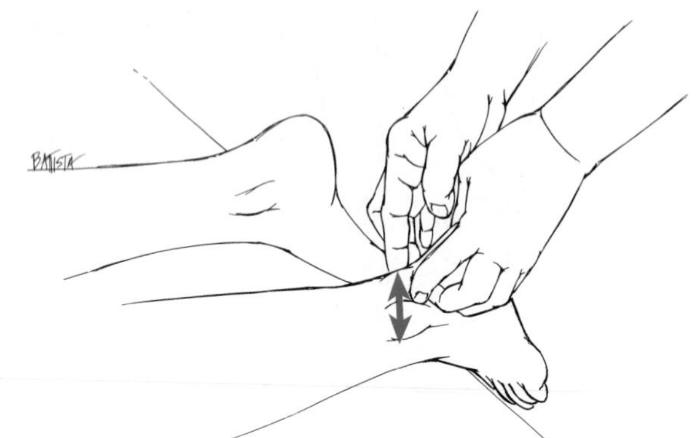

Figure 9-39. Fingertips used to perform back-and-forth strokes in the Achilles A–P plane.

4. Release of the Muscles of the Dorsum of the Foot and of the Ligaments of the Ankle

- *Anatomy*: Dorsal interossei, extensor digitorum longus and brevis, EHL and brevis (Fig. 9-40), deltoid ligament, anterior talofibular ligament, and calcaneofibular ligament (see Figs. 9-8 and 9-9).
- *Dysfunction*: The tendons and their associated retinacula are susceptible to irritation as they travel under the retinacula on the dorsum of the foot. Ligamentous injuries are usually inversion stresses from an acute episode. The most commonly injured ligament is the anterior talofibular.

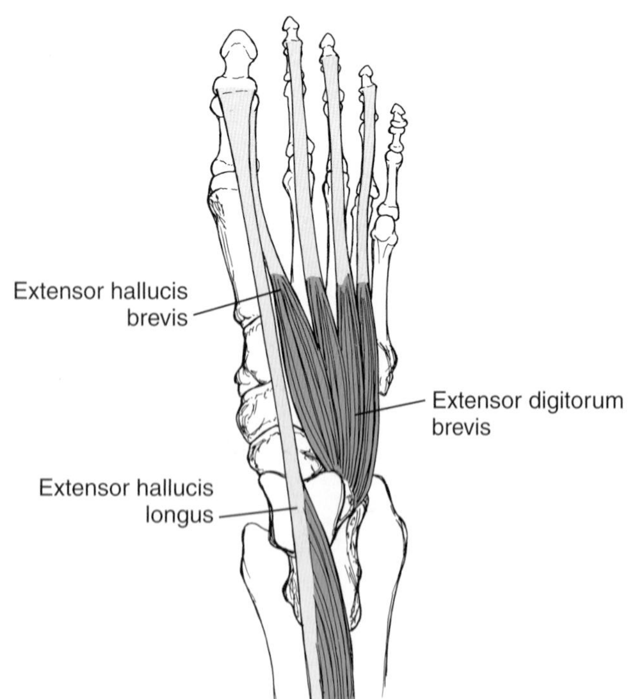

Figure 9-40. Intrinsic muscles on the dorsum of the foot include the extensor hallucis brevis and the extensor digitorum brevis.

Position

- TP—standing
- CP—supine

Strokes

1. Using double thumbs on the midline of the foot, perform a spreading motion to part the midline of the retinacula and fascia on the dorsum of the foot (Fig. 9-41).

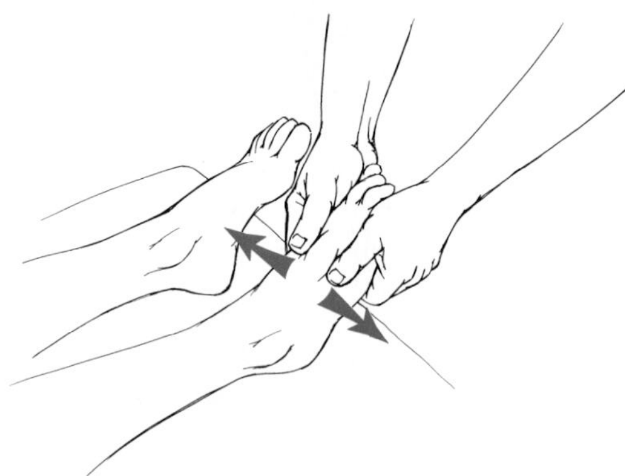

Figure 9-41. Double-thumb technique used to perform a series of spreading strokes on the fascia on the dorsum of the foot.

2. To release the extensor digitorum brevis and extensor hallucis brevis on the dorsum of the foot, begin by placing both thumbs at the anterolateral calcaneus as your hands hold the foot. Using double-thumb technique, oscillate the foot rhythmically into supination as you perform short, scooping strokes in an M–L direction (Fig. 9-42). Continue these transverse scooping strokes on the entire dorsum of the foot to the toes to release the tendons of the tibialis anterior, EHL, and extensor digitorum longus on the dorsum of the foot.

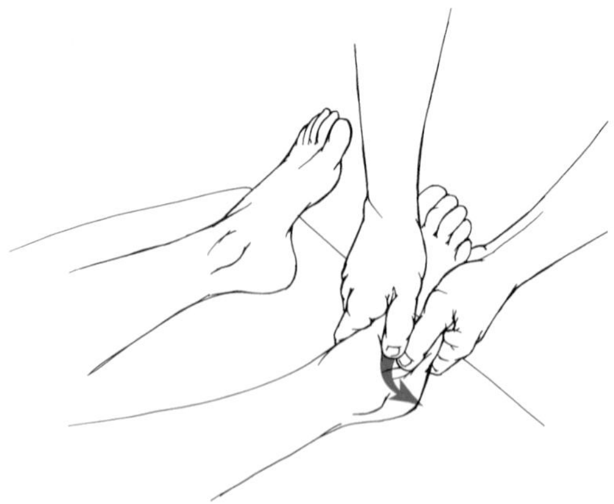

Figure 9-42. Double-thumb technique used to perform M–L scooping strokes to release the extensor hallucis brevis and extensor digitorum brevis.

3. Using a thumb or finger, perform short, longitudinal strokes on the dorsal interossei in between the metatarsals (Fig. 9-43). Put the fingertips of your supporting hand underneath where you are working to spread the metatarsals open as you stroke.

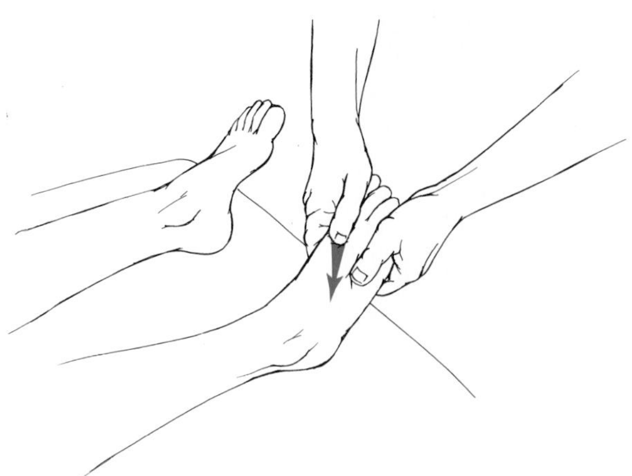

Figure 9-43. Single-thumb technique used to perform scooping strokes toward the heel in the area between the metatarsals.

4. To release the ligaments of the ankle, work in the same area as the retinacula but at a deeper level. Using your fingertips, single- or double-thumb technique, perform back-and-forth strokes on the anterior talofibular ligament from the anterior portion of the distal fibula to the talus with back-and-forth strokes in the M–L and A–P planes (Fig. 9-44). Next, release the calcaneofibular ligament from the inferior aspect of the fibula to the calcaneus. Finally, using the same tools, release the deltoid ligaments from the distal end of the medial malleolus to the heel in the A–P plane. Rock the entire foot with these strokes in an oscillating rhythm.

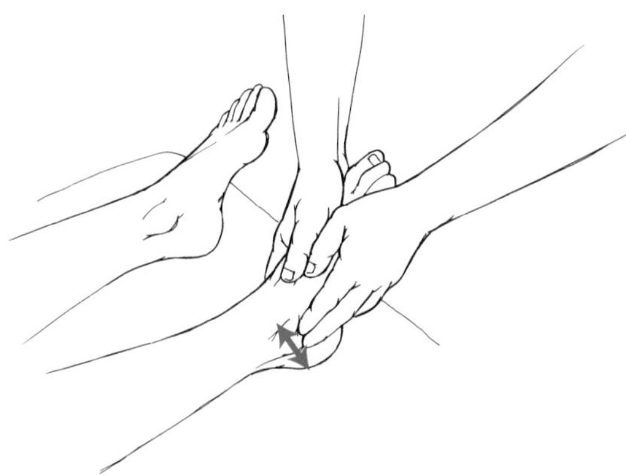

Figure 9-44. Fingertips used to perform transverse strokes on the anterior talofibular ligament.

5. **Release of the Plantar Fascia and the Muscles of the First Layer of the Foot**

- ***Anatomy:*** Plantar aponeurosis, abductor hallucis, flexor digitorum brevis, and abductor digiti minimi (Fig. 9-45**A** and **B**).
- ***Dysfunction***: The plantar aponeurosis is similar to a guy wire that adds significant support to the longitudinal arch. Static stresses, such as jobs that require long periods of standing, thicken and dry out the aponeurosis. The muscles are susceptible to fatigue from excessive static weight bearing. The fascia and muscles are prone to overuse and acute injury in runners, dancers, and those who play racquet sports.

Position

- TP—standing for first stroke, sitting for other strokes
- CP—supine; an optional position is prone, with foot over the edge of the table

Strokes

CAUTION: **Do not perform deep strokes on the feet of pregnant women, as some theories suggest this may stimulate uterine contraction.**

1. Sit or stand at the foot of the table and use a broad fist to perform a series of slow, continuous strokes on the plantar aponeurosis from the base of the toes to the heel (Fig. 9-46). Emphasize the pressure at the index knuckle. Use lotion to reduce the friction, but you want some drag to stretch the superficial fascia.
2. Sit at the foot of the table. Using single-, double-, or braced-thumb technique, part the midline of the plantar aponeurosis in short, spreading strokes. Begin just below the toes, taking the lateral tissue more laterally and the medial more medially. Continue inch by inch to the heel.
3. Turn your body to face the medial aspect of the foot. Using single- or double-thumb technique, perform short, scooping strokes on the abductor hallucis in the medial direction, supinating the foot with each stroke (Fig. 9-47). Begin your strokes at the anterior part of the medial calcaneus and continue inch by inch to the base of the great toe.
4. Release the flexor digitorum brevis in the middle of the foot with short scooping strokes in a lateral to medial direction while supinating the foot. Begin at the middle part of the anterior calcaneus and continue to the toes.
5. Using single-, double-, or braced-thumb technique, release the abductor digiti minimi with short scoop-

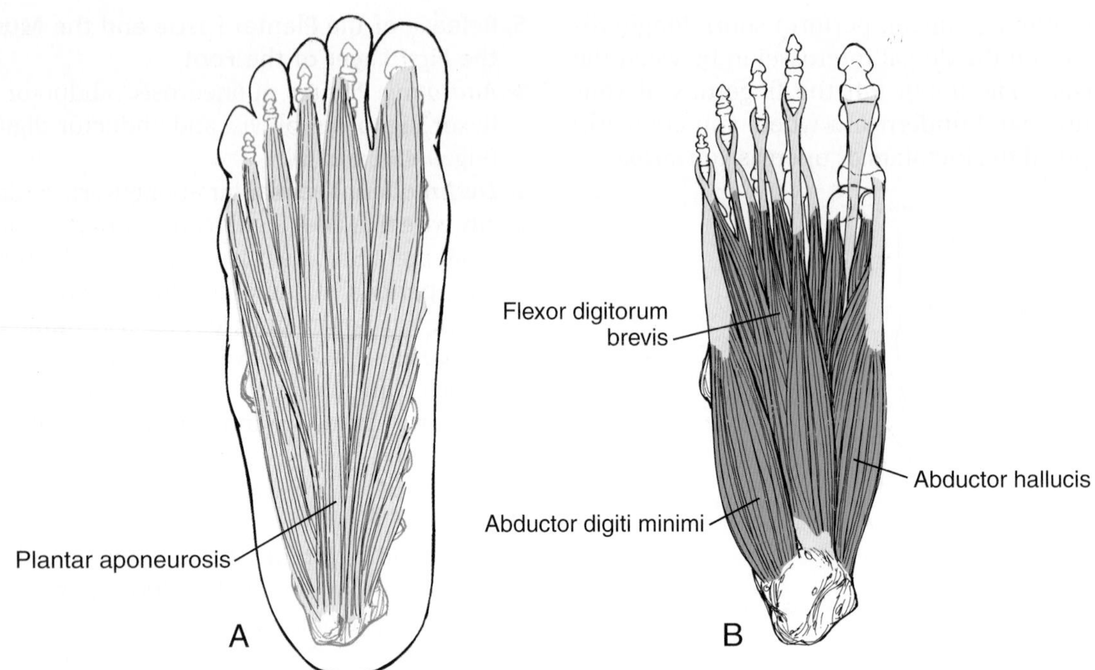

Figure 9-45. A. Plantar aponeurosis is a thickening of the deep fascia on the sole of the foot. **B.** First layer of muscles on the plantar aspect of the foot includes the abductor hallucis, flexor digitorum brevis, and the abductor digiti minimi.

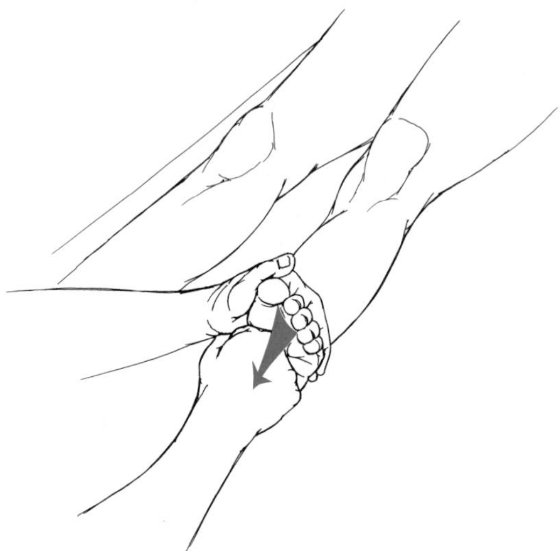

Figure 9-46. Broad-fist technique to stretch the plantar fascia.

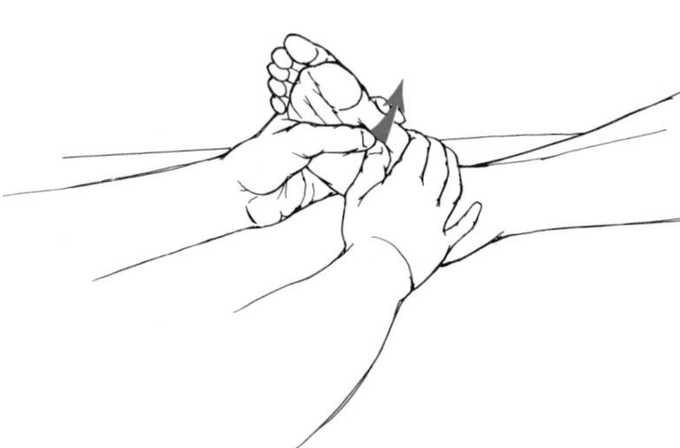

Figure 9-47. Double-thumb technique used to perform scooping strokes for the abductor hallucis.

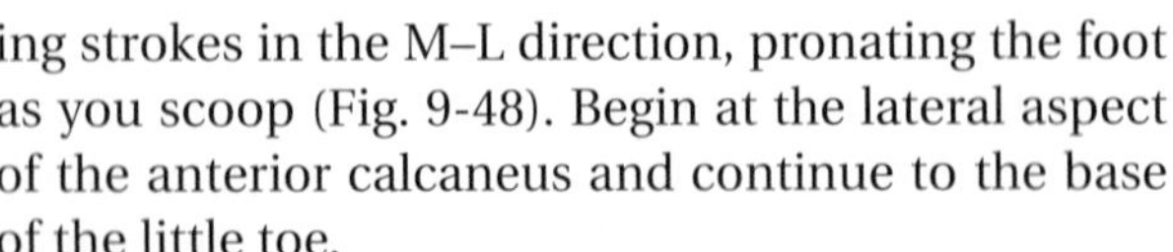

ing strokes in the M–L direction, pronating the foot as you scoop (Fig. 9-48). Begin at the lateral aspect of the anterior calcaneus and continue to the base of the little toe.

6. Release of the Second, Third, and Fourth Layers of the Foot

- *Anatomy*: Adductor hallucis (oblique and transverse heads); flexor hallucis brevis; flexor and opponens digiti minimi; lumbricals, which arise from the flexor digitorum longus tendons; and quadratus plantae (Fig. 9-49**A** and **B**).
- *Dysfunction*: Foot muscles are often held in a sustained contraction, predisposing them to ischemia and fibrosis. Static or dynamic stresses contribute to cumulative or overuse injuries. Sustained contraction of the adductor hallucis contributes to hallux valgus.

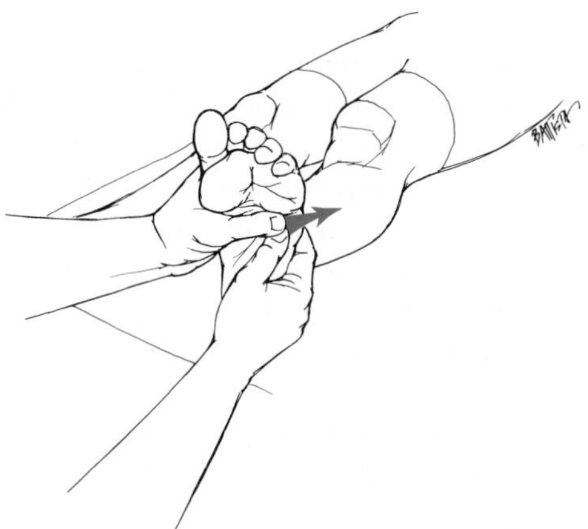

Figure 9-48. Double-thumb technique used to perform scooping strokes for the abductor digiti minimi.

Position

- TP—sitting
- CP—supine

Strokes

1. Deep to the flexor digitorum brevis is the quadratus plantae. Using double-thumb technique, release the quadratus plantae with a series of short scooping or back-and-forth strokes in the M–L plane. Begin at the anterior aspect of the calcaneus and continue to the midfoot where it attaches to the flexor digitorum longus tendon.
2. Using single- or double-thumb technique, perform a series of deep scooping posterior to anterior (P–A) strokes and back-and-forth strokes in the M–L plane on each of the flexor digitorum longus and flexor hallucis longus tendons (Fig. 9-50). Perform the same strokes on either side of the tendons to release the lumbricals. Begin in the midfoot and continue to the ends of each of the four lateral toes. Dorsiflex the foot and extend the toes to bring the tendons closer to the surface for easier work. Continue to the end of the toes.
3. Release the oblique head of the adductor hallucis, which originates in the midfoot underneath the flexor digitorum longus tendons. Using single- or double-thumb technique, perform short scooping strokes transverse to the line of the fiber from the midfoot to the lateral side of the great toe.
4. Release the transverse head of the adductor hallucis, which attaches to the deepest aspect of the ball of the foot (Fig. 9-51). Using a double-thumb technique, perform short scooping P–A strokes, beginning at the medial aspect of the fifth MTP joint and continuing inch by inch to the lateral aspect of the big toe.

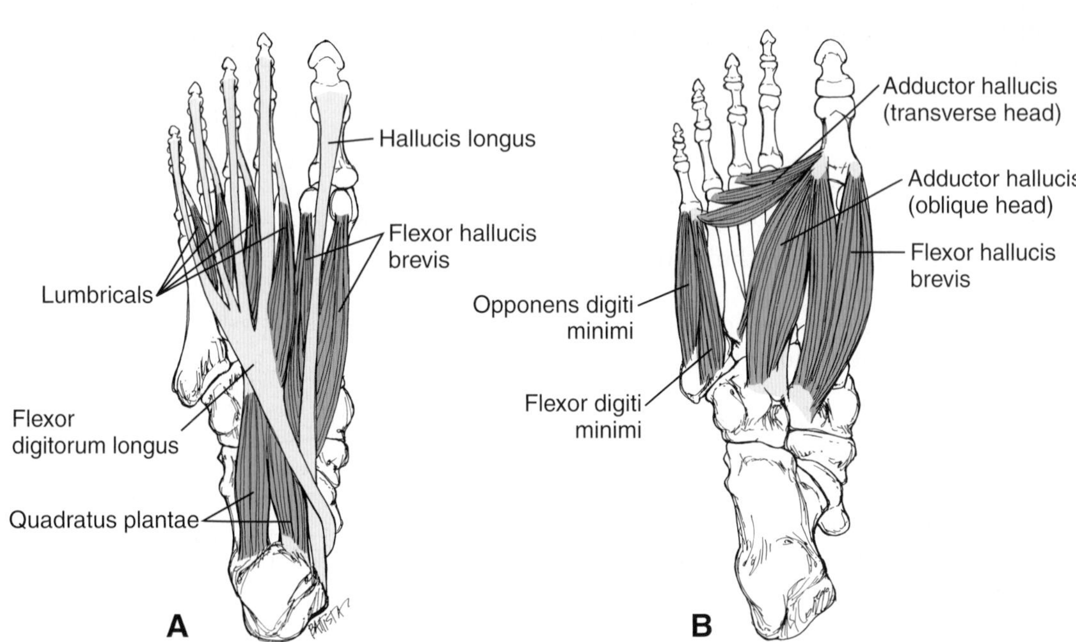

Figure 9-49. A. Second layer of plantar muscles includes the quadratus plantae and the four lumbrical muscles. **B.** Third layer of muscles on the bottom of the foot includes the flexor hallucis brevis, flexor digiti minimi, opponens digiti minimi, and the oblique and transverse heads of the adductor hallucis.

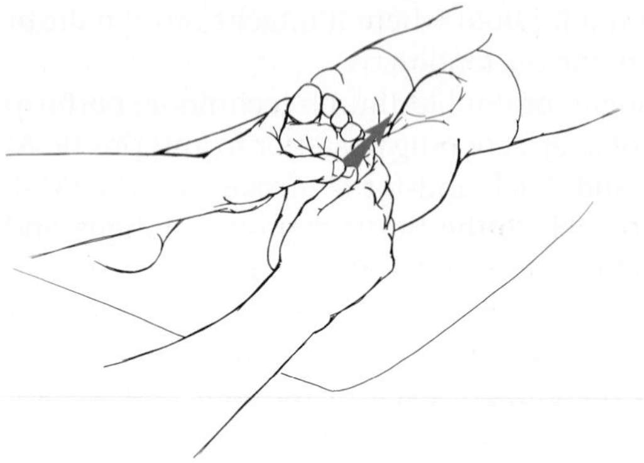

Figure 9-50. Single-thumb technique to release the lumbricals and tendons of the flexor digitorum longus and flexor hallucis longus.

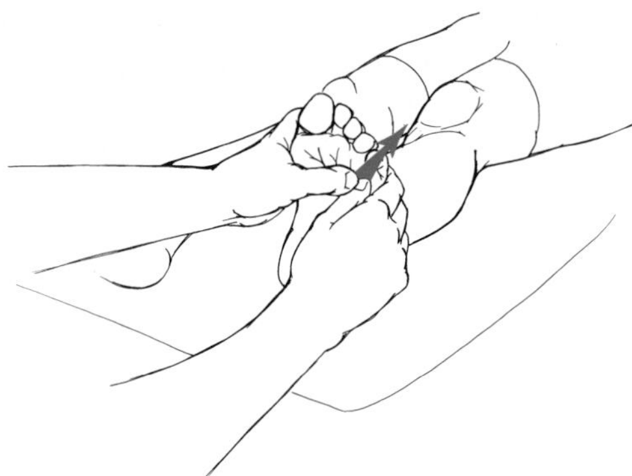

Figure 9-51. Double-thumb technique used to perform P–A scooping strokes on the attachments of the transverse head of the adductor hallucis.

Level II—Leg

1. Release of Muscle Attachments in the Anterior and Lateral Compartments

- *Anatomy*: Tibialis anterior, extensor digitorum longus, EHL, and peroneus longus and brevis (Fig. 9-52).
- *Dysfunction*: Chronic compartment syndromes are believed to be microtrauma to muscles, often exercise induced, that leads to a myositis and eventual fibrosis. The muscles and connective tissue tend to dehydrate and lose their lubricant. Chronic inflammation of the periosteum and planter fascia thickens the tissue at the site of injury.

Position

- TP—standing, or sitting on the table
- CP—supine, knee flexed, foot on the table

Strokes

You may stand or sit to perform these strokes. If you are standing, wrap your hands around the leg, holding and stabilizing the leg. If you are sitting on the table, gently sit on the client's foot to help stabilize the leg. Perform back-and-forth strokes in the M–L and the A–P planes with double-thumb technique on the myotendinous junctions, and perform brisk, transverse friction strokes on the tenoperiosteal attachments to the bone as needed.

1. While sitting or standing, use double-thumb technique to perform short, back-and-forth strokes in the M–L and the A–P planes to release the attachments of the tibialis anterior on the lateral surface of the proximal tibia. Follow this muscle down to the ankle and with special attention to the myotendinous junction approximately 6 inches above the ankle.

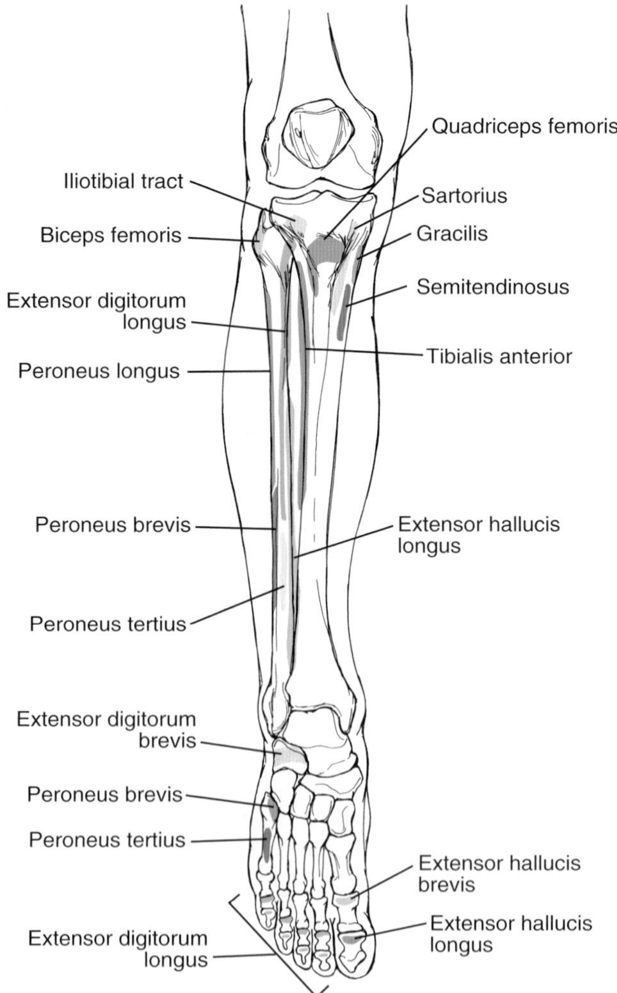

Figure 9-52. Muscle attachments on the anterior leg, ankle, and foot.

2. Using the same technique, release the attachments of the extensor digitorum longus on the lateral condyle of the tibia and the anterior medial crest of the fibula (Fig. 9-53).

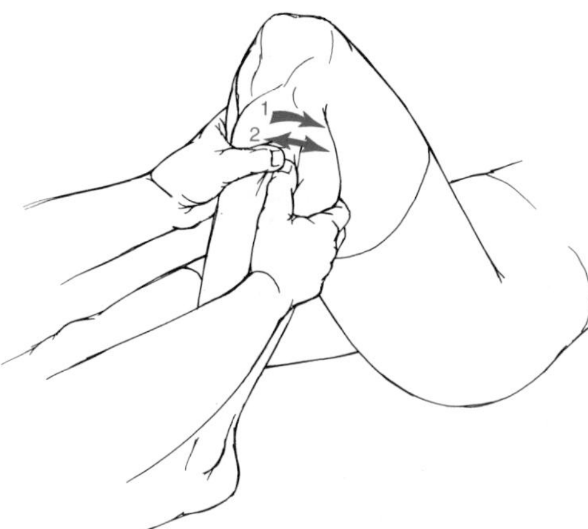

Figure 9-53. Double-thumb technique used to perform either (1) short scooping strokes in an M–L direction or (2) back-and-forth strokes in the M–L plane.

3. The EHL is deep to the tibialis anterior and the extensor digitorum longus. Using double-thumb technique, perform short, back-and-forth strokes in the M–L and the A–P plane, with the intention of penetrating through the more superficial muscles to the EHL.
4. Using double-thumb technique, perform either short, scooping strokes or back-and-forth strokes in the M–L and the A–P plane to release the peroneus longus from the upper two-thirds of the lateral aspect of the fibula and the peroneus brevis from the lower one-third (Fig. 9-54). Follow the tendons to the ankle with special attention to the myotendinous junction several inches above the ankle. Perform a brisk, transverse stroke at these sites if they feel fibrotic.

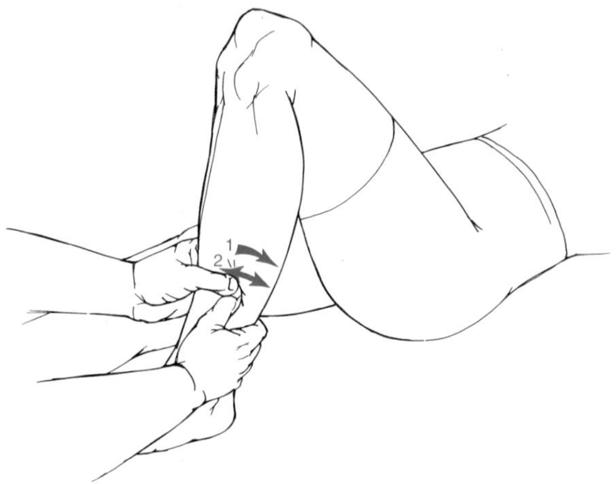

Figure 9-54. Double-thumb technique used to perform either (1) short scooping strokes in an M–L direction or (2) back-and-forth strokes in the M–L plane on the distal aspect of the tibia and fibula.

2. Release of the Tendons Crossing the Ankle and the Deep Peroneal and Posterior Tibial Nerves

- *Anatomy*: Deep peroneal nerve (see Fig. 9-4) and posterior tibial nerve (see Fig. 9-3), peroneus longus and brevis, tibialis anterior, EHL, extensor digitorum longus, tibialis posterior, and flexor digitorum longus and flexor hallucis longus (Fig. 9-55 **A** and **B**).
- *Dysfunction*: The tendons and their associated sheaths are susceptible to tenosynovitis where they cross the ankle through the fibro-osseous tunnels formed by the retinaculum. These nerves are susceptible to injury from an acute sprain of the ankle, a chronic overuse injury, or positional dysfunction such as pronated ankles. The tarsal tunnel describes the superficial and deep layers of the flexor retinaculum at the medial ankle and the posterior tibial nerve that travels between them.

Position

- TP—standing, facing your work
- CP—supine

Strokes

1. Release the tendons and tendon sheaths of the tibialis anterior, EHL, and extensor digitorum longus. Place both thumbs on the dorsum of the foot, while you hold the foot with both hands (see Fig. 9-42). Perform short, scooping strokes in an M–L direction with your thumbs, while you supinate the foot in an oscillating rhythm. With the same strokes, release the deep peroneal nerve under the inferior extensor retinaculum at the joint line of the ankle just lateral to the tendon of the EHL.
2. Release the posterior tibial nerve in the tarsal tunnel and the posterior tibialis, flexor digitorum longus, and flexor hallucis longus tendons at the medial ankle using double-thumb technique (Fig. 9-56). Perform short, scooping strokes while pronating the foot in an oscillating rhythm under the medial malleolus by scooping toward the heel, taking the nerve and tendons away from the bone.
3. Using double-thumb technique, release the calcaneal branch of the posterior tibial nerve by performing a series of gentle, scooping strokes toward the Achilles tendon between the medial malleolus and the center of the heel, inverting the foot with each stroke.

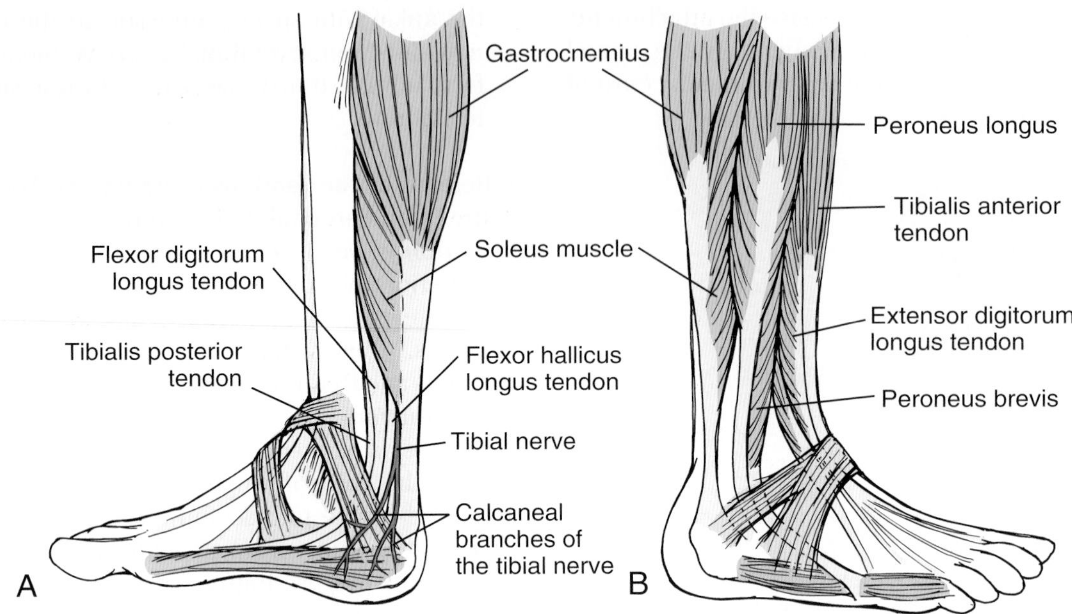

Figure 9-55. **A.** Medial leg, ankle, and foot showing the tendons of the tibialis posterior, flexor digitorum longus, flexor hallucis longus, and the tibial nerve. **B.** Lateral leg, ankle, and foot showing tendons of peroneus longus and brevis, tibialis anterior, and extensor digitorum longus.

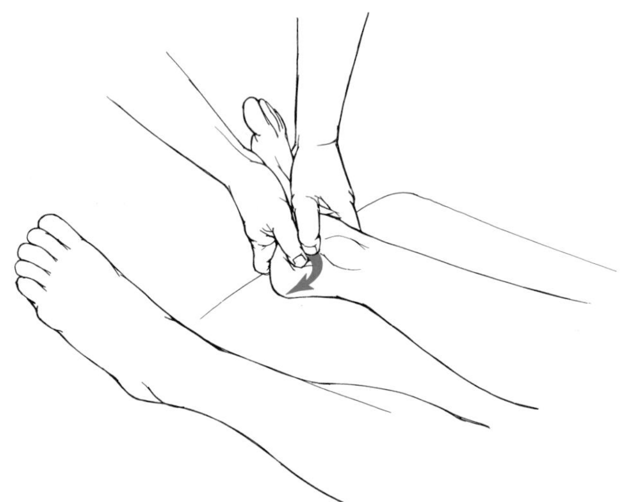

Figure 9-56. Double-thumb technique used to perform gentle scooping strokes to release the posterior tibial nerve in the tarsal tunnel.

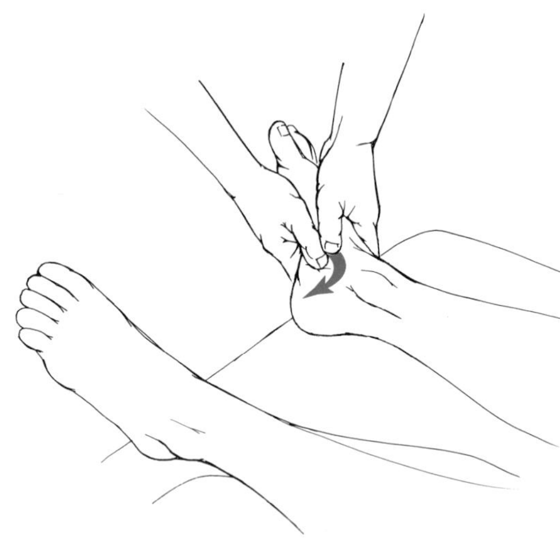

Figure 9-57. Double-thumb technique used to perform gentle scooping along the medial arch.

4. To release the medial and lateral plantar nerves and the abductor hallucis, use double-thumb technique and perform short, scooping strokes toward the plantar surface of the medial arch under the navicular and proximal first metatarsal (Fig. 9-57). Pronate the foot with each stroke.

5. Release the peroneal tendons and their associated tendon sheaths from the lateral malleolus (Fig. 9-58). Using fingertips or single thumb, scoop the tendons away from the malleolus as you supinate the foot. Begin your series a few inches proximal to the ankle, and continue to the base of the fifth metatarsal.

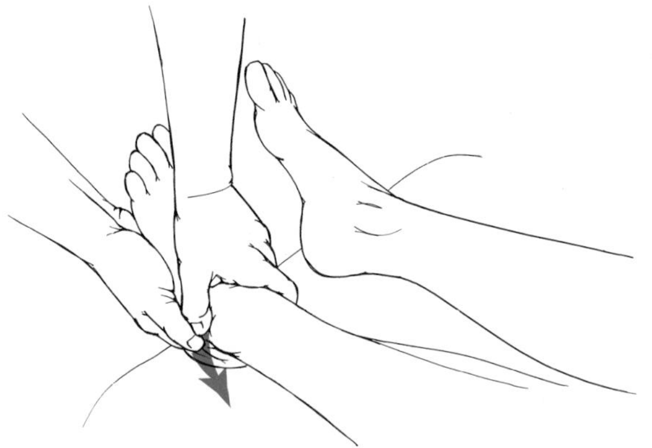

Figure 9-58. Double-thumb technique used to perform gentle scooping on the peroneal tendons.

3. Release of the Muscles and Attachments in the Posterior Compartments

- *Anatomy*: Soleus, tibialis posterior, popliteus, flexor hallucis longus, and flexor digitorum longus (Fig. 9-59).

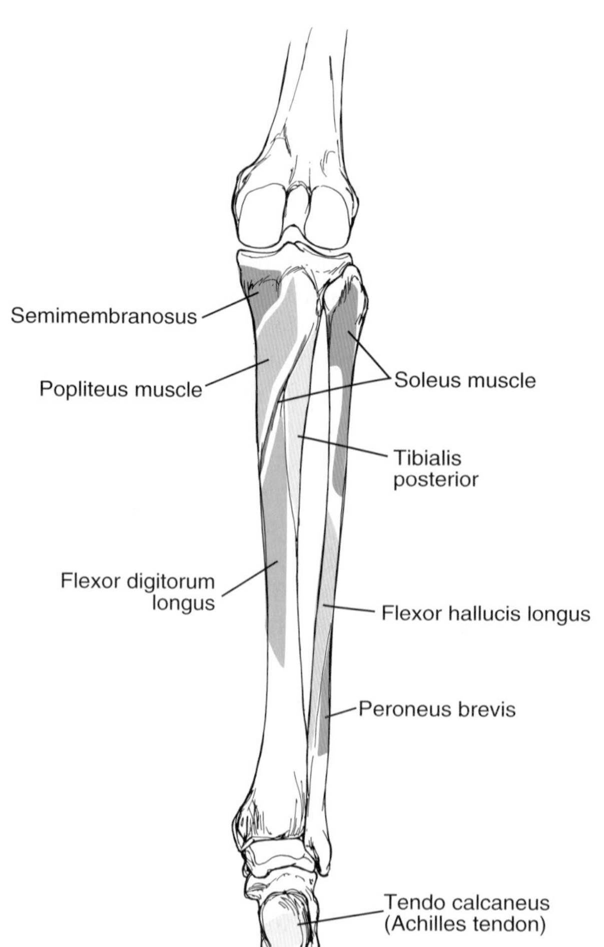

Figure 9-59. Muscle attachment sites on the posterior leg and foot.

- *Dysfunction*: Injuries to the medial leg, particularly tibialis posterior shin splints, are the most common shin splints in runners and dancers. The muscles tend to shorten and become fibrotic after overuse or acute injury.

Position

- TP—standing, facing headward or facing the table with the client prone, or sitting with client supine
- CP—There are two possible positions: (1) prone, with knee flexed to 90° or knee flexed with leg resting on your flexed leg on the table and (2) supine with the knee flexed, foot on the table

Strokes

The intention is to "look" with your hands for any fibrosis or hypertonicity. This thickened or knotted feel may be in the muscle belly, in the myotendinous junction, or at the tenoperiosteal attachment to the bone.

1. Stand, facing the table, with the client prone and the client's leg resting on your thigh. To release the soleus, flexor hallucis longus, and peroneus brevis from the posterior fibula, use braced- or double-thumb technique and perform a series of back-and-forth strokes in an M–L plane from the proximal portion of the posterior fibula and continue these strokes to the posterior surface of the lateral malleolus (Fig. 9-60). Move the tissue aside to make contact with the bone. An alternate position is to have the client supine, knee flexed, foot on the table, and use the fingertips of one or both hands to perform the same strokes (Fig. 9-61).

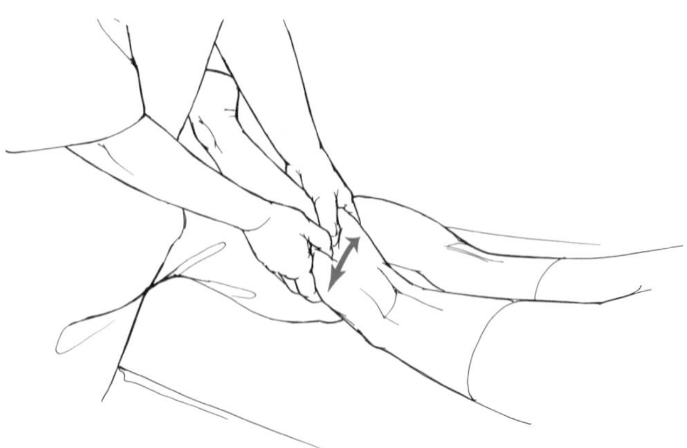

Figure 9-60. Double-thumb release of the muscle attachments on the posterior leg.

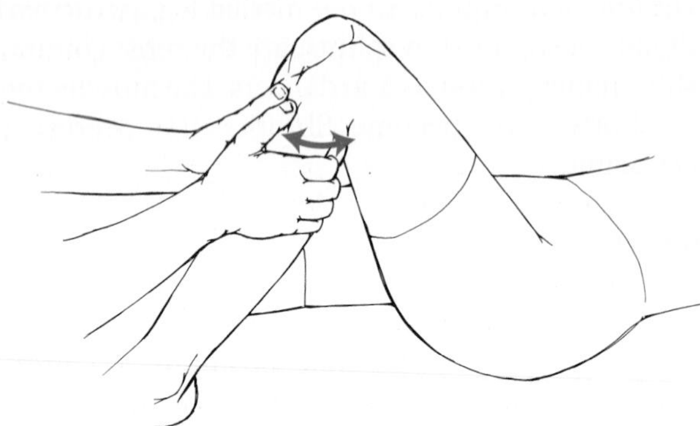

Figure 9-61. Supine technique to release the muscle attachments on the posterior leg. The fingertips of one or both hands are performing back-and-forth strokes in the M–L plane.

2. Perform a series of back-and-forth strokes in an M–L plane in the deepest aspect of the center of the calf to release the tibialis posterior and soleus from the interosseus membrane and the adjacent tibia. Use the fingertips of one or both hands if the client is supine, or use braced- or double-thumb technique if the client is prone. Again, continue these strokes down to the posterior aspect of the tibia. Perform more brisk transverse friction strokes if the area feels fibrotic.
3. To release the popliteus and flexor digitorum longus, use the same hand positions described above to perform back-and-forth strokes or brisk transverse friction strokes on the posterior tibia. Continue these strokes down the medial leg to the medial malleolus, scanning the area for any fibrosis.

4. Release of the Muscles and Ligaments that Attach to the Calcaneus and Heel Spurs

- *Anatomy*: Abductor hallucis, flexor digitorum brevis, abductor digiti minimi, quadratus plantae, and long plantar ligament (Fig. 9-62).
- *Dysfunction*: Plantar fasciitis is an acute or chronic strain that can arise from prolonged standing or from overuse such as excessive running. Activities such as running create a repetitive pulling on the periosteal attachment to the calcaneus and can create a traction spur, one type of heel spur. Another type of heel spur arises in response to static stress, which creates a microinflammation of the periosteum creating a bony spur.

Position

- TP—sitting
- CP—supine

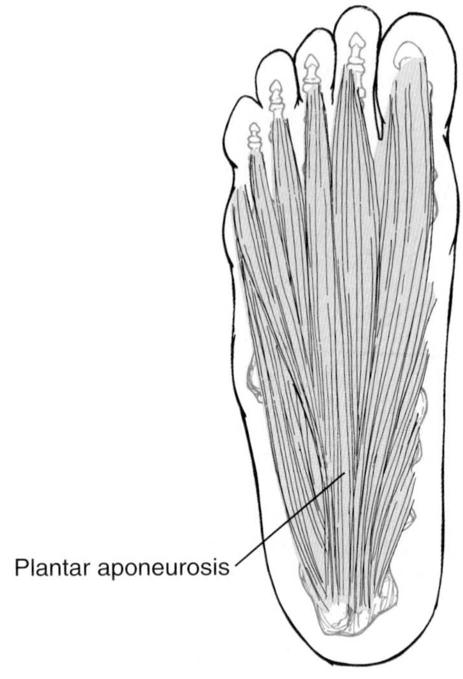

Figure 9-62. Plantar aponeurosis is a thickening of the deep fascia on the sole of the foot.

Strokes

The intention is to both dissolve the fibrosis in the plantar fascia associated with chronic irritation, and to "clean the bone" of the heel. It is possible to dissolve small calcium crystals (spicules) that are embedded in the fascia. It is also possible to clean the surface of larger, pedunculated (rounded) spurs of these small mineral deposits and fibrous depositions. The intention is not to dissolve the larger spur, but rather to release any fibrous adhesions attaching to the bone. This can be painful with plantar fasciitis or heel spurs. Remember to work only within the comfortable limits of the client. The successful outcome of these treatments often takes 6 to 12 sessions. Work a little deeper each session if possible. The healthy heel is not sensitive to deep pressure.

1. Using the knuckle (MCP joint) of your flexed index or middle finger, the PIP joint of your index finger, or a blunt instrument such as a T bar, perform deep back-and-forth strokes in the M–L plane on the entire plantar aspect of the heel (Fig. 9-63). Cover the medial, posterior, and lateral sides, as well as the center. Rock your body and translate that into a rocking of the foot with each stroke.
2. Perform a series of brisk, back-and-forth strokes in the M–L plane on the medial, middle, and lateral aspects of the anterior calcaneus. This releases the

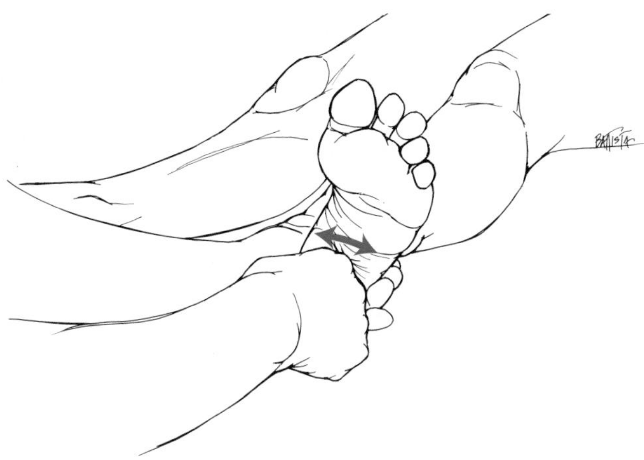

Figure 9-63. Use of the index knuckle to perform transverse friction strokes on the heel.

attachments of the abductor hallucis, flexor digitorum brevis, quadratus plantae, abductor digiti minimi, and long plantar ligament.

3. If you find a heel spur, perform brisk, friction strokes on the spur. Only work for approximately 5 seconds on any one painful spot. Move to another spot, if only a few millimeters away. Work for approximately 5 minutes each session directly on the bone, as too much work bruises the area.

5. Release of the Attachment Points and the Joint Capsule and Ligaments of the Metatarsophalangeal and Interphalangeal Joints

- *Anatomy*: Joint capsule and ligaments of the MTP and IP joints (Fig. 9-64), superficial and deep layers of the transverse metatarsal ligaments, annular and cruciate ligaments, plantar digital nerve, tibialis posterior and anterior, and peroneus brevis and longus.
- *Dysfunction*: The joint capsules and ligaments are typically thickened and fibrotic as a result of disuse,

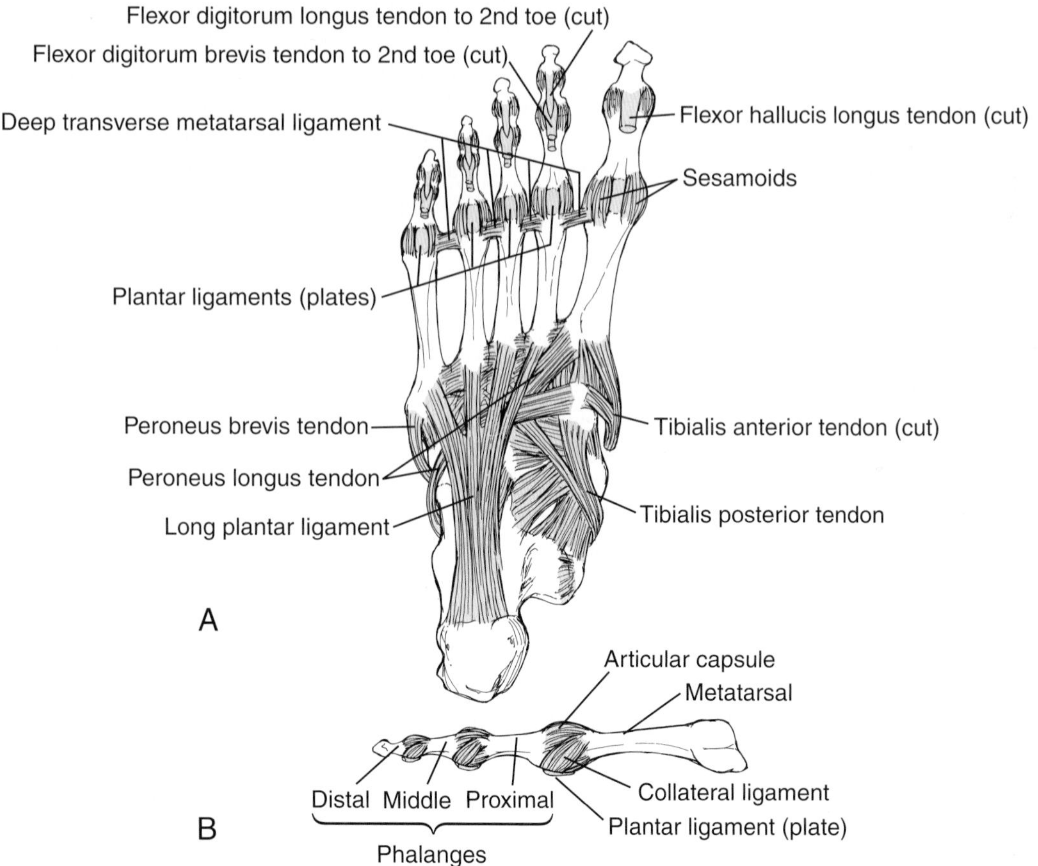

Figure 9-64. A. Ligaments and tendon insertions on the plantar aspect (bottom) of the foot. **B.** Joint capsule and collateral ligaments of the MTP and IP joints. Note that the fibers of the joint capsule are aligned parallel to the shaft of the bone and that the collateral ligaments are angled in a dorsal to plantar direction.

static stress, or inflammation from injury. This fibrosis decreases joint motion, leading to potential degeneration. With excessive running or chronic weight distribution problems, tendon attachment points become fibrotic. Work all the attachment points that have become fibrotic. The ones listed below are the most common.

Position

- TP—sitting in a chair or on the table
- CP—supine

Strokes

1. Using double- or braced-thumb, perform a series of 1-inch, back-and-forth strokes on the tuberosity of the plantar surface of the navicular, first cuneiform, and base of the first metatarsal to release the attachments of the tibialis posterior and tibialis anterior (Fig. 9-65).

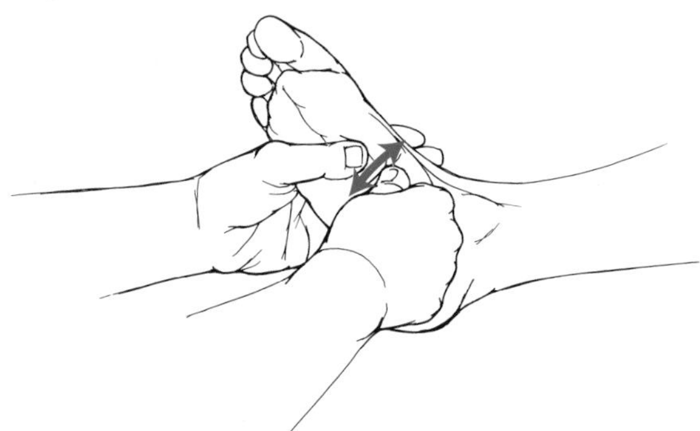

Figure 9-65. Braced-thumb technique used to perform back-and-forth strokes on the plantar surface of the navicular.

2. Using double- or braced-thumb, release the base of the fifth metatarsal with short, back-and-forth strokes in the M–L plane to release the abductor digiti minimi, the flexor digiti minimi, and the peroneus brevis. Release the peroneus longus tendon with scooping strokes in the P–A direction from the area just proximal to the base of the fifth metatarsal, and perform a series of strokes following the tendon to its attachment to the lateral surface of the base of the first metatarsal.
3. Release of the dorsal and plantar interossei. These muscles lie in between and on the plantar surface of the lateral four metatarsals, from the midfoot to the base of the toes. Perform a series of 1-inch, scooping strokes in the P–A (heel-to-toe) direction. The intention is to create space in between the metatarsals. Place your fingertips on the dorsum of the foot opposite your working thumb to act as a counterforce.
4. Use single-thumb or fingertip technique and perform back-and-forth strokes on the medial and lateral aspect of each toe, concentrating at the IP joints (Fig. 9-66). Work transverse to the shaft of each toe to release the collateral ligaments and joint capsule.

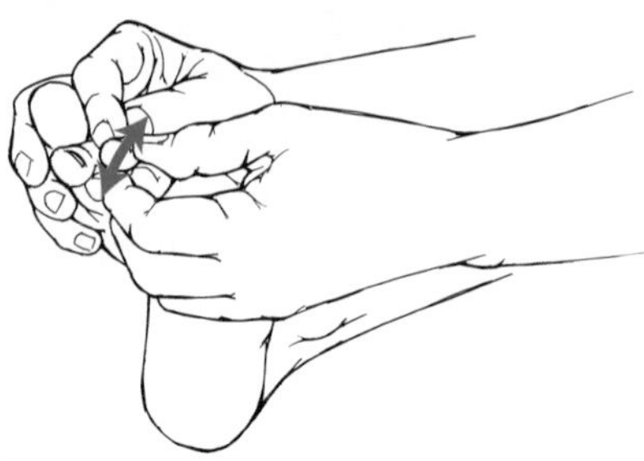

Figure 9-66. Fingertip of the right index finger is used to perform back-and-forth strokes on the IP joints, transverse to the shaft of the bone, to release the medial collateral ligament of the third toe.

5. The plantar digital nerve can become entrapped between the superficial and the deep layers of the transverse metatarsal ligament, which runs between the two metatarsal heads. We first release the ligament by using single-thumb technique to perform back-and-forth stokes in the A–P plane on the medial and lateral aspect of each MTP joint. Then, to release the nerve from potential entrapment, use a single-thumb technique to perform a series of scooping strokes in the M–L plane transverse to the nerve in between each MTP joint (Fig. 9-67).

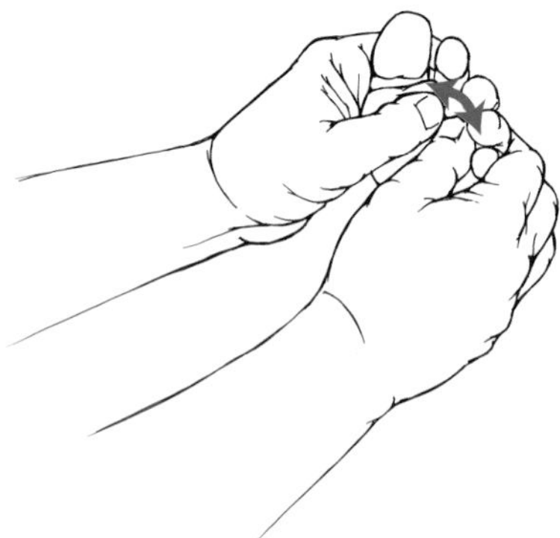

Figure 9-67. Right thumb is used to perform gentle scooping strokes in the M–L plane to release the plantar digital nerve in between the heads of the metatarsals.

6. Mobilization of the Ankle and Foot

- *Anatomy*: The tarsus consists of seven bones: talus, calcaneus, navicular, cuboid, and three cuneiform bones. The metatarsus consists of five metatarsals. Digits are formed by the phalanges (Fig. 9-68).

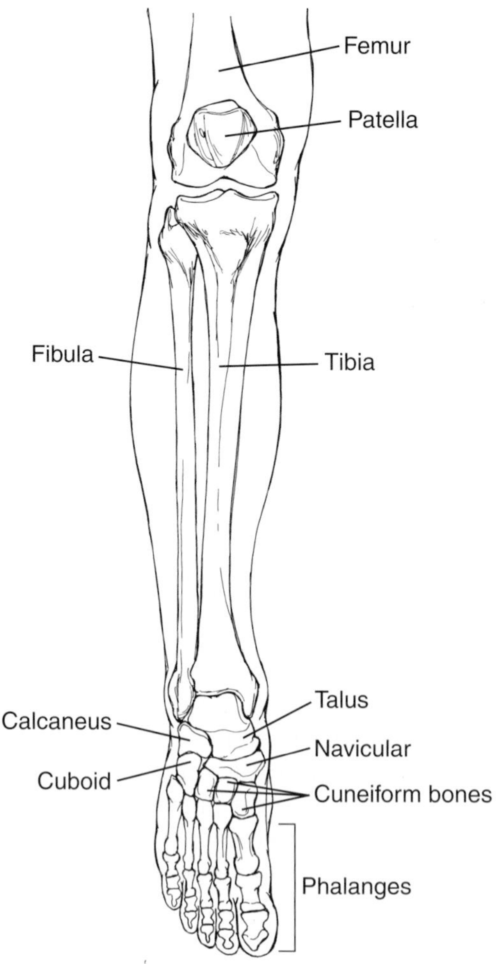

Figure 9-68. Bones and joints of the ankle and foot.

- ***Dysfunction***: Acute injury or chronic overuse tends to inhibit the normal gliding characteristics of the joints, causing joint dysfunction and subsequent soft-tissue compensations. These compensations include sustained contraction or weakening in the muscles or fibrosis in the joint capsule and ligaments. The toes often have a thickening of the joint capsules and a loss of the normal glide.

Position

- TP—sit on end of table, facing away from the client, with client's leg resting on your thigh and a pillow under the client's knee
- CP—supine

Strokes

1. Mobilization of the first metatarsal and first MTP joint. Stabilize the ankle with your hand closest to the table. Grasp the area of the client's first MTP joint with your other hand, with your thumb on the dorsal surface, fingertips underneath. Perform a clockwise circle on client's right foot, with the outside line of the circle being described by the MTP joint (Fig. 9-69). Repeat many times to hydrate the joint. As you create the circle, plantar flex the foot, pronating it; then roll it into dorsiflexion, supinating it. Perform a counterclockwise circle on the left.

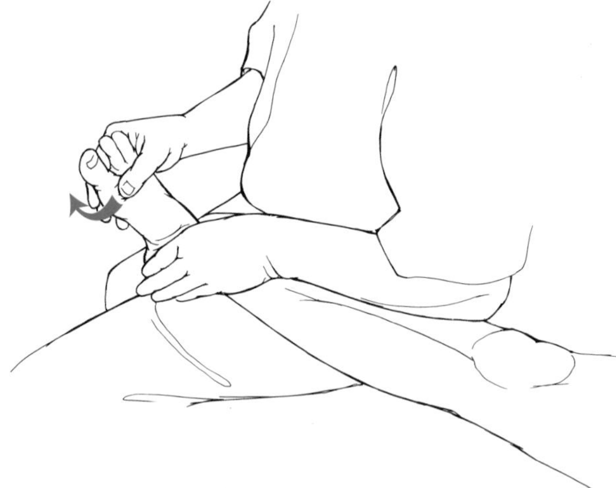

Figure 9-69. Mobilization of the forefoot and first MTP joint.

2. Hold adjacent metatarsals with opposite hands and move the hands in opposite directions in a dorsal-plantar shearing motion. Repeat many times in an oscillating motion. Repeat for each metatarsal.
3. To release the joint capsule of the great toe, use double- or single-thumb technique or fingertips and perform back-and-forth strokes transverse to the shaft of the bone. Work around the entire circumference of the first MTP joint, concentrating on the dorsal and medial surface (Fig. 9-70).

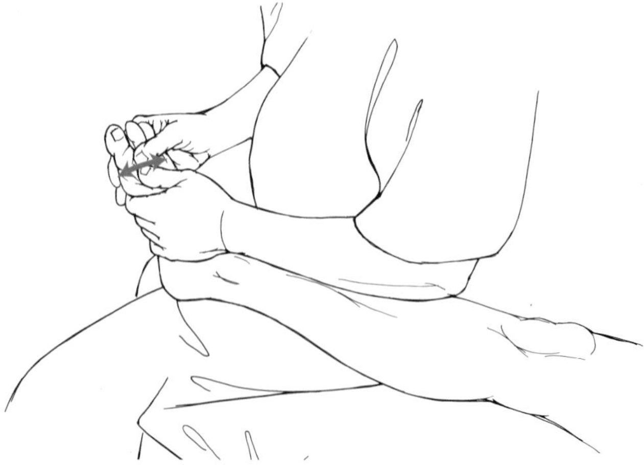

Figure 9-70. Double-thumb technique used to perform brisk, transverse strokes on the joint capsule of the first MTP joint.

4. To mobilize the toes, stabilize the distal end of one metatarsal with one hand, and grasp the proximal portion of the phalange with the other. Mobilize the toes first in a dorsal-plantar and a M–L glide and then in circumduction (Fig. 9-71). Perform the same dorsal-plantar and M–L glide on the IP joints by stabilizing the proximal phalange and moving the distal phalange.

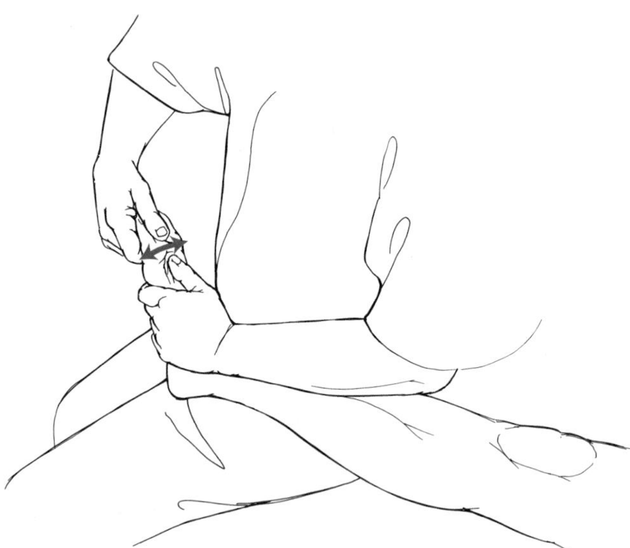

Figure 9-71. Mobilization of the MTP and IP joints. The left hand is stabilizing the proximal joint, and the distal hand is moving the distal bone.

5. To correct the position of the sesamoid bones of the great toe, flex the toe to give some slack. Then, using the flat surface on the lateral aspect of the index finger, place it deep in the tissue on the lateral side of the sesamoid under the MTP joint of the great toe. Keep tension in the index finger as you pull the toe into extension; then pull the sesamoid medially as you move the great toe medially. Continue a medial pull on the sesamoid as you pull the toe laterally, to normalize the sesamoid's position (Fig. 9-72).

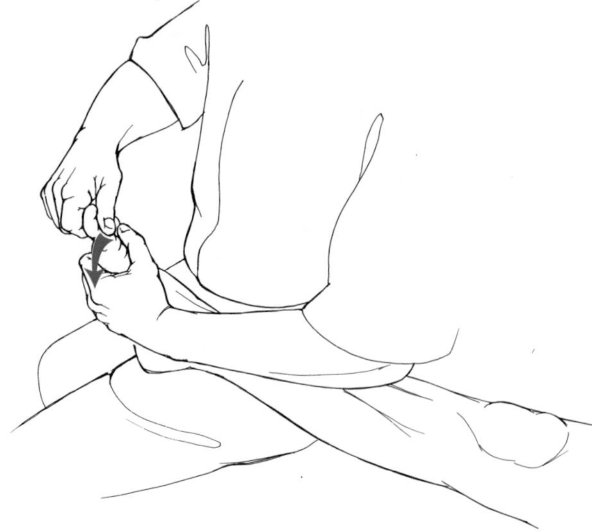

Figure 9-72. Mobilization of the sesamoids. The index finger of the right hand pulls the sesamoid medially in coordination with moving the great toe.

6. Mobilization of the ankle. Cup the heel with one hand, and hold the dorsum of the foot with the other hand. Passively move the ankle into dorsiflexion. Lean back to traction the ankle. Rock the leg (hip) into adduction and abduction as you cock the ankle into pronation and supination in rhythmic oscillations. As you adduct the leg, pronate the ankle, and as you abduct the hip, supinate the ankle. This stimulates the cartilage of the ankle joint to increase cellular synthesis and promotes hydration of the joint. Repeat for approximately 10 seconds (Fig. 9-73).

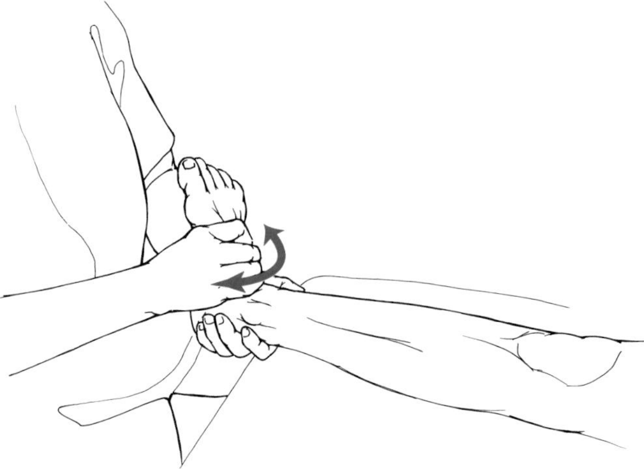

Figure 9-73. Mobilization of the ankle includes three movements: One, dorsiflex the ankle; two, traction the ankle by pulling at the heel; and three, pronate and supinate the ankle.

CASE STUDY

KB is a 55-year-old, 5'7', 180-lb, female realtor who presented to my office complaining of pain and stiffness in the right foot and ankle. The pain began approximately 2 years earlier when her foot "turned and collapsed." She saw her medical doctor who recommended ibuprofen, a podiatrist who made orthotics and recommended exercises, and an acupuncturist. She reported that the pain is mostly an ache, but that it becomes worse with driving, that it can become stiff if she sits for more than a few minutes, and that she can experience stabbing pain if she has been on it for awhile. She has been unable to hike due to the pain, which was her favorite form of exercise.

Examination revealed that the patient walked with a slight limp. In standing, the ankles were pronated, and the feet were flat, with flatness greater in the right than in the left. Active ROM was moderately reduced in dorsiflexion on the right. Plantar flexion was slightly limited, eliciting a pain at the anterior ankle. Active inversion was painful at the lateral ankle. Passive dorsiflexion was limited, and passive plantar flexion was painful at the navicular. Isometric testing elicited pain at the navicular with resisted inversion and weakness of the dorsiflexors. Extensive crepitation was produced at the ankle when the ankle was mobilized with it fully dorsiflexed and then pronated and supinated. This indicated extensive degeneration in the ankle. To palpation there was extensive fibrosis at the lateral and anterior ankle, sustained contractions in the posterior calf muscles and peroneals, and fibrosis in the plantar fascia.

A diagnosis was made of pronation, fibrosis of the anterolateral ligaments, and osteoarthritis of the ankle. Treatments were recommended on a weekly basis for 4 weeks. Treatments began with the patient supine. PIR MET was performed for the gastrocnemius and soleus to lengthen those muscles and to allow for greater dorsiflexion. CR MET was performed for the posterior tibialis and peroneals to reduce their hypertonicity and to decrease the fibrosis at the tenoperiosteal attachments of those muscles. CR MET was then performed to strengthen the tibialis anterior. OM was performed, with concentration on the thickened tissue at the anterior joint line, the lateral malleolus, and the navicular. The ankle was then mobilized for several minutes with the ankle held in dorsiflexion, and then the heel and ankle were pronated and supinated in an oscillating rhythm. This motion elicited audible "crunching" sounds, although it was not painful. This technique reduces calcium deposits on the articular surfaces.

The patient returned 1 week later and reported that the pain was reduced 80%. The same treatment described above was repeated. The mobilization elicited much less crepitation, indicating that the calcium deposits were reduced. KB returned for her next two visits reporting continuing improvement and elected to continue care on a weekly basis. At her eleventh visit, approximately 3 months after her initial treatment, she reported that she was completely pain free and that she was now able to hike without pain. I saw the patient occasionally after that, approximately one time per month. Six months after her initial visit she took a walking trip to Europe and reported that she had no pain during or after her trip.

STUDY GUIDE

Level I—Leg

1. Describe the MET for an acute ankle.
2. List the ligaments that comprise the lateral collateral ligament of the ankle.
3. List the compartments of the leg, and list which muscles are in each compartment.
4. Describe the MET for the muscles of the leg, ankle, and foot.
5. Describe which muscles tend to be short and tight and which muscles tend to be weak in the leg, ankle, and foot.
6. Describe the signs and symptoms for the first eight dysfunctions and injuries in the chapter.
7. List the names of the intrinsic muscles in each layer of the foot.
8. Describe two common dysfunctions in the knee and foot that are associated with pronation.
9. Describe the functions of the ligaments of the ankle.
10. Describe two possible outcomes of an ankle ligament sprain.

Level II—Leg

1. List the main nerves to the leg, ankle, and foot, their function, their common entrapment sites, and the direction of the stroke to treat them.
2. Describe the attachment sites for the anterior talofibular ligament and the direction of the strokes to treat it.

3. List which muscles are typically tight and short and which muscles are weak in hammer toes and claw toes.
4. Describe the assessment findings in pronation. Describe which muscles are typically short and tight and which muscles are typically weak in pronation.
5. List the tendons that pass behind the medial and lateral ankle and on the dorsum of the foot, and list the stroke direction to treat them.
6. Describe the signs and symptoms of the less common dysfunctions and injuries of the leg, ankle, and foot.
7. Describe how much extension the first MTP joint must have for normal gait. Why?
8. Describe the direction of dysfunction of the sesamoids of the great toe and the stroke direction to treat them.
9. Describe the movement direction for mobilization of the ankle and foot.
10. Describe the stroke direction to treat the collateral ligaments of the toes.

REFERENCES

1. Garrick J, Webb D. Sports Injuries. 2nd Ed. Philadelphia: WB Saunders, 1999.
2. Andrews J. Overuse syndromes of the lower extremity. Clin Sports Med 1983;2:137–148.
3. McPoil T. The foot and ankle. In: Malone T, McPoil T, Nitz A, eds. Orthopedic and Sports Physical Therapy. St. Louis: Mosby, 1997:261–293.
4. Cailliet R. Foot and Ankle Pain. 3rd Ed. Philadelphia: FA Davis, 1997.
5. Garrett JC. The lower leg. In: Scott WN, Nisonson B, Nicholas J, eds. Principles of Sports Medicine. Baltimore: Williams & Wilkins, 1984:342–347.
6. Windsor R, Chambers K. Overuse injuries of the leg. In: Kibler WB, Herring SA, Press JM, eds. Functional Rehabilitation of Sports and Musculoskeletal Injuries. Gaithersburg: Aspen, 1998:265–272.
7. Hertling D, Kessler R. The lower leg, ankle, and foot. In: Management of Common Musculoskeletal Disorders. Baltimore: Lippincott Williams & Wilkins, 1996: 379–443.
8. Freeman MAR, Wyke B. Articular reflexes at the ankle joint: an electromyographic study of normal and abnormal influences of ankle-joint mechanoreceptors upon reflex activity in the leg muscles. Br J Surg 1967; 54: 990–1001.
9. Freeman MAR, Dean MRE, Hanham IWF. The etiology and prevention of functional instability of the foot. J Bone Joint Surg Br 1965;47:669–677.
10. Platzer W. Locomotor System. 4th Ed. Vol. 1. New York: Thieme Medical, 1992.
11. Norkin C, Levangie P. The ankle-foot complex. In: Joint Structure and Function. Philadelphia: FA Davis, 1992: 379–418.
12. Corrigan B, Maitland GD. Practical Orthopaedic Medicine. London: Butterworths, 1983.
13. Hammer W. Functional Soft Tissue Examination and Treatment by Manual Methods. 2nd Ed. Gaithersburg: Aspen, 1999.
14. Hoppenfeld S. Physical Examination of the Spine and Extremities. New York: Appleton-Century-Crofts, 1976.
15. Magee D. Lower leg, ankle, and foot. In: Orthopedic Physical Assessment. Philadelphia: WB Saunders, 1997: 599–672.
16. Janda V. Evaluation of muscular imbalance. In: Liebenson C, ed. Rehabilitation of the Spine. Baltimore: Williams & Wilkins, 1996:97–112.

SUGGESTED READINGS

Cailliet R. Foot and Ankle Pain. 3rd Ed. Philadelphia: FA Davis, 1997.

Corrigan B, Maitland GD. Practical Orthopaedic Medicine. London: Butterworths, 1983.

Cyriax J, Cyriax P. Illustrated Manual of Orthopedic Medicine. London: Butterworths, 1983.

Garrick J, Webb D. Sports Injuries. 2nd Ed. Philadelphia: WB Saunders, 1999.

Greenman PE. Principles of Manual Medicine. 2nd Ed. Baltimore: Williams & Wilkins, 1996.

Hammer W. Functional Soft Tissue Examination and Treatment by Manual Methods. 2nd Ed. Gaithersburg: Aspen, 1999.

Hertling D, Kessler R. The lower leg, ankle, and foot. In: Management of Common Musculoskeletal Disorders. Baltimore: Lippincott Williams & Wilkins, 1996:379–443.

Hoppenfeld S. Physical Examination of the Spine and Extremities. New York: Appleton-Century-Crofts, 1976.

Kendall F, McCreary E, Provance P. Muscles: Testing and Function. 4th Ed. Baltimore: Williams & Wilkins, 1993.

Magee D. Lower leg, ankle, and foot. In: Orthopedic Physical Assessment. Philadelphia: WB Saunders, 1997:599–672.

McPoil T. The foot and ankle. In: Malone T, McPoil T, Nitz A, eds. Orthopedic and Sports Physical Therapy. St. Louis: Mosby, 1997:261–293.

Norkin C, Levangie P. The ankle-foot complex. In: Joint Structure and Function. Philadelphia: FA Davis, 1992:379–418.

Reid DC. Sports Injury and Assessment. New York: Churchill Livingstone, 1992.

Windsor R, Chambers K. Overuse injuries of the leg. In: Kibler WB, Herring SA, Press JM, eds. Functional Rehabilitation of Sports and Musculoskeletal Injuries. Gaithersburg: Aspen, 1998:265–272.

The Elbow, Forearm, Wrist, and Hand

Soft tissue injuries to the elbow often involve the muscle attachments to the lateral and medial elbow, called "tennis elbow" and "Little Leaguer's (Golfer's) elbow," respectively.[1,2] Nerve compression is also common in the elbow, wrist and hand region. The most frequently occurring peripheral nerve compression in the body is carpal tunnel syndrome, a compression of the median nerve at the wrist.[3] The ulnar nerve can also become entrapped at the elbow, a condition called cubital tunnel syndrome.[4] Trauma to the wrist is the most common injury in the upper extremity, followed by injuries to the interphalangeal (IP) joints of the hand are the next most common.[5]

Overview of the Elbow, Forearm, Wrist, and Hand

The bones of the upper limb are the **humerus** (the arm), the **radius** and **ulna** (the forearm), the **carpals** (the wrist), and the **metacarpals** and **phalanges** (the hand). The elbow is the articulation of the distal humerus with the proximal radius and ulna. Flexion and extension occur between the humerus and the ulna, and pronation and supination occur between the radius and the ulna. The wrist consists of 8 bones in two rows, and 15 muscles cross the wrist, 9 on the extensor surface (dorsum) and 6 on the anterior (palmar) surface. The hand consists of 19 bones and 19 joints.

Anatomy, Function, and Dysfunction of the Elbow and Forearm

BONES AND JOINTS OF THE ELBOW AND FOREARM

See Figure 10-1.

Humerus

- *Structure*: The distal end of the humerus expands into the medial and the lateral epicondyles. The

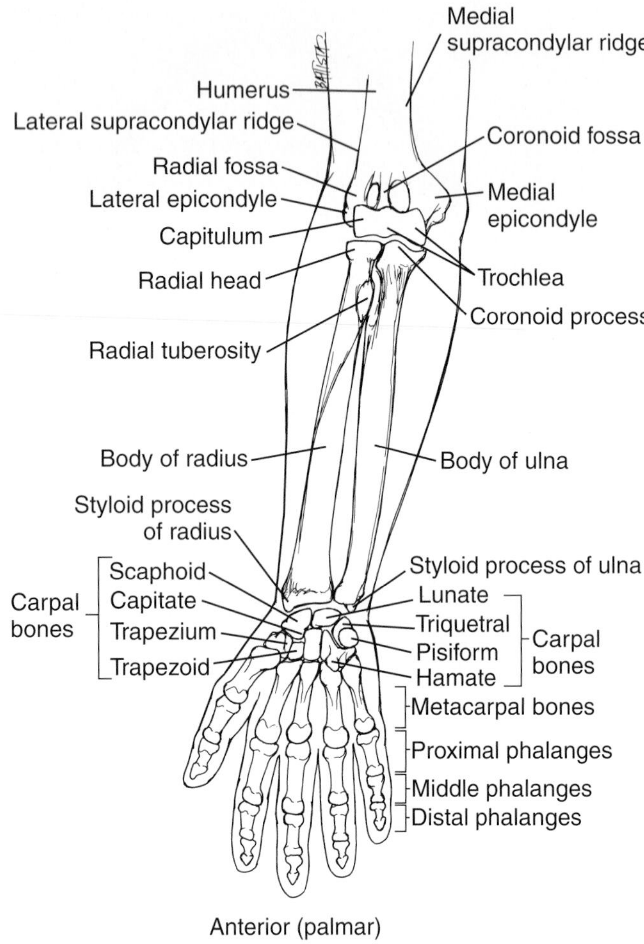

Figure 10-1. Bones of the elbow, forearm, wrist, and hand.

trochlea and the capitulum of the humerus form condyles that articulate with the radius and ulna, respectively. On the posterior surface is a large indentation, the olecranon fossa, to accept the olecranon process of the ulna during extension. On the medial side of the trochlea is a groove (sulcus) for the ulnar nerve. The radial nerve travels in a groove on the posterior surface of the humerus.

Ulna

- ***Structure***: The ulna has a large hook-shaped proximal end called the olecranon process, to which the triceps attaches. The anterior surface is the cartilage-lined trochlear notch, which articulates with the humerus to form the humeroulnar joint. The proximal portion of the ulna has a small curved surface, the radial notch, for articulation with the radius, forming the proximal radioulnar joint.

Radius

- ***Structure***: The proximal end of the radius is called the head and articulates with the capitulum of the humerus on its superior side and with the ulna on its medial side. The radius carries most of the load from the arm to the hand and therefore widens at its distal end and articulates with the first row of carpal bones. On the medial aspect of the proximal shaft is the radial tuberosity, which serves as the attachment site for the biceps brachii.

Joints of the Elbow and Forearm

- ***Structure***: The three bones of the arm and forearm form four joints at the elbow and forearm. The four joints are the humeroulnar and humeroradial joints and the proximal and distal radioulnar joints. The first three joints form the elbow, and the distal radioulnar joint is proximal to the wrist.
  - The **humeroulnar joint** is the articulation between the trochlea of the humerus and the trochlear notch of the ulna.
  - The **humeroradial joint** is the articulation between the capitulum of the humerus and the head of the radius.
  - The **proximal radioulnar joint** is the articulation between the head of the radius and the radial notch of the ulna.
  - The **distal radioulnar joint** is the articulation between the head of the ulna and the ulnar notch of the radius.
- ***Function***: Flexion and extension occur at the humeroulnar and humeroradial joints. Pronation and supination involves the rotation of the radius around the ulna. This motion occurs at the proximal and the distal radioulnar joints. The relaxed, open position of the elbow joint is slight flexion, and the closed position is extension.
- ***Dysfunction and injury***: Dysfunctions and injuries of the elbow are not nearly as common as soft-tissue injuries. The elbow may develop traumatic arthritis and consequent degeneration after a fall directly on the elbow or on an outstretched hand. If the elbow is injured and swells, it assumes a position of slight flexion to accommodate the excess fluid. If the elbow is immobilized or if joint motion is restricted due to pain, it may develop capsular fibrosis and stiffen in this flexed position. In passive motion assessment, flexion will be more restricted than extension.

- *Treatment implications*: Loss of joint motion is treated initially with muscle energy technique (MET). Orthopedic massage (OM) is performed on the periarticular soft tissue to dissolve adhesions and to allow for greater extensibility. Postisometric relaxation (PIR) MET is performed on the short and tight muscles that may be inhibiting the joint's normal range of motion (ROM). Finally, mobilization is performed to stimulate the nutritional exchange in the cartilage and to help dissolve calcium deposits on the articular surfaces.

SOFT-TISSUE STRUCTURES OF THE ELBOW AND FOREARM

Joint Capsule and Ligaments of the Elbow and Forearm

- *Structure*: The joint capsule of the elbow is thin and lax. It encloses the joint surfaces, but it does not enclose the medial and lateral epicondyles. Strong **radial** and **ulnar collateral ligaments** blend with the capsule, reinforcing it.
  - The **ulnar collateral ligament** usually has two portions, the anterior portion traveling from the medial epicondyle to the coronoid portion of the ulna and the posterior portion traveling from the medial epicondyle to the olecranon. The ulnar nerve travels under the fibers to the olecranon.
  - The **radial collateral ligament** travels from the lateral epicondyle of the humerus to the annular ligament, which encloses the radial head. The radial collateral ligament is interwoven with the superficial extensor muscles.[6]
  - The **annular ligament of the radius** attaches to the ulna and encircles the radial head. It is lined with cartilage on its inner surface to reduce friction as the head of the radius turns in pronation and supination.
  - As in the leg, an **interosseous membrane** connects the radius and ulna, strengthening the two bones and providing a site for muscle attachments.
- *Function*: As in the other joints of the body, the ligaments and joint capsule provide passive stability to the joints of the elbow. These structures also provide a neurosensory role and have reflex connections with the surrounding muscles. The joint capsule interweaves with the fascia of the brachialis, triceps, and anconeus muscles.[7] To prevent pinching of the joint capsule between the articular surfaces during extension, these muscles contract and pull the capsule out of the joint space.
- *Dysfunction and injury*: A thickening of the ligaments of the elbow typically follows cumulative stress or an acute injury. Passive supination is restricted with fibrosis of the annular ligament, and passive medial and lateral glide are reduced with fibrosis of the lateral and medial collateral ligaments. Weakness or sustained contraction of the triceps and brachialis potentially cause an impingement of the joint capsule.
- *Treatment implications*: If the ligaments have become fibrotic and thickened because of the deposit of excessive collagen after an injury, perform contract-relax (CR) MET to the muscles that attach to the capsule and ligaments, including the triceps, brachialis, and superficial extensors or the wrist and hand. Next, perform OM, including transverse friction massage, to the body (midportion) and attachment points of the ligaments. This process helps dissolve the adhesions and restores normal extensibility. If the ligaments have become too slack and the elbow is unstable, exercise rehabilitation is recommended to restore stability.

Fascia

- *Structure*: The fascia of the arm is called the brachial fascia and forms two compartments, the **anterior compartment,** which contains the flexors of the elbow, and the **posterior compartment,** which contains the extensors of the elbow.

  The fascia of the forearm is called the antebrachial fascia and forms three compartments: the **anterior,** which contains the flexors; the **posterior,** which contains the extensors; and the **radial,** which contains a muscle of elbow flexion, the brachioradialis, and two extensors of the wrist, the extensor carpi radialis longus (ECRL) and the extensor carpi radialis brevis (ECRB).

Nerves

- *Structure*: The nerves that exit from the neck and travel into the arm are called the **brachial plexus.** After they travel under the clavicle, they form seven long nerves into the arm, forearm, and hand. We consider the three main nerves, the **ulnar, median,** and **radial nerves,** because they are commonly in-

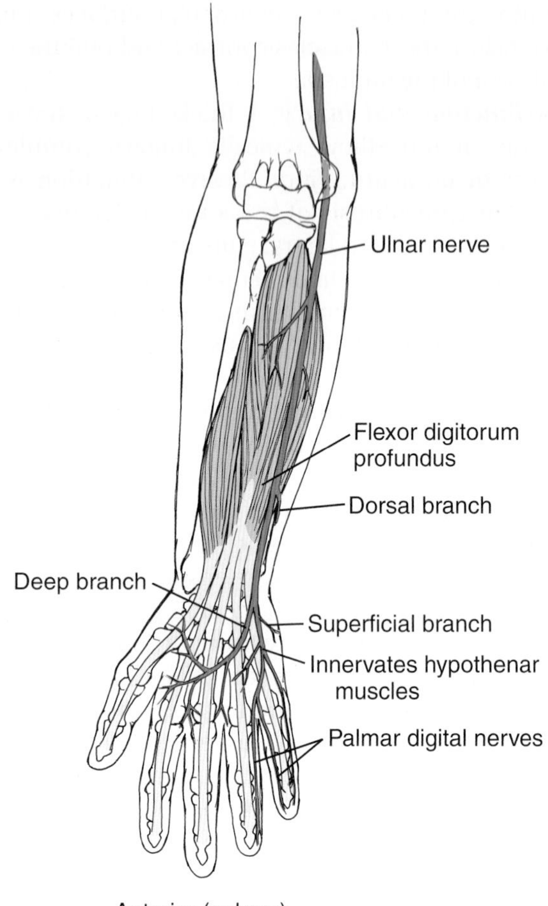

Figure 10-2. Course of the ulnar nerve through the elbow, forearm, wrist, and hand.

volved clinically. The ulnar and median nerves travel along the medial side of the arm between the two heads of the biceps muscle in a groove called the median bicipital sulcus. The radial nerve travels on the posterior side of the humerus in the groove for the radial nerve under the lateral head of the triceps. At the elbow, each of the nerves can become entrapped at the following sites:

- The **ulnar nerve** travels through the **cubital tunnel** formed by the ulnar collateral ligament and a fascial expansion of the flexor carpi ulnaris. It then travels through the two heads of the flexor carpi ulnaris (Fig. 10-2).
- The **median nerve** travels through a fibro-osseous tunnel on the anterior-medial surface of the distal end of the humerus, beneath the edge of the aponeurosis of the biceps called the lacertus fibrosis, and then between the two heads of origin of the pronator teres (Fig. 10-3).
- The **radial nerve** travels from the extensor compartment to the flexor compartment between the brachialis and the brachioradialis. It then passes under the fibrous origin of the ECRB and then enters the supinator canal approximately 2 inches distal to the lateral epicondyle under a fibrous arch called the arcade of Frohse (Fig. 10-4).

- *Function*: The three main nerves, the ulnar, median, and radial nerves function as follows:
  - The **ulnar nerve** supplies the ulnar flexors in the forearm, hand, and skin on the ulnar side of the hand and fourth and fifth fingers.
  - The **median nerve** innervates most of the flexors of the arm, forearm, and hand, as well as the skin of the wrist, the thenar eminence, the palm, the flexor side of the thumb, and the index and the middle fingers.
  - The **radial nerve** innervates all the extensors of the arm and the skin on the extensor side of the arm and hand.

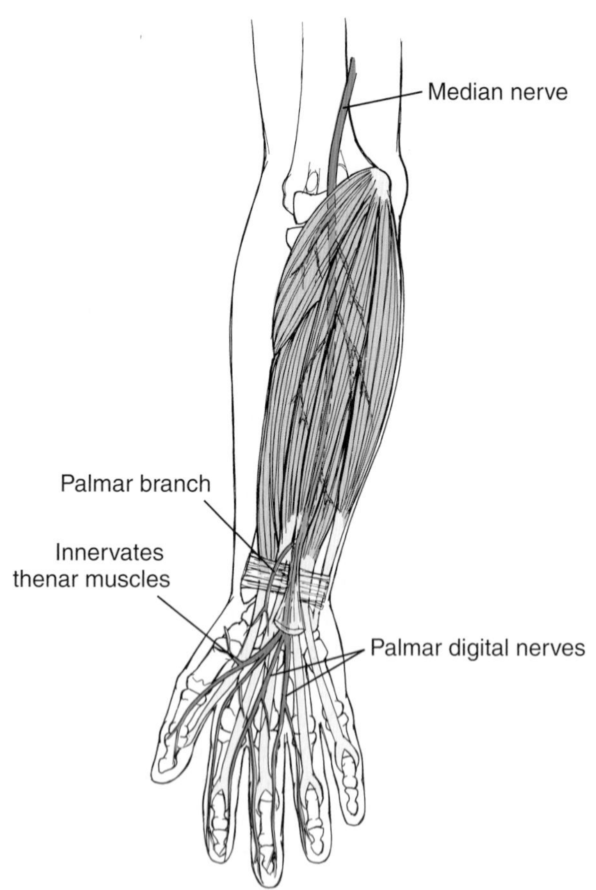

Figure 10-3. Course of the median nerve through the elbow, forearm, wrist, and hand.

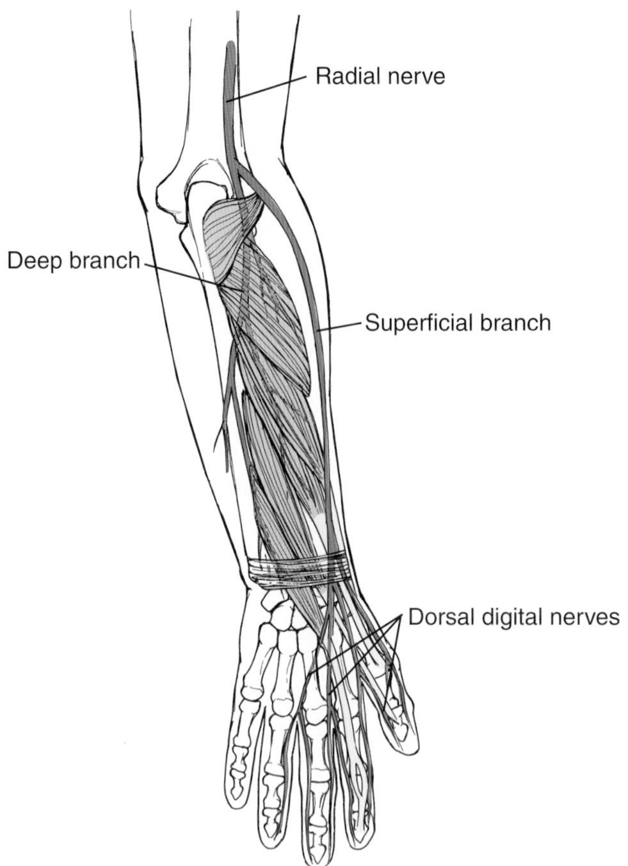

Figure 10-4. Course of the radial nerve through the elbow, forearm, wrist, and hand.

- ***Dysfunction and injury***: The nerves of the elbow may be injured as a result of any trauma to the elbow or cumulative stress. The **ulnar nerve** is often irritated with repetitive elbow flexion, which narrows the cubital tunnel, or from sustained elbow flexion, which commonly occurs with sleeping. The **median nerve** is often irritated due to repetitive pronation or pronation and flexion of the elbow. The **radial nerve** can be irritated by a repeated pronation, elbow extension, and wrist flexion (wringing motion) or overuse of the extensor muscles. The nerves may also become entrapped in the sustained contraction of overused muscles, which creates a thickening in the fascia at its attachment sites, or in the fibro-osseous tunnel through which the nerve travels. The specific anatomy of the entrapment sites are described above in the section "Structure."
- ***Treatment implications***: The treatment protocol for nerve entrapment is for the therapist first to perform MET to the muscles that interweave with the particular tunnel to reduce the hypertonicity in the muscles and to increase the length and extensibility of the connective tissue forming the tunnel. For example, to release the cubital tunnel, perform MET to the flexor carpi ulnaris, as its fascial expansion interweaves with the cubital tunnel. Next, perform manual release of the nerve by gentle, scooping strokes transverse to the line of the nerve. This dissolves the adhesions surrounding the nerve and releases the tension in the fascia suspending the nerve. Deep OM strokes, including transverse friction massage, are often needed to release the fibrosis in the fascia that forms the tunnels. The specific treatment protocol for the common entrapment sites is listed in the "Technique" section.

Muscles

- ***Structure***: The muscles that move the elbow are three flexors and two extensors. The flexors are the brachialis, biceps brachii, and the brachioradialis. The two extensors are the triceps and the anconeus.

The forearm has 19 muscles, 11 in the extensor and radial compartments and 8 in the flexor compartment. Of these 19, 6 forearm muscles move only the wrist and 9 additional muscles move the thumb and fingers and act secondarily at the wrist.

- The **superficial anterior compartment** includes the pronator teres, the flexor digitorum superficialis, the flexor carpi radialis, the flexor carpi ulnaris, and the palmaris longus, which is frequently absent (Fig. 10-5**A**).
- The **deep anterior compartment** includes the pronator quadratus, the flexor digitorum profundus, and the flexor pollicis longus (Fig.10-5**B**).
- The **radial compartment** includes the brachioradialis, the ECRL, and the ECRB (Fig. 10-6**A**).
- The **superficial posterior compartment** includes the extensor digitorum, the extensor digiti minimi, and the extensor carpi ulnaris (Fig. 10-6**B**).
- The **deep posterior group** includes the supinator, the abductor pollicis longus, the extensor pollicis brevis, the extensor pollicis longus, and the extensor indicis (Fig. 10-6**C**).
- Two muscles are involved in pronation, the pronator teres and the pronator quadratus, and two muscles are involved in supination, the biceps brachii and the supinator.
- Forearm muscles may also be categorized by the location of their attachments. The medial and the lateral epicondyles of the distal end of the humerus

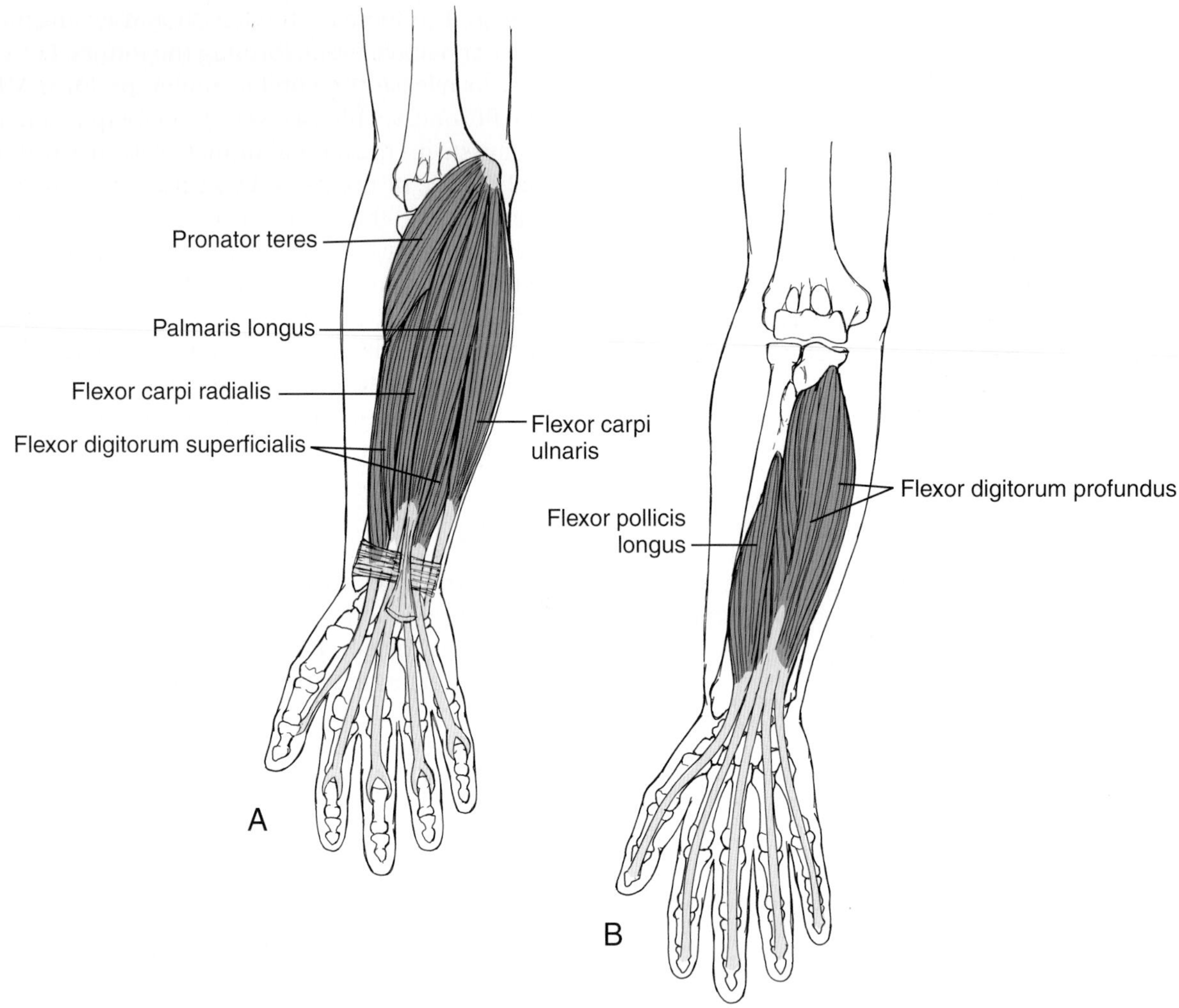

Figure 10-5. Forearm muscle compartments. **A.** Superficial anterior. **B.** Deep anterior.

are the attachment points for many of the muscles that move the wrist and hand.

- Muscles attaching to the medial epicondyle of the humerus are the common flexor tendon, including the flexor carpi radialis, flexor carpi ulnaris, palmaris longus, flexor digitorum superficialis, and flexor digitorum profundus.
- Muscles attaching to the lateral epicondyle of the humerus are the extensors of the wrist and hand, including the ECRL, ECRB, extensor carpi ulnaris, and extensor digitorum.

- *Function*: The muscles that cross the elbow and forearm are essential to movement of the hand in all activities of daily living and for recreation and sport. The hand and wrist muscles also help to reinforce the joint capsule of the elbow and produce a compressive force to the elbow during muscle contraction; therefore, these muscles contribute to joint stability.[8] Many of the muscles that move the wrist and hand attach to the humerus because it provides a much more stable base than the forearm. Co-contraction of the flexor and extensor muscles of the elbow, wrist, and hand provides stability to the elbow and forearm for movements of the wrist and hand.
- ***Dysfunction and injury***: Dysfunction and injuries to the muscles and associated fascia attaching in the elbow region are common. **Tennis elbow,** or lateral epicondylitis, is considered an acute manifestation of a chronic condition. The acute episode is a tenoperiosteal tear of the wrist extensors, most commonly the ECRB. The chronic problem is a degenerative disorder caused by tissue fatigue from repetitive gripping. Tennis players, musicians, massage therapists, and carpenters are all susceptible to overuse of gripping motions. **Golfer's elbow (Little Leaguer's elbow),** or medial epicondylitis, is considered a tenoperiosteal tear of the wrist flexors and the

pronator teres. It is caused by repetitive wrist flexion and pronation (e.g. golf, throwing, gripping).

- *Treatment implications*: Perform CR MET to reduce the hypertonicity in the involved muscle. Lengthen the myofascia with PIR MET. Perform OM to the involved muscles, including transverse friction massage at the attachment sites.

Anatomy of the Muscles of the Elbow, Forearm, Wrist, and Hand

See Muscle Table 10-1.

Muscular Actions of the Elbow and Forearm

See Table 10-2.

Anatomy, Function, and Dysfunction of the Wrist

BONES AND JOINTS OF THE WRIST

- *Structure*: The wrist is composed of eight carpal bones in two rows (see Fig. 10-1). The two joints of the wrist are the **distal radiocarpal** and **midcarpal joints.** The distal radiocarpal joint is the articulation of the distal end of the radius and an articular disc (meniscus) called the triquetral fibrocartilage complex (TFCC) with the proximal row of carpal bones. The midcarpal joint is the articulation of the proximal and distal rows of the carpal bones.
  - The proximal row of carpal bones, from lateral to medial, are the navicular (scaphoid), lunate, tri-

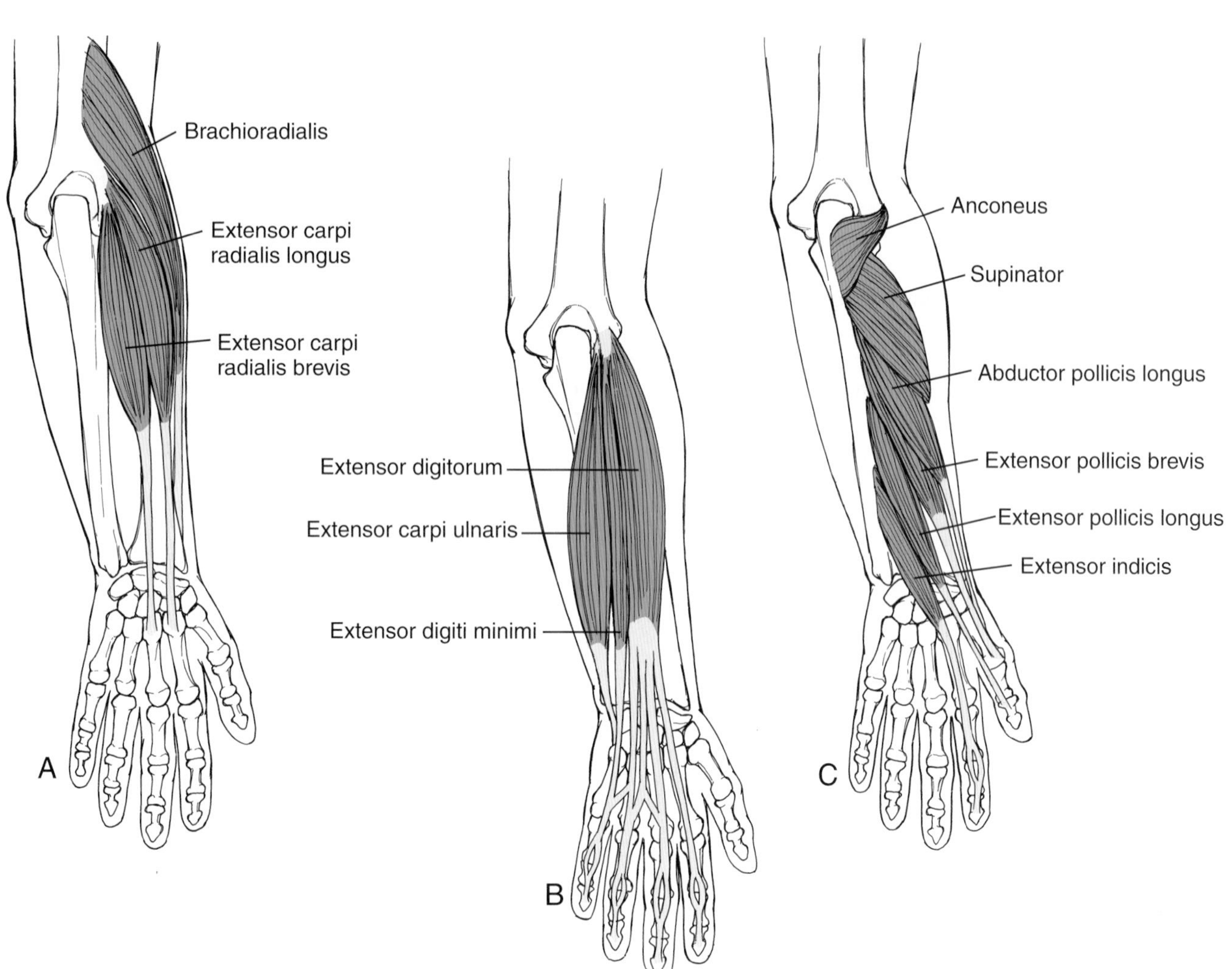

Figure 10-6. Compartments of forearm muscles. **A.** Radial. **B.** Superficial posterior. **C.** Deep posterior.

TABLE 10-1 ANATOMY OF THE MUSCLES OF THE ELBOW, FOREARM, WRIST, AND HAND

Anterior Compartment Muscles of the Arm

Muscle	*Origin*	*Insertion*	*Action*
Biceps brachii	Two heads—short head from the coracoid process; long head from the upper lip of the glenoid fossa (supraglenoid tubercle).	Tuberosity of the radius; bicipital aponeurosis inserts into the fascia of the forearm.	Flexion and supination of the elbow; flexion and abduction of the arm.
Brachialis	Distal 1/2 of the anterior portion of the humerus.	Coronoid process of the ulna and the joint capsule.	Flexion of the elbow.

Posterior Compartment Muscles of the Arm

Muscle	*Origin*	*Insertion*	*Action*
Triceps brachii	Long head—lower edge of the glenoid cavity (infraglenoid tubercle); Lateral head—upper 1/3 of the posterior surface of the humerus; Medial head—lower 2/3 of the posterior surface of the humerus;	Olecranon process of the ulna and the posterior joint capsule.	Extension of the elbow and assistance in extension of the shoulder joint.
Anconeus	Posterior surface of the lateral condyle of the humerus.	Posterior surface of the proximal ulna and lateral aspect of olecranon.	Extension of the forearm and tension of the capsule of the elbow.

Anterior Group of the Forearm: Superficial Layer

Muscle	*Origin*	*Insertion*	*Action*
Pronator teres	Two heads—humeral head from the medial epicondyle of the humerus; ulnar head from the coronoid process of the ulna;	On the pronator tuberosity on the middle 1/3 of the radius.	Pronation of forearm and flexion of the elbow.
Flexor digitorum superficialis	Humeral head—medial epicondyle of the humerus; Ulnar head—medial coronoid process; Radial head—radial tuberosity area.	Split tendons attach to the sides of the middle phalanx of the four fingers (palmar surface); between the heads is a tendinous arch through which the medial nerve, as well as the ulnar artery and vein, travels.	Flexion of the PIP joints of the second to the fifth digits; assists in flexion of MCP joints and the wrist.
Flexor carpi radialis	Medial epicondyle of the humerus.	Base of the second and the third metacarpals (palmar surface).	Flexion and radial deviation of the wrist; weak flexion of the elbow.
Palmaris longus (may be absent)	Medial epicondyle of the humerus.	Palmar surface of the hand into the palmar aponeurosis.	Palmar surface of the hand into the palmar aponeurosis.
Flexor carpi ulnaris	Humeral head—medial epicondyle of the humerus Ulnar head—olecranon and posterior margin of the ulna.	Pisiform bone and the base of the fifth metacarpal; extends to the pisohamate ligament and the hamate bone.	Flexion and ulnar deviation of the wrist; weak flexion of the elbow.

TABLE 10-1 ANATOMY OF THE MUSCLES OF THE ELBOW, FOREARM, WRIST, AND HAND—cont'd

Anterior Group of the Forearm: Deep Layer

Muscle	*Origin*	*Insertion*	*Action*
Pronator quadratus	Lower 1/4 of the anterior side of the ulna.	Lower 1/4 of the anterior side of the radius.	Pronation of the forearm.
Flexor digitorum profundus	Proximal 3/4 of the ulna and interosseous membrane.	Base of the anterior surface of the distal phalanges of the second to the fifth fingers.	Flexion of DIP joints of the fingers 2–5 and assists in flexion of PIP, MCP, and wrist; forms most of the muscle bulk at the medial forearm next to ulna and can be palpated when the distal phalanges are flexed.
Flexor pollicis longus	Middle anterior surface of the radius.	Base of the distal phalanx of the thumb (palmar surface).	Flexion of the IP joint of the thumb; assists in flexion of the wrist.

Radial Group of Forearm Muscles

Muscle	*Origin*	*Insertion*	*Action*
Extensor carpi Radialis brevis	Lateral epicondyle of the humerus, the radial collateral ligament, and the annular radial ligament.	Base of the third metacarpal (dorsal surface).	Extension and radial deviation of the hand.
Extensor carpi Radialis longus	Distal 1/3 of the lateral supracondylar crest of the humerus proximal to the brevis.	Base of the second metacarpal.	Extension of the wrist.
Brachioradialis	Proximal 2/3 of the lateral supracondylar crest of the humerus.	Lateral surface of the styloid process of the radius.	Brings forearm into neutral and flexes elbow from this position.

Posterior Group of the Forearm: Superficial Layer

Muscle	*Origin*	*Insertion*	*Action*
Extensor digitorum	Posterior surface of the lateral epicondyle of the humerus, the radial collateral ligament, and the annular ligament.	Four tendons to the bases of the second and the third phalanges of the four fingers on the dorsal surfaces; forms the dorsal aponeurosis of fingers 2–5.	Extension and spreading of the fingers, wrist, and forearm; strongest dorsiflexor of the wrist.
Extensor digiti minimi	Arises together with the extensor digitorum at lateral epicondyle.	Dorsal aponeurosis of the fifth digit.	Extends the fifth digit and assists ulnar deviation of hand.
Extensor carpi ulnaris	Posterior surface of the lateral epicondyle of the humerus.	Base of the fifth metacarpal (dorsal surface).	Extension of the wrist; ulnar deviation of the wrist together with the flexor carpi ulnaris; and extension of the forearm.

TABLE 10-1 ANATOMY OF THE MUSCLES OF THE ELBOW, FOREARM, WRIST, AND HAND—cont'd

Posterior Group of the Forearm: Deep Layer

Muscle	*Origin*	*Insertion*	*Action*
Supinator	Lateral epicondyle of the humerus and supinator crest of the ulna.	Outer surface of the upper 1/3 of the radius.	Supination of the forearm.
Abductor pollicis longus	Posterior surface of the ulna; distal to supinator crest of the ulna.	Base of the first metacarpal, radial side.	Abduction and extension of the CMC joint of the thumb.
Extensor pollicis brevis	Posterior surface of the radius and ulna, distal to abductor pollicis longus.	Base of the proximal thumb.	Extension of the MCP joint of the thumb; extension and abduction of the CMC joint of the thumb.
Extensor pollicis longus	Posterior surface of the ulna, from the medial midshaft, extending distally and laterally on the ulna.	Base of the distal phalanx of the thumb (dorsal surface).	Extension of the IP joint of the thumb; extension of the wrist.
Extensor indicis	Distal 1/3 of the dorsal surface of the ulna.	Dorsal aponeurosis of the index finger.	Extension of the index finger.

quetrum, and the pisiform, which sits on the triquetrum.

- The distal row, from lateral to medial, are the trapezium, trapezoid, capitate, and hamate.

- *Function*: The radius carries approximately 80% of the load from the arm to the hand. The radius of the forearm is analogous to the tibia in the leg, which carries approximately 80% of the load to the foot. The main function of the wrist is precise control of the hand position for fine motor control and optimum strength. Achieving optimum strength is possible by maintaining control of the length–tension relationship of the extrinsic muscles of the hand.[8]

The wrist has four basic movements: radial abduction, ulnar abduction, flexion, and extension. These movements can be combined to perform circumduction. The pisiform bone functions as a sesamoid for the flexor carpi ulnaris.

- *Dysfunction and injury*: A fall on an outstretched hand (FOOSH) injury typically involves a position of extension of the wrist and the elbow. As the radius carries the majority of the load, its distal end is a common site of fracture, called a Colles' fracture. A FOOSH injury is also a common cause of ligamentous sprains.

- *Treatment implications*: A posttraumatic injury to the wrist, especially one that has been immobilized due to fracture, typically has a significant loss of motion. To treat this type of injury, perform MET to increase the joint ROM. Then perform PIR MET to lengthen the shortened myofascia and interweaving ligaments. Perform OM, including transverse friction massage, to help dissolve the adhesions. Mobilize the wrist to help reduce calcium deposits and rehydrate the cartilage.

SOFT-TISSUE STRUCTURES OF THE WRIST

Joint Capsule and Ligaments

- *Structure*: The distal radioulnar joint has a strong capsule and is strengthened by ligaments. The midcarpal joint depends primarily on ligaments for support. The ligaments also provide significant passive control of wrist motion. As in the foot, the carpal bones of the wrist form a transverse and longitudinal arch that is concave anteriorly. This bony arch is covered with the dense **flexor retinaculum (transverse carpal ligament)** and forms the **carpal tunnel** through which the **median nerve** travels, along with the nine tendons of the fingers and thumb (see the section "Muscles").

The joint capsule of the wrist is reinforced by the flexor and extensor retinaculum, which is a thickening of the fascia of the forearm, and an extensive system of ligaments, including the radial and ulnar collateral ligaments, the palmar and dorsal radiocarpal ligaments, and the pisohamate ligament.

- ***Function***: The wrist ligaments help transmit the forces that move through the wrist and hand, stabilize the carpal bones, and perform a neurosensory role. The arches in the hand are created by the bones, which are suspended and reinforced by the flexor retinaculum and the intercarpal ligaments. Increase in the arch can occur through the action of the palmaris longus, flexor carpi ulnaris, and the intrinsic muscles of the hand. Contraction of the flexor carpi ulnaris tightens the proximal portion of the flexor retinaculum.
- ***Dysfunction and injury***: Injuries to the ligaments of the wrist are common and are usually the result of an acute injury rather than a cumulative stress. A FOOSH is a common injury that sprains the wrist, either the dorsal or palmar ligaments. The flexor retinaculum can thicken in response to cumulative use of the finger flexors, contributing to a narrowing of the carpal tunnel and compression of the median nerve, called **carpal tunnel syndrome** (see the section "Nerves").
- ***Treatment implications***: To treat the wrist ligaments, first perform CR MET to the muscles that interweave with the involved ligaments. On the anterior wrist these muscles are the flexors of the wrist, fingers, and thumb, and on the posterior wrist these muscles are the extensors of the wrist, fingers, and thumb. This treatment creates a contracting and relaxing force, which helps realign the healing fibers, and acts as a pump to promote nutritional exchange. Next, perform OM, including gentle scooping strokes in the more acute phase and transverse friction massage in the chronic phase, to dissolve thick and fibrotic tissue.

TABLE 10-2 MUSCULAR ACTIONS OF THE ELBOW AND FOREARM

Flexion

- Biceps brachii—flexes and supinates the forearm
- Brachialis
- Brachioradialis—pronates forearm if supinated; supinates if pronated
- Pronator teres—pronates forearm and flexes the elbow
- Palmaris longus—weak flexor of elbow and wrist
- Flexor carpi ulnaris—flexes elbow; flexes and adducts wrist
- Flexor carpi radialis—flexes wrist and elbow; abducts wrist and pronates forearm
- Flexor digitorum superficialis—flexes forearm; flexes middle phalanges of four middle fingers

Extension

- Triceps brachii—also extends and adducts arm
- Anconeus—also responsible for pulling the synovial membrane out of the way of the olecranon process during extension

Supination

- Supinator
- Biceps brachii

Pronation

- Pronator teres—also flexes elbow
- Pronator quadratus

Ligaments of the Wrist

See Table 10-3.

Nerves

See Figures 10-2 to 10-4.

- ***Structure***: After traveling through the tunnels at the elbow, the **ulnar, median** and **radial nerves** travel through the forearm to the wrist area and hand.
  - The **ulnar nerve** travels with the flexor carpi ulnaris to the wrist, where it travels on top of (anterior) the flexor retinaculum on the radial side of the pisiform. It divides into superficial and deep branches that then travel under the pisohamate ligament, which is a fibro-osseous space between the pisiform and the hook of the hamate called the **tunnel of Guyon.**[9] It contributes branches called the interdigital nerves to the fingers (see the section "Nerves of the Hand").
  - The **median nerve** exits the elbow region between the two humeral heads of the pronator teres and then travels between the superficial and the deep flexors. It continues in the midline of the palmar aspect of the wrist through the **carpal tunnel** formed by the carpal bones and the flexor retinaculum.
  - The **radial nerve** divides into superficial and deep (interosseous) branches distal to the elbow. The deep branch travels between the superficial and the deep layers of the extensors and under

TABLE 10-3 WRIST LIGAMENTS

Ligament	*Origin*	*Insertion*
Transverse carpal ligament distal flexor retinaculum	Navicular (scaphoid) and tubercle of the trapezium	Pisiform and hook of the hamate
Pisohamate ligament	Pisiform bone	Hook of the hamate
Ulnar collateral ligament	From the distal end of the styloid process of the ulna	Medial side of the triquetral and pisiform bones
Radial collateral ligament	Distal end of the styloid process of the radius	Radial side of the scaphoid bone

the extensor pollicis longus. The superficial radial nerve travels under the skin on the distal aspect of the radius to the dorsum of the thumb and index finger.

- *Function*: The ulnar, median, and radial nerves provide sensory and motor functions to the hand.
  - The **ulnar nerve** has muscular branches to the flexor carpi ulnaris and the ulnar portion of the deep flexors of the fingers, the hypothenar muscles, the interossei, the adductor pollicis, and the deep head of the flexor pollicis brevis. It is sensory to the ulnar side of the hand, most specifically at the tip of the little finger.
  - The **median nerve** supplies most of the flexors of the forearm and the thenar muscles. It is sensory to the lateral portion of the palm and thenar eminence. Its innervation is most specific at the tip of the index finger.
  - The **radial nerve** has muscular branches that innervate all the extensors and has a sensory to the dorsum of the hand, most specifically at the webspace between the thumb and the index fingers.
- *Dysfunction and injury*:
  - Compression of the **median nerve** at the wrist is called **carpal tunnel syndrome.** A common cause is overuse of the finger flexors, which can create inflammation and swelling. Chronic irritation leads to fibrosis or thickening of the sheath and thickening of the transverse carpal ligament, narrowing the tunnel. Other causes include previous injury, subluxation of the lunate, edema from pregnancy, and osteoarthritis (OA).
  - The **ulnar nerve** may be trapped as it passes through the **tunnel of Guyon,** which is formed by the pisohamate ligament between the pisiform and the hook of the hamate. Or, it may be irritated from swelling of the flexor carpi ulnaris at the insertion into the pisiform.
- *Treatment implications*: To treat carpal tunnel syndrome, perform CR MET to the wrist and finger flexors to reduce their hypertonicity and to increase the extensibility of the fascia of the wrist and hand attaching to these muscles. Next, perform CR MET to the muscles that attach to the transverse carpal ligament (flexor retinaculum) to increase the extensibility of the ligament. Then perform a gentle distraction of the flexor retinaculum. For chronic conditions, perform OM strokes to the attachment points of the flexor retinaculum.
  - For the ulnar nerve, perform CR MET to the flexor carpi ulnaris to release the tension in the pisohamate ligament. Next perform OM, transverse to the line of the ligament. Then, perform gentle scooping strokes transverse to the line of the nerve in the tunnel of Guyon.

Muscles

- *Structure*: Six muscles have tendons crossing the anterior wrist. Three of these act only on the wrist: the palmaris longus, flexor carpi radialis, and flexor carpi ulnaris. The other three flex the fingers and thumb and act secondarily on the wrist: the flexor digitorum superficialis, flexor digitorum profundus, and flexor pollicis longus. In addition to the median nerve, nine tendons pass through the carpal tunnel: the flexor pollicis longus and the four tendons each of the flexor digitorum superficialis and profundus.

Nine muscles cross the dorsum of the wrist. Three of these muscles are wrist muscles: ECRB, ECRL, and extensor carpi ulnaris. The other six are finger and thumb muscles and act secondarily on the wrist: the extensor digitorum, extensor indicis, extensor digiti minimi, extensor pollicis longus, extensor pollicis brevis, and the abductor pollicis longus.

The tendons that cross the wrist are stabilized and lubricated to ensure precise control of movement and smooth gliding. The structures that stabilize the tendons are the retinaculum of the wrist and the fibrous connective tissue holding the flexor tendons to the fingers and thumb called annular (vaginal) ligaments. The flexor tendons are lubricated by synovial sheaths in the palm and fingers.

- *Function*: The primary roles of the muscles that cross the wrist are to provide strength and stability for the hand and to allow fine positional movements. Achieving this strength and stability is possible by maintaining the optimal length–tension relationship of the extrinsic muscles of the fingers and thumb (see "Muscles of the Hand" section below).[8]
- *Dysfunction and injury*: Tendinitis at the attachment points of the wrist, called insertional tendinitis, is common from injury and overuse. These include the ECRB and the ECRL, the extensor carpi ulnaris, the flexor carpi radialis, and the flexor carpi ulnaris. Another common dysfunction is **stenosing tenosynovitis (De Quervain's tenovaginitis)** of the extensor pollicis brevis and the abductor pollicis longus. These two muscles travel together through a fibro-osseous tunnel formed by the extensor retinaculum over the radial styloid. Repetitive gripping motions cause the tendons to rub against each other, creating irritation and inflammation. This inflammation creates swelling in the acute stage and fibrosis in the chronic stage. Both conditions narrow the tunnel and create pain with movement using the muscles.
- *Treatment implications*: For De Quervain's tenovaginitis, perform CR MET to the involved tendons, and perform OM, using gentle scooping strokes transverse to the line of the tendons. Deeper friction strokes are indicated if thickened, fibrotic tissue is palpated in the chronic condition. For insertional tendinitis, perform CR MET for the involved tendon to reduce the hypertonicity, to lengthen the myofascia, and to increase the resilience of the fascia at the tenoperiosteal junctions. Perform OM for the entire length of the muscle and transverse friction massage at the insertion points.

Muscular Actions at the Wrist

See Table 10-4.

Anatomy, Function, and Dysfunction of the Hand

BONES AND JOINTS OF THE HAND

The hand has 19 bones and 19 joints (see Fig.10-1). There are five metacarpals and three phalanges for each of the four fingers, and two phalanges for the thumb.

Carpometacarpal Joints

- *Structure*: The articulations between the distal row of carpal bones and the base of the metacarpals are called the carpometacarpal (CMC) joints. The thumb is the first CMC joint and is the articulation of the first metacarpal and the trapezium.
- *Function*: The CMC joints of the second, third, and fourth fingers are synovial joints with simple flexion and extension movements. The second and third CMC joints are nearly immobile, which provides a stable base for the cupping and holding motions of the palm. The fifth CMC (the little finger) has the capability of a slight amount of abduction and adduction in addition to flexion and extension.

The first CMC joint (the thumb) is described as a saddle joint and has a wide variety of movements, including flexion and extension, abduction and adduction, and some axial rotation. The thumb faces the palm instead of anteriorly like the other fingers, which allows it to touch the other fingers (called opposition), an essential motion in holding, gripping, and pinching.

- *Dysfunction and injury:* The hand is a common site for arthritis, both the degenerative and the systemic type, such as rheumatoid arthritis (RA). Hereditary factors may be related to arthritis of the fingers and thumb. OA typically manifests as joint swelling at the distal IP (DIP) joints, called Heberden's nodes, or at the proximal IP (PIP) joints, called Bouchard's nodes. The CMC joint of the thumb is one of the most commonly arthritic joints in the body. OA is common in the DIP joints, less common in the PIP joints, and fairly rare in the metacarpophalangeal (MCP) joints.[3]

Degenerative arthritis is related to overuse and inflammation leading to capsular fibrosis, loss of the normal synovial fluid, and cartilage degeneration. Of-

TABLE 10-4 MUSCULAR ACTIONS AT THE WRIST

Two compound joints compose the wrist: the radiocarpal and the midcarpal joints. There are four basic motions: flexion, extension, radial deviation (abduction), and ulnar deviation (adduction). Six muscles of the forearm move only the wrist. Nine additional muscles that move the thumb and fingers also move the wrist.

Wrist

Flexion

- Flexor carpi ulnaris
- Flexor carpi radialis
- Palmaris longus

Extension

- Extensor carpi ulnaris
- ECRL
- ECRB

Radial Deviation (Abduction)

- ECRL
- ECRB
- Flexor carpi radialis
- Palmaris longus

Ulnar Deviation (Adduction)

- Flexor carpi ulnaris
- Extensor carpi ulnaris

---

ten, predisposing factors such as subluxation or fixation of the normal gliding characteristics of the joint are present. The most common cause of swelling at the PIP is collateral ligament tears.[10] The thumb is also a common site of sesamoiditis, an inflammation of the sesamoid bones.

- ***Treatment implications***: The treatment protocol for OA of the hand is MET for the finger flexors and extensors to help stimulate the normal joint lubrication by tensing the joint capsule through its attachment to the muscles. Perform OM to release adhesions in the annular ligaments of the flexor tendons and at the tenoperiosteal attachments of the flexors to the thumb and fingers. Perform transverse friction massage to the ligament system of the fingers and thumb, concentrating on transverse strokes to the collateral ligaments and transverse metacarpal ligaments. Then perform joint mobilization to the involved joint.

Metacarpophalangeal Joints

- ***Structure***: MCP joints are the articulations of the convex heads of the metacarpals and the concave bases of the phalanges (fingers). They are synovial joints with a joint capsule and three ligaments: the palmar, transverse metatarsal, and collateral. The MCP joint of the thumb has two sesamoid bones embedded within the joint capsule and the flexor pollicis brevis tendon.
- ***Function***: The MCP joint has four possible motions: flexion, extension, adduction, and abduction.
- ***Dysfunction and injury:*** MCP dysfunction and injury are the same as those of the CMC joint.
- ***Treatment implications***: Treatment for MCP injuries are the same as that for the CMC joint.

Interphalangeal Joints

- ***Structure***: The IP joints are the articulations between the proximal and distal phalanges. Each of these joints has a joint capsule, two collateral ligaments, and a fibrocartilage palmar plate (see the section "Joint Capsules and Ligaments of the Interphalangeal Joints").
- ***Function***: IP joints are synovial hinge joints with two possible motions, flexion and extension. The flexion of these joints toward the palm allows the holding and gripping action of the hand.
- ***Dysfunction and injury:*** IP joint dysfunction and injury are the same as those of the CMC joint.
- ***Treatment implications***: Treatment for IP dysfunction is the same as that for the CMC joint.

SOFT-TISSUE STRUCTURES OF THE HAND

Joint Capsules and Ligaments

The clinically important ligaments of the hand may be described by location (Fig. 10-7**A** and **B**).

Joint Capsules and Ligaments of the Carpometacarpal Joints

- All CMC joints of the hand have transverse and longitudinal ligaments. The CMC joint of the thumb has a loose joint capsule, reinforced by radial, ulnar, palmar, and dorsal ligaments. An intermetacarpal ligament exists between the first and the second metacarpals.

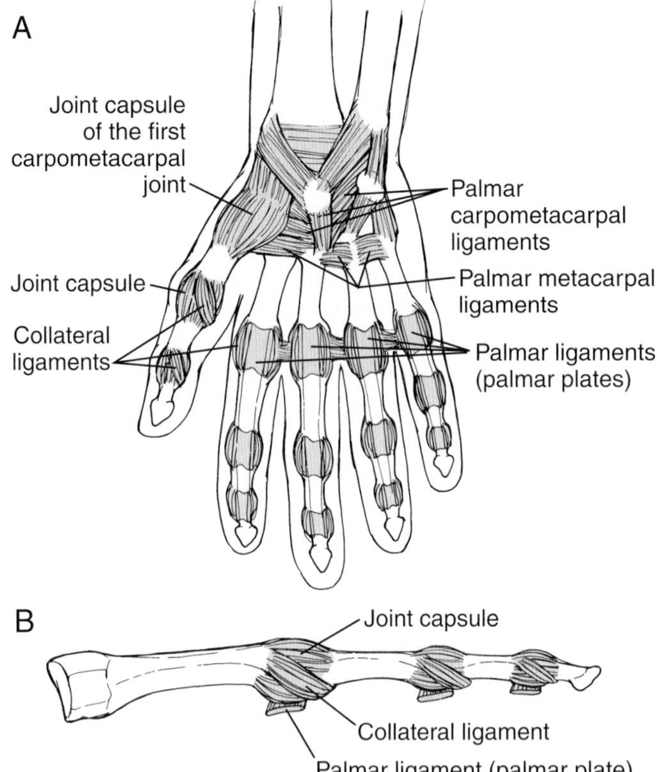

Figure 10-7. **A.** Joint capsule, collateral ligaments, deep transverse metacarpal ligaments, and palmar ligaments of the MCP and IP joints. **B.** Lateral view of the joint capsule and collateral ligaments of the MCP and IP joints.

Joint Capsules and Ligaments of the Metacarpophalangeal Joints

- The **joint capsules** of the MCP joints are interwoven with medial and lateral collateral ligaments; transverse metacarpal ligaments; and the palmar ligament, a thick, dense fibrocartilage structure.
- The **collateral ligaments** of the MCP joints are thick, rounded cords on the sides of the joints.
- The **transverse metacarpal ligaments** interweave with the joint capsules of the MCP joints and the palmar plates. They have a deep and superficial portion, and the palmar digital nerve travels through the two layers of these ligaments.
- The **palmar ligaments (palmar or volar plates)** are embedded in the walls of the joint capsules on the palmar side of the MCP joints. They are attached to the heads of the metacarpals and the proximal phalanges of the MCP joints. The distal portion of these ligaments has a cartilage lining, and the proximal portion is membranous. They have a groove in them for the flexor tendons of the fingers and are interwoven with the transverse metacarpal and collateral ligaments of the MCP joints.

Joint Capsule and Ligaments of the Interphalangeal Joints

- The **joint capsule** of the IP joints is reinforced with two collateral ligaments and a palmar ligament. The flexor tendons of the fingers interweave with the joint capsules of the IP joints.
- The **collateral ligaments** of the IP joints connect the IP joints. The fibers are oriented in a proximal to distal direction following the shaft of the bone. They help guide the flexion and extension movement of the IP joints.
- The **palmar ligaments (palmar or volar plates)** are embedded in the walls of the joint capsules on the palmar side of the IP joints of the fingers and the thumb. They are attached from the proximal to the distal portion of the IP joints. They are interwoven to the joint capsule and collateral ligaments and have a groove in them for the flexor tendons of the fingers.
- The flexor tendons are held in place by a fibrous sheath called the **annular or vaginal ligament,** which creates a fibro-osseous tunnel with the bone.

- *Function*:
  - The **joint capsule** has a fibrous and synovial layer that provides passive stability to the joint, guides joint motion, provides lubrication to the joint through stimulation of the synovial layer, and plays a neurosensory role. The joint capsule also contains mechanoreceptors and pain receptors that provide information about movement, position, pressure, and pain, as well as reflex connections to the surrounding muscles.
  - The **collateral ligaments** of the IP joints stabilize the articulating bones and suspend the palmar plate and flexor sheath.[11]
  - The **transverse metacarpal ligament** holds the heads of the metacarpals together.
  - The **palmar plate** functions to expand the articular surface for the metacarpal head and prevents the long flexor tendons from impinging into the joint.[8]
- *Dysfunction and injury:*
  - A fibrosis of the collateral ligaments and joint capsule of the fingers is common as a consequence of acute trauma; after cumulative stresses, such as

repetitive gripping motions; or in degenerative conditions of the joints.

- Acute injury of the PIP joints is the most commonly injured joint of the hand.[11] The incident typically involves jamming a finger, which hyperextends the joint, spraining the joint capsule and collateral ligaments. A chronic microtearing of the IP collateral ligament is also common, especially at the PIP joint. This tearing creates swelling in the acute stage and can cause joint degeneration by preventing the normal gliding of the joint surfaces.[10] Injury to the collateral ligaments of the MCP joints can lead to adhesions that result in decreased flexion of that joint. Injury to the medial (ulnar) collateral ligament of the thumb is a common ski injury caused by forceful hyperextension or abduction of the thumb.
- A thickening of the deep transverse metacarpal ligaments is common with acute or degenerative conditions. Shortening, which is subsequent to the ligament thickening, compresses the metacarpal heads together, leading to dysfunction and pain at the MCP joints. With thickening also comes decreased space for the palmar digital nerve, and this may lead to pain, numbing, and tingling in the fingers.
- The annular ligament may thicken and shorten from excessive use of the flexor tendons, such as keyboard work, or from repetitive gripping motions. Increased friction of the flexor tendons develops at the tunnel formed by these ligaments, especially at the MCP joints. This increased friction creates irritation, inflammation, and potential fibrosis of the ligament.
- The palmar ligament may thicken as a result of degenerative arthritis, or they may become injured from a FOOSH. When the hand is immobilized after an injury, the membranous portion of the ligament may retract and develop adhesions, leading to flexion contracture of the joint.[12]

- ***Treatment implications***: Treat the ligaments of the hand by first performing MET to the muscles that interweave with the ligaments. As the most involved ligaments are usually on the palmar side, concentrate the MET on the flexors of the fingers and thumb. Next, perform OM to the involved ligaments, transverse to the line of the fiber. If the ligament is thickened, use transverse friction strokes. If the finger is held in sustained flexion, release the torsion in the collateral ligaments by performing a palmar to dorsal scooping motion on the ligaments. Finally, mobilize the joints in the area of the involved ligament, to help normalize neurologic function and to hydrate the area of the ligament. To treat the palmar ligaments, use a scooping stroke in a proximal to distal direction to reduce adhesions and tethering in the membranous portion of the ligament.

Fascia

- ***Structure***: The antebrachial fascia of the forearm is strengthened on the extensor surface of the wrist by the extensor retinaculum, which continues as the dorsal fascia of the hand. On the palmar surface, the antebrachial fascia thickens into the **palmar fascia,** which is interwoven into the aponeurosis of the palmaris longus muscle. The fascia continues as the fascia covering the thenar and hypothenar eminences, and interweaves with the flexor retinaculum at the wrist. It continues distally and interweaves with the transverse metacarpal ligament and the flexor tendon sheaths.
- ***Dysfunction***: Thickening and nodular formation of the palmar fascia can occur spontaneously for unknown reasons, a condition called Dupuytren's disease. It can create a severe disability of the hand owing to flexion contracture of the tendons of the fingers.

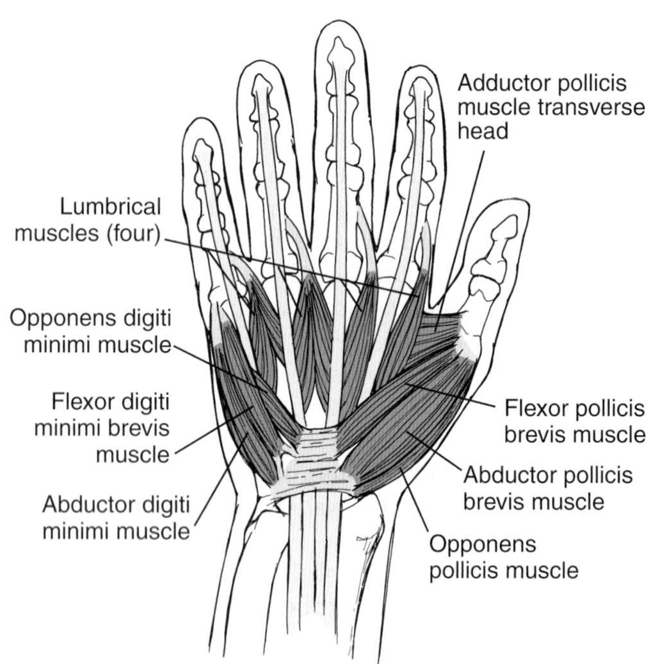

Figure 10-8. Muscles and flexor tendons of the hand.

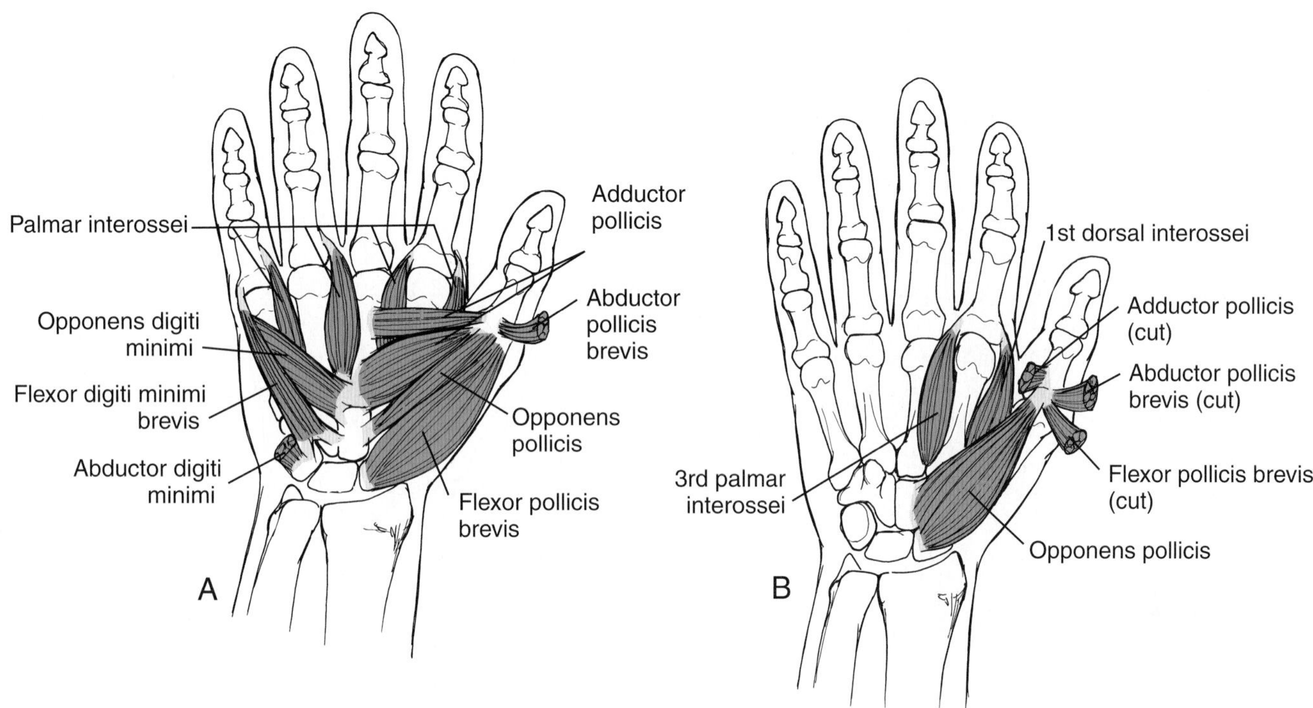

Figure 10-9. A. Deep layer of hand muscles. **B.** Deep layers of the hand muscles with both heads of the adductor pollicis sectioned to reveal the interossei underneath.

- ***Treatment implications***: Symptoms from Dupuytren's disease may be relieved somewhat through deep longitudinal and transverse work on the palmar fascia. This condition typically requires surgical intervention.

Nerves of the Hand

- ***Structure***: The median and ulnar nerves have terminal branches called the **palmar digital nerves (interdigital nerves).** Palmar digital nerves travel between the superficial and the deep layers of the transverse metacarpal ligament between the heads of the metacarpals. In the fingers and thumb, they travel along the sides of the long flexor tendons, outside the fibrous sheaths (see Figs. 10-2 to 10-4).
- ***Function***: Each palmar digital nerve gives off sensory branches to the skin on the front and sides of the fingers, as well as articular branches to the MCP and IP joints.
- ***Dysfunction and injury***: Interdigital nerves can become entrapped in between the superficial and the deep layers of the transverse metacarpal ligament. The ligaments thicken because of injury, overuse, or disease. The hand is typically held in sustained flexion, compressing the metacarpal heads and the interdigital nerves.
- ***Treatment implications***: To treat the interdigital nerves, perform OM to first release the transverse metacarpal ligament. Then perform gentle scooping strokes perpendicular to the line of the nerve in between the heads of the metacarpals.

Muscles of the Hand

- ***Structure***: The hand has 18 intrinsic muscles, and 9 extrinsic muscles (Figs. 10-8 to 10-10). The fingers have two extrinsic flexors and three extensors. The thumb has four extrinsic muscles, one on the palmar side and three on the dorsal side. Most of the intrinsic muscles of the hand are contained in two distinct pads, the thenar eminence at the base of the thumb and the hypothenar eminence at the base of the fifth finger. In addition to these pads the intrinsic muscles include the lumbricals and the dorsal and palmar interossei.

As the flexor tendons travel over the MCP and IP joints, they are enclosed within a lubricated tendon sheath, sometimes called a bursa, allowing the ten-

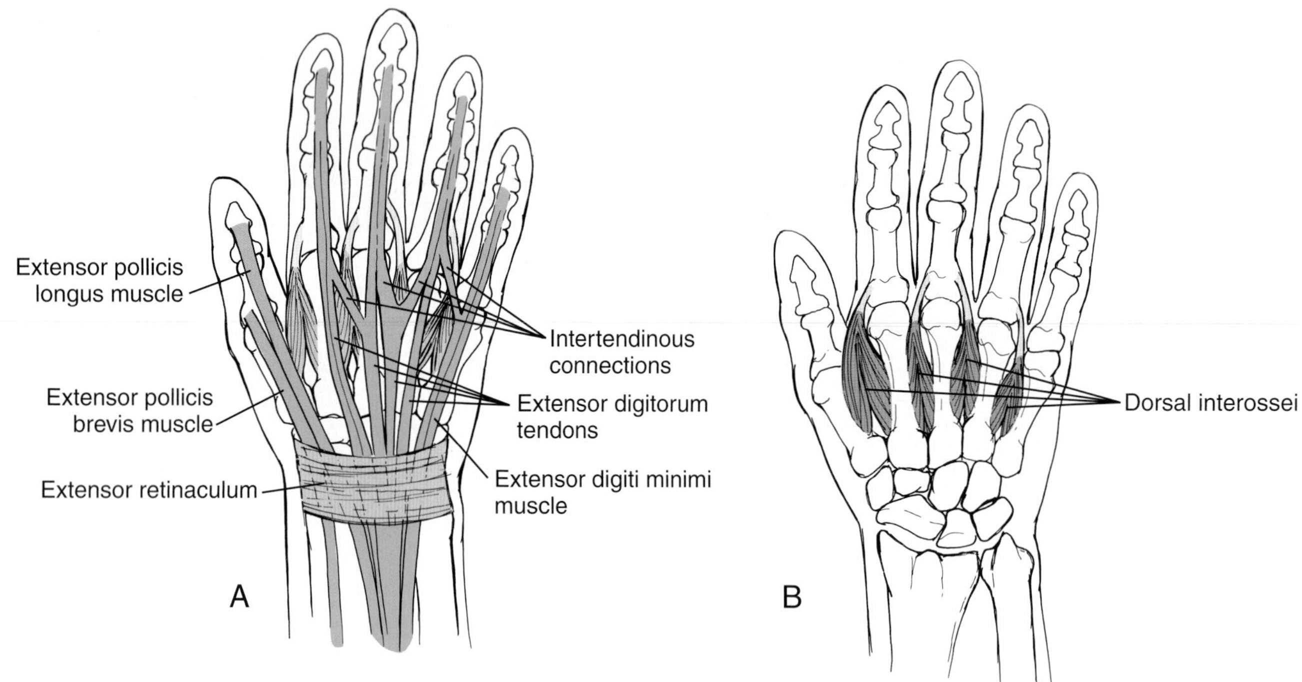

Figure 10-10. A. Muscles and tendons of the dorsum of the hand. **B.** Dorsal interossei muscles.

dons to slide freely within them. The annular ligaments form a fibro-osseous tunnel that encloses the flexor tendons and their sheaths to the heads of the metacarpals in the fingers and the thumb. These ligaments act like a retinaculum, stabilizing and guiding the movement of the tendons.

The extensors pass under the extensor retinaculum, are enclosed within their own tendon sheaths, and form an extensor hood on the dorsal surface of each digit that replaces the posterior portion of the joint capsule. This hood wraps around the joint and attaches to the transverse metacarpal ligament.

- *Function*: Extension of the fingers is caused by the combined action of the extensors and the intrinsics. The lumbrical muscles have been described as functioning as the primary organ of sensory feedback in the hand. These muscles have more muscle spindles than any other muscle in the body.[5]

The wrist and the hand have an optimum position in which all the extrinsic muscles of the hand are under equal tension and that provides the finger flexors and thumb with optimum power. This is called the **"position of function"** of the wrist and hand. In this position the wrist is held in neutral, and the fingers are moderately flexed at the MCP joints and slightly flexed at the PIP and DIP joints.

- *Dysfunction and injury*: The hand is susceptible to acute and chronic dysfunctions and injuries. Tearing of the tendon away from the bone (avulsion) of the extensor tendon at the end of the finger is the most common closed-tendon (does not cut the skin) injury to athletes.[5] The incident involves a forceful impact on the tip of the finger.

Chronic dysfunctions are often of the fatigue type. Through overuse the muscles are held in a sustained contraction and build up metabolic waste products, creating an acidic environment and decreased oxygen. This manifests as ischemic pain which leaves the muscles sensitive to modest pressures. Weakness of the intrinsic muscles and sustained contraction of the finger extensors produce a clawing of the fingers. The tendons of the finger flexors can develop a thickening of their tendon sheath, causing a nodule to form that can become entrapped in the annular ligament, creating a "trigger finger." The flexor pollicis longus can become irritated because of repetitive gripping motions or acute trauma, such as a FOOSH. The dorsal and palmar interossei and lumbricals can become irritated because of repetitive fine motor movements of the fingers, such as done by musicians.

- *Treatment implications*: The basic protocol is first to perform CR or PIR MET to the involved muscles and fascia to increase their extensibility and to help restore normal neurologic function. Next, perform OM with scooping strokes, transverse to the line of the fiber. Transverse friction strokes may be used if fibrosis is palpated. Mobilization of the associated joint is performed to help normalize the articular and periarticular nerves that communicate with the muscle.

Muscle Imbalances of the Elbow, Wrist, and Hand

- **Muscles that tend to be tight and short:** The pronator teres, the flexor carpi ulnaris, the flexors of the fingers, and the muscles of the thenar eminence
- **Muscles that tend to be weak and inhibited:** The finger extensors, the lumbricals, and the interossei

Positional Dysfunction of the Muscles of the Elbow, Wrist, and Hand

- The muscles of the forearm tend to develop a torsion toward pronation. The muscles of the hand develop a torsion that folds the thenar and hypothenar muscles toward the midline of the palm and the fingers into a sustained flexed position.

Intrinsic Muscles of the Hand

See Muscle Table 10-5.

Muscular Actions of the Hand

See Table 10-6.

Dysfunction and Injury of the Elbow, Forearm, Wrist, and Hand

FACTORS PREDISPOSING TO ELBOW, FOREARM, WRIST, AND HAND PAIN

- Repetitive gripping, such as playing tennis or hammering, can fatigue and weaken the wrist and finger flexors and extensors, predisposing them to an acute tear at their tenoperiosteal attachments at the elbow and wrist.
- Repetitive or prolonged use of finger flexors, such as keyboard work, can cause a tendinitis, leading to localized pain, swelling, or both at the wrist, leading to carpal tunnel syndrome.
- Repetitive elbow flexion and extension, such as carpentry work or playing instruments such as the violin, can cause elbow pain.
- Repetitive elbow extension, such as throwing a ball, irritates the muscle attachments at the elbow.
- Repetitive pronation or supination (twisting) motions.
- Previous injury to the joints can cause a thickening of the joint capsule and collateral ligaments, limiting joint motion, leading to degeneration of the cartilage and OA.
- A subluxation of the lunate in the wrist can cause carpal tunnel syndrome. A fixation of the MCP or IP joint can lead to degeneration and OA.
- Immobility
- Fatigue

DIFFERENTIATION OF ELBOW, FOREARM, WRIST, AND HAND PAIN

It is important to realize that pain in the elbow, wrist, and hand can come from disease processes rather than from injuries and dysfunctions to the neuromusculoskeletal system. See the section "Contraindications to Massage Therapy: Red Flags" in Chapter 2, "Assessments & Technique" for guidelines on when massage is contraindicated and when to refer the client to a doctor.

The elbow, wrist, and hand are common areas where a combination of pain, numbing, and tingling may be referred from the cervical spine. As mentioned in Chapter 5, "Cervical Spine," one type of referred pain is caused by muscle, ligament, joint capsule, disc, or dura mater. These tissues elicit what is called **sclerotomal** pain when they are injured. Usually the sclerotomal pain is described as deep, aching, and diffuse. A second type of referred pain, called **radicular** pain is caused by an irritation of the spinal nerve root. If the sensory (dorsal) root is irritated, there is sharp pain, numbing, or tingling that is well-localized in what are called dermatomes. A dermatome is an area of the skin supplied by the sensory root of a single spinal nerve (see Chapter 3, "Lumbosacral Spine" for a figure of the dermatomes). If there is compression of the motor (ventral) nerve root, in addition to the pain, numbing, and tingling, there may be weakness in the muscles supplied by that nerve root, called the **myotome.** The relevant myotomes of the elbow, wrist, and hand are as follows: C6 is wrist extension; C7 is wrist flexion; and C8 is thumb extension. The entrapment of a peripheral nerve in the area of the elbow, wrist, and hand may also lead to some combination of pain, numbing, or weakness. In peripheral entrapment, manual pressure over the entrapped nerve typically increases the intensity of

TABLE 10-5 INTRINSIC MUSCLES OF THE HAND

Thenar Eminence

Muscle	*Origin*	*Insertion*	*Action*
Abductor pollicis brevis	From the flexor retinaculum and the tubercles of the navicular and trapezium and the tendon of abductor pollicis longus.	Radial side of the proximal phalanx and radial sesamoid of the MP joint; lies superficial to opponens pollicis and partly superficial and lateral (radial) to the flexor pollicis brevis.	Draws the thumb forward in a plane at right angles to the palm and rotates it medially.
Opponens pollicis	Deep to the abductor pollicis brevis, arises from the tubercle of the trapezium and the flexor retinaculum.	Attaches the entire length of the lateral border and lateral half of the palmar surface of the first metacarpal.	Bends it medially across the palm and rotates it medially (i.e., in opposition); abducts, flexes, and rotates first metacarpal.
Flexor pollicis brevis	Partly overlapped by abductor pollicis, the flexor arises by a deep and superficial part; superficial part arises from the distal border of the flexor retinaculum; and the deep part arises from the tubercle of the trapezium, passing along the radial side of the tendon of the flexor pollicis longus.	Radial sesamoid bone of the MCP joint of the thumb.	Flexes the proximal phalanx of the thumb; flexes the MCP joint and rotates it medially in cooperation with opponens.
Adductor pollicis	Arises by transverse and oblique heads: Oblique head—capitate, bases of the second and the third metacarpals; Transverse head—entire length of the shaft of the third metacarpal bone.	Ulnar sesamoid bone of the MCP joint of the thumb.	Produces adduction and assists in opposition and flexion of the thumb on the first phalanx; produces slight flexion, ulnar deviation, and lateral rotation.

Hypothenar Eminence

Muscle	*Origin*	*Insertion*	*Action*
Abductor digiti minimi	Arises from the pisiform bone, the tendon of the flexor carpi ulnaris, and the pisohamate ligament.	Into the base of the proximal phalanx (ulnar side) of the fifth digit.	Abducts the little finger.
Flexor digiti minimi	Lies on the radial side of the abductor digiti minimi, and mostly deep to it, arising from the hook of the hamate and the palmar surface of flexor retinaculum.	On the ulnar side of the base of the proximal phalanx along with abductor digiti minimi; separated at its origin from abductor digiti minimi by the deep branches of ulnar artery and nerve.	Flexes the little finger at its MCP joint.

TABLE 10-5 INTRINSIC MUSCLES OF THE HAND—cont'd

Hypothenar Eminence—cont'd

Muscle	*Origin*	*Insertion*	*Action*
Opponens digiti minimi	Deep to the abductor and flexor digiti minimi, arising from the hook of the hamate and flexor retinaculum.	Into the entire length of the ulnar margin of the fifth metacarpal.	Draws the fifth metacarpal forward and laterally (radially) at the same time, rotating it about its axis so that its anterior surface comes to face the thumb in opposition.
Lumbricals (I–IV)	Arise from the radial side of the tendons of the flexor digitorum profundus.	Each passes to the radial side of the corresponding finger and to the joint capsules of the MCP joint.	Act in association with the interossei to flex the digits at the MCP joints, thus causing traction of the tendons of the flexor digitorum profundus.
Dorsal interossei	Four bipennate muscles, each arising from adjacent sides of the two metacarpal bones.	Attach to the bases of the proximal phalanges and the dorsal digital expansion; first attaches to the radial side of the proximal phalanx of the index finger; the second and the third attach to the sides of the proximal phalanx of the middle finger; and the fourth attaches to the ulnar side of the ring finger.	Abduct the finger from the axis of the middle finger.
Palmar interossei	Smaller and less powerful than the dorsal, they arise from the palmar surfaces of the second, the fourth, and the fifth metacarpals instead of between them; except for the first, each of the four arises from the entire length of the metacarpal.	Attach to corresponding phalanges.	Adduct the fingers to the midaxis.

the symptoms' temporarily. This increased intensity of symptoms' is an indication for treatment. The OM techniques that release peripheral nerve entrapment are highly effective. If symptoms do not resolve after several treatments, refer the client to a chiropractor or osteopath for spinal evaluation.

Differentiation of other conditions may be categorized according to the region involved. An ache at the medial and lateral epicondyles that is increased with gripping or isometric challenge of the wrist flexors, pronators, or extensors is typically a tenoperiosteal tear of the muscle attachments. Pain in the same region also may be a nerve entrapment. Unlike tendinitis or a tenoperiosteal tear, an entrapment is not typically aggravated by isometric challenge.

Pain in the anterior forearm may be a bicipital or pronator teres tendinitis. Both conditions are often painful with isometric challenge. Pain at the wrist may be a tendinitis at the insertion points of the wrist flexors and extensors. With tendinitis, flexors and extensors are tender to palpation and painful with isometric challenge. Pain at the wrist may also

TABLE 10-6 MUSCULAR ACTIONS AT THE HAND

The hand consists of 19 bones and 19 joints. Nine muscles from the forearm move the fingers or thumb, and the hand has 18 intrinsic muscles. For clarity, the actions of the fingers and thumb are differentiated.

Fingers

Flexion

- Flexor digitorum superficialis
- Flexor digitorum profundus
- Flexor digiti minimi
- Lumbricals and interossei assist flexion

Extension

- Extensor digitorum
- Extensor indices
- Extensor digiti minimi

Adductors

- Long finger flexors are principal adductors, assisted by palmar interossei

Abductors

- Dorsal interossei, assisted by long extensors
- Abductor digiti minimi

Thumb

Flexion

- Flexor digitorum longus (extrinsic)
- Flexor pollicis brevis (intrinsic)

Extension

- Extensor pollicis longus
- Extensor pollicis brevis

Abduction

- Abductor pollicis longus (extrinsic)
- Abductor pollicis brevis (intrinsic)

Adduction

- Adductor pollicis, oblique and transverse heads

Opposition

- Opponens pollicis
- Opponens digiti minimi

be a ligament sprain. Sprains are often associated with an acute injury. They are not painful to isometric challenge, but they are painful to passive stretch. Numbing and tingling in the thumb and the index and middle fingers may be carpal tunnel syndrome. Phalen's test (pressing the dorsum of the hands together in front of the chest for 1 minute) is usually positive. Aching and stiffness in the thumb joints or in the fingers may be OA. With OA, there is a loss of normal joint play and thickened and tender joint capsule and collateral ligaments.

COMMON DYSFUNCTIONS AND INJURIES OF THE ELBOW, FOREARM, WRIST, AND HAND

Lateral Epicondylitis (Tennis Elbow)

- ***Causes:*** Lateral epicondylitis, or tennis elbow, is considered an acute manifestation of a chronic condition. The acute episode is a tenoperiosteal tear of the wrist extensors, most commonly the ECRB. The chronic problem is a degenerative disorder caused by tissue fatigue from repetitive gripping. Tennis players, musicians, massage therapists, and carpenters are susceptible to overuse of gripping motions.
- ***Symptoms:*** A gradual or intermittent mild ache often develops insidiously. Usually, the most tender area is at the anterior portion of the lateral epicondyle at the tenoperiosteal junction of the wrist extensors, particularly the ECRB. The client may also feel pain in the body of the tendon over the radial head or at the musculotendinous junction of the extensors several inches distal to the radial head. The ache can increase to severe pain and progress down the back of the forearm to the wrist and hand.
- ***Signs:*** Clients experience increased pain with gripping motions and resisted wrist extension. They also experience pain on resisted extension of the middle finger, with their elbow extended. Pain may occur with passive flexion of the wrist and with pronation of the forearm as the ECRB is stretched over the proximal radial head, making the muscle susceptible to injury.
- ***Treatment:*** Perform CR MET for the wrist and finger extensors, especially the ECRB. Perform OM, including transverse friction massage, on the attachment points.

Medial Epicondylitis (Little Leaguer's or Golfer's Elbow)

- *Causes:* Repetitive wrist flexion and pronation (e.g. golfing, throwing, and gripping) can lead to medial epicondylitis. This condition is common to massage therapists, carpenters, golfers, and tennis players.
- *Symptoms:* Medial epicondylitis symptoms are pain at the medial side of the elbow at the tenoperiosteal junction of the pronator teres and at the flexor carpi radialis on the anterior medial epicondyle of the humerus and possible pain at the musculotendinous junction of flexors just distal to the medial epicondyle. Usually this condition has little radiation, but it may involve an ulnar nerve entrapment.
- *Signs:* Clients experience painful resisted wrist flexion with the elbow in extension and supination. Pain may be elicited on resisted pronation, implicating pronator teres.
- *Treatment:* Perform PIR MET for the wrist and the finger flexors by increasing wrist extension, with the client's elbow extended and forearm supinated.

Cubital Tunnel Syndrome (Entrapment of Ulnar Nerve at Elbow)

- *Causes:* Repetitive elbow flexion, which narrows the cubital tunnel, or sustained elbow flexion, which commonly occurs with sleeping, are cubital tunnel syndrome causes. The ulnar nerve can be entrapped at several locations: at the fascia of the subscapularis (see Chapter 6, "The Shoulder"); at the distal third of the medial arm; and at the cubital tunnel. The ulnar nerve may also be entrapped between the two heads of the flexor carpi ulnaris or at the tunnel of Guyon (see the section "Wrist").
- *Symptoms:* Clients experience pain, tingling, and numbing to the fourth and the fifth fingers. They may also experience medial elbow ache, which can extend to the forearm.
- *Signs:* Cubital tunnel syndrome signs include weakness of the intrinsic muscles of the hand and wasting of the hypothenar eminence which is innervated by the ulnar nerve. Digital pressure over the ulnar nerve behind the medial epicondyle, sustained passive flexion of the elbow for 1 minute, or resisted wrist flexion with ulnar deviation reproduce ulnar nerve entrapment symptoms.
- *Treatment:* Perform MET to the flexor carpi ulnaris to reduce the hypertonicity, and increase the length and extensibility of the fascia forming the cubital tunnel. Then perform manual release of the nerve with gentle, scooping strokes transverse to the line of the nerve. Deep OM strokes, including transverse friction massage, are often needed to release the fibrosis in the area of the cubital tunnel.

Carpal Tunnel Syndrome

- *Causes:* Carpal tunnel syndrome symptoms are elicited by median nerve compression, which leads to decreased circulation and therefore decreased oxygen. Causes of this condition include overuse of finger flexors (e.g., keyboard work, building trades, and massage therapy), which can cause inflammation of the tendon sheaths, which can develop into fibrosis or thickening of the flexor tendon and fibrosis of the transverse carpal ligament. Carpal tunnel syndrome may also occur because of previous injury or other chronic microtrauma, subluxation of the lunate, edema from pregnancy, and OA.
- *Symptoms:* Clients experience insidious onset of numbing and tingling in the first three fingers. Symptoms are worse at night or upon arising in the morning and usually relieved by moving the hand ("shaking it out"). There may be pain at the wrist that may radiate to the elbow.
- *Signs:* Pressing the dorsum of the hands together in front of the chest for 1 minute (Phalen's test) reproduces carpal tunnel syndrome symptoms. If flexor tendinitis is an underlying factor, resistive testing of the finger flexors increases symptoms.
- *Treatment:* Perform CR MET to the muscles that attach to the transverse carpal ligament (flexor retinaculum) to increase the extensibility of the ligament. These muscles include the palmar longus, the muscles of the thenar and hypothenar eminence, and the flexor carpi ulnaris. Next, perform a gentle distraction of the flexor retinaculum. For chronic conditions, perform OM strokes to the attachment points of the flexor retinaculum.

Ligamentous Wrist Sprains

- *Cause:* A common cause of a wrist sprain is a fall on an outstretched hand (FOOSH).
- *Symptoms:* Pain is usually well-localized to the site of injury. The most common ligaments involved are the lunocapitate on the dorsal side and the radiolunate on the palmar side.[3]

- *Signs:* Passive wrist flexion yielding pain on the dorsum of the wrist typically indicates lunocapitate ligament. Leaning on an extended wrist is painful for the dorsal lunocapitate and the palmar radiolunate ligaments.
- *Treatment:* Perform CR MET to the muscles that attach to the ligaments, either the flexors or the extensors. Next, perform OM, including transverse friction massage, to the body and attachment points of the ligaments. If the ligaments have become too slack and the wrist is unstable, exercise rehabilitation is recommended to restore stability.

Abductor Pollicis Longus and Extensor Pollicis Brevis Tenovaginitis (De Quervain's Tenovaginitis)

- *Causes:* Repetitive gripping motions cause the tendons to rub against each other creating irritation and inflammation. This irritation and inflammation creates swelling in the acute stage and fibrosis in the chronic stage. Both conditions narrow the tunnel and create pain with movement using the muscles.
- *Symptoms:* A tenovaginitis symptom is the insidious onset of pain at the anatomic "snuff-box," the area over the scaphoid bounded by the tendons of the abductor pollicis longus and the extensor pollicis brevis and the extensor pollicis longus on the other side. Another possible symptom is pain in the distal lateral forearm, especially with gripping activities.
- *Signs:* Resisted thumb extension and resisted thumb abduction increase pain. Have the client flex his or her thumb, wrap his or her fingers around the thumb, and ulnar deviate the wrist (Finkelstein's test). A positive test elicits pain at the snuff-box.
- *Treatment:* Perform MET to the involved tendons and OM, with gentle scooping strokes transverse to the line of the tendon. Deeper friction strokes are indicated if thickened, fibrotic tissue is palpated in the chronic condition.

Osteoarthritis of the Thumb and Fingers

- *Causes:* Hereditary factors related to arthritis of the fingers may be a cause of thumb and finger OA. Degenerative arthritis is related to overuse and inflammation leading to capsular fibrosis, loss of the normal synovial fluid, and cartilage degeneration. Often, predisposing factors such as subluxation or fixation of the normal gliding characteristics of the joint are present.
- *Symptoms:* OA of the thumb has pain at the CMC joint with thumb movements, especially gripping. There is often crepitation and weakness. With OA of the fingers, there is pain and loss of ROM at the involved joint.
- *Signs:* With OA of the thumb, clients experience pain on passive abduction of the thumb and painful crepitation in mobilization of the first CMC joint. With OA of the fingers, clients experience pain and limited flexion of the MCP, PIP, and DIP joints, with a thickened feel to the joint capsule and ligaments.
- *Treatment:* The treatment protocol for arthritis of the hand is MET for the finger flexors and extensors to help stimulate the normal joint lubrication by tensing the joint capsule through its attachment to the muscles. Perform OM to release adhesions in the annular (vaginal) ligaments of the flexor tendons and at the tenoperiosteal attachments of the flexors to the thumb and fingers. Perform transverse friction massage to the ligament system of the fingers and thumb, concentrating on transverse strokes to the collateral ligaments and transverse metacarpal ligaments. Then perform joint mobilization to the involved joint.

LESS COMMON DYSFUNCTION AND INJURIES

Bicipital Tendinitis at the Elbow

- *Causes:* Repetitive throwing and repetitive pronation or supination are causes of bicipital tendinitis at the elbow.
- *Symptom:* Pain, usually well-localized to either the lower myotendinitis junction in the middle of the cubital fossa, just proximal to the elbow crease, or at the lower tenoperiosteal junction between the radial tuberosity and ulna, is a bicipital tendinitis symptom.
- *Signs:* Clients experience painful resisted elbow flexion with their forearm supinated or with resisted supination.
- *Treatment:* Perform MET for the biceps, and OM at the above named sites.

Triceps Tendinitis at the Elbow

- *Causes:* Repetitive elbow extension, as in tennis backhand, or repetitive or excessive arm pressing, as in the handstands of gymnastics, cause triceps tendinitis at the elbow.

- *Symptom:* Pain at the tenoperiosteal insertion of the olecranon of the elbow is a symptom of triceps tendinitis at the elbow.
- *Sign:* Clients experience pain with resisted elbow extension.
- *Treatment:* Perform MET for the triceps, and OM for the tenoperiosteal attachment.

Entrapment of the Median Nerve at the Elbow

- *Causes:* Repetitive pronation or pronation and flexion of the elbow cause median nerve entrapment at the elbow. The nerve may be entrapped in a fibro-osseous tunnel on the anterior-medial surface of the distal end of the humerus, beneath the edge of the aponeurosis of the biceps (lacertus fibrosis) or between the two heads of the origin of the pronator teres (pronator syndrome).
- *Symptoms:* Similar to those of carpal tunnel, symptoms of median nerve entrapment at the elbow are numbing and tingling of the first three fingers.
- *Signs:* Symptoms may be aggravated by full passive pronation of the elbow or by digital pressure at anterior-medial surface of distal humerus. If entrapment is severe, clients experience a loss of strength pinching the tip of the thumb with the index finger, called Froment's sign.
- *Treatment:* Perform MET to the biceps and pronator to reduce the hypertonicity and to increase the length and extensibility of the connective tissue. Perform manual release of the nerve with gentle, scooping strokes transverse to the line of the nerve.

Radial Tunnel Syndrome (Entrapment of Radial Nerve at the Elbow)

- *Causes:* Repeated pronation, elbow extension, and wrist flexion (wringing motion) or overuse of extensor muscles are often causes of radial tunnel syndrome. This condition is found in musicians, tennis and golf players, and massage therapists. The nerve may be entrapped at the anterolateral aspect of the distal humerus as the nerve travels between the brachialis and the brachioradialis, as it passes under the fibrous origin of the ECRB, and as it enters the supinator canal approximately 2 inches distal to the lateral epicondyle under a fibrous arch called the arcade of Frohse.[13]
- *Symptoms:* Deep, dull ache and paresthesias at the lateral epicondyle and posterior aspect of the proximal forearm are symptoms of radial nerve entrapment. Extensor muscle weakness might also occur.
- *Signs:* Clients experience increased pain on resisted supination of the forearm or with passive extension and pronation of the elbow and flexion of the wrist. Grip weakness also occurs.
- *Treatment:* Perform MET to the brachialis, brachioradialis, ECRB, and supinator. Perform manual release of the nerve with gentle, scooping strokes transverse to the line of the nerve.

Extensor Carpi Radialis Brevis and Longus Tendinitis

- *Cause:* Repetitive wrist extension causes ECRB and ECRL tendinitis.
- *Symptoms:* Localized pain or a vague deep ache on the dorsum of the hand are symptoms of this condition. The usual sites are the tenoperiosteal junction at the base of the second metacarpal (for ECRL) or the base of the third metacarpal (for ECRB).
- *Signs:* Clients experience pain with resisted wrist extension with radial deviation.
- *Treatment:* Perform MET for the ECRB and ECRL. To reduce the hypertonicity, lengthen the myofascia and increase the resilience of the fascia at the tenoperiosteal junctions. Perform OM for the entire length of the muscle, and perform transverse friction massage at the insertion points.

Extensor Carpi Ulnaris Tendinitis

- *Causes:* Playing tennis and racquet sports and excessive keyboard work are common causes of extensor carpi ulnaris tendinitis.
- *Symptoms:* Localized pain or vague deep ache at the ulnar styloid, between the ulna and triquetral, or at the base of the fifth metacarpal are symptoms of this condition.
- *Signs:* Clients experience pain with resisted ulnar deviation of the wrist and pain with wrist extension.
- *Treatment:* Perform MET for the extensor carpi ulnaris, and perform OM at the muscle bellies, the myotendinous junctions, and the attachment points.

Flexor Carpi Ulnaris Tendinitis

- *Cause:* Repetitive wrist flexion, such as excessive keyboard work or massage therapy, causes flexor carpi ulnaris tendinitis.

- *Symptoms:* Localized pain or vague ache at the tenoperiosteal junction on the pisiform (palmar surface) or at the base of the fifth metacarpal are symptoms of this condition.
- *Sign:* Clients may experience increased pain with resisted wrist flexion with ulnar deviation.
- *Treatment:* Perform MET for the flexor carpi ulnaris, and perform OM at the muscle bellies, the myotendinous junctions, and the attachment points.

Flexor Carpi Radialis Tendinitis

- *Cause:* Repetitive wrist flexion causes flexor carpi radialis tendinitis.
- *Symptoms:* Localized pain or ache at tenoperiosteal insertion of palmar surface at the base of the second metacarpal that may radiate to the elbow.
- *Signs:* Clients may experience increased pain with resisted wrist flexion with radial deviation.
- *Treatment:* Perform MET for the flexor carpi radialis, and perform OM at the muscle bellies, the myotendinous junctions, and the attachment points.

Ulnar Nerve Compression at the Wrist (Handlebar Palsy)

- *Causes:* Prolonged pressure on the hypothenar eminence and a FOOSH injury cause ulnar nerve compression at the wrist. The ulnar nerve passes through the tunnel of Guyon, which is formed by the pisohamate ligament between the pisiform and the hook of hamate, and may be compressed in the tunnel or may be irritated from swelling of the flexor carpi ulnaris at its insertion into the pisiform.
- *Symptoms:* Symptoms include numbing and tingling to the ring and little finger if the superficial branch is affected or deep aching pain in the palm of hand if deep branch of ulnar nerve is affected.
- *Signs:* Digital pressure over the nerve near the pisiform increases the intensity of symptoms.
- *Treatment:* Perform MET to the flexor carpi ulnaris to release the tension in the pisohamate ligament. Perform OM strokes, transverse to the ligament, and then gentle, scooping strokes perpendicular to the line of the nerve at the tunnel.

Flexor Pollicis Longus Tendinitis

- *Cause:* Repetitive gripping, such as done in racquet sports, causes flexor pollicis longus tendinitis.
- *Symptoms:* The symptoms of this condition are a deep ache most commonly at the thenar eminence as the tendon runs along the extent of the first metacarpal or at the tenoperiosteal insertion on the palmar surface at the base of the distal phalanx.
- *Sign:* Clients experience pain that increases with resisted thumb flexion at IP joint.
- *Treatment:* Perform MET for the flexor pollicis longus, and perform OM at the muscle belly, the myotendinous junctions, and the attachment points.

Dorsal and Palmar Interosseous Tendinitis

- *Cause:* Repetitive fine motor movements of the fingers, such as those done by musicians, cause dorsal and palmar interosseous tendinitis.
- *Symptom:* Pain between the metacarpal shafts is a symptom of this condition.
- *Signs:* Clients experience pain on resisted abduction (dorsal) or adduction (palmar).
- *Treatment:* Perform MET for the interossei, which is resisted abduction and adduction, and OM in between the shafts of the metacarpals.

Stenosing Tenosynovitis of Digits (Trigger Finger)

- *Causes:* Repetitive forceful gripping causes a thickening of the tendon sheath and a nodule to form on the tendons. Hereditary factors may also be a cause.
- *Symptom:* Stenosing tenosynovitis' symptoms are fingers locking in flexion and needing to be passively extended or extended with a snap that can be painful.
- *Sign:* Observation of this above mentioned snapping is a sign of this type of tenosynovitis.
- *Treatment:* This condition may be unresponsive to manual therapies, but treatment may reduce intensity and frequency of symptoms. Perform transverse and longitudinal strokes on the tendon, the involved tendon sheath, and the annular ligament that suspends the tendon to the bone.

Entrapment Neuropathy of Interdigital Nerve

- *Causes:* The interdigital nerves can become entrapped in between the superficial and the deep layers of the transverse carpal ligament. The ligaments thicken because of injury or repetitive gripping motions. The hand is typically held in sustained flexion, compressing the metacarpal heads and the nerves.

- *Symptoms:* Burning pain in one or more fingers, with either increased or decreased sensation and cold fingers are symptoms of this condition.
- *Signs:* Clients may experience acute tenderness of the palmar surface of the webspace between the metacarpal heads. Hyperextension of the finger may increase pain at this site.
- *Treatment:* Perform OM to first release the transverse metacarpal ligament. Then perform gentle, scooping strokes perpendicular to the nerve, in between the heads of the metacarpals.

Assessment of the Elbow, Wrist, and Hand

BACKGROUND

Pain at the elbow is often localized to the lateral and medial epicondyles and usually represents a tendinitis of the muscle attachments at those sites. Examination reveals pain with isometric testing and with passive stretch of the involved muscles. The elbow is also the site of neurologic symptoms referred from C6 to C7 nerve-root irritation. The pain is deep and gripping and often is present even at rest. The examination findings typically include painless weakness of the wrist extensors and flexors. This finding requires a referral to a chiropractor or an osteopath.

Pain at the wrist has traumatic and cumulative origins. A FOOSH can sprain the ligaments, as well as fracture the distal end of the radius, a common injury. Pain at the wrist is also commonly associated with chronic overuse, such as the tendinitis associated with retail clerks, carpenters, and massage therapists. Either history can lead to neurologic symptoms, or conditions such as carpal tunnel syndrome. Conditions of traumatic and cumulative origin are fairly easy to assess.

Pain and disability in the hand is one of the most common complaints presented to the therapist. The thumb is one of the most common sites for OA and can lead to great disability. The fingers are also common sites for arthritis of the degenerative and the rheumatoid types. The hand is a common site for referral of numbing and tingling from the C6 to C8 nerves. Such referral leads to painless weakness, unlike the pain with isometric contraction of an involved musculotendinous unit.

HISTORY QUESTIONS FOR THE CLIENT WHO HAS ELBOW, FOREARM, WRIST, AND HAND PAIN

- When Does It Hurt?

Local problems in the elbow, wrist, and hand usually involve pain with use, with some notable exceptions. For example, carpal tunnel and cubital tunnel syndromes cause numbing and tingling at night. Referral of pain from the cervical spine exists independent of movement of the extremity. It is important to realize that you may have a client who has both a local and a referred problem overlapping.

ELBOW

Inspection and Observation

- *Position:* Client must be suitably undressed so that you can observe the skin. Have the client stand in front of you, in the anatomical position (i.e., arms at sides, palms facing forward).
- *Observation:* Note the position of the neck and shoulders, as well as the elbows, and compare sides. A sustained deviation of the neck may indicate a cervical problem. Note any redness, heat, swelling, scars, etc. about the elbow. Normally, the forearms have approximately a 10° to 15° lateral deviation relative to the arm; this deviation is called the **carrying angle.** A deviation from the normal side may indicate a previous trauma.

Active Movements

Flexion and Extension

- *Position:* Client stands facing you.
- *Action:* Instruct the client to follow your movements. First, abduct the arms to 90° with the palms up to compare elbow extension (Fig. 10-11). Next, place your fingertips on your shoulders to compare elbow flexion (Fig. 10-12).
- *Observation:* The normal range for extension is 0° (i.e., fully straight), although you may observe some hyperextension in women and children. Inability to fully extend the elbow often indicates a joint problem. The typical ROM for elbow flexion is 140° to 160°.

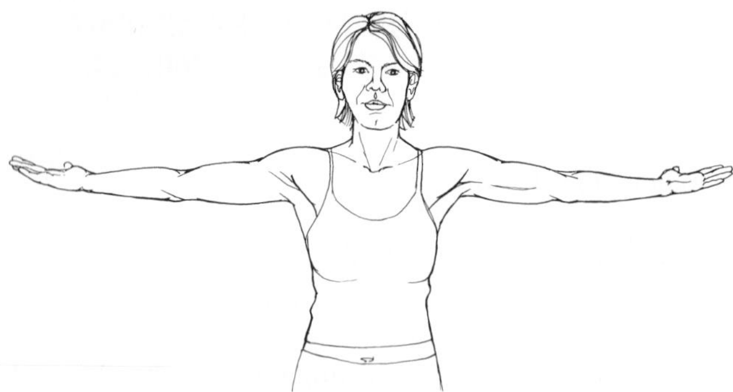

Figure 10-11. Active elbow extension is best observed with the client's arms abducted to 90°.

Pronation and Supination (Fig. 10-13A and B)

- *Position:* Client stands facing you, with elbows against his or her body and flexed 90° and with thumb facing up (i.e., with the forearm in neutral).
- *Action:* Ask the client to turn his or her palms down fully and then turn both palms up fully.
- *Observation:* Inability to supinate fully may indicate fixation of the proximal or distal radioulnar joints, shortened forearm flexors, or OA.

Passive and Resisted Movements

Flexion, Extension, Pronation, and Supination

- *Position:* Client is sitting.
- *Action:* Place one hand on the elbow and the other hand on the distal forearm. Take the joint to the limit of pain, tissue tension, or both. If it is not painful, move the joint with some overpressure to assess the end feel.
- *Observation:* Flexion range is approximately 160°. Normally, there is a soft-tissue end feel. If there is decreased motion and a thick, leathery end feel, it

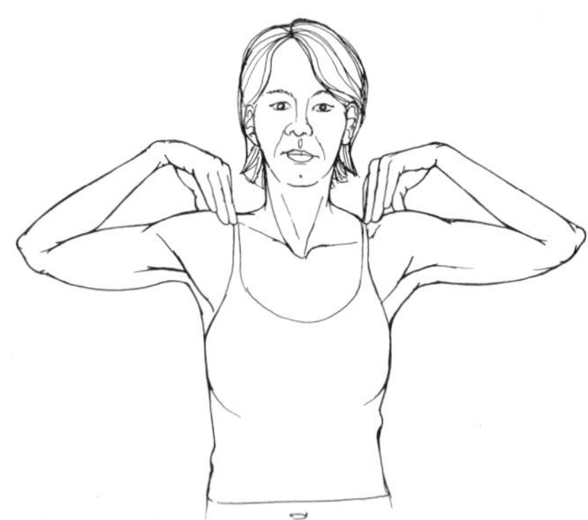

Figure 10-12. Active elbow flexion is done by having the client attempt to touch the shoulders with the fingertips.

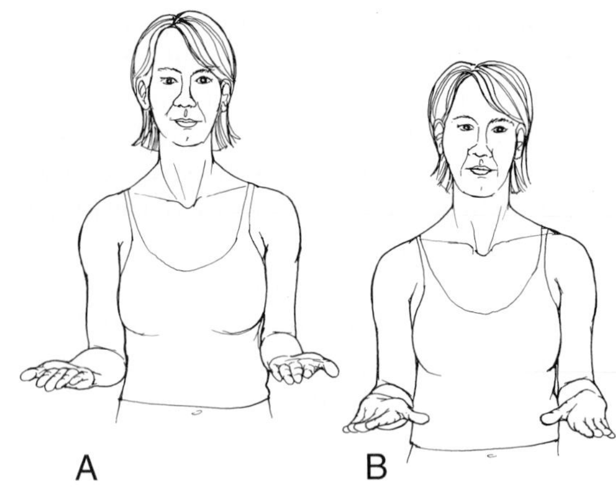

Figure 10-13. **A.** Active supination. **B.** Active pronation, with the thumbs abducted, which allows for an easy measure of the ROM.

indicates fibrosis of the capsule. Decreased flexion is the capsular pattern of the elbow and is an early sign of arthritis. If there is a decreased range and a bony end feel, it indicates arthritis.

A mushy end feel during extension indicates swelling in the joint.

Inability to supinate fully may indicate a fixation of the proximal or the distal radioulnar joints, shortened forearm flexors, or OA.

Tests for Lateral Epicondylitis

- *Position:* Client is sitting.
- *Action:* Two tests are common for lateral epicondylitis. In test one, the client's elbow is in extension and his or her forearm is pronated. Press the wrist into flexion and ulnar deviation (Fig. 10-14**A**). In test two, the client's elbow and wrist are extended and the forearm is pronated. Have the client resist as you attempt to press the wrist into flexion (Fig. 10-14**B**).
- *Observation:* The first test places maximum stretch on the common extensor tendon. The second test isometrically challenges the wrist extensors. These tests are typically painful with lateral epicondylitis. The first position is also used for PIR MET to lengthen the extensors in a chronically shortened condition.

Tests for Medial Epicondylitis

- *Position:* Client is sitting.
- *Action:* Two tests are common for medial epicondylitis. In test one, the client's elbow is extended and the forearm is supinated. Press the wrist into extension (Fig. 10-15**A**). In test two, the

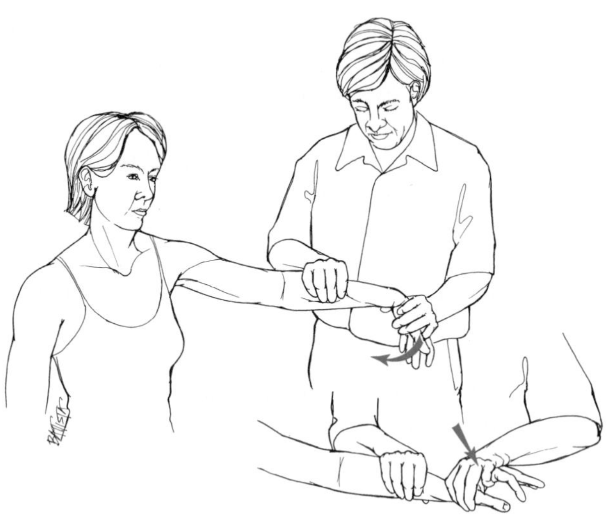

Figure 10-14. *Left and upper right.* One test for lateral epicondylitis is to extend the elbow and then press the wrist into flexion. *Lower right.* A second test for lateral epicondylitis is to have the client resist as you attempt to flex the wrist.

client's elbow and wrist are extended and the forearm supinated. Have the client resist as you attempt to press the wrist into further extension (Fig. 10-15**B**).

- *Observation:* The first test places maximum stretch on the common flexor-pronator tendon. The second test isometrically challenges the wrist flexors. These tests are typically painful with medial epicondylitis. The first position is also used for PIR MET to lengthen the flexors in a chronically shortened condition.

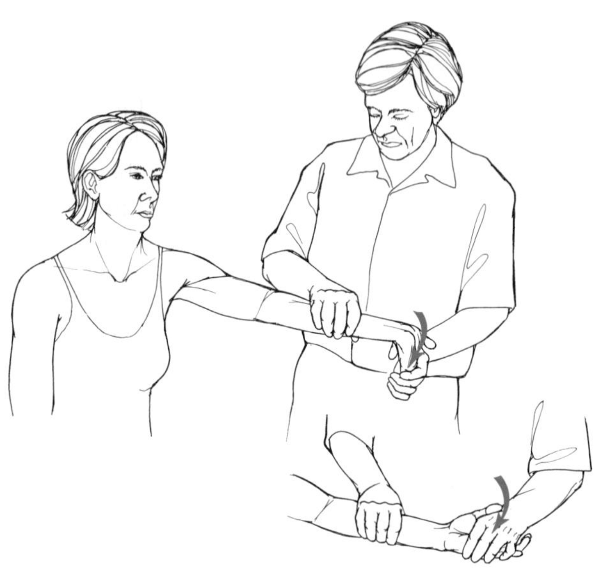

Figure 10-15. *Left and upper right.* One test for medial epicondylitis is to extend the elbow and then passively stretch the wrist into extension. *Lower right.* A second test is to have the client resist as you attempt to press the wrist into extension.

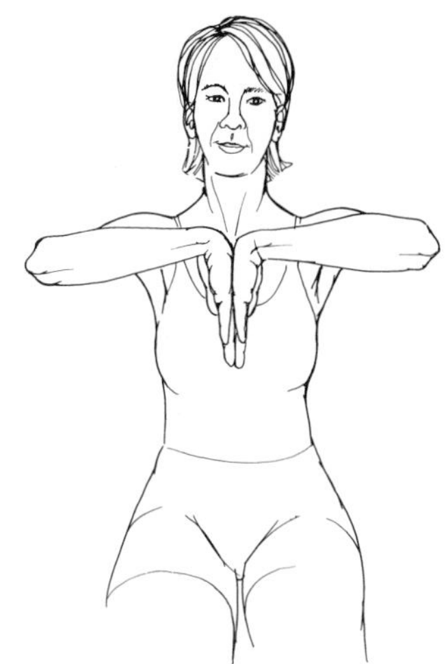

Figure 10-16. Active flexion of the wrist is performed by having the client place the backs of the hands together. This allows easy comparison of both sides. If this position is held for 1 minute, is it called Phalen's Test, a test for carpal tunnel syndrome.

WRIST

Active Movements

Flexion

- *Position:* Client is sitting and is asked to follow your movements.
- *Action:* Have the client bring the back of the hands together in front of the chest with the forearms parallel to the floor (Fig. 10-16).
- *Observation:* Note whether the backs of the hands can touch each other equally and whether the forearms are at the same level. Loss of flexion manifests either as the inability to touch the back of the other hand or as the elbow being higher on the involved side.

Carpal Tunnel Syndrome Test (Phalen's Test)

- *Position:* If the position described above is held for 1 minute or until numbing or tingling arise in the thumb, index, or middle fingers, you are testing whether there is a compression of the median nerve in the carpal tunnel. This is called the **Phalen's test.**
- *Observation:* The client reports a numbing and tingling in the thumb and the index and middle fingers that is elicited or worsened if he or she began the test with these symptoms.

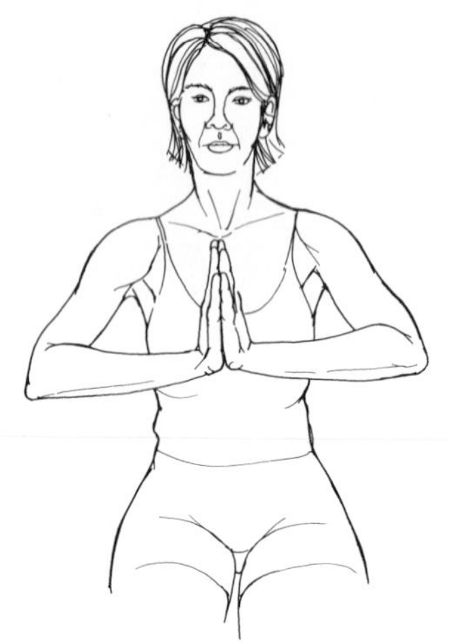

Figure 10-17. Active extension of the wrists. Comparison of both sides.

Extension

- *Position:* Client is sitting and asked to follow your movements.
- *Action:* Bring the palms together in a "prayer position" in front of the chest with the forearms parallel to the floor (Fig. 10-17).
- *Observation:* Note whether the forearms are at the same level. Loss of extension manifests as the elbow being lower on the involved side. The range is 60° to 70°, tests the joint capsule and ligaments on the palmar surface, and is most limited in joint injuries or dysfunction, as extension is the close-packed position for the wrist.

Functional Screening Test for the Wrist

- *Position:* Client is sitting.
- *Action:* Have the client rest his or her hand on the table and attempt to lean his or her weight to that side on the extended wrist.
- *Observation:* A sharp, localized pain at the dorsum of the wrist usually indicates a joint problem, whether a fixation or subluxation of one of the carpals, or an arthritic joint. A positive funding may also indicate a sprain. Inability to perform this motion may indicate a fracture.

Passive Movements: Note the Range of Motion and the End Feel

Flexion, Extension, and Radial or Ulnar Deviation

- *Position:* Client is sitting.
- *Action:* Stabilize the forearm with one hand, hold the client's hand with the other hand, and move the wrist into the four motions. Note that radial and ulnar deviations are done with the wrist in 0° of flexion and extension.
- *Observation:*
  - Flexion tests ligaments on the dorsum of the hand and the joint capsule.
  - Extension tests the joint capsule and ligaments on the palmar surface and is most limited in joint injuries or dysfunction, as extension is the close-packed position for the wrist.
  - Radial deviation tests ulnar collateral ligament.
  - Ulnar deviation tests the radial collateral ligament and compresses the TFCC.

HAND

Hand Inspection

- *Position:* If the wrist or hand is the area of complaint, have the client sit, and place both his or her hands on the thighs. Inspect these areas for swelling and scars and feel the hands for temperature differences from one side to the other.
- *Observation:* Note any nodular swellings on the MCP, PIP, or DIP joints, which may indicate OA. If there is a single or a few joints involved, it is usually a result of OA. If there are multiple swollen joints, primarily at the MCP joints and they are fairly uniform bilaterally, it usually indicates RA. Note if the fingers have an ulnar deviation, which is typical of RA.

Thumb Movements

- In anatomical position, abduction of the thumb occurs by moving the thumb perpendicular to the palm, and adduction moves it toward the palm. Extension moves the thumb laterally, and flexion moves the thumb across palm. Opposition is considered full when the tip of the thumb can touch the base of the little finger.

Active Movements

Flexion, Extension, Adduction, Abduction, and Opposition

- *Position:* Client is sitting, with hands resting on the thighs and asked to follow your movements.
- *Action:* For easy comparison, have client perform the following movements with both hands: flexion, extension, adduction, abduction, and opposition.

- ☐ ***Observation:*** Abduction and extension are painful in capsulitis and OA of the first CMC joint.

Abduction

- ☐ ***Position:*** Client is sitting. Have the client reach his or her arms out in front, with forearms supinated and hands together, and have the client place the palms up.
- ☐ ***Action:*** Have the client abduct both thumbs to their full range. Compare sides.
- ☐ ***Observation:*** A clinically significant motion of the thumb to assess is abduction. An injured or arthritic thumb has decreased abduction, extension, and opposition.

Test for Tenovaginitis of the Thumb (Finkelstein's Test)

- ☐ ***Position:*** Client is sitting. Have the client flex his or her thumb to the palm and wrap the fingers around the thumb.
- ☐ ***Action:*** Have the client cock his or her wrist into ulnar deviation (Fig. 10-18).
- ☐ ***Observation:*** Pain at the radial styloid, anatomical snuff-box, or both indicates the presence of a tenovaginitis of the extensor pollicis brevis and abductor pollicis longus tendons.

Passive Movements

Abduction and Extension

- ☐ ***Position:*** Client is sitting. Sit next to the client.
- ☐ ***Action:*** Stabilize the hand, and gently pull the thumb into abduction and then into extension. Always do the painful side last.

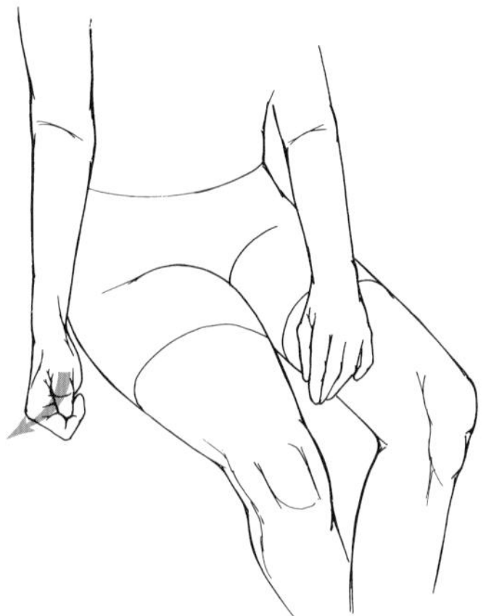

Figure 10-18. Finkelstein's Test, to rule out stenosing tenosynovitis of the extensor pollicis brevis and abductor pollicis longus.

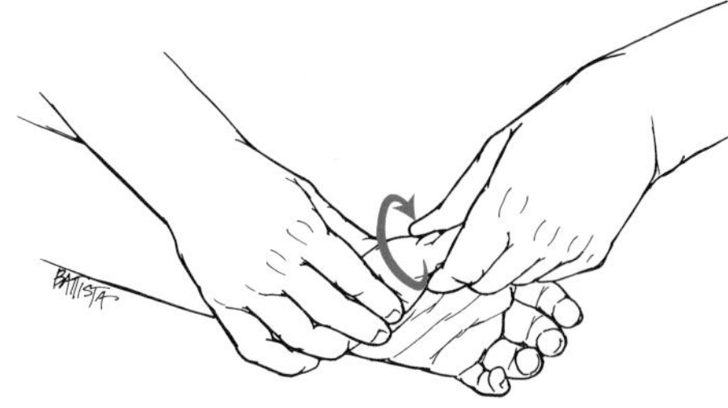

Figure 10-19. To assess the function of the first CMC joint, hold the joint between your thumb and index finger and gently circumduct the thumb.

- ☐ ***Observation:*** Abduction and extension stretch the anterior capsule and are painful in capsulitis, arthritis, or arthrosis of the first CMC joint. Painful, crepitus, limitation of motion indicates OA. The range of passive abduction may be increased with an injury and consequent insufficiency of the ulnar collateral ligament, a common injury in skiers.

Test to Assess Whether a Client Has Osteoarthritis of the Thumb

- ☐ ***Position:*** Client is sitting. Sit next to the client. Hold the client's thumb below the CMC joint with your thumb in the distal part of the snuff-box and your index finger in the thenar pad opposite the thumb.
- ☐ ***Action:*** Holding the shaft of the thumb with your other hand, gently circumduct the thumb (Fig. 10-19).
- ☐ ***Observation:*** Pain and crepitation indicates OA of the first CMC joint. As in the patellar grinding test, this test is also used as a treatment. Gently mobilize the CMC articulation to "clean" the surfaces of spicules of calcium that have deposited. Only perform this for a few minutes per session and only within the client's comfortable limits.

Fingers

Active Movements

Flexion and Extension

- ☐ ***Position:*** Client is sitting.
- ☐ ***Action:*** First, have the client make a fist and attempt to touch the tips of the fingers to the distal palmar crease (Fig. 10-20). Second, have the client fully extend the fingers.
- ☐ ***Observation:*** If the client cannot touch the fingertips to the palm, note the distance from the fin-

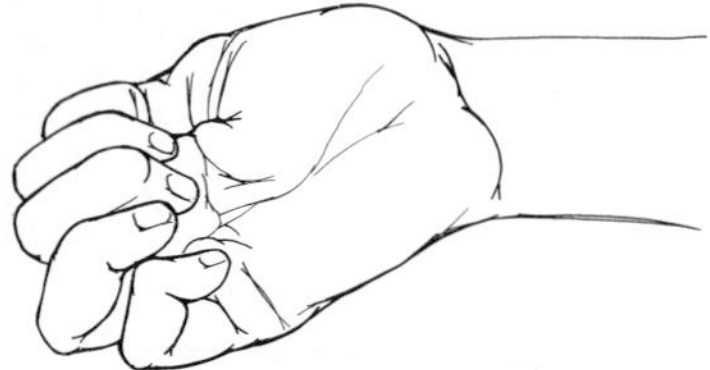

Figure 10-20. Active finger flexion. Notice the ring finger's inability to touch the palm.

gertip to the palm, and reevaluate after your treatment to see if the client can get closer. In the second movement, note whether the fingers can extend all past neutral, which is the normal range. Inability to flex fully is caused by joint capsule fibrosis, lumbricals, or OA of the joint.

PASSIVE MOVEMENTS

Flexion of the Metacarpophalangeal, Proximal Interphalangeal, and the Distal Interphalangeal Joints

- *Position:* Client is sitting.
- *Action:* Passively flex the MCP, the PIP and the DIP joints one at a time.
- *Observation:* In capsular fibrosis and degenerative joint disease (DJD) passive flexion is limited.[13] If passive flexion is limited in the MCP joint, perform the **Bunnel-Littler Test** to differentiate whether the restriction is from tight lumbricals and interossei or from a tight joint capsule. The MCP joint is held in slight extension as you attempt to move the PIP into flexion. If the PIP joint is difficult to flex, next move the MCP joint into slight flexion, as this relaxes the intrinsic muscles. If the PIP joint is still tight, the capsule is restricting the movement.

Techniques

MUSCLE ENERGY TECHNIQUE

As mentioned, the CR METs serve not only as therapeutic techniques but as assessment tools. It is important to realize that the muscles in the elbow, wrist, and hand are often weak because of an irritation, injury, or dysfunction of the nerves in the cervical spine. This is also true for the muscles of the leg, ankle, and foot, which are myotomes for nerves from the lumbar spine (see Chapter 9, "The Leg, Ankle, and Foot").

Muscle Energy Technique for Acute Elbow, Wrist, and Hand Pain

1. Contract-Relax Muscle Energy Technique for Acute Elbow Pain

- *Intention:* The intention is to contract and relax the muscles of flexion and extension of the elbow. This pumps the waste products and swelling out of the injured area, increases the nutritional exchange, and helps realign the healing fibers.

CAUTION: **This technique is performed only within pain-free limits. There are beneficial effects with only grams of pressure.**

- *Position:* Client is supine, with elbow in 90° of flexion. Hold the distal forearm in one hand and place the other hand on the anterior arm to stabilize it (Fig. 10-21).
- *Action:* Have the client resist as you slowly and gently press the elbow toward flexion for approximately 5 seconds. Relax for a few seconds. Have the client resist as you slowly and gently pull the forearm, attempting to extend the elbow. Relax, and repeat cycle several times.

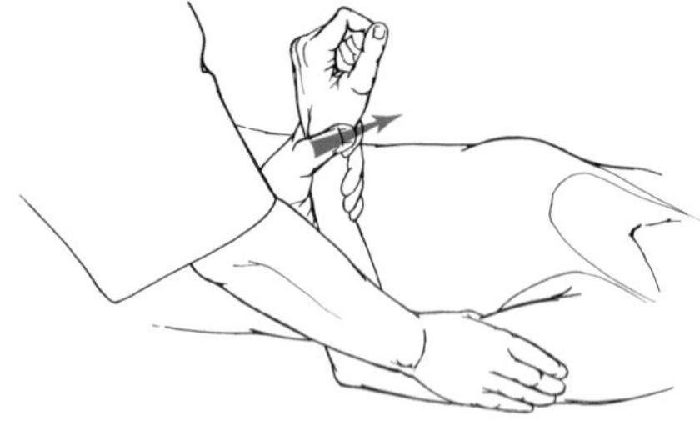

Figure 10-21. CR MET for acute elbow pain.

2. Contract-Relax Muscle Energy Technique for Acute Wrist Pain

- *Intention:* The intention is to contract and relax the muscles of flexion and extension of the wrist. This pumps the waste products and swelling out of an injured area, increases the nutritional exchange, and helps realign the healing fibers.

CAUTION: **This technique is performed only within pain-free limits. There are beneficial effects with only a few grams of pressure.**

- ***Position:*** Client is supine with the arm resting on the table. The elbow is slightly flexed, and the wrist and hand are in the position of function (i.e., with the wrist in slight extension and the MCP and IP joints in slight flexion). Place a stabilizing hand on the proximal forearm and the other hand on the dorsum (top) of the wrist (Fig. 10-22).
- ***Action:*** Have the client resist as you slowly and gently press the top of the wrist toward flexion for approximately 5 seconds. Relax for a few seconds. Place the fingertips of your working hand on the client's palm and have the client resist as you slowly and gently pull up on the palm toward wrist extension. Relax, and repeat cycle several times.

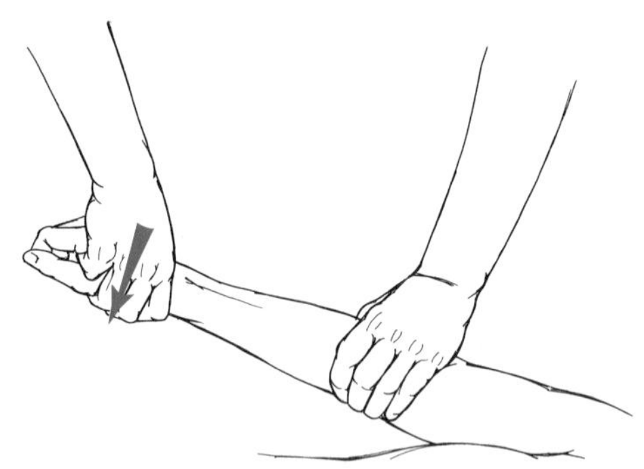

Figure 10-22. CR MET for acute wrist pain.

3. Contract-Relax Muscle Energy Technique for Acute Finger and Thumb Pain

- ***Intention:*** The intention is to contract and relax the fingers and thumb muscles of flexion and extension. This pumps the waste products and swelling out of an injured area, increases the nutritional exchange, and helps realign the healing fibers.

CAUTION: **This technique is performed only within pain-free limits. There are beneficial effects with only grams of pressure.**

- ***Position:*** Client is supine with the arm resting on the table. The elbow is slightly flexed, and the wrist and hand in the position of function (i.e., with the wrist in slight extension and the MCP and IP joints in slight flexion). Place a stabilizing hand on the proximal forearm. For the fingers, place the other hand on the dorsum of the fingers. For the thumb, place the other hand on the dorsum of the thumb.
- ***Action:*** *For the fingers,* have the client resist as you slowly and gently press the top of the fingers toward flexion for approximately 5 seconds (Fig. 10-23**A**). Relax for a few seconds. Place the fingertips of the working hand on the palmar aspect of the client's fingers and have client resist as you slowly and gently pull the fingers up, toward finger extension (Fig. 10-23**B**). Relax, and repeat cycle several times. *For the thumb,* have the client resist as you slowly and gently press the top of the thumb toward flexion (toward the palm) for approximately 5 seconds (Fig. 10-23**C**). Relax for a few seconds. Place the fingertips of the working hand on the palmar aspect of the client's thumb and have the client resist as you slowly and gently pull the thumb up, toward extension (Fig. 10-23**D**).

Muscle Energy Technique for Elbow, Forearm, Wrist and Hand Muscles

4. Contract-Relax Muscle Energy Technique for the Brachioradialis

- ***Intention:*** The intention is to reduce the hypertonicity or to facilitate (strengthen) and bring sensory awareness to this muscle. This muscle is often short and tight and contributes to entrapment of the radial nerve.
- ***Position:*** Client is supine with the elbow in slight flexion and the forearm in neutral (i.e., with the palm facing the client's body). Place the working hand on the distal forearm (Fig. 10-24).
- ***Action:*** Have the client resist as you attempt to extend the elbow for approximately 5 seconds. Relax and repeat several times. For sensory awareness, tap lightly on the muscle belly.

5. Contract-Relax and Postisometric Relaxation Muscle Energy Technique for the Extensor Carpi Radialis Brevis and Longus

- **Intention:** The intention is to reduce the hypertonicity, to facilitate (strengthen) and bring sensory awareness, or to lengthen the myofascia of these muscles. These muscles are commonly involved in lateral epicondylitis (tennis elbow) and are part of the myotome of the C6 nerve root.

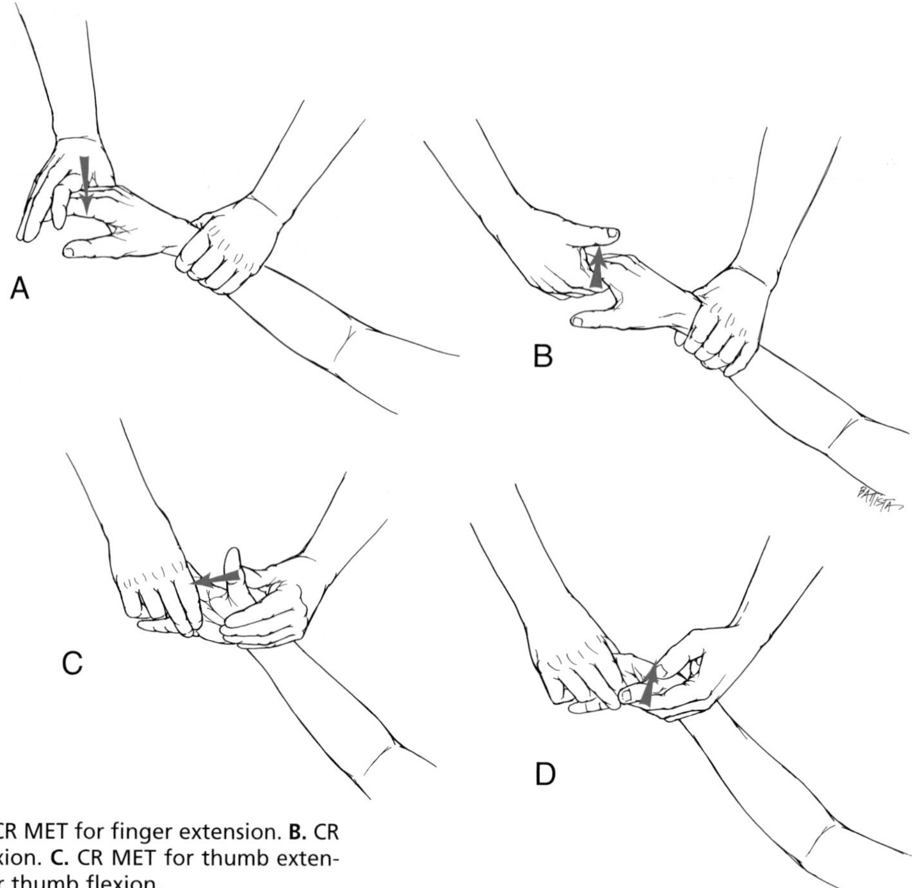

Figure 10-23. **A.** CR MET for finger extension. **B.** CR MET for finger flexion. **C.** CR MET for thumb extension. **D.** CR MET for thumb flexion.

- ***Position:*** Client is supine with the elbow extended, the wrist in slight extension, and the hand in the position of function. Place the palm of the working hand on the dorsum of the hand.
- ***Action:*** For CR MET, have the client resist as you press on the dorsum of the hand toward wrist flexion for approximately five seconds (Fig. 10-25**A**). Relax and repeat several times. For PIR MET, move wrist into greater flexion, and have client resist as you press toward flexion (Fig. 10-25**B**). Relax and repeat CR–lengthen cycle several times.
- ***Observation:*** Painless weakness implicates a problem with the C6 nerve root. Pain at the lateral elbow implicates lateral epicondylitis.

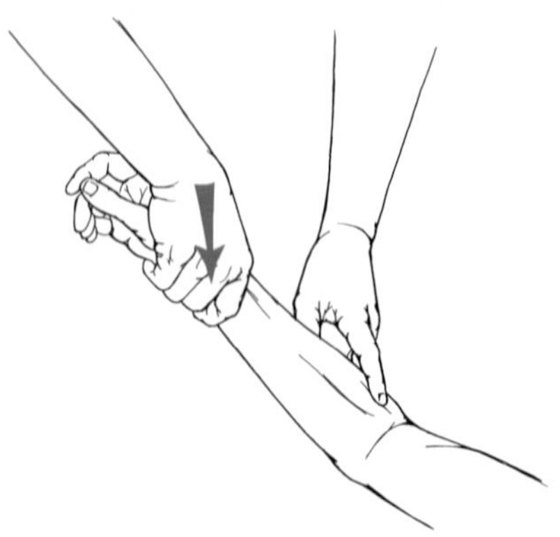

Figure 10-24. CR MET for the brachioradialis.

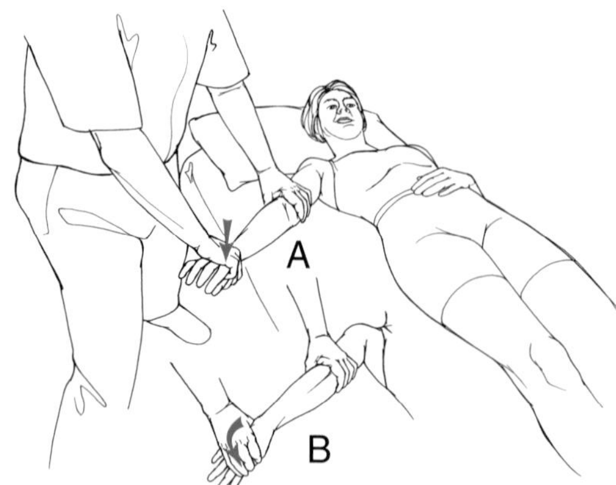

Figure 10-25. **A.** *Left and upper right.* CR MET for the ECRB and ECRL. **B.** *Bottom and center.* PIR MET for the ECRB and ECRL.

6. Contract-Relax Muscle Energy Technique for the Extensor Digitorum, Extensor Indicis, and Extensor Digiti Minimi

- *Intention:* The intention is to reduce the hypertonicity, to facilitate (strengthen) and bring sensory awareness, or to lengthen the myofascia of these muscles. The extensor digitorum is also commonly involved in lateral epicondylitis (tennis elbow).
- *Position:* Client is supine with the elbow extended, the wrist in slight extension, and the fingers extended. Place the palm of the working hand on the dorsum of the fingers (Fig. 10-26).
- *Action:* Have the client resist as you press on the dorsum of the fingers toward finger flexion for approximately 5 seconds. Relax and repeat several times.

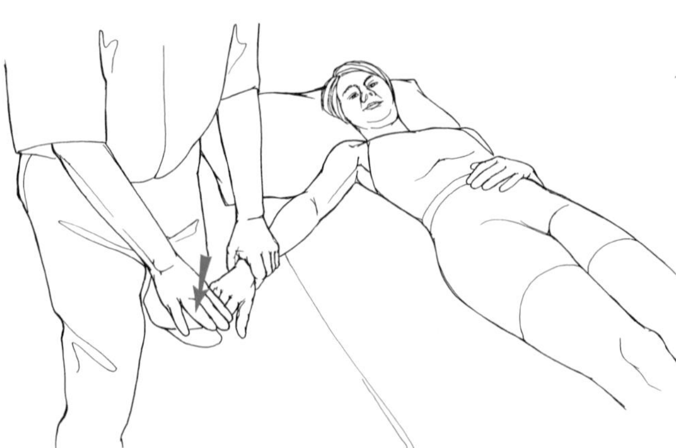

Figure 10-26. CR MET for the extensor digitorum, extensor indicis, and extensor digiti minimi.

7. Contract-Relax and Postisometric Relaxation Muscle Energy Technique for the Pronator Teres

- *Intention:* The intention is to reduce the hypertonicity, to facilitate (strengthen) and bring sensory awareness, or to lengthen the myofascia of the pronator teres. This muscle is often short and tight and contributes to entrapment of the median nerve.
- *Position:* Client is supine with the elbow against the client's body and the forearm in neutral (i.e., with the palm facing the client's body). Instruct the client to avoid using the finger flexors (e.g., the client should not make a fist). Place the palm of the working hand on the flexor surface of the distal forearm (Fig. 10-27).
- *Action:* For CR MET, have the client resist as you attempt to turn the forearm into supination for approximately 5 seconds. Relax and repeat several times. For PIR MET, move the forearm into greater supination, and have the client resist as you attempt to turn the forearm into greater supination. Relax, and repeat CR–lengthen cycle several times.

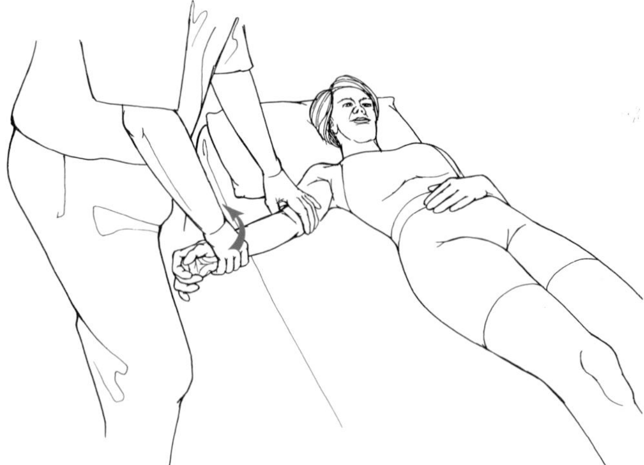

Figure 10-27. CR and PIR MET for the pronator teres.

8. Contract-Relax Muscle Energy Technique for the Flexor Carpi Radialis and the Flexor Carpi Ulnaris

- *Intention:* The intention is to reduce the hypertonicity, to facilitate (strengthen) and bring sensory awareness, or to lengthen the myofascia of these muscles. The flexor carpi ulnaris is typically short and tight and is commonly involved in compression of the ulnar nerve (cubital tunnel syndrome).
- *Position:* Client is supine with the elbow extended, the forearm supinated, the wrist slightly flexed, and the fingers relaxed. For the flexor carpi radialis, place your hand on the thenar eminence. For the flexor carpi ulnaris, place your hand on the hypothenar eminence.
- *Action:* For the flexor carpi radialis, flex the wrist toward the radial (thumb) side and have the client resist as you press the wrist toward wrist extension toward the ulnar (pinkie) side (Fig. 10-28**A**). Relax and repeat several times. For the flexor carpi ulnaris, flex the wrist toward the ulnar side and have the client resist as you press the wrist toward wrist extension toward the radial (thumb) side (Fig. 10-28**B**).

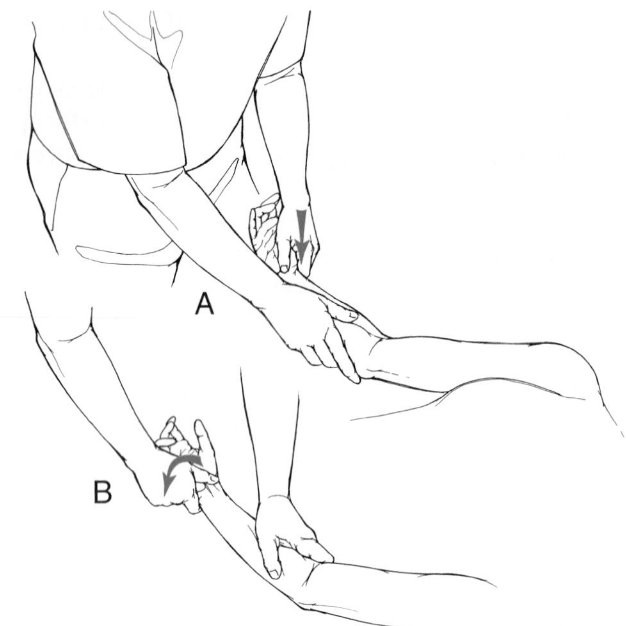

Figure 10-28. **A.** *Upper.* CR MET for the flexor carpi radialis. **B.** *Lower.* CR MET for the flexor carpi ulnaris.

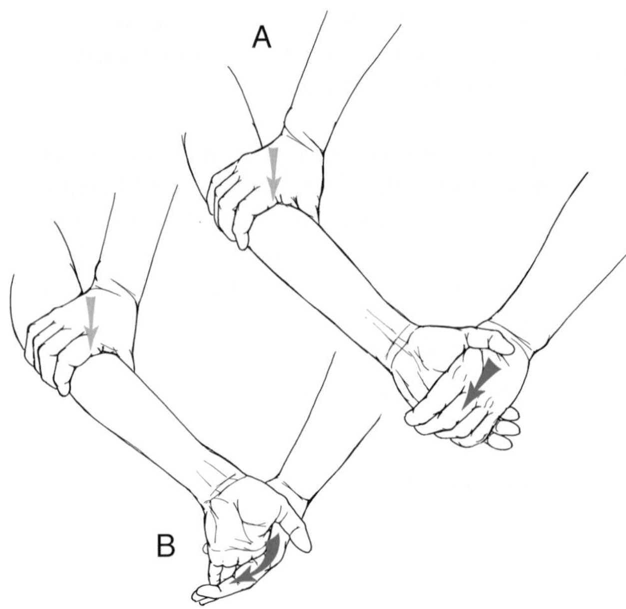

Figure 10-29. **A.** *Upper and right.* CR MET for the flexor digitorum superficialis and profundus. **B.** *Lower and left.* PIR MET for the flexor digitorum superficialis and profundus.

- ***Observation:*** Painless weakness of the wrist flexors implicates a problem with the C7 nerve root. Pain at the medial elbow implicates medial epicondylitis.

9. Contract-Relax and Postisometric Relaxation Muscle Energy Technique for the Flexor Digitorum Superficialis and the Flexor Digitorum Profundus

- ***Intention:*** The intention is to reduce the hypertonicity, to facilitate (strengthen) and bring sensory awareness, or to lengthen the myofascia of these muscles. These flexors are typically short and tight.
- ***Position:*** Client is supine with the elbow extended, the forearm supinated, and the wrist over the edge of the table. Place your fingers on the palmar surface of the fingers, and place your stabilizing hand on the distal forearm.
- ***Action:*** For CR MET, have the client resist as you press the fingers toward finger extension (Fig. 10-29**A**). Relax and repeat several times. For PIR MET, after the relaxation phase, press fingers toward greater extension and have the client resist as you press toward greater finger extension (Fig. 10-29**B**).

Muscle Energy Technique for Chronic Loss of Wrist Motion

10. Muscle Energy Technique for Loss of Range of Motion in the Wrist

- ***Intention:*** The wrist is typically limited in its ROM after a traumatic injury, such as a Colles' fracture to the distal radius. This MET is focused on increasing joint motion, rather than muscle length.
- ***Position:*** Client is supine with the elbow flexed to 90°. To increase extension, place one hand on the palm of the hand and bend the wrist into the comfortable limit of extension. To increase flexion, place your hand on the dorsum of the client's hand and flex the wrist to its comfortable limit.
- ***Action:*** To increase extension, move the wrist into its comfortable limit of extension. Have the client resist as you press toward greater extension (Fig. 10-30). Relax, and as the client relaxes, press the wrist into greater extension. Repeat the CR–lengthen-cycle several times. To increase flexion, have the client resist as you press toward wrist flexion for approximately 5 seconds. Relax, and when the client is relaxed, press the wrist into greater flexion. Repeat the CR–lengthen-cycle several times.

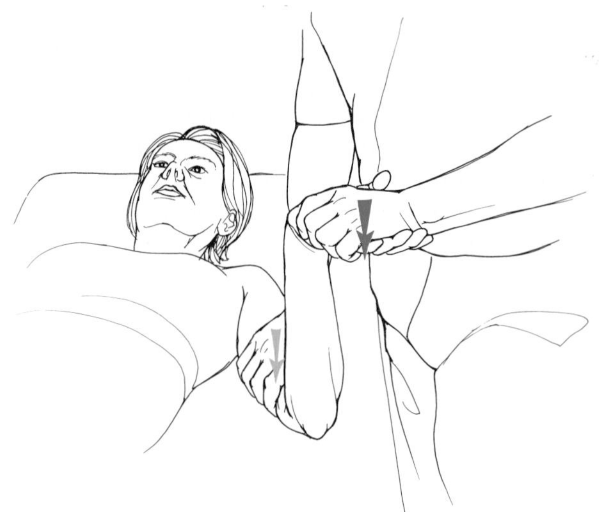

Figure 10-30. MET to increase the wrist extension ROM.

ORTHOPEDIC MASSAGE

Level I—Elbow, Forearm, Wrist, and Hand

1. Release of the Superficial and the Deep Fascia of the Forearm

- *Anatomy*: Antebrachial fascia and the flexors and extensors of wrist and fingers (Fig. 10-31**A** and **B**).
- *Dysfunction*: Chronic dysfunction of the forearm involves chronic shortening of the fascia of the arm, forearm, and hand. The fascia surrounding the muscles (epimysium) and the fascicles (perimysium) may develop fibrosis (thickening) owing to repetitive microtrauma, as in carpentry, massage therapy, and computer work.

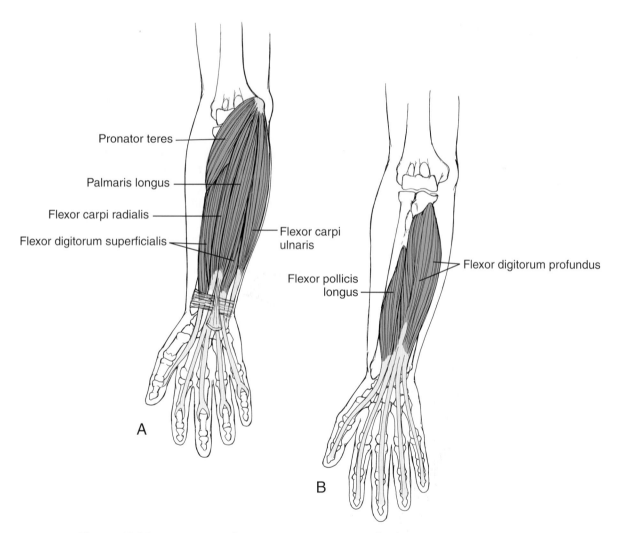

Pronator teres
Palmaris longus
Flexor carpi radialis
Flexor digitorum superficialis
Flexor carpi ulnaris
A
Flexor pollicis longus
Flexor digitorum profundus
B

Figure 10-31. Forearm muscle compartments. **A.** Superficial anterior. **B.** Deep anterior.

Position

- TP—standing
- CP—supine

Strokes

CAUTION: **These first three strokes are contraindicated for acute conditions in which there is swelling and heat and for atrophied tissue.**

1. Using a soft fist, perform a series of long, continuous strokes starting at the wrist and continuing to the elbow (Fig. 10-32). Use a small amount of lotion to avoid skin burn. Keep your wrist in neutral, and let your hand mold gently to the client's arm. Begin with the client's forearm supinated. Repeat over the entire flexor surface of the forearm, and continue the strokes on the flexor surface of the humerus, including the biceps, brachialis, and brachioradialis. Repeat the stroke several times, until you feel a relaxation in the soft tissue.

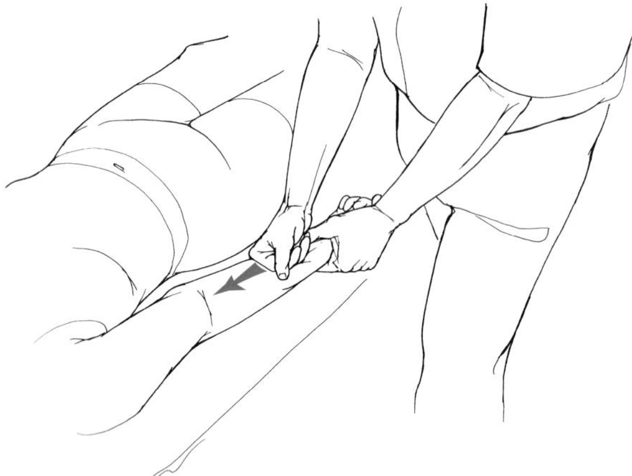

Figure 10-32. Soft-fist technique to stretch the antebrachial fascia.

2. Perform this same series of strokes (as described in stroke 1) on the extensor surface, with the client's forearm pronated.
3. Place the client's forearm in supination and perform a series of spreading strokes with your fingertips or thumbs to "part the midline" (Fig. 10-33). Begin just above the elbow and work down to the wrist. Cover the entire flexor compartment. Then place the client's arm in pronation, and perform the same spreading strokes to release the entire extensor compartment.
4. For acute conditions, flex the elbow to relax the muscles and perform gentle, transverse, scooping strokes using the same positions that are illustrated in the sections "Release of Sustained Contraction in the Flexor and Extensor Muscles" (see Fig. 10-38), "Release of the Torsion in the Flexor and Extensor Muscles" (see Fig. 10-39), and "Release of Attachments at the Medial Epicondyle and the Ulnar and Median Nerves" (see Figs. 10-61 and 10-62).

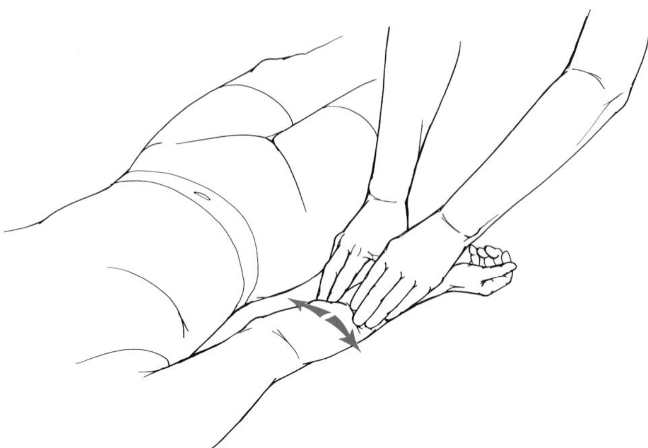

Figure 10-33. Fingertip technique spreading the antebrachial fascia.

2. Release of Sustained Contraction in the Flexor and Extensor Muscles

- ***Anatomy***: Flexors and extensors of the wrist and fingers (Fig. 10-34**A** and **B**).
- ***Dysfunction***: If muscles remain in a sustained contraction, the fascia that covers the muscle, fascicles, and fibers themselves may develop adhesions. A tight muscle is often a weak muscle, and it fatigues easily. Sustained contraction also causes acidic buildup from metabolic wastes and decreases oxygen, leading to ischemic pain.

Position

- TP—standing
- CP—supine

Strokes

1. To release the fascial coverings of the flexors of the wrist and hand and to help separate the individual muscles from one another, first place the client's forearm in supination. Using either a single- or a double-thumb technique, perform long, slow, longitudinal strokes from the midforearm to the elbow, covering the entire flexor surface (Fig. 10-35). Flex your thumb slightly by gently squeezing the client's forearm as you stroke. This allows the thumb joint

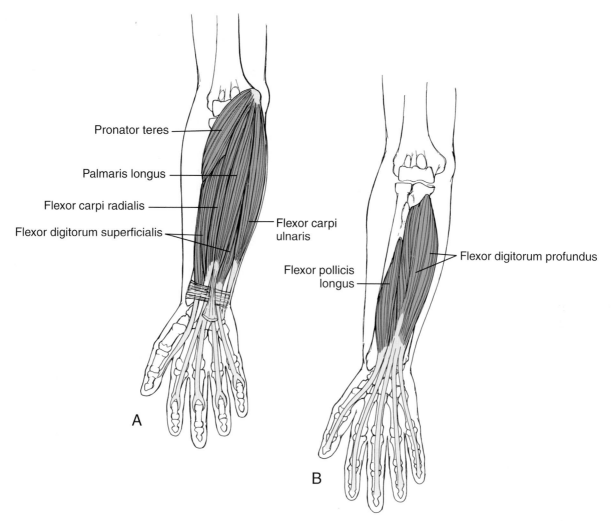

Figure 10-34. Compartments of forearm muscles. **A.** Superficial anterior. **B.** Deep anterior.

to stay open and disperses the force through your entire hand. Be careful not to push the arm into the glenoid fossa, which would compress the shoulder.

2. To release the brachioradialis place the forearm in neutral (i.e., with the client's thumb pointed toward the ceiling). Using either a single- or a double-thumb technique, begin at the radial styloid and perform long, slow, longitudinal strokes, continuing to the supracondylar ridge above the elbow (Fig. 10-36). Perform longitudinal and transverse strokes on the ridge. If you are using a single-thumb technique, you may start this series of strokes with the client's elbow in flexion, and as you stroke, move the client's elbow into extension, as this increases the stretch of the fascia.
3. Place the client's forearm in pronation. Using either a single- or a double-thumb technique, perform long, slow, longitudinal strokes to release the wrist and

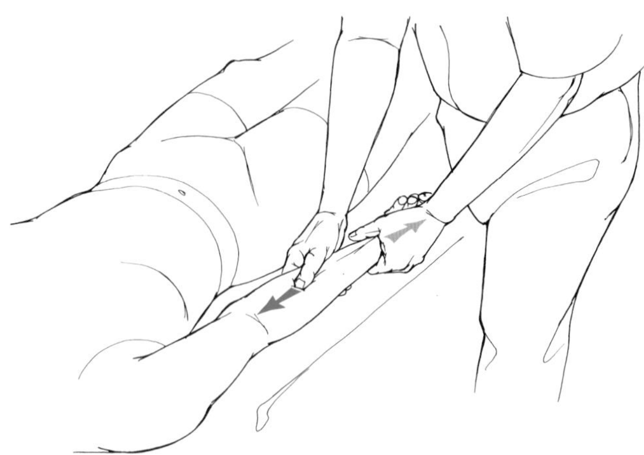

Figure 10-35. Thumb release of the forearm muscles.

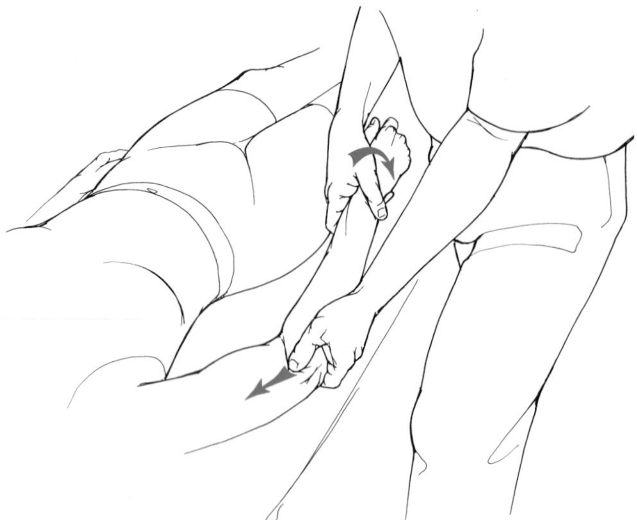

Figure 10-36. Thumb release of the brachioradialis. Extend the client's elbow as you stroke the brachioradialis.

hand extensors from their myotendinous junctions in the midforearm to their attachments at the elbow.

3. Release of the Torsion in the Flexor and the Extensor Muscles

- ***Anatomy***: Flexors and extensors of wrist and fingers and thumb (Fig. 10-37**A** and **B**) and superficial radial nerve (see Fig. 10-4)
- ***Dysfunction***: Muscles that undergo sustained contraction develop torsion. Sustained tension on the ventral (anterior) surface pronates the wrist; excessive tension on the dorsal surface tends to supinate the wrist. The superficial radial nerve can become entrapped in the fascia in the distal forearm. The extensor pollicis brevis and abductor pollicis longus cross over the ECRL and ECRB in the distal forearm, a site of potential irritation (called "intersection syndrome").

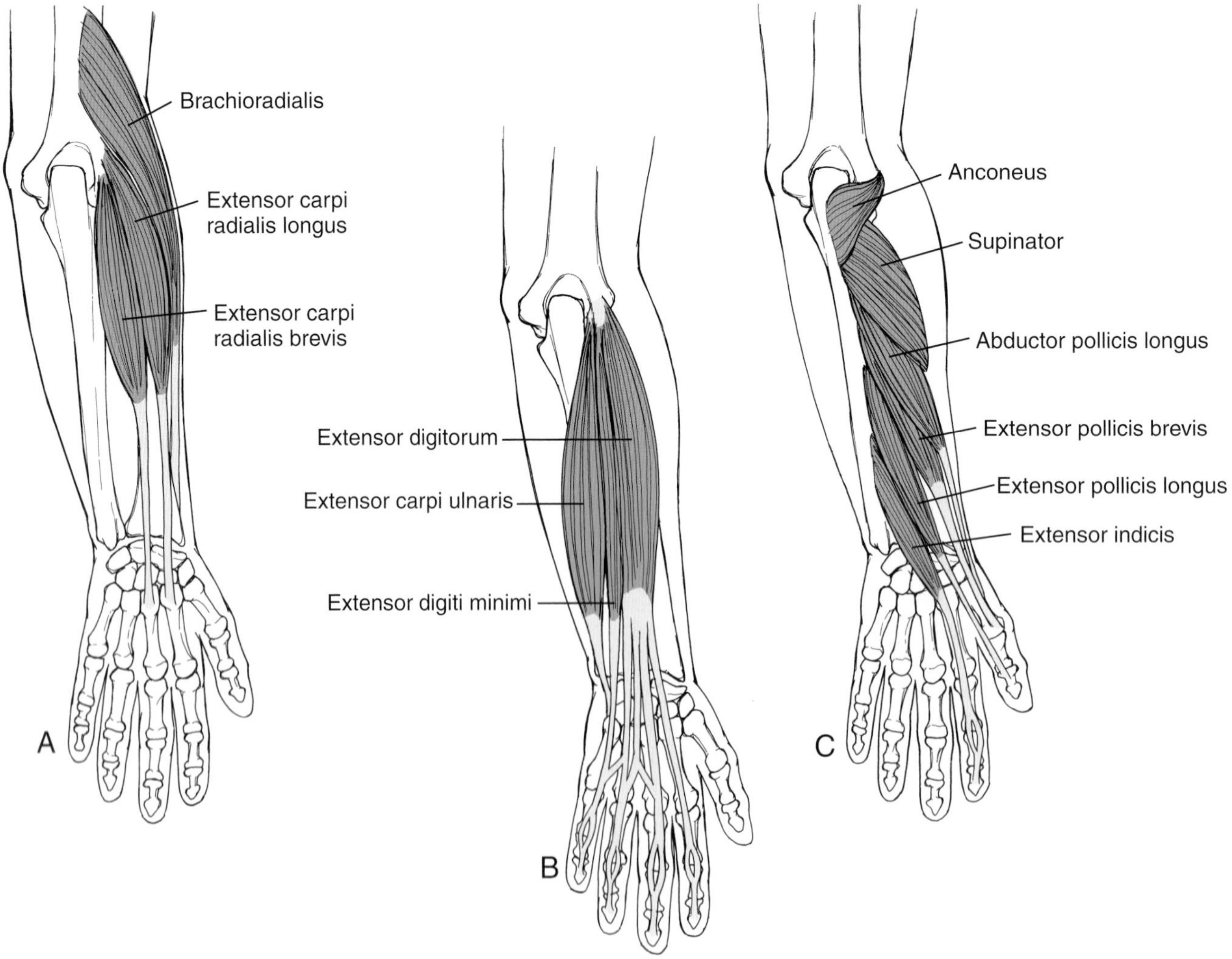

Figure 10-37. Forearm muscle compartments. **A.** Radial. **B.** Superficial posterior. **C.** Deep posterior.

Position

- TP—standing for the first three strokes and sitting for the fourth stroke
- CP—supine, with the client's elbow in slight flexion; or sitting

Strokes

1. These strokes involve releasing the torsion in the forearm muscles by scooping the flexors medially and the extensors laterally. If you are on the client's right side, hold the distal forearm with your right hand. Your left thumb should rest on the lateral epicondyle (Fig. 10-38). Perform short, scooping strokes by flexing your left thumb toward your palm. Pronate the forearm with each stroke in an oscillating rhythm of approximately 1 to 2 cycles per second. Repeat this motion to cover the entire surface of the dorsal and radial aspects of the forearm. These are gentle strokes and should be comfortable for the client.

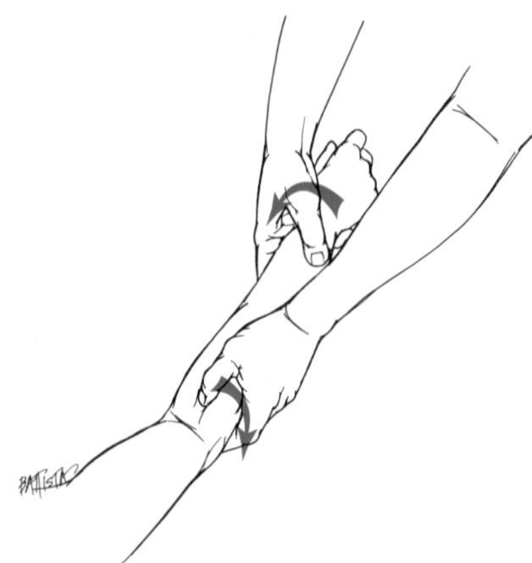

Figure 10-38. Roll the extensors laterally as you pronate the forearm.

As you stroke on the distal third of the dorsum and lateral aspects of the radius, you are releasing the superficial radial nerve and the site of intersection syndrome.

2. Switch hand positions so that your right hand is on the origin of his flexor-pronator group at the medial epicondyle. Your left hand is on the distal aspect of his lateral forearm (Fig. 10-39). Perform a series of short, scooping strokes beginning on the medial epicondyle with the thumb of one hand as you supinate the forearm with the other hand. Continue this series of strokes on the entire flexor compartment. Follow the pronator teres to its insertion on the middle of the radius.

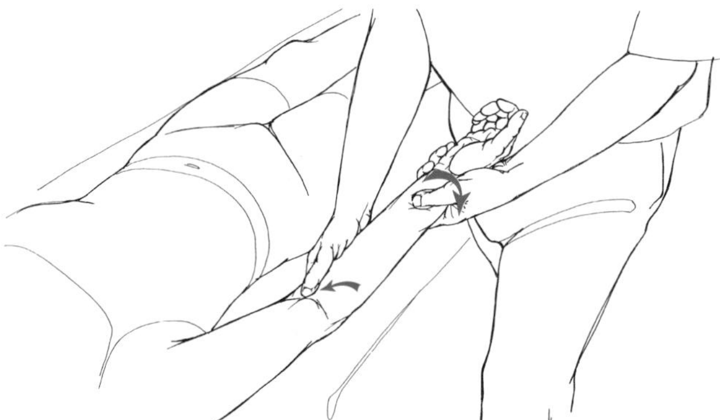

Figure 10-39. Roll the flexors medially as you supinate the forearm.

3. An alternate method for patients who have bulky forearms is for you to sit on the table and place the patient's forearm on your thigh (Fig. 10-40). Using a double- or a braced-thumb technique, roll the radial and extensor muscles laterally. For the flexors, face the table and place the patient's arm on the table, and use the same double- or braced thumb technique to roll the flexors medially.

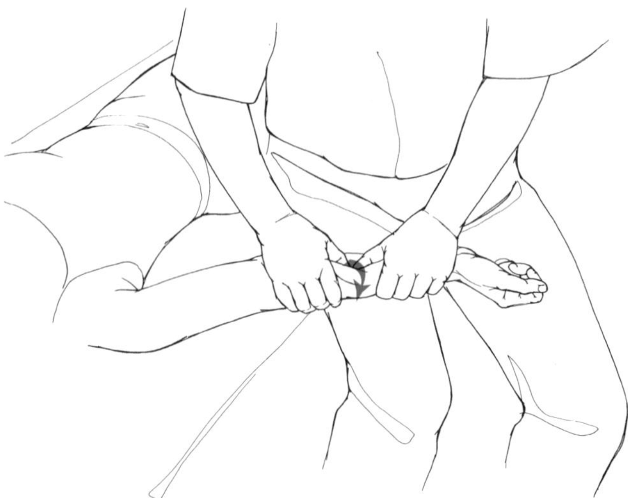

Figure 10-40. Double-thumb release of the forearm flexors.

4. Release of the Dorsum of the Hand and the Webspace of the Thumb

- *Anatomy*: The extensor muscles of the wrist and hand, the dorsal interossei, the adductor pollicis, and the intermetacarpal ligament (Fig. 10-41).
- *Dysfunction*: The tendinous insertion points of the extensor muscles tend to develop fibrosis with injury or overuse. The thumb tends to be held is an adducted and flexed position, which shortens the adductor pollicis, the first dorsal interossei, and the intermetacarpal ligament.

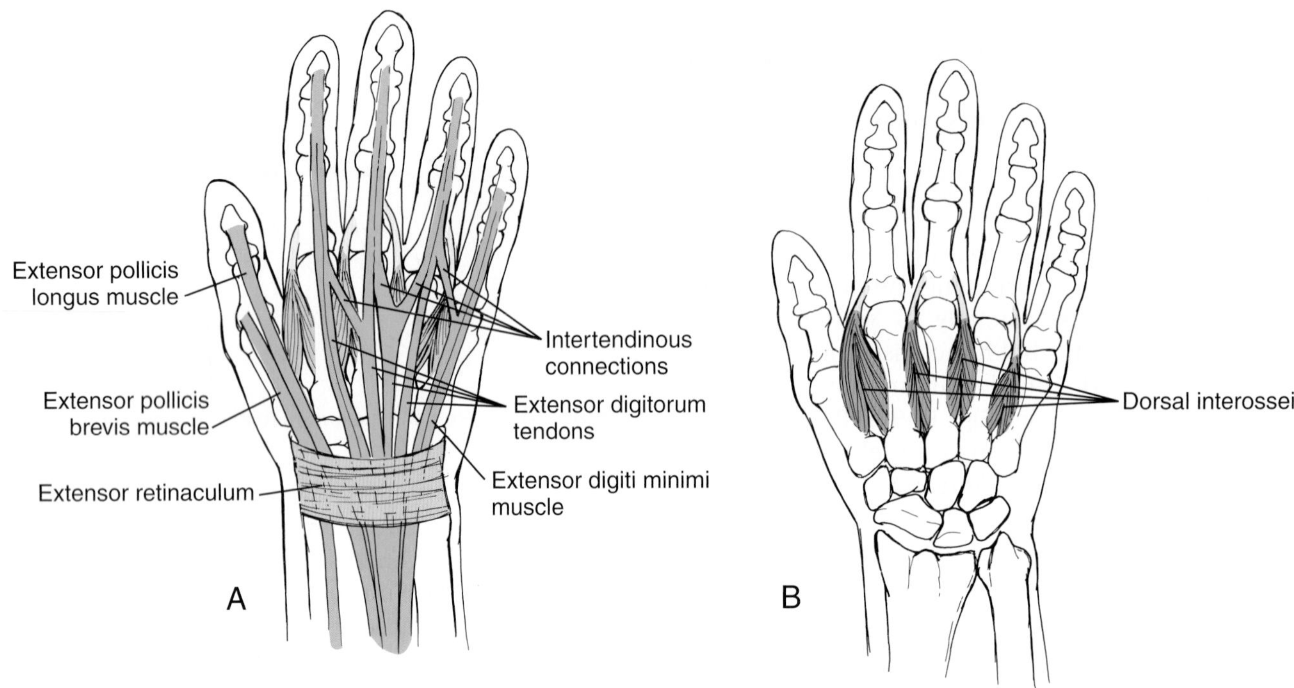

Figure 10-41. **A.** Muscles and tendons of the dorsum of the hand. **B.** Dorsal interossei muscles.

Position

- TP—standing, or sitting on the table or in a chair
- CP—supine

Strokes

1. Facing headward, perform superficial, spreading strokes with your thumbs on the dorsum of the hand to release the superficial fascia, the extensor retinaculum, and extensor digitorum tendons. Begin at the wrist, and continue to the base of the fingers (Fig. 10-42).
2. Use a soft thumb to perform 1-inch scooping strokes between the metacarpals to release the dorsal interossei (Fig. 10-43). Support the hand from the palmar surface with your fingertips resting between the metacarpals you are working on to wedge the bones apart as you work. Continue these scooping strokes in between the MCP joints.

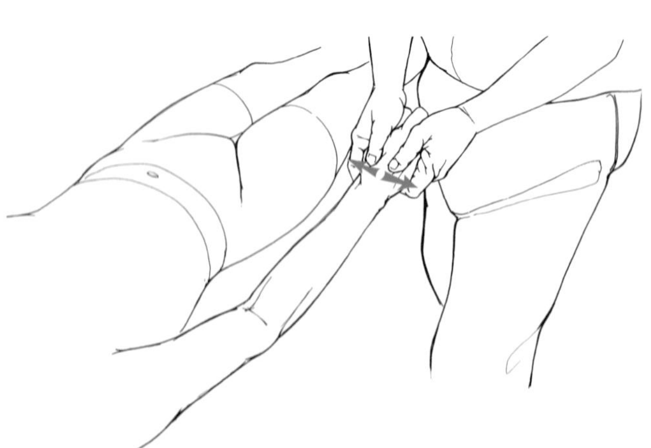

Figure 10-42. Thumbs are spreading the fascia of the dorsum of the hand.

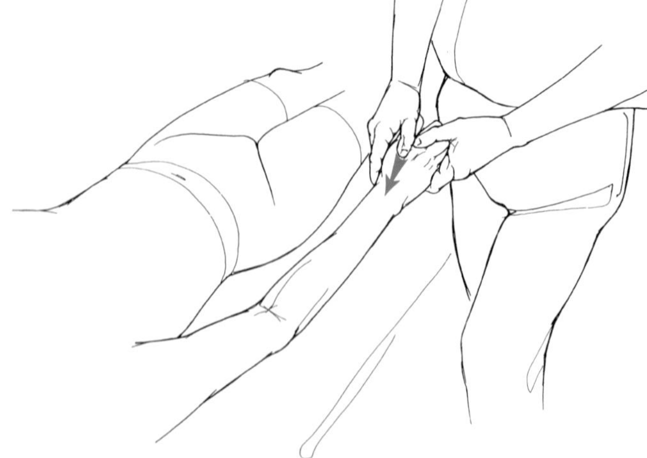

Figure 10-43. Single-thumb release of the dorsal interossei between the metacarpals.

CAUTION: Do not perform the following stroke deeply on a pregnant woman. There is a theory that deep stimulation on pressure points in this area may stimulate uterine contraction.

3. While sitting or facing footward, release the first dorsal interossei, the adductor pollicis, and the intermetacarpal ligament at the webspace between the thumb and the index finger. Perform longitudinal and transverse scooping strokes. First, perform a series of short, longitudinal, scooping strokes in the proximal to distal direction. Begin along the shaft of the thumb, then in midbelly, and finally next to the shaft of the index finger (Fig. 10-44). Place your index finger under the muscle you are working on to add a counterforce. This stroke may also be done as a shearing stroke, with the working finger moving in one direction, and the finger underneath moving in the opposite direction as you stroke.

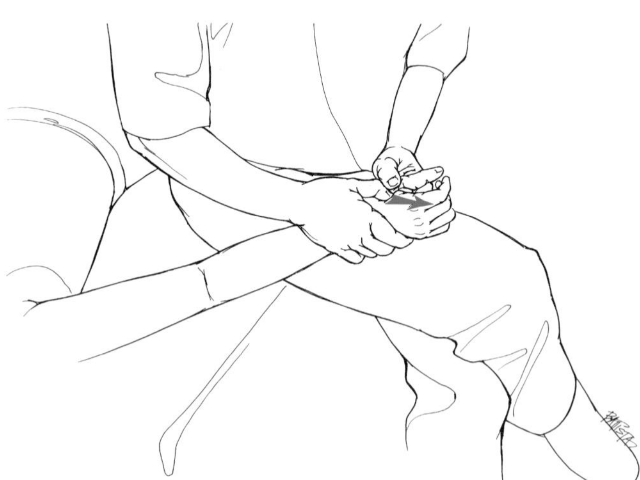

Figure 10-44. Single-thumb technique of longitudinal strokes on the first dorsal interossei, the adductor pollicis, and the intermetacarpal ligament.

4. Next, begin a series of short, scooping strokes on the dorsal-medial surface of thumb transverse to the shaft, taking the tissue "off the bone" (Fig. 10-45).
5. Now stand facing the table and place a flexed knee on the table. With the client's hand resting on your thigh, perform a series of short, scooping strokes along the dorsal-lateral surface of the index finger. Take the tissue off the bone toward the thumb (Fig. 10-45).

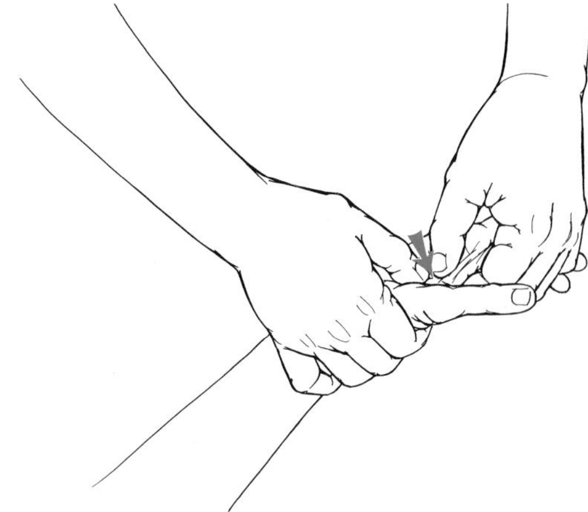

Figure 10-45. Double-thumb release of the first dorsal interossei.

5. Release of the Thenar and the Hypothenar Eminences

- ***Anatomy***: *Thenar muscles*—abductor pollicis brevis, flexor pollicis brevis (superficial and deep heads), adductor pollicis (transverse and oblique heads), opponens pollicis; *hypothenar muscles*—abductor digiti minimi, flexor digiti minimi brevis, opponens digiti minimi; and palmar aponeurosis (Fig. 10-46).
- ***Dysfunction***: The hand tends to move into sustained flexion in chronic dysfunction, after injury, or because of arthritis. This rolls the thenar muscles into medial torsion and the hypothenar muscles into a

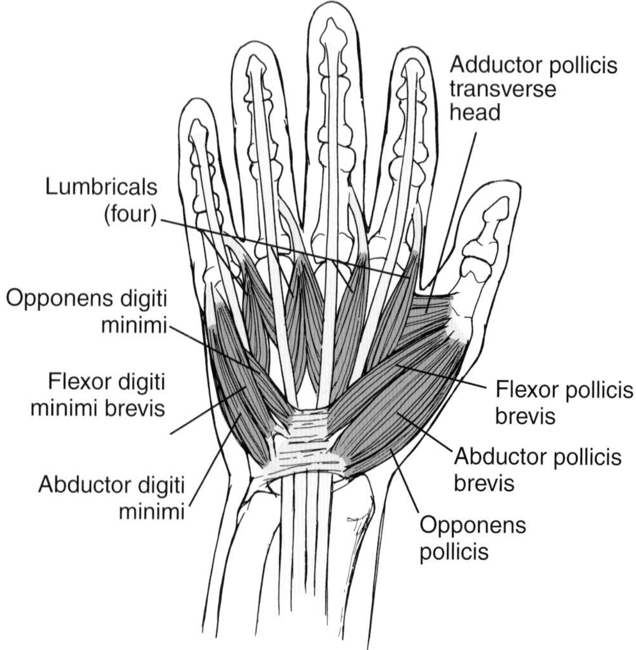

Figure 10-46. Muscles and flexor tendons of the hand.

lateral torsion, which folds these muscular pads toward the center of the palm.

Position

- TP—standing; or sitting on the table or in a chair, resting the client's hand on your thigh
- CP—supine

Strokes

1. To release the palmar aponeurosis, place your thumbs on the midline of the palm and your fingers on the dorsum of the hand. Perform a series of slow, spreading strokes with your thumbs to part the midline of the palm. Repeat many times, and cover the entire palm (Fig. 10-47).

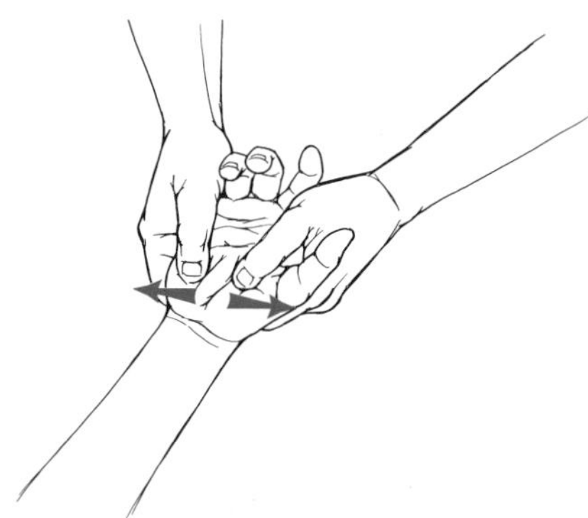

Figure 10-47. Double-thumb release of the palmar interossei.

2. Sit on the table and rest your client's hand on your thigh. Using a double-thumb technique perform short, scooping strokes in the medial to lateral (M–L) direction on the thenar eminence (Fig. 10-48). Begin at the proximal portion of the most lateral aspect of the thenar for the opponens pollicis and the abductor pollicis brevis. Continue to the MCP joint. Begin a second line of M–L scooping strokes closer to the palm for some of the fibers of the abductor pollicis brevis and for the superficial head of the flexor pollicis. Again, continue to the MCP joint. Support your strokes by placing your fingertips on the back of the thumb. Rock your body into each stroke, and externally rotate the thumb with each stroke.

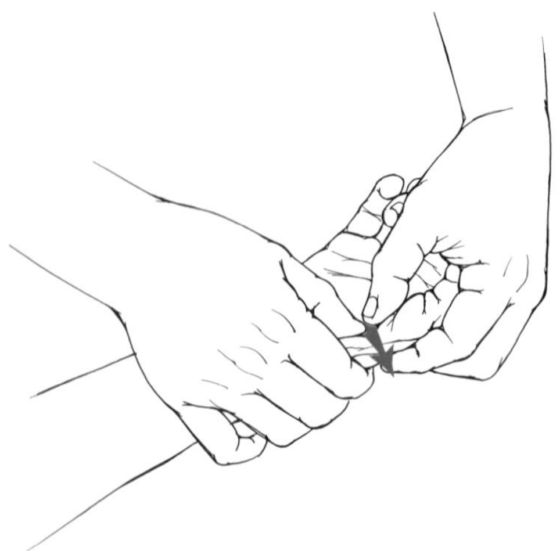

Figure 10-48. Double-thumb technique with scooping strokes on the thenar eminence.

3. To release the hypothenar eminence, stand facing the table. Place the client's hand on the table or rest it on your thigh, which is resting on the table. Use the same strokes as we did in the thenar work, except roll the muscles from lateral to medial (Fig. 10-49). Begin at the pisiform and perform short, scooping strokes with the thumbs for the abductor digiti minimi, flexor digiti minimi, and opponens digiti minimi. Continue to the fifth MCP joint.

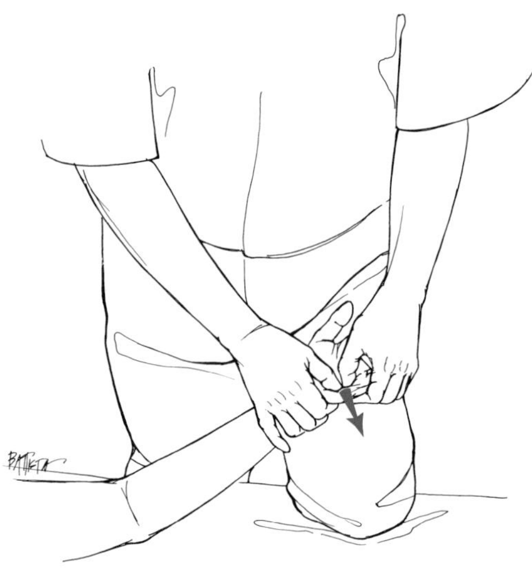

Figure 10-49. Double-thumb technique with scooping strokes on the hypothenar eminence.

6. Transverse and Longitudinal Release of Palmar Aspect of Fingers

- *Anatomy*: Flexor digitorum superficialis and profundus, lumbricals, palmar and dorsal interossei, joint capsule, medial and lateral collateral ligaments, transverse metacarpal ligament, and palmar ligament (Fig. 10-50A–C).
- *Dysfunction*: The flexors of the fingers tend to shorten and become fibrotic with overuse or injury, keeping the fingers in a sustained flexion. The joint capsule and collateral ligaments also become fibrotic and shorten as a result of inflammation from overuse, injury, or arthritis, and they hold the joint in a sustained flexion. The collateral ligament's posi-

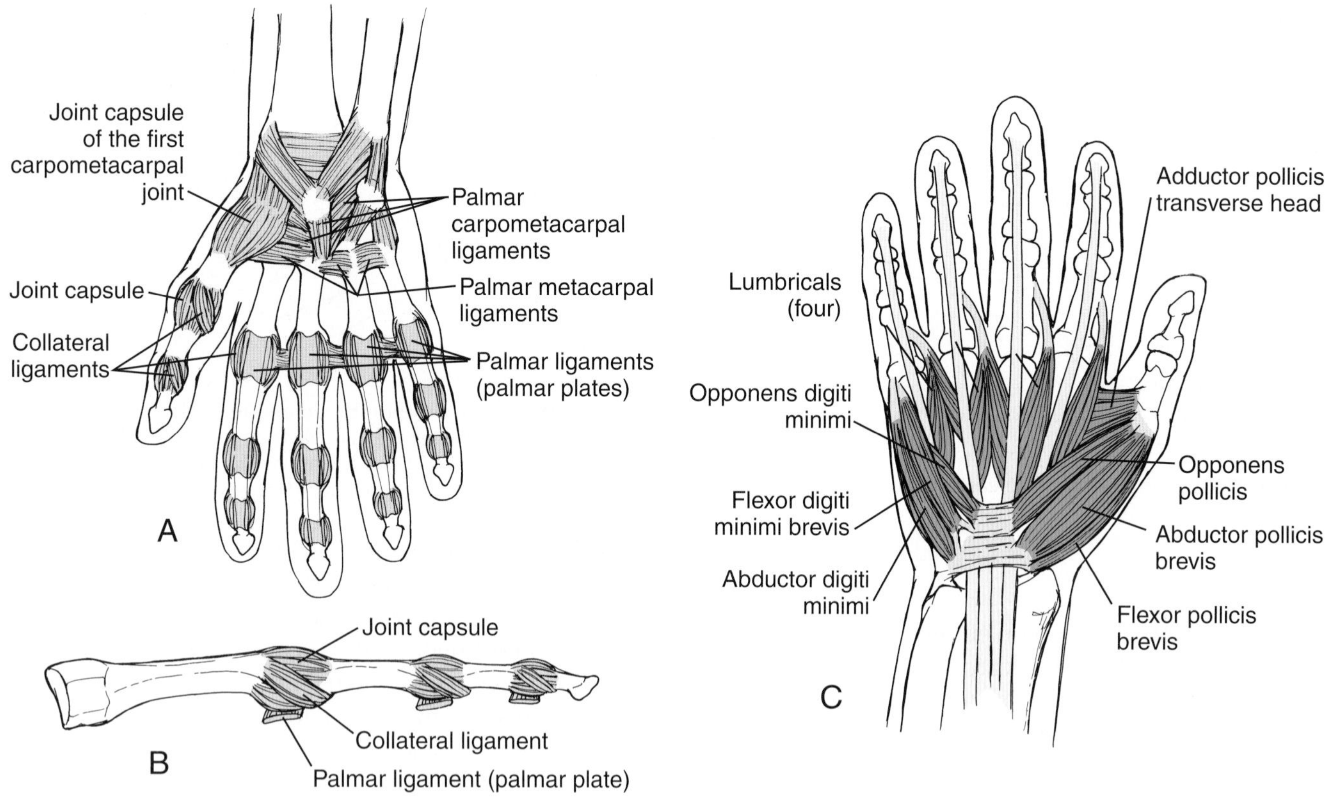

Figure 10-50. **A.** Joint capsule, collateral ligaments, deep transverse metacarpal ligaments, and palmar ligaments of the MCP and IP joints. **B.** Lateral view of the joint capsule and collateral ligaments of the MCP and IP joints. **C.** Muscles and flexor tendons of the hand.

tion of dysfunction is to "fall" into an anterior torsion (toward the palm) with the MCP or IP joints becoming fixed toward a sustained flexed position. The membranous portion of the palmar ligament may develop adhesions if the joint is held in a sustained flexion.

Position

- TP—standing, with your flexed knee on the table and supporting the client's hand on your thigh; or sitting in a chair or on the table, resting the client's hand on your thigh
- CP—supine

Strokes

1. Release the tendons of the flexor digitorum superficialis and profundus. Using a single- or a double-thumb technique, perform short, back-and-forth strokes in the M–L plane transverse to the line of the tendons. Begin at the base of the hand and continue to the tip of each finger and thumb (Fig. 10-51).
2. To release the lumbricals and the interossei underneath, perform a series of short, scooping strokes with the tip of your thumb in the distal to proximal direction on the radial side of the flexor digitorum tendons and between the metacarpals (Fig. 10-52). Place your fingertips on the back of her hand to stabilize your work.
3. Release the transverse metacarpal ligament by performing short back-and-forth strokes in the proxi-

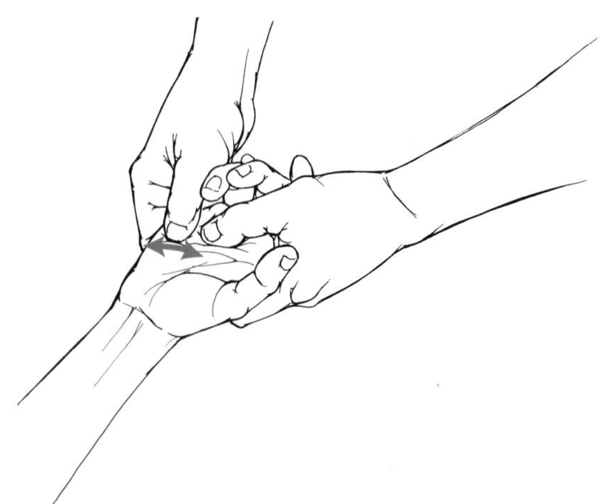

Figure 10-51. Single-thumb technique with transverse strokes on the flexor tendons.

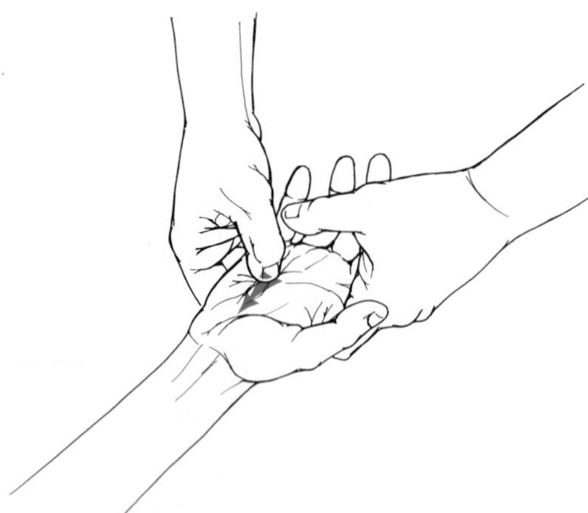

Figure 10-52. Single-thumb release of the lumbricals and palmar interossei.

mal to distal direction on either side of the heads of the second to fifth metacarpals (Fig. 10-53). Release the interdigital nerve by gently scooping back-and-forth in the M–L plane between the heads of the metacarpals.

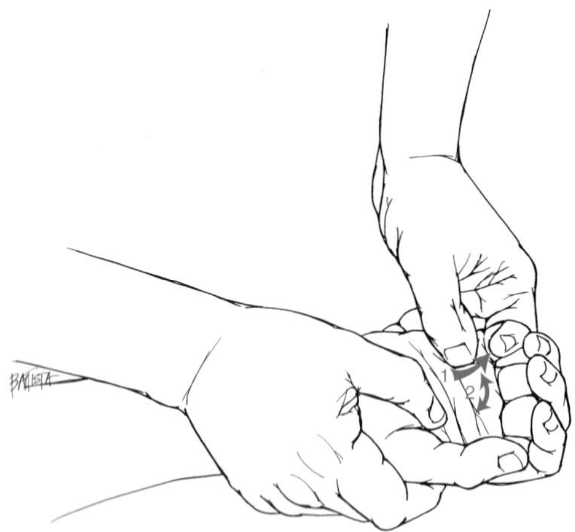

Figure 10-53. Single-thumb technique with (1) short back-and-forth strokes in the proximal to distal plane for the transverse metacarpal ligament and (2) gentle scooping strokes in the M–L place to release the interdigital nerve.

4. Release the joint capsule and collateral ligaments by using a single- or a double-thumb technique and by performing short, back-and-forth strokes transverse to the shaft on the medial and lateral side of each finger and thumb (Fig. 10-54).

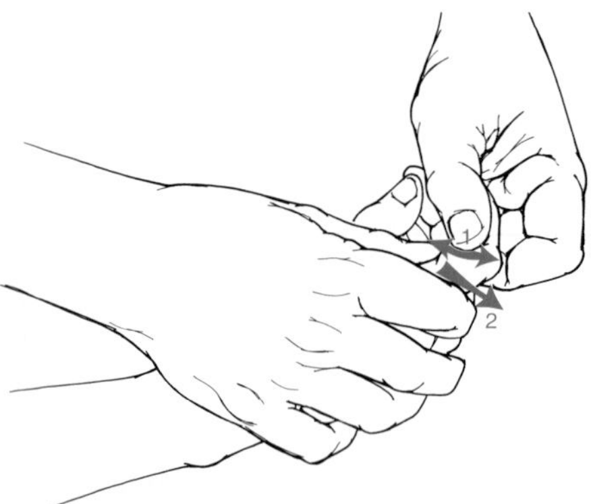

Figure 10-54. Single-thumb technique with (1) a series of back-and-forth strokes transverse to the collateral ligaments and joint capsule and (2) a lifting of the collateral ligaments dorsally as you extend the client's finger.

5. To help normalize the position of the medial and lateral collateral ligaments, turn the client's hand so that it is resting palm down on your thigh. Place your index finger on the medial or lateral side of the IP joint. Begin with the IP joint in flexion, and lift the ligaments in a palmar to dorsal direction as you extend the finger (see Fig. 10-54).
6. To release adhesions in the membranous portion of the palmar plate, first place the lateral portion of your index finger into the flexor surface, proximal to the IP or the MCP joint while the joint is flexed. Perform a scooping stroke in a proximal to distal direction, tractioning the tissue as you extend the finger. Repeat several times (Fig. 10-55).

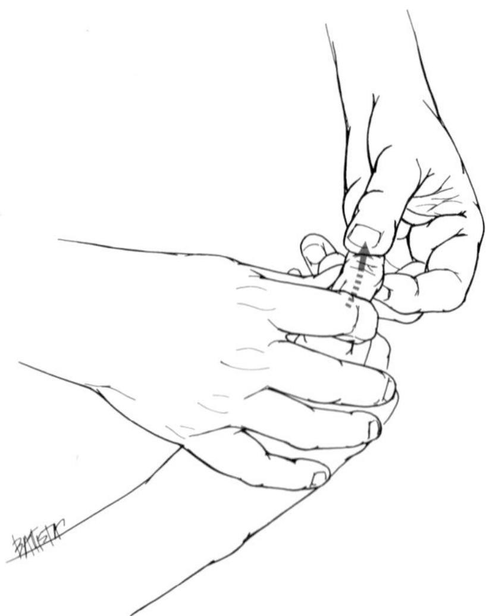

Figure 10-55. To release any adhesions in the membranous portion of the palmar ligament, the lateral portion of the index finger presses into the flexor surface proximal to the IP joint while it is flexed. As you extend the finger, the index finger scoops distally, tractioning the tissue.

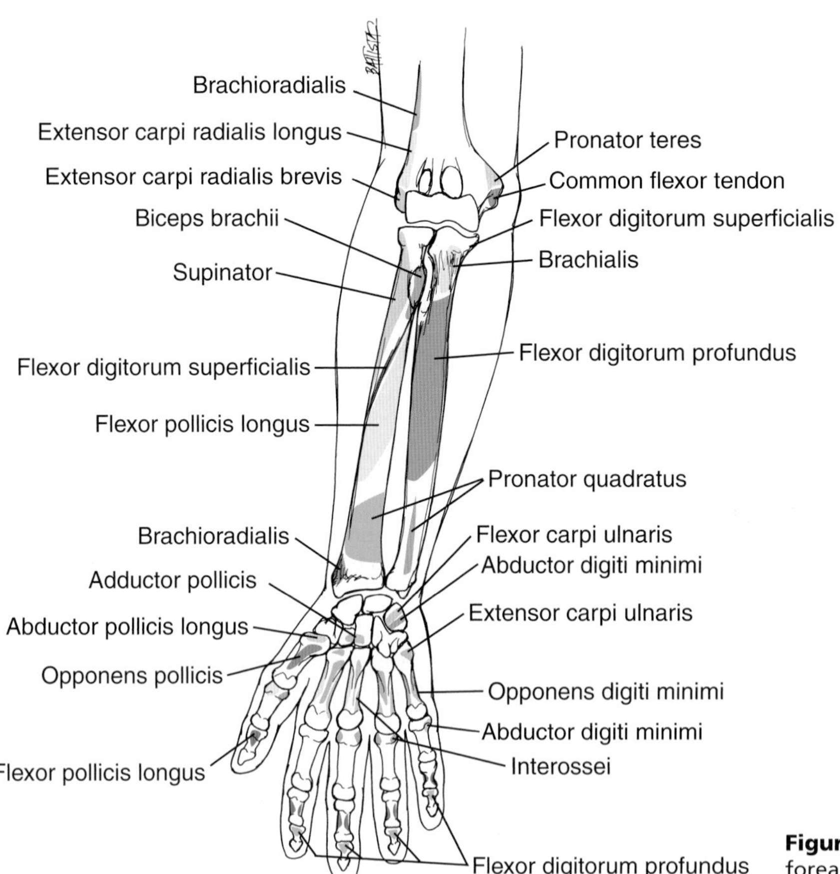

Figure 10-56. Muscle attachments on the anterior forearm, wrist, and hand.

Level II—Elbow, Wrist, and Hand

1. Release of the Attachments at the Lateral Epicondyle and the Radial Nerve

- *Anatomy*: Extensor muscles of the wrist and hand, the brachioradialis, the supinator, and the radial nerve (Fig. 10-56).
- *Dysfunction*: The lateral epicondyle is the site of tennis elbow, an overuse or acute strain of the origins of the extensor tendons of the wrist and hand, especially the ECRB. Radial tunnel syndrome is an entrapment of the radial nerve at the elbow.

Position

- TP—standing
- CP—supine

Strokes

1. Tuck the client's arm into your axilla, and hold the arm with both hands. Your thumbs will be together at the distal third of the lateral arm. Using a double-thumb technique, perform a series of short posterolateral scooping strokes on the distal humerus (Fig. 10-57). You have two intentions. One intention is to release the radial nerve as it passes between the brachialis and the brachioradialis. The second intention is to release the attachments of the brachioradialis and ECRL from the supracondylar ridge. Begin your strokes just lateral to the biceps, and push the biceps medially slightly to make your tissue

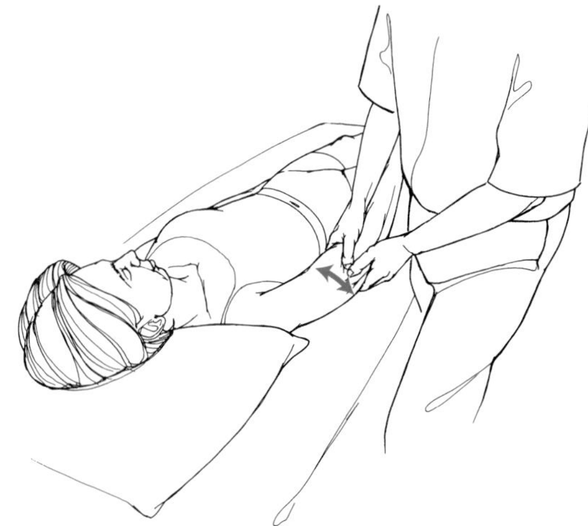

Figure 10-57. Double-thumb release of the attachments on the lateral epicondyle and release of the radial nerve.

contact. Have the client's elbow in midflexion, and flex it more as you stroke. Add a slight external rotation of the humerus with each stroke.

2. Holding the distal forearm in one hand, use a single-thumb technique to release the attachments of the ECRB, common extensor tendon at the lateral epicondyle (Fig. 10-58). Release the radial collateral ligament and joint capsule from the posterior surface of the lateral epicondyle with back-and-forth strokes using your flexed index finger.
3. Using the single thumb technique described in the stroke above, release the radial nerve below the lateral epicondyle. Perform a series of gentle, scooping strokes transverse to the nerve in the M–L plane just distal and medial to the lateral epicondyle where the nerve travels through the fibrous origin of the ECRB. Using your index finger, release the nerve as it enters the supinator canal as it pierces the supinator muscle on the posterolateral portion of the radial head.

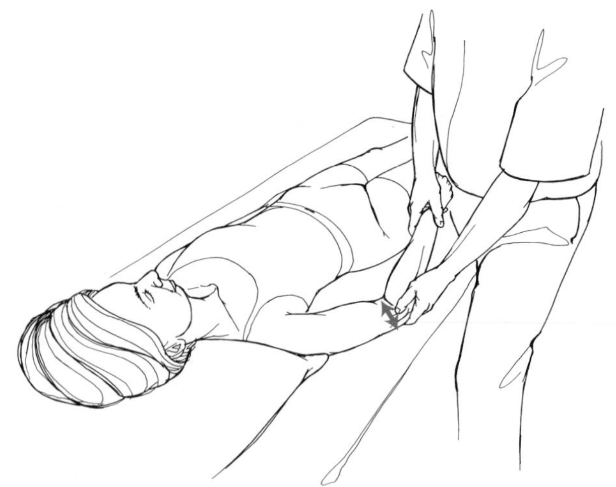

Figure 10-58. Single-thumb release of the attachments on the lateral epicondyle and release of the radial nerve.

2. Release of Attachments at the Medial Epicondyle and the Ulnar and Median Nerves

- *Anatomy*: Pronator teres, flexor carpi radialis, ulnaris, flexor digitorum superficialis and profundus, flexor pollicis longus, palmaris longus, biceps (Fig. 10-59), and ulnar and median nerves (see Figs. 10-2 and 10-3).
- *Dysfunction*: The medial epicondyle is the site of golfer's elbow (little leaguer's elbow), which is a strain of the tenoperiosteal junction of the pronator

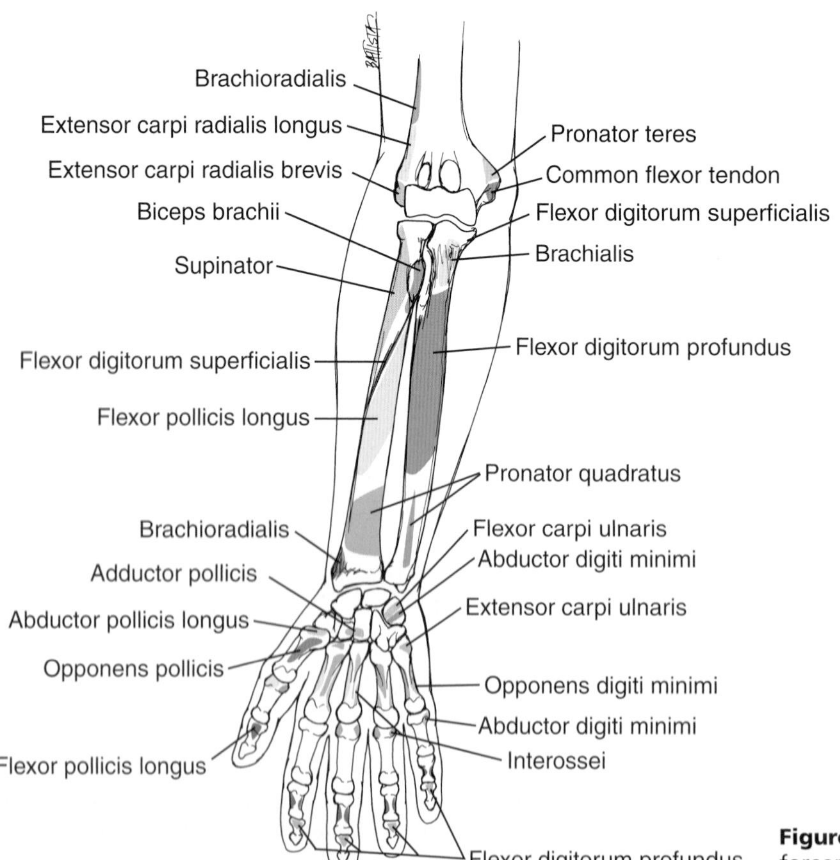

Figure 10-59. Muscle attachments on the anterior forearm, wrist, and hand.

teres and the flexor carpi radialis. The myotendinous junctions of the wrist and fingers flexors are also involved. The flexors and pronator teres are typically short and tight. The ulnar and median nerves may be entrapped in the elbow region.

Position

- TP—standing
- CP—supine or sitting

Strokes

1. Release the biceps attachment to the radial tuberosity by placing your thumb on the biceps tendon at that site. Hold your thumb on the tendon as you oscillate the entire arm into pronation and supination to provide transverse friction to the tendon (Fig. 10-60). Keep moving the thumb onto different sites after a few oscillations.

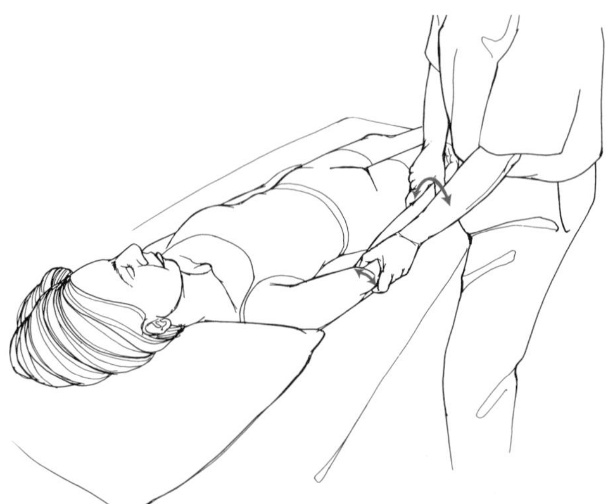

Figure 10-60. Release of the bicipital attachments on the proximal radius.

2. To release the flexor pollicis longus, flexor digitorum superficialis, and flexor digitorum profundus attachments, flex the client's elbow to 90° and have her wrist and fingers relaxed to bring the muscles into slack. Facing the table and with the client's forearm in neutral, use your fingertips to perform deep back-and-forth strokes in the M–L plane on the radius and ulna as your supporting hand pronates the forearm (Fig. 10-61).
3. Release the ulnar nerve at two sites. At the first site, tuck the client's arm into your axilla, as shown previously. First, use fingertips to scoop in the posterior to anterior (P–A) and the M–L planes first at the medial aspect of the distal humerus where the nerve travels through the fibrous expansion of the common flexor tendon (called the "cubital tunnel"). Next, to release the ulnar nerve as it travels through the ulnar and humeral heads of the flexor carpi ulnaris, turn to face the foot of the table and flex the client's elbow to 90° (Fig. 10-62). Hold the distal forearm with one hand, and use the fingertips of your superior hand to scoop a P–A, M–L direction two finger-widths distal to the medial epicondyle as you pronate the forearm.

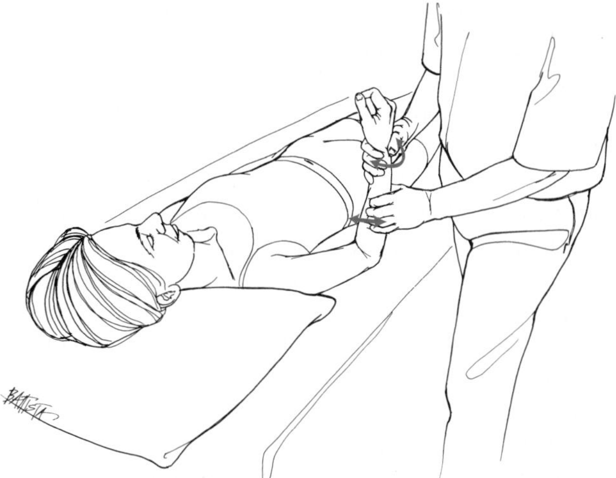

Figure 10-61. Fingertip release of the flexor surface of the forearm. The support hand pronates and supinates the forearm as the fingertips scoop back-and-forth on the soft tissue.

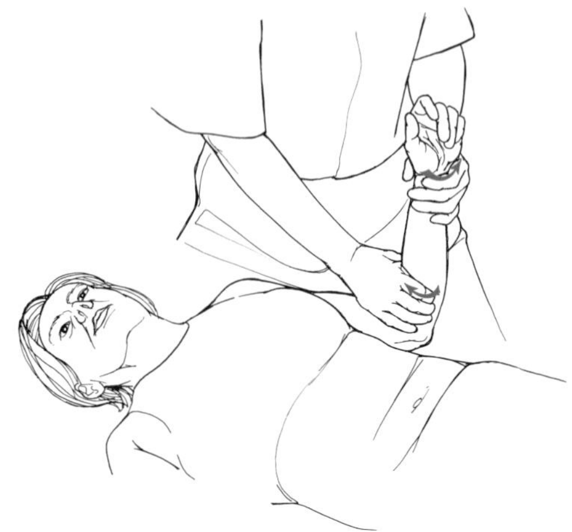

Figure 10-62. Fingertip release of the ulnar nerve at the proximal forearm.

4. To release the median nerve, turn your body toward the head of the table. Keep the client's elbow flexed to 90°. Using fingertips, perform gentle, scooping strokes perpendicular to the shaft of the forearm as you pronate the client's forearm with each stroke (see Fig. 10-61). Release the nerve at two sites. First,

release it at the anterior middle surface of the distal humerus medial to the bicipital tendon. Second, release the nerve between the two heads of the pronator teres, immediately distal to the medial epicondyle and more toward the midbody of the muscle.

3. Release of the Extensor Attachment Points and the Ligaments on the Dorsum of the Wrist

- ***Anatomy***: ECRL and ECRB, extensor pollicis longus and brevis, abductor pollicis longus, extensor carpi ulnaris, ulnar and radial collateral ligaments, dorsal radiocarpal ligament, brachioradialis, and superficial radial nerve (Fig. 10-63).
- ***Dysfunction***: Tenoperiosteal junctions tend to become fibrotic with overuse or acute injury. The ligaments on the dorsum of the wrist shorten and become fibrotic after a FOOSH injury, predisposing the wrist to arthritis.

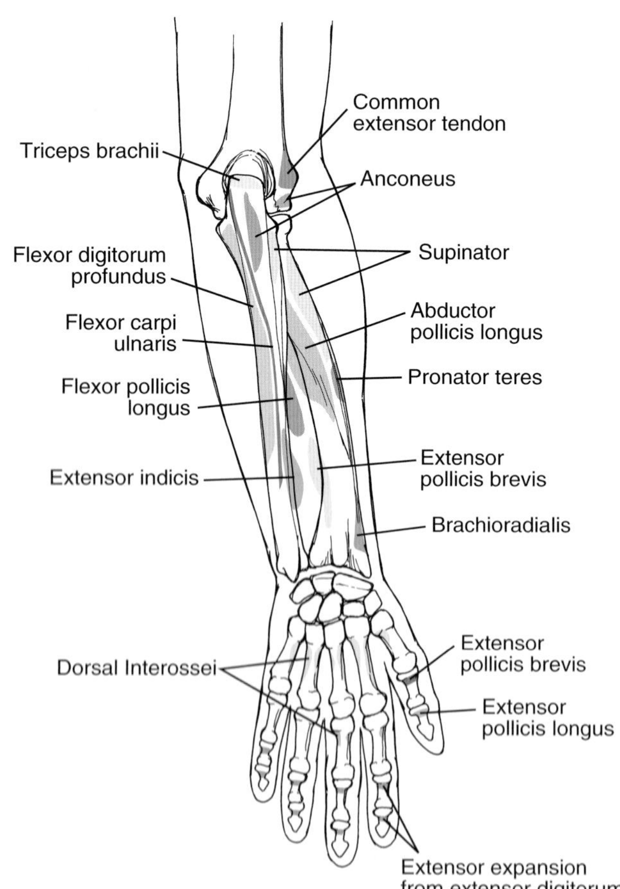

Figure 10-63. Attachments on the posterior surface of the forearm, wrist, and hand.

Position

- TP—standing, facing headward for strokes on the hand and wrist; or sitting
- CP—supine

Strokes

1. Release the ECRB and ECRL with back-and-forth strokes in the M–L plane, from the base of the third and the second metacarpal, respectively, and the dorsal radiocarpal ligament underneath. Use a double- or a single-thumb technique if you are standing or a fingertips technique if you are sitting (Fig. 10-64). Oscillate the forearm in a radioulnar glide as you perform these strokes.

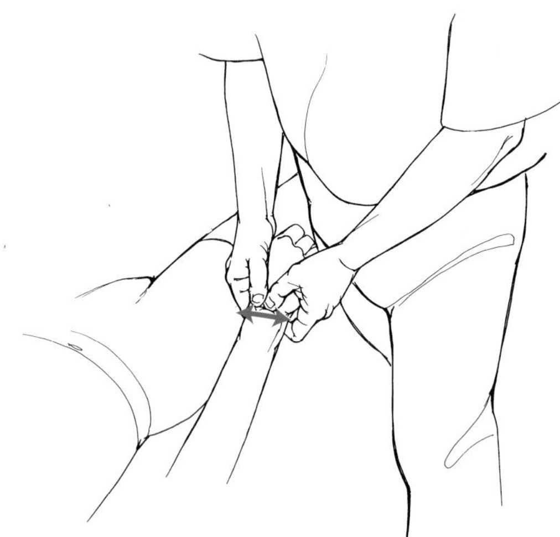

Figure 10-64. Double-thumb release of the extensor attachments at the wrist.

2. Release the extensor carpi ulnaris and the ulnar collateral ligament by performing short, back-and-forth strokes in the M–L plane, from the ulnar styloid to the base of the fifth metacarpal. Cover the dorsum and medial aspect of the wrist. Oscillate the wrist in short arcs of a radioulnar glide as you perform these strokes. Using your index finger, perform back-and-forth strokes in the anterior to posterior (A–P) plane between the ulnar styloid and the pisiform to release the ulnar collateral ligament.
3. Perform gentle, back-and-forth strokes with a single-, a double-thumb, or a fingertips technique in the area of the anatomical snuff-box. Turn the client's wrist so that it is in neutral, and perform a series of strokes from the lateral aspect of the radial styloid process to the base of the first metacarpal (Fig. 10-65). You are releasing the extensor pollicis brevis

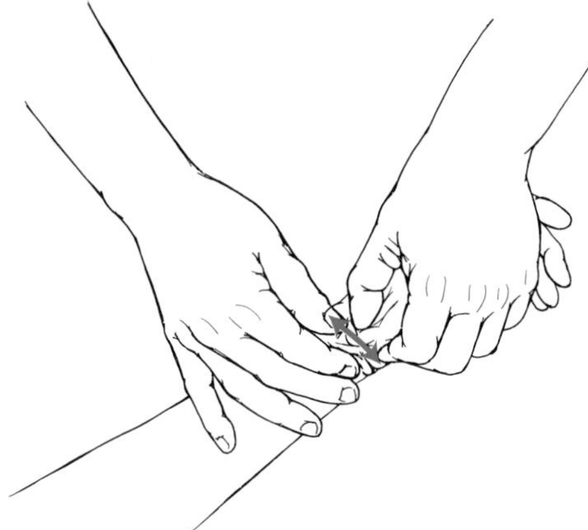

Figure 10-65. Double-thumb release of the extensor pollicis brevis and abductor pollicis longus.

and the abductor pollicis longus, the potential site of tenovaginitis; the brachioradialis attachment; and the radial collateral ligament. Begin another series of strokes at Lister's tubercle, a bony prominence on the dorsum of the radius, and continue to the distal aspect of the dorsum of the thumb.

4. Release of Wrist Flexor Insertion Points and the Median and Ulnar Nerves at the Wrist

- ***Anatomy***: Flexor carpi radialis, flexor carpi ulnaris, median and ulnar nerves, flexor retinaculum, ulnar collateral ligament, and pisohamate ligament (Fig. 10-66).
- ***Dysfunction***: The wrist flexors tend to thicken at their insertion points at the wrist as a result of the muscles being overworked in gripping, holding, and keyboard work. The flexor retinaculum may thicken due to irritation or inflammation of the finger flexors. The pisohamate ligament may thicken because of injury or overuse of the flexor carpi ulnaris.

Position

- TP—standing
- CP—supine

Strokes

1. Using a double-thumb technique, perform a series of back-and-forth strokes in the M–L plane from the palmar aspect of the distal radius to the base of the

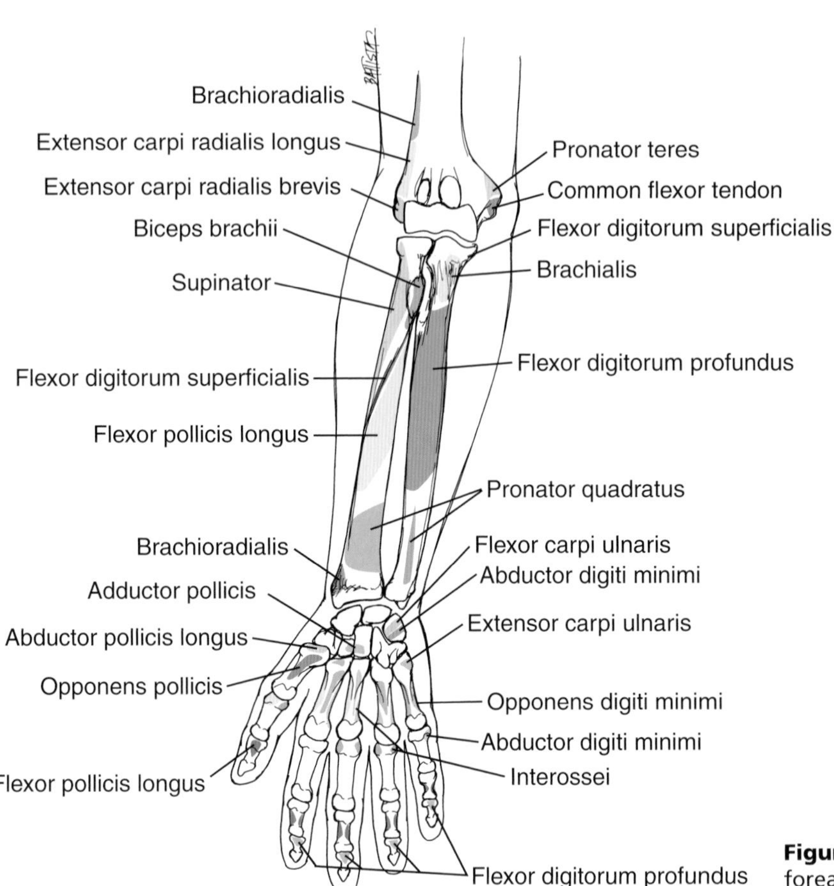

Figure 10-66. Muscle attachments on the anterior forearm, wrist, and hand.

second and the third metacarpals (Fig. 10-67). You are releasing the flexor carpi radialis, the lateral side of the flexor retinaculum, and the base of the thenar pad. Oscillate the wrist in gentle arcs of radial and ulnar glide as you perform these strokes.

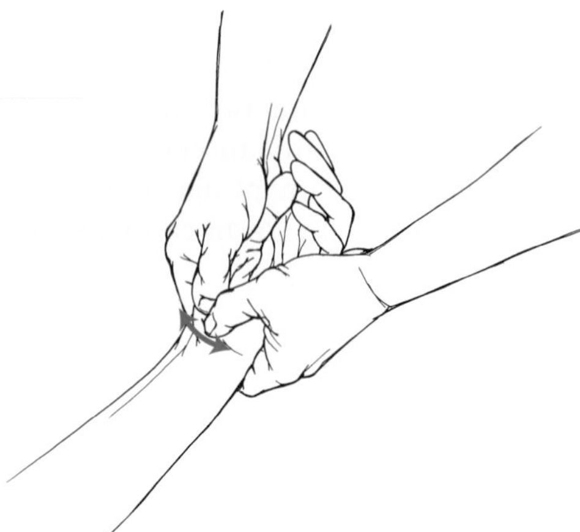

Figure 10-67. Double-thumb release of the attachments of the flexor carpi radialis, the lateral side of the flexor retinaculum, and the muscle attachments on the base of the thenar pad.

2. Using a double-thumb technique, perform a series of back-and-forth strokes in the M–L plane from the ulnar styloid to the pisiform and the fifth metacarpal. You are releasing the flexor carpi ulnaris and the medial aspect of the flexor retinaculum (Fig. 10-68). Oscillate the wrist in gentle arcs of radial and ulnar deviation as you perform these strokes. To release the ulnar collateral ligament, place your index finger just distal to the medial aspect of the ulnar styloid process and perform back-and-forth strokes in the A–P plane as you rock the wrist in pronation and supination to shear the tissue.

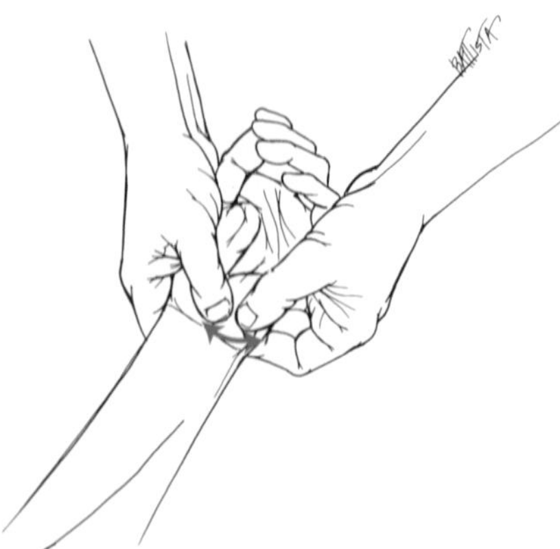

Figure 10-68. Double-thumb release of the flexor carpi ulnaris and the medial aspect of the flexor retinaculum.

3. To release the carpal tunnel in acute conditions, stretch the flexor retinaculum with a myofascial-holding technique. Place your thumbs at the bases of the thenar and hypothenar eminences (Fig. 10-69). Apply a gentle spreading pressure away from the midline and hold this for approximately 1 minute. This lengthens the flexor retinaculum.

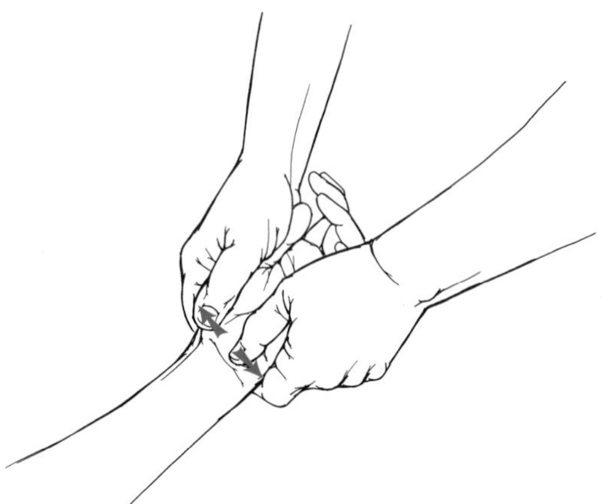

Figure 10-69. Myofascial-holding technique to stretch the flexor retinaculum for acute conditions of carpal tunnel syndrome.

4. In subacute and chronic carpal tunnel syndrome, perform back-and-forth strokes in an inferior to superior (I–S) plane on the attachments of the transverse carpal ligament at two sites: on the lateral side of the pisiform and hook of the hamate and on the medial side of the tubercles of the navicular and trapezium (Fig. 10-70).

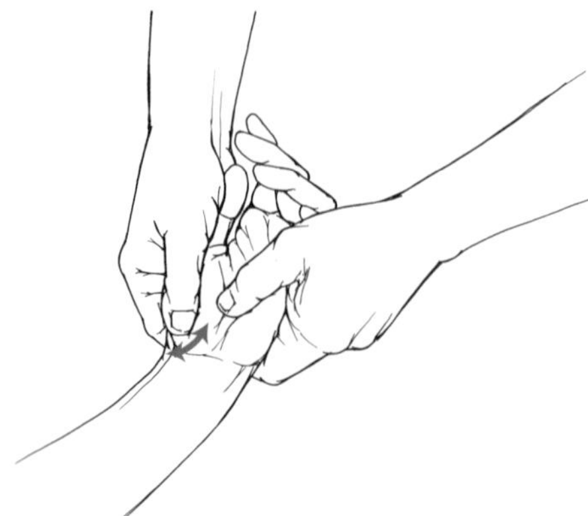

Figure 10-70. Single-thumb release of the attachment points of the flexor retinaculum on the tubercles of the navicular and the trapezium.

5. Using a single-thumb technique, perform gentle back-and-forth strokes in the I–S plane in between the pisiform and the hook of the hamate to release the pisohamate ligament (Fig. 10-71). Next, release the ulnar nerve as it travels under this ligament through the tunnel of Guyon with gentle, back-and-forth strokes in the M–L plane between these two bony landmarks.

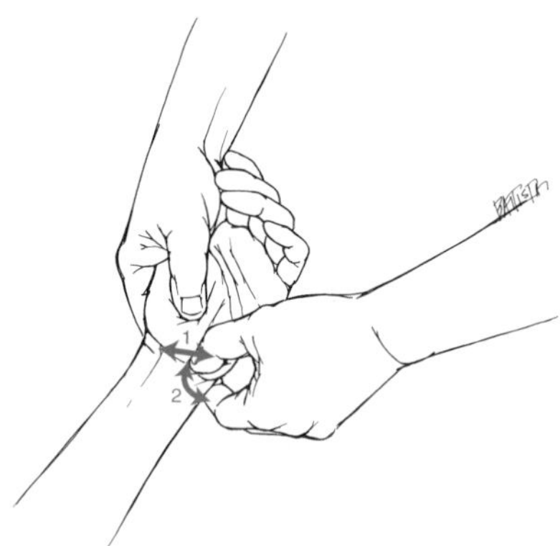

Figure 10-71. (1) Release of the pisohamate ligament. (2) Release the ulnar nerve traveling through the tunnel of Guyon.

5. Release of the Joint Capsule and Ligaments of the Thumb and Mobilization of the Thumb

- *Anatomy*: Flexor pollicis brevis; flexor pollicis longus; joint capsule of the thumb; flexor pollicis longus; deep head of flexor pollicis brevis; first CMC joint; and palmar and dorsal CMC ligaments, which strengthen the joint capsule (Fig. 10-72).

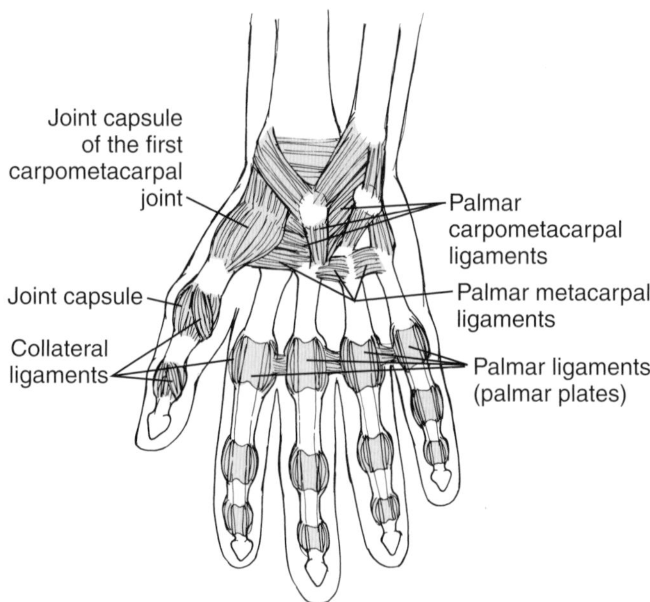

Figure 10-72. Joint capsule, collateral ligaments, deep transverse metacarpal ligaments, and palmar ligaments of the MCP and IP joints.

- *Dysfunction*: The CMC joint of the thumb is one of the most commonly arthritic joints of the body. The joint capsule thickens, decreasing the normal glide of the articulating surfaces. Aching in the thenar pad may be caused by these degenerative changes.

Position

- TP—sitting or standing
- CP—supine, with palm up

Strokes

1. Sit on the table, and place the client's hand on your thigh, palm up. Using a single- or a double-thumb technique, perform scooping strokes in the M–L direction and then back-and-forth strokes in the M–L plane to release the deep head of the flexor pollicis brevis, the flexor pollicis longus tendon, and the palmar joint capsule and ligaments (Fig. 10-73). Cover the entire thenar pad and work until you can penetrate through the muscles to the bone without pain. This may take many sessions.

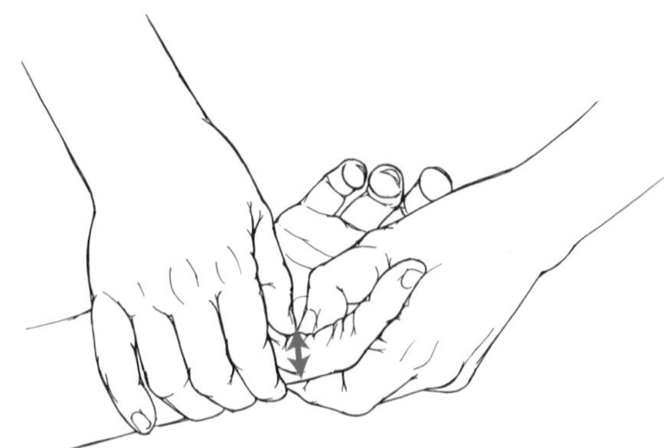

Figure 10-73. Double-thumb release of the deepest layers of the thenar muscles and the anterior joint capsule.

2. To release any fibrosis in the dorsal aspect of the joint capsule of the first CMC joint, stand and place the client's forearm in neutral. Using a single- or a double-thumb technique, perform back-and-forth strokes in the M–L plane (Fig. 10-74). Oscillate the forearm in pronation and supination while performing the strokes.
3. To mobilize the first CMC joint, place your flexed knee on the table and rest the client's hand on your thigh. Hold the client's thumb at the CMC joint with your thumb in the distal part of the snuff-box and your index finger on the thenar pad opposite the thumb. Holding the shaft of the client's thumb with your other hand, gently circumduct the thumb (see Fig. 10-19). Always work within your client's comfortable limit. The client should be able to relax

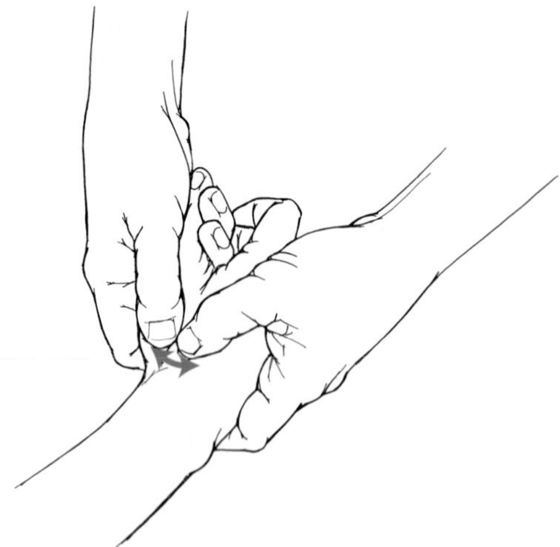

Figure 10-74. Release of the joint capsule of the dorsal surface of the thumb (the first CMC joint).

completely into this mobilization. It is normal to hear and feel some grinding (crepitation) if the joint is arthritic. Only perform this for a few minutes each session. This mobilization can help dissolve spicules of calcium on the joint surfaces and can clean larger spurs on the rims of the joint.

6. Joint Play of the Metacarpals, Phalanges, and Elbow

- *Anatomy*: Joints of the elbow, wrist, and hand (see Fig. 10-1).
- *Dysfunction*: Loss of joint play from chronic tension, overuse, or injury decreases the normal gliding characteristics of the joint. Because of this loss of motion, the joint capsule and ligaments thicken, causing further loss of motion. As the joint loses motion, sensory nerves (mechanoreceptors) from the soft tissue surrounding the joint stimulate reflexes to the surrounding muscles, resulting in either weakness (inhibition) or sustained contraction. This is called the arthrokinetic reflex. The intention of the treatment is to help normalize the joint motion.

Position

- TP—standing or sitting
- CP—sitting

Strokes

1. To mobilize the elbow, grasp the client's elbow by placing your flexed index fingers between the medial and lateral epicondyles and the olecranon, while resting your thumbs on the anterior cubital fossa (Fig. 10-75). Tuck the client's distal arm into your axilla. Mobilize the elbow by first flexing the client's elbow slightly as you rock it up and laterally while increasing the pressure of your lateral and medial index fingers in the joint space. Bring the elbow down and in toward the client's body, and repeat these movements several times to normalize the joint capsule function and the articular surfaces. Then have the client lean back to add some traction, and gently bring the elbow into full extension.
2. To release potential calcium deposits from the joint space, bring the client's elbow to full extension, squeeze the joint with your hands, and rock it back-and-forth in an M–L glide.
3. To mobilize the wrist, place the client's forearm in pronation. Wrap your hands around the wrist such that one hand is holding the distal forearm, and your index finger and webspace of the other hand is wrapped around the wrist. Gently oscillate your hands in opposite directions to perform an A–P glide (Fig. 10-76).

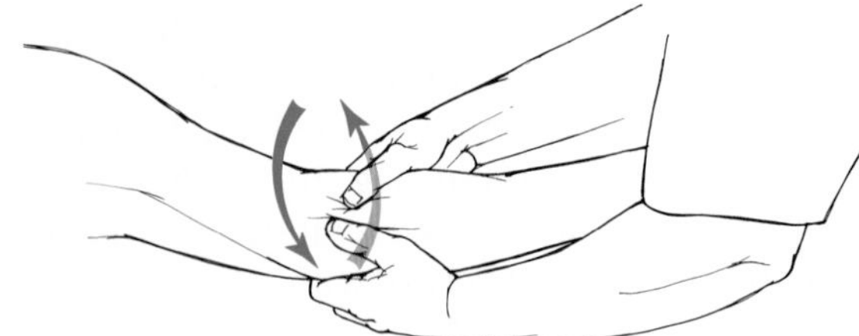

Figure 10-75. Mobilization of the elbow.

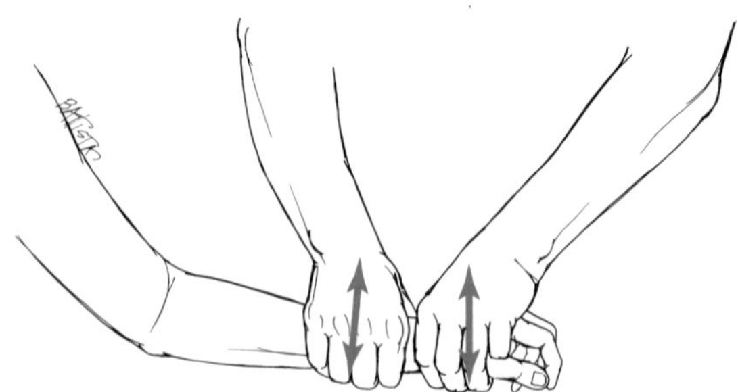

Figure 10-76. Mobilization of the wrist. Hands move in opposite directions.

4. To perform dorsal-palmar glide of metacarpals, grasp the adjacent metacarpals with your thumbs on the dorsal surface and your fingertips underneath. Shear the metacarpals in opposite directions in short, oscillating strokes (Fig. 10-77).

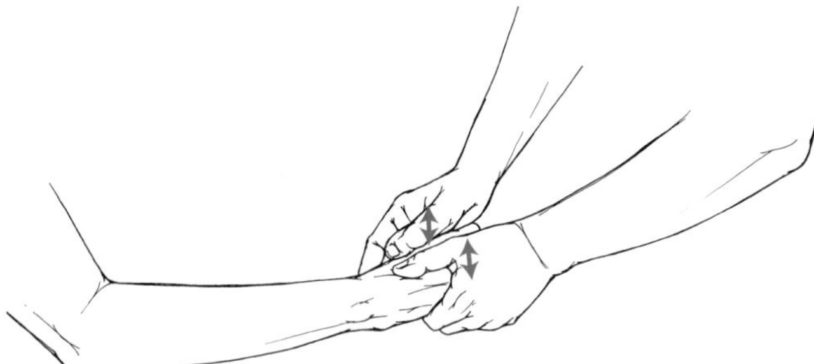

Figure 10-77. Dorsal-palmar glide of the metacarpals. Move the adjacent metacarpals in opposite directions.

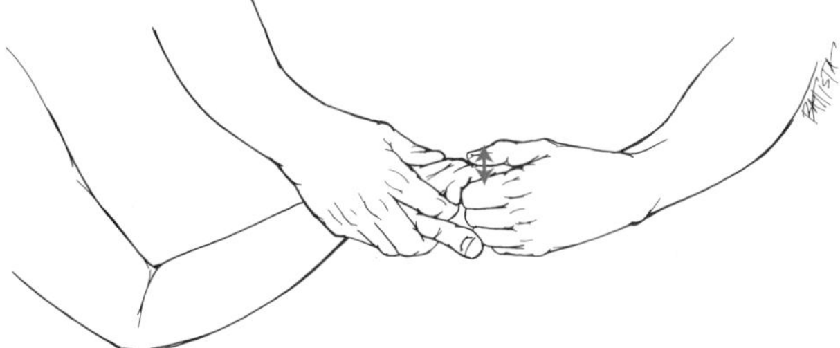

Figure 10-78. Dorsal-palmar glide of the MCP, PIP, and DIP joints.

5. To perform M–L and dorsal-palmar glide of the MCP, PIP, and DIP joints, stabilize the proximal portion of the joint. Grasp the distal portion with your thumb and forefinger, performing the glide to the distal portion of the joint in short, oscillating strokes (Fig.10-78).

6. To have the client perform self-care for the fingers, instruct him or her to wrap their entire hand around one finger, place the hand in the pronated position, then move the hand in an M–L, back-and-forth motion to mobilize IP joints into lateral bending. This helps clean the lateral rim of the joint, the first site of calcium deposits.

CASE STUDY

RK is a 65-year-old, 5'2", 115-lb, female administrative assistant who presented to my office with a chief complaint of pain at the left wrist. She stated that she fractured the wrist when she fell on her outstretched hand approximately 10 weeks prior to her visit. She was diagnosed with a Colles' fracture, a fracture to the distal radius, and surgery was performed to fixate the displaced bone. After surgery she was referred to physical therapy, but she stated that it was difficult for her to continue because the treatments seem to make the pain worse. At the time of her visit, she described the pain as aching and burning with any movement of the wrist and said that the pain can become sharp with certain motions.

Upon examination, active ROM was approximately 2° of motion in flexion, extension, supination, pronation, and radial and ulnar deviation. Passive motion was minimally greater than active motion and had a capsular end feel initiallyw, with a bony end feel at the end range. Isometric testing was weak and painful in wrist and finger extension, radial and ulnar deviation, and pronation and supination. Grip strength was 35 pounds on the left and 70 pounds on the right. The patient is right-handed. To palpation, there was a thickened, fibrous feel to the tissue on the dorsum of the wrist. Touching the area of the fracture was emotionally distressing for the patient.

A diagnosis was made of posttraumatic arthropathy and capsular fibrosis. Recommendations were made for four treatments, with a reevaluation after the fourth visit.

Treatment began with the patient supine, with her elbow at 90° of flexion. CR MET was performed for the wrist flexors and extensors; and to increase radial and ulnar deviation, as well as pronation and supination. Light pressures were used. The patient was instructed in how to perform these techniques at home. OM was performed with light scooping strokes at the radiocarpal, midcarpal, and CMC joints. There was extreme tenderness over the fracture site, but the patient tolerated the work well.

RK returned to the office 1 week later and reported that she did not flare up after our session. Upon examination, there was a slight increase in wrist extension. The same treatment described above was performed. Slight increases in the pressure were applied, in the MET and in the manual work. On her next visit, she stated that she was feeling a slight decrease in pain. Active ROM was approximately 10° in all ranges. MET and OM, including transverse friction massage, were performed. The manual work concentrated on the soft tissue over the fracture site. After her sixth visit, she stated that the pain was reduced 50% and that she was using the hand more in daily activities. The patient was seen for 12 visits over a 6-month period. At the time of our last visit, she was pain-free, and she stated that her hand and wrist were functioning normally. Her ROM was normal, except in flexion and supination, which were reduced 25%. Grip strength was 60 pounds on the left and 70 pounds on the right.

STUDY GUIDE

Level I—Elbow, Forearm, Wrist, and Hand

1. Describe the "position of function" of the wrist and hand.
2. List the names of the muscles in the thenar and the hypothenar groups.
3. Describe the origins and insertions of the following: flexor carpi ulnaris, ECRB, pronator teres, and extensor carpi ulnaris.
4. Describe the signs and symptoms for seven common dysfunctions and injuries in the elbow, wrist, and hand.
5. Describe the MET for acute elbow, wrist, and hand pain.
6. Describe the treatment protocol for injured ligaments.
7. Describe the stroke direction to release the thenar and the hypothenar eminences.
8. List the muscles in the five fascial compartments of the forearm.
9. Describe the stroke direction to release the collateral ligaments of the fingers.
10. Describe the implication if your client has painless weakness while attempting to perform MET.

Level II—Elbow, Forearm, Wrist, and Hand

1. Describe the direction of mobilization in self-care for the fingers.
2. List the origins and insertions of the muscles of the thenar and the hypothenar eminence.
3. Describe the signs and symptoms of the less common injuries and dysfunctions of the elbow, wrist, and hand.
4. Describe the common entrapment sites of the median, radial, and ulnar nerves at the elbow.
5. Describe the two muscles involved in De Quervain's tenovaginitis at the wrist and describe the treatment protocol.
6. Describe the attachment sites for the transverse carpal ligament and the treatment protocol for carpal tunnel syndrome.
7. Describe the common entrapment sites of the median and ulnar nerves at the wrist.
8. Describe the MET for the muscles of the elbow, wrist, and hand.
9. Describe the mobilizations of the elbow, wrist, and hand.
10. Describe the treatment protocol for degenerative arthritis of the hand.

REFERENCES

1. Parkes J. Common injuries about the elbow in sports. In: Scott WN, Nisonson B, Nicholas J, eds. Principles of Sports Medicine. Baltimore: Williams & Wilkins, 1984:140–155.
2. Garrick J, Webb D. Sports Injuries. 2nd Ed. Philadelphia: WB Saunders, 1999.
3. Szabo R, Madison M. Carpal tunnel syndrome. Orthop Clin North Am 1992; 23:103–109.
4. Hertling D, Kessler R. The elbow and forearm. In: Management of Common Musculoskeletal Disorders. Baltimore: Lippincott Williams & Wilkins, 1996:217–242.
5. Wadsworth C. The wrist and hand. In: Malone T, McPoil T, Nitz A, eds. Orthopedic and Sports Physical Therapy. St. Louis: Mosby, 1997:327–378.
6. Platzer W. Locomotor System, vol 1. 4th Ed. New York: Thieme Medical, 1992.
7. Frick H, Leonhardt H, Starck D. Human Anatomy, vol. 1. New York: Thieme Medical, 1991.
8. Norkin C, Levangie P. The elbow complex. In: Joint Structure and Function. Philadelphia: F.A. Davis, 1992:241–261.
9. Pecina M, Krmpotic-Nemainic J, Markiewitz A. Tunnel Syndromes. Boca Raton: CRC Press, 1991.
10. McRae R. Clinical Orthopedic Examination. 2nd Ed. Edinburgh: Churchill Livingstone, 1983.
11. Posner M. Wrist injuries. In: Scott WN, Nisonson B, Nicholas J, eds. Principles of Sports Medicine. Baltimore: Williams & Wilkins, 1984:156–177.
12. Cailliet R. Hand Pain and Impairment. 4th Ed. Philadelphia: FA Davis, 1994.
13. Hammer W. Functional Soft Tissue Examination and Treatment by Manual Methods. 2nd Ed. Gaithersburg: Aspen, 1999.

SUGGESTED READINGS

Cailliet R. Hand Pain and Impairment, 4th Ed. Philadelphia: F.A. Davis, 1994.

Corrigan B, Maitland GD. Practical Orthopaedic Medicine. London: Butterworths, 1983.

Cyriax J, Cyriax P. Illustrated Manual of Orthopedic Medicine. London: Butterworths, 1983.

Garrick J, Webb D. Sports Injuries. 2nd Ed. Philadelphia: WB Saunders, 1999.

Greenman PE. Principles of Manual Medicine. 2nd Ed. Baltimore: Williams & Wilkins, 1996.

Hammer W. Functional Soft Tissue Examination and Treatment by Manual Methods. 2nd Ed. Gaithersburg: Aspen, 1999.

Hertling D, Kessler R. The elbow and forearm. In: Management of Common Musculoskeletal Disorders. Baltimore: Lippincott Williams & Wilkins, 1996:217–242.

Hoppenfeld S. Physical Examination of the Spine and Extremities. New York: Appleton-Century-Crofts, 1976.

Kendall F, McCreary E, Provance P. Muscles: Testing and Function. 4th Ed. Baltimore: Williams & Wilkins, 1993.

Magee D. Orthopedic Physical Assessment. 3rd Ed. Philadelphia: WB Saunders, 1997.

Norkin C, Levangie P. Joint Structure and Function. 2nd Ed. Philadelphia: FA Davis, 1992.

Platzer W. Locomotor System, vol 1. 4th Ed. New York: Thieme Medical, 1992.

Reid DC. Sports Injury and Assessment. New York: Churchill Livingstone, 1992.

Wadsworth C. The wrist and hand. In: Malone T, McPoil T, Nitz A, eds. Orthopedic and Sports Physical Therapy. St. Louis: Mosby, 1997:327–378.

INDEX

Page numbers in italics followed by f denote figures; those followed by t denote tables.

Q

R